The Developing Brain

The Developing Brain

Michael Brown

University of Oxford

Roger Keynes

University of Cambridge

Andrew Lumsden

King's College London

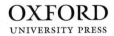

OXFORD

UNIVERSITY PRESS

OXFORD

UNIVERSITY PRESS

Great Clarendon Street, Oxford OX2 6DP

Oxford University Press is a department of the University of Oxford.
It furthers the University's objective of excellence in research, scholarship,
and education by publishing worldwide in
Oxford New York

Athens Auckland Bangkok Bogotá Buenos Aires Cape Town
Chennai Dar es Salaam Delhi Florence Hong Kong Istanbul Karachi
Kolkata Kuala Lumpur Madrid Melbourne Mexico City Mumbai
Nairobi Paris São Paulo Singapore Taipei Tokyo Toronto Warsaw
with associated companies in Berlin Ibadan

Published in the United States
by Oxford University Press Inc., New York

First published 2001

A catalogue record for this book is available from the British Library

Library of Congress Cataloging in Publication Data
(data applied for)

ISBN 0 19 854793 5

Typeset by Newgen Imaging Systems (P) Ltd.,
Printed in Great Britain
on acid-free paper by
The Bath Press, Bath

Preface

IF, as has been suggested, the mammalian brain is the most improbable of all cell aggregates, the problems posed by its development might seem formidable. After a century of steady progress, and with foundations laid by pioneers such as Santiago Ramón y Cajal, Ross Harrison, Hans Spemann, Viktor Hamburger, Roger Sperry and Rita Levi-Montalcini, the past two decades have seen a truly remarkable acceleration. With it has come the realization that the same molecular pathways that evolved to build less complicated nervous systems, in animals such as worms and flies, also construct the basic layout of our own brains. Much of this book's focus is on these early developmental stages and their cellular and molecular basis, integrating recent discoveries with a synthesis of the classical literature. But differences are as significant as similarities, and perhaps entirely novel mechanisms are needed to generate the patterns of connectivity underlying human faculties such as language or a sense of humour. Here, we remain ignorant, not surprisingly, but significant advances in understanding the plasticity of synaptic interactions in the mammalian brain have given us some insights and are covered towards the end of the book. We have also included a final chapter on regeneration and repair, in the belief that the intractable nature of many human brain disorders will eventually yield to a deeper knowledge of brain development. We have kept the technical detail in the text deliberately brief, opting instead for an extensive reference list for further consultation, and each chapter is supplemented with a summary of key points.

This introductory book is intended for anyone studying the physical aspects of brain development, from molecule to morphology, and should suit final-year undergraduates, graduate students and postdoctoral research scientists, as well as teachers in the field. We have stopped short of behavioural and cognitive development, where many fascinating questions regarding links with the developing brain are still to be explored, but we hope that the book will also inform those interested in this area.

Further reading

Hamburger, V. Ontogeny of neuroembryology. *J. Neurosci.* **8**, 3535–40 (1988).
Bateson, P. and Martin, P. *Design for a life. How behaviour develops* (Jonathan Cape, London, 1999).

September 2000
Oxford   M.B.
Cambridge   R.K.
London   A.L.

Contents

1

Model Systems and Review of Early Morphogenesis

Model systems for the study of neural development

There is good reason to believe that many of the mechanisms underlying neural development are fundamentally similar in vertebrates and invertebrates such as worms and insects, whose multicellular common ancestor almost certainly possessed a nervous system.[1] Experiments on neural development are therefore carried out using a variety of invertebrate and vertebrate species, usually in the hope that they will illuminate general principles. As always, the art is to pick the right species for the right question and the results, not surprisingly, meet with varying success. Each species has its own particular advantages; those used most frequently, and the main reasons for using them, are discussed below.

Among the *invertebrates* are insects such as the grasshopper and the fruitfly, *Drosophila melanogaster*. The grasshopper embryo provides large cells that can be readily labelled, for example with fluorescent dye, which allows their lineal descendants and differentiating axons to be followed during subsequent development. It turns out that the anatomical ground-plan of the grasshopper nervous system is replicated in miniature in *Drosophila*,[2] and the well-advanced molecular genetics of this species have been exploited in recent years with great success. It is possible, for example, to carry out mutant screens for some feature of neural development, such as axon guidance or neuromuscular synapse formation, and subsequently clone the relevant genes and analyse their function *in vivo* by gene perturbation experiments.

Two further invertebrates have also been studied intensively, the nematode worm, *Caenorhabditis elegans*, and the medicinal leech, *Hirudo medicinalis*. The adult *C. elegans*

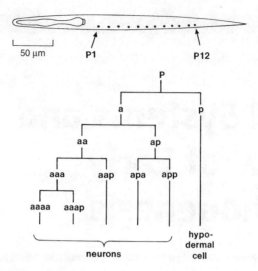

Figure 1.1 *Above*: nematode worm after hatching, showing the positions of the 12 'P' precursor cells of the ventral cord. *Below*: stereotyped lineage of descendants of each P cell (a, anterior; p, posterior). The daughter cells of a particular P cell have different phenotypes, but cells at identical positions in each of the 12 lineages have similar phenotypes. After Brown *et al.*[60]

has less than 1000 cells overall, and about 300 of these are neurons. Direct observation of living cells using differential interference contrast (Nomarski) optics, in combination with serial electron micrographs of fixed material, has identified every cell at post-hatching stages of development, revealing stereotyped, invariant patterns of cell division and differentiation (Fig. 1.1).[3] Such anatomical precision, combined with the sophisticated molecular genetics available in this species, has made the worm a powerful experimental system, particularly in the analysis of axon guidance and nerve cell death (see, respectively, Chapters 9 and 13). The large, easily labelled cells of the developing segmental ganglia of the leech have also allowed a detailed study of the cell–cell interactions during early neural development,[4] and although its genetics are not at present as advanced as in the worm or the fly, it remains a good model system for combining analysis at the cellular and molecular levels.[5] Lastly, the nervous systems of primitive invertebrates, such as *Hydra attenuata*, contain relatively simple nerve nets that undergo continuous remodelling throughout life, and their study at the cellular level has shown the importance of regional signals within the organism in determining neuronal fate.[6] The accessibility of individual neurons and synapses to microelectrode recording in certain invertebrate systems, particularly the sea slug *Aplysia californica*, has also been important in elucidating the synaptic basis of learning, as described in Chapter 15.

Several *vertebrates* have provided popular experimental systems. Among lower vertebrates, the zebrafish *Danio rerio* has been increasingly prominent in recent years, with the recognition that it combines excellent cellular resolution with the ability to carry out large-scale mutant screens and, on the horizon, cloning and functional analysis of novel genes.[7,8] The large eggs of the South African clawed frog *Xenopus laevis* are ideal for the injection of mRNA, and this, together with the accessibility of its early embryo to *in vitro* manipulation, has made it particularly useful for studies of neural induction in vertebrates (see Chapter 2).

Among the higher vertebrates (amniotes: reptiles, birds and mammals), the chick embryo (*Gallus domesticus*) is a time-honoured subject for developmental neurobiologists, largely because its accessibility to surgical manipulation and grafting experiments is much greater than for mammals. The transplantation of cells and tissues from the Japanese quail embryo into the chick, which can then be identified by Feulgen staining for nucleolar RNA or with quail-specific monoclonal antibodies, has added a very useful and stable lineage marker for constructing regional fate maps or the analysis of migratory cell populations such as the neural crest.[9]

The mouse and rat continue to be the most popular species for studying mammalian neural development. Many spontaneously occurring neural mutations have been described in the mouse, affecting for example the development of cerebral and cerebellar cortex. Their molecular analysis, combined with transgenic technology to achieve ectopic gene expression and targeted gene ablation, has made the mouse the mammal of choice for molecular genetic studies of early development. The rat, on the other hand, provides larger neonates and easier surgical access for analysing the later, postnatal stages of development, and for the same reason it is also useful for studies of regeneration and transplantation in the mature mammalian nervous system. Finally, higher mammals are needed to model the development and plasticity of the human cerebral cortex, for which purpose the ferret, cat and monkey have been used (see Chapter 14).

Comparative and descriptive features of nervous system morphogenesis

The major comparative and descriptive features of the early stages of *morphogenesis* of the nervous system will now be considered. By 'morphogenesis' is meant the way in which the constituent cells of the nervous system are organized *en masse*, and the manner in which they undergo the complex movements and shape changes to arrive at the morphology of the mature nervous system. The aim here is not to provide a detailed descriptive topographical embryology of the nervous system, which is available in many textbooks, but to introduce and define certain key structures that will be discussed in more depth in the following chapters. The fine-tuning of morphogenesis in the nervous system, involving the processes of cell migration, axon guidance, synapse formation, cell death and synapse elimination, will also be discussed later.

Comparative aspects of early neural development in vertebrates and invertebrates

Comparative zoologists speculate that the common ancestor of the vertebrates and insects might have been a worm-like organism showing bilateral symmetry, a ventral nerve plexus or an aggregated nerve 'cord', and a tubular gut with an anterior mouth (Fig. 1.2) [*note*: the term *anterior* is commonly used by zoologists and developmental biologists to denote the direction of the head (*cranial*) or beak (*rostral*), in contrast to the *posterior* or tail (*caudal*) end; this can be confusing to those schooled in the nomenclature of human anatomy, where (with the body posture erect) anterior usually denotes *ventral* rather than cranial/rostral]. Traditionally, zoologists have placed the mouth of both vertebrates and insects on the ventral side of the body, facing the substratum on which the animal lies, which means in turn that the nerve cord is placed dorsally in vertebrates and ventrally in insects. Alternatively, however, as pointed out last century and again more recently, if the *nerve cord* is taken as the fixed ventral reference point, the mouth is placed dorsal in vertebrates and ventral in insects, so one is inverted compared with the other, and we humans are back to front.

Recent molecular genetic studies on the development of dorsoventral polarity in early embryos suggest that the scheme based on the anatomical fixity of the nerve cord, rather than the mouth, is probably the correct way of comparing vertebrates with insects. The homologues of genes that are ventral determinants in vertebrates (e.g. *Bmp4*, a member of the TGFβ superfamily) have turned out to be dorsal determinants in the fly (e.g. *dpp*) and vice versa (e.g. *chordin* is a dorsal determinant in vertebrates while its fly homologue, *sog*, is a ventral determinant),[10,11] strongly

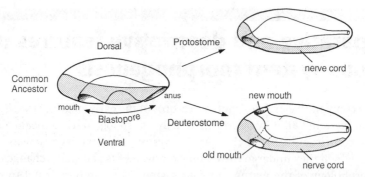

Figure 1.2 In the common ancestor of protostomes and deuterostomes (*left*), the neurogenic region (*shaded*) and mouth are together placed ventrally. This arrangement is retained in the protostomes (most invertebrates), while in deuterostomes (vertebrates, other chordates and echinoderms) the mouth shifts to open dorsally, perhaps to collect food filtering down from above. This means that the vertebrate body must have flipped over at some later stage to produce the modern form with a ventral mouth and a dorsal neural tube. After Lacalli.[61]

suggesting that insects and vertebrates are indeed dorsoventrally inverted with respect to each other.[12] Just how this took place during evolution is of course uncertain, but one possible scenario is outlined in Fig. 1.2.

The presence of a nerve cord in the common ancestor of insects and vertebrates is strongly suggested by the remarkably similar regional expression of homologous sets of pattern-regulating genes in the early developing brains of flies and vertebrates, and by the patterns of early axon growth.[13] The central nervous system (CNS) of both insects and vertebrates appears, therefore, to be built according to a common ground-plan, with morphological similarities representing true homology rather than the fortuitous result of convergent evolution (see Chapter 4). Similar homology deriving from common ancestry has also been argued for the evolution of animal limbs.[14] This ground-plan will be considered later, after the major features of CNS morphogenesis have been reviewed.

Morphogenesis of the invertebrate nervous system

The adult insect CNS comprises the supraoesophageal and suboesophageal ganglia in the head, interconnected by paired circumoesophageal connectives, and the segmental ganglia for the posterior body segments that are interconnected both longitudinally and transversely across the midline (Fig. 1.3). In the early embryo, neural progenitor cells (neuroblasts) first appear in the *neurogenic ectoderm*, where they segregate and delaminate from the surrounding ectoderm cells, moving deeper into the body to form the stem cells of the CNS primordium. The neuroblasts comprising the most anterior part of the insect brain (the future supraoesophageal ganglion) are subdivided into three main groupings (proto-, deuto- and tritocerebrum, Fig. 1.3), while the posterior brain (the future suboesophageal ganglion) comprises the paired ganglia of the gnathal segments (mandibular, maxillary and labial) which later fuse. Extensive morphogenetic movements of the brain neuroblast populations take place during head development, as in vertebrates (see below), and this contrasts with the relatively immobile development of cells constituting the segmental ganglia of the body regions.

One region of the insect peripheral nervous system, the stomatogastric nervous system (SNS), shows a striking resemblance to the vertebrate autonomic nervous system. It consists of a chain of ganglia surrounding the foregut, whose activity it controls, and derives from a small neuroectodermal thickening, or *placode*, located in the foregut region and separate from the main neurogenic ectoderm. From here, like the vertebrate neural crest cells (see below), SNS precursor cells migrate considerable distances to reach their final destinations and differentiate into ganglia.[15]

Morphogenesis of the vertebrate nervous system

During vertebrate gastrulation, cell–cell interactions between the dorsal endo-mesoderm and the overlying ectoderm define the region of the ectoderm that will

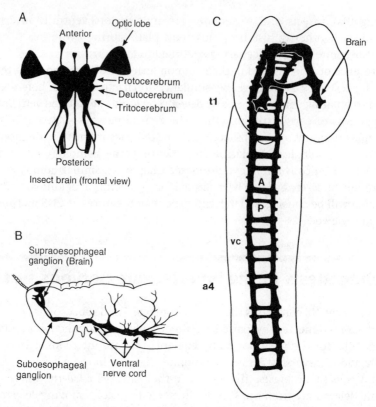

Figure 1.3 Scheme of the insect CNS. (A) Frontal view of the insect brain showing the three main component regions of the supraoesophageal ganglion, the largest being the protocerebrum with associated optic lobes. (B) Lateral view. (C) Developing ventral nerve cord (vc) showing arrangement of segmental ganglia; each pair is interconnected across the midline by anterior (**A**) and posterior (**P**) connectives. t1, first thoracic segmental level; a4, fourth abdominal segment. A,B after Reichert and Boyan;[37] C after Campos-Ortega and Hartenstein.[62]

form the nervous system and establish its principal axes. The nervous system is first apparent when, as a result of further cell–cell interactions constituting the process of *neural induction* (see Chapter 2), the ectoderm on the dorsal side of the embryo (*neural ectoderm*, or *neurectoderm*) thickens to form a keyhole-shaped structure, the *neural plate* (see Fig. 2.1). From its inception at neural induction, the nervous system is organized along two principal axes: the rostrocaudal (anteroposterior) axis, or *neuraxis*, which corresponds with the main body axis, and the mediolateral axis. The expanded anterior end of the neural plate is the anlage (primordium) of the brain, while its narrower posterior portion is the future spinal cord. Cell shape changes during the subsequent stage of *neurulation* (see below) then convert the flat neural plate into a hollow *neural tube* that sinks within the embryo and becomes covered dorsally by ectoderm and, later, mesoderm cells. The basal surface of the neural plate is lined by a *basal lamina* containing extracellular matrix molecules; after neurulation, this envelops the outside surface of the neural tube.

The neural tube gives rise directly to the entire CNS and indirectly to the major part of the peripheral nervous system (PNS). The latter originates largely from the *neural crest*, a ridge of cells that arises at the interface between neural and epidermal ectoderm (the *neural folds*). The crest cells later detach and migrate extensively within the embryo (see below). Other components of the PNS, such as the sensory epithelia of nose and ear, and the neurons of certain cranial ganglia, are derived from *placodes*, epithelial thickenings that form in otherwise *epidermal ectoderm* around the margins of the anterior neural plate. In this early phase, therefore, the ectoderm is divided into distinct regions, each differentially fated to form neural tissue, neural crest, placodes or epidermis.

Neurulation

Immediately following neural induction there is a period of morphogenesis that involves the rapid elongation of the neurectoderm, accompanied by changes in the morphology of the cell sheet associated with cell movement, rearrangement and changes in individual cell shape. Throughout the neurectoderm, cells lose the simple cuboidal/columnar morphology characteristic of embryonic epithelia and take on a tall columnar, pseudostratified arrangement. Those at specialized regions, such as the midline of the neural plate, undergo prominent shape changes, causing the plate to buckle inwards, elevating the margins (the *neural folds*) on either side. The bending of the plate is followed by a spectacular morphogenetic process, neurulation, in which the folds meet each other in the dorsal midline and pinch off from the surrounding ectoderm, so that a separate primordium, the neural tube, is formed (Fig. 1.4). A similar process of invagination and segregation takes place during the formation of placodal structures such as the ear (otic) vesicle and the lens of the eye (see Chapter 8). Although these processes are critical for the early formation of the nervous system, there are pronounced variations in the way neurulation proceeds in different vertebrate classes. How neurulation is controlled at the molecular level remains poorly understood.

Neurulation in higher vertebrates

Neurulation in higher vertebrates can be divided into a primary phase, during which the neural plate changes rapidly in shape and rolls into a tube,[16] forming the brain and rostral (anterior) spinal cord, and a secondary phase, during which the caudal (posterior) region of the spinal cord is formed. Failure of proper neural tube bending and/or closure can result in a relatively common class of human malformations known as neural tube defects, in which the neural tube remains open, locally (spina bifida), or in the cranial region (exencephaly, anencephaly or craniorachischisis), or throughout the entire neuraxis (craniorachischisis totalis).

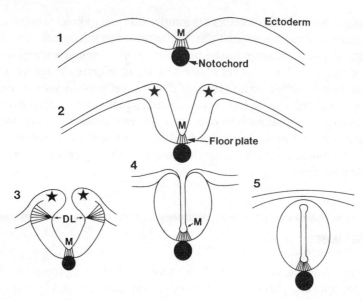

Figure 1.4 The main morphogenetic events of neurulation. 1. Midline ventral furrow formed by wedging of cells at median hinge point (M, future floor plate). 2. Elevation of the neural folds (asterisks), brought about by the movements of convergence–extension plus further bending of the neural plate at the midline, and cell intercalation in the surrounding ectoderm. 3. Cells may wedge at additional dorsolateral hinge points, allowing the neural folds to converge. 4,5. The neural folds fuse at the dorsal midline, and the neural tube segregates from epidermal ectoderm. After Schoenwolf and Alvarez.[63]

Some of the mutations associated with these defects are discussed at the end of this chapter.

The morphogenetic processes underlying primary neurulation have been difficult to dissect in terms of assigning particular steps to particular cellular activities. One reason is that neurulation probably results from complex tissue interactions produced from coordinated changes in cell shape and cell movements within subregions of the neuroepithelium, as well as from changes in cell behaviour outside the neural plate. Along the midline of the neural plate, a longitudinal furrow forms through the basal widening and apical narrowing (wedging) of neuroepithelial cells that acts as a *hinge point* around which the plate bends (Fig. 1.4). Just how this wedging takes place, and what triggers it, remain uncertain. Embryonic epithelial cells possess circumferential apical microfilaments, which could generate wedging by constriction, although it is unaffected by disruption of these microfilaments using cytochalasins. A further possibility is that the bases of these cells expand due to an alteration in the timing of interkinetic nuclear migration (see below).[17] As they change shape, the midline cells remain closely associated with the underlying midline axial mesoderm (the *notochord*), and will form the definitive *floor plate* of the neural tube. Indeed, in birds both populations derive from the same earlier source during gastrulation, Hensen's node.[18] The notochord and floor plate are co-extensive as far as the mid-diencephalon of the forebrain (see below); rostral to this, the mesoderm ventral to the neural tube (*prechordal mesoderm*) and the overlying ventral midline cells of the neuroepithelium show similar molecular properties to the notochord–floor plate complex.[19,20]

Secondary hinge points form in the midlateral parts of the neural plate, at the level of the future brain and caudal spinal cord in the chick embryo. This gives the folding plate the appearance of four subplates linked together, and the closing tube develops a rhombic shape in cross-section (Fig. 1.4). Concurrent with initial bending, the shape of the neural plate changes dramatically as its cells undergo an active rearrangement process called *convergence–extension*. Cell intercalation during convergence–extension narrows the mediolateral axis of the neural plate and extends the rostrocaudal axis of the plate. The movements of convergence–extension, coupled with the bending of the neural plate at flexure points and cell intercalation in the surrounding ectoderm, bring the neural folds together. They then fuse at the dorsal midline, forming the *roof plate*, so creating the tube that segregates deeper into the embryo from non-neural, epidermal ectoderm (Fig. 1.4). Factors extrinsic to the neural epithelium assist in driving this process as the neural plate fails to fold when separated from the adjacent ectoderm, endoderm and mesoderm; of these, the expansion of the epidermal ectoderm appears to be the most important.[21]

Secondary neurulation

The morphogenetic movements of neurulation also appear to be important in setting up the different regions of the neuraxis. For instance, the neural tube is wider at its rostral end, where the brain forms, than at the caudal end, the future spinal cord. This difference in shape arises partly because the movements of convergence–extension, which narrow the neural plate in the mediolateral axis but extend it on the rostrocaudal axis, are much more pronounced in posterior parts of the neural plate, presumably as a result of early patterning events. In addition, the neuroepithelium in some regions of the tube undergoes significant changes in shape and cell movement to establish particular portions of the nervous system. One of the most obvious examples of these more specialized regional movements involves the eye. Eye formation is first evident morphologically during neurulation, when the neuroepithelium at the level of the prospective caudal forebrain (diencephalon) evaginates to form the bilaterally paired optic vesicles. Contact between the lateral surface of the optic vesicle and surface ectoderm results in formation of the lens (see Chapter 8). At the point where the neural tube and eye vesicle are coextensive, the neuroepithelium narrows to form the optic stalk, eventually extinguishing the lumen to form the optic nerve. At the same time, the eye vesicle becomes invaginated laterally to form a cup whose inner layer gives rise to the neural retina and whose outer layer forms the pigmented epithelium (Fig. 1.5). Thus, eye formation requires a unique series of morphogenetic processes to shape the neuroepithelium into a structure appropriate for its regional differentiation.

A further example of secondary neurulation is seen in higher vertebrate embryos, where the lumen of the most caudal levels of the neural tube is formed through

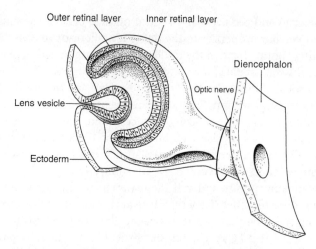

Figure 1.5 Development of the vertebrate eye. The optic vesicle, developing as an evagination from the diencephalon, is shown in cross-section. The inner retinal layer of cells is the future neural retina, while the outer retinal layer will form the pigment epithelium. After Drews.[64]

coalescence of multiple cavities appearing in a solid cord of midline neurogenic cells.[22] This begins at the site of closure of the posterior end of the neural tube, the *posterior neuropore*, and corresponds to the upper sacral level of the human spinal cord.

Neurulation in fishes

The neural tube of teleost fishes does not form through bending of the neural plate but through convergence–extension movements that cause cells to pile up along the midline and bulge ventrally, creating a structure called the *neural keel*. This later cavitates, like secondary neurulation in the caudal neural tube of bird embryos, producing a hollow neural tube very similar in appearance to that of tetrapod embryos. As in tetrapods, the neural crest forms from cells intermediate in position between the neurectoderm and surface ectoderm, but in fish they delaminate directly into the mesoderm without ever forming a part of the neural keel (see Chapter 5). A similar situation prevails in the head region of mammalian embryos, where the neural crest leaves the ectoderm before neural tube closure.

The early brain vesicles and neuromeres

The early neural plate resembles a homogeneous sheet of epithelial cells. As it rolls up and closes into a tube, a series of constrictions subdivides the rostral part into vesicles representing the primordia of the forebrain (*prosencephalon*), midbrain (*mesencephalon*) and hindbrain (*rhombencephalon*) (Fig. 1.6). Further subdivision generates a series of segment-like swellings, or *neuromeres*, within each of these regions (Fig. 1.7), while caudal to the hindbrain the neural tube remains a uniformly narrow cylinder, the precursor of the spinal cord. These early morphological features of the neural tube reflect the overall plan of the CNS and, as discussed in Chapter 3, predict its later regional specializations.

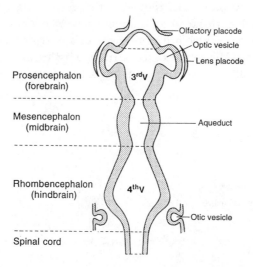

Figure 1.6 Schematic diagram of the three primary vesicles of the vertebrate brain. The olfactory and lens placodes are associated with the forebrain, and the otic vesicle with the hindbrain. The cavities of the forebrain and hindbrain vesicles are the future ventricles (3rdV, third ventricle; 4thV, fourth ventricle), and the cavity of the midbrain forms the aqueduct. After Drews.[64]

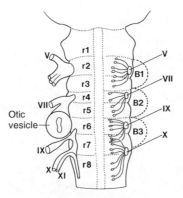

Figure 1.7 Neuromeres in the developing hindbrain (rhombomeres, r1–r8). Rostral is uppermost. In the chick embryo, successive pairs of rhombomeres supply motor innervation (through cranial nerves V, VII, IX, X) to the muscles of successive branchial arches (B1, B2, B3).

Concurrent with segmentation, the neural tube undergoes pronounced bending movements to become sharply flexed (Fig. 1.8). The earliest flexure is in the region of the midbrain (the *cephalic flexure*), and results in the forebrain swinging posteriorly beneath the hindbrain. Another flexure appears more caudally (the *cervical flexure*) in the same direction, in the region of the future hindbrain/spinal cord junction. The hindbrain then flexes in the opposite direction, about the future pontine/medullary junction (the *pontine flexure*), causing the dorsal surface of the hindbrain neural tube to broaden at the flexure point. The roof plate that forms this surface gapes widely, giving the neural folds of this region a rhombic shape when seen from the dorsal side. These dramatic flexures, which bring otherwise distant regions into proximity (such as the forming eye and the source of its extrinsic muscles, alongside the hindbrain), probably depend on differential cell proliferation between ventral and dorsal regions of the neural tube.

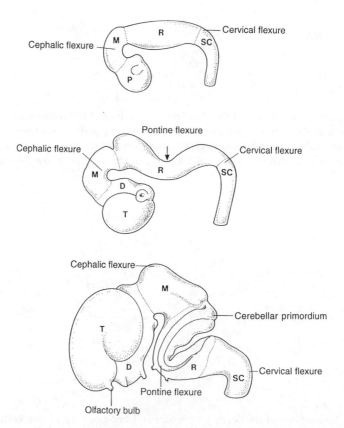

Figure 1.8 Sequential development of human brain flexures (top to bottom) as described in the text. P, prosencephalon; M, mesencephalon; R, rhombencephalon; SC, spinal cord; T, telencephalon; D, diencephalon. After Drews.[64]

Definitive parts of the vertebrate brain

The degree of complexity of the brain in different vertebrate species reflects, of course, its evolution.[23] The appearance of the brain in early chordate evolution accompanied the development of the organs of special sense, and one of the earliest known chordates, *Pikaia*, had a bilobed head with a pair of tentacles and, presumably, a primitive brain.[24] The CNS of the tadpole of the ascidian *Ciona intestinalis*, which is widely regarded as the most distant living relative of the vertebrates, consists of an anterior brain vesicle containing sensory and motor neurons, and a posterior neural tube. The CNS of the living primitive chordate *Amphioxus*, on the other hand, consists largely of a spinal cord.[25] The basic subdivisions of forebrain, midbrain and hindbrain are seen in all vertebrates, and during evolution the most striking changes have taken place in the rostral part of the forebrain, which gives rise to the *olfactory bulb* and the *telencephalon* (Fig. 1.9). Compared with the comparative simplicity of the fish telencephalon, the mammalian telencephalon undergoes remarkable expansion, proliferation and folding during development to generate the basal ganglia and cerebral cortex of the adult brain (see Chapter 7; Fig. 1.10).

The caudal forebrain, or *diencephalon*, lies between the developing telencephalic vesicles. It becomes enveloped by them as they proliferate and expand, and generates the nuclei of the thalamus and hypothalamus. Its most rostral limit (the *lamina terminalis*) is the site of closure of the rostral end of the neural tube, the *anterior neuropore*. The dorsal midbrain forms the *tectum* of lower vertebrates, which subdivides into a rostral part for vision and a caudal part for processing auditory and vestibular information; the mammalian equivalents are, respectively, the *superior* and *inferior colliculi*. Lastly, the hindbrain, which includes the motor and sensory nuclei for innervation of the neighbouring *branchial arches*, becomes further subdivided into the rostral *metencephalon*, the future pons, and the caudal *myelencephalon*, the future medulla (Fig. 1.9). Together with a contribution from the midbrain, the metencephalon gives rise to the cerebellum (see Chapter 7).

The spinal cord

After neural tube closure, the spinal cord continues to be a polarized epithelium (*neuroepithelium*). The basal poles of the cells secrete the basal lamina lining the external surface of the tube, and the apical poles are linked by junctional complexes bordering the tube's *central canal*. In the dorsoventral axis, the tube is subdivided dorsally into two (left and right) *alar plates*, joined in the midline by the *roof plate*, and ventrally into two *basal plates* united in the midline by the floor plate (Fig. 1.11). An often inconspicuous furrow called the *sulcus limitans* forms between alar and basal plates. Such subdivision of the vertebrate spinal cord is the morphological

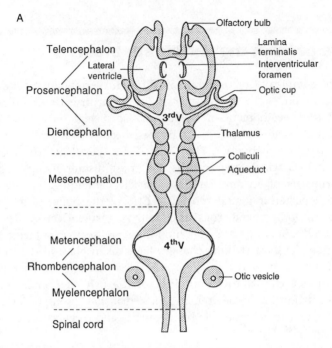

A

Olfactory bulb

Telencephalon

Lamina
terminalis

Lateral
ventricle

Interventricular
foramen

Prosencephalon

Optic cup

3rd V

Diencephalon

Thalamus

Colliculi

Aqueduct

Mesencephalon

Metencephalon

4th V

Rhombencephalon

Otic vesicle

Myelencephalon

Spinal cord

Definitive regions of the brain

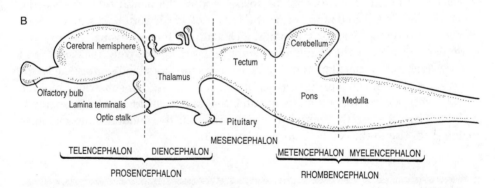

B

Cerebral hemisphere

Cerebellum

Tectum

Thalamus

Olfactory bulb

Lamina terminalis

Pons

Medulla

Optic stalk

Pituitary

MESENCEPHALON

TELENCEPHALON   DIENCEPHALON

METENCEPHALON MYELENCEPHALON

PROSENCEPHALON

RHOMBENCEPHALON

Figure 1.9 (A) Schematic longitudinal section through the developing vertebrate brain to show the main regions. After Drews.[64] (B) Side view showing the main subdivisions of the developing vertebrate brain. After Romer and Parsons.[65]

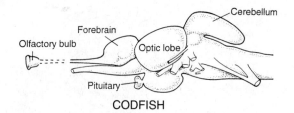

CODFISH

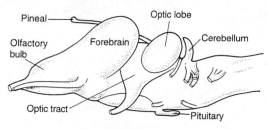

FROG

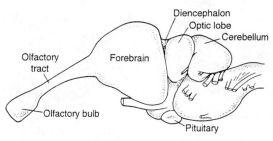

ALLIGATOR

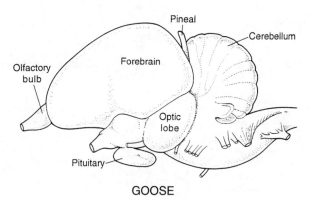

GOOSE

Figure 1.10

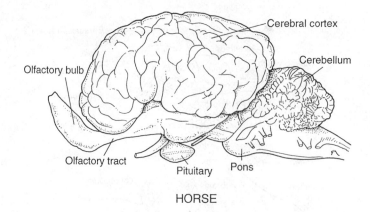

HORSE

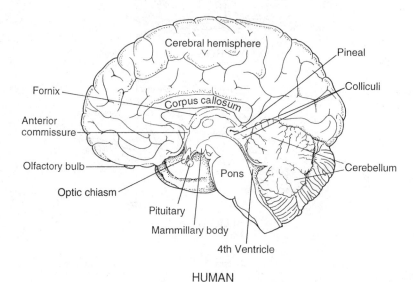

HUMAN

Figure 1.10 Comparative anatomy of external features of vertebrate brains. After Romer and Parsons.[65]

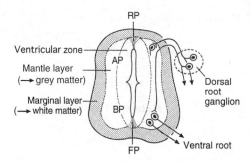

Figure 1.11 Transverse section through the early spinal cord to show main regions. RP, roof plate; AP, alar plate; BP, basal plate; FP, floor plate.

counterpart of the dorsoventral regionalization created by expression of patterning genes (see Chapter 3). Restricted expression of such genes in ventral (e.g. *HNF-3β*, midline) and dorsal (e.g. *snail*) cell lineages is also detectable in ascidian larvae, and may have been present in the common ancestor of both vertebrates and ascidians.[26]

Cell division within the neural tube

Within the tube, neuroepithelial cells show a characteristic sequence of morphological changes as they progress through successive cell cycles (*mitosis*) and rounds of cell division (*cytokinesis*): just before mitosis, at the end of G2, the cells detach their basal processes from the basal lamina, round up and divide, and then extend the basal processes out again during G1 to the basal lamina (Fig. 1.12). During all early divisions and some later ones, the axis of the mitotic spindle is tangential to the long axis of the neural tube and the plane of cytokinetic cleavage is radial; after division, the two daughter cells lie side by side and each re-enters the cell cycle. Later on, however, the cleavage planes are no longer strictly radial, and some of the daughter cells drop out of the cell cycle to become post-mitotic and differentiate. In so doing, they migrate along *radial glial cells*, spanning the radial thickness of the neuroepithelium, to accumulate in the *mantle layer* (the future grey matter, Fig. 1.11) of the developing

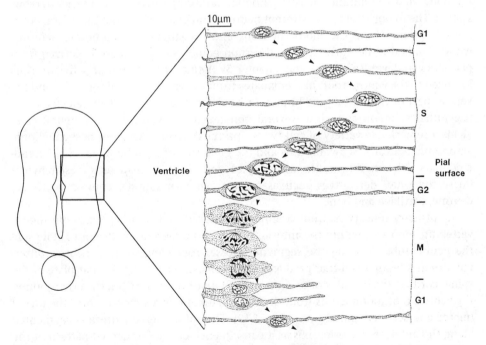

Figure 1.12 Cell division and interkinetic nuclear migration in the developing spinal cord. The stages of the cell cycle are indicated on the right. After Sauer.[27]

spinal cord and many brain regions (the process of migration in the developing cerebral and cerebellar cortex is discussed in Chapter 7). The axon tracts then develop on the outer aspect of the mantle layer, forming the *marginal layer* or future white matter (Fig. 1.11).

Also characteristic of neuroepithelial development is the *interkinetic nuclear migration*, first described in light microscope studies:[27] during G1–S–G2, the nucleus migrates from an apical position towards the basal surface and then processes back again towards the apical pole of the cell before mitosis (Fig. 1.12). This apical–basal shuttling of the nucleus during the cell cycle is seen in many columnar, pseudostratified epithelia during development, other examples being the otic and lens placodes and vesicles, the nasal pit epithelium, the early somites and the coelomic and gut epithelium.[28] It is possible that shuttling exposes the nucleus to regional variations in cytoplasmic determinants within the cell which effect critical changes in gene expression, but its precise biological significance is unclear.

The neural crest and morphogenesis of the peripheral nervous system in vertebrates

The peripheral nervous system combines the primary motor and sensory neurons of the body, and the autonomic (sympathetic, parasympathetic and enteric) nervous system. The majority of its constituent neurons and glia derive from the neural crest, the exceptions being the motor neurons and preganglionic autonomic neurons, whose cell bodies lie in the CNS, and certain cranial sensory neurons derived from placodal ectoderm (see below and Chapter 5). A small population of Schwann cells localized to the ventral roots also emanates from the ventral neural tube,[29,30] and the ventral part of the developing hindbrain has been shown to contribute cells to the trigeminal ganglion as well as several non-neuronal tissues.[31,32] The neural crest yields a remarkable variety of cell types—primary sensory neurons, post-ganglionic autonomic neurons, Schwann cells and the glial cells of peripheral ganglia, adrenomedullary (chromaffin) cells, melanocytes and, in the head, ectomesenchymal (mesectodermal) derivatives such as vascular smooth muscle, connective tissue, dentine, cartilage and bone.[9,33]

The primary sensory neurons originate from crest cells that aggregate (in higher vertebrate embryos) within the anterior halves of the mesodermal somites alongside the neural tube, forming the segmental dorsal root ganglia. Each neuron differentiates as a bipolar cell that produces two axons, one entering the alar plate of the spinal cord via the dorsal root to connect with neurons in the CNS, the other joining the ventral root motor axons from the basal plate motor neurons to form the mixed (motor and sensory) spinal nerve (Fig. 1.13). The spinal nerve pattern is segmented along the anterior–posterior axis as a consequence of the segmented pattern of the somites. If, for example, the somites are reversed in anterior–posterior orientation by surgical grafting in chick embryos, the polarized pattern of spinal nerve outgrowth

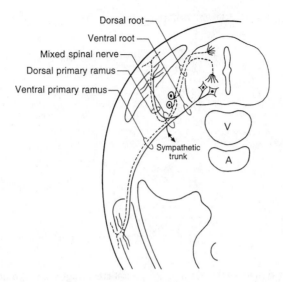

Dorsal root
Ventral root
Mixed spinal nerve
Dorsal primary ramus
Ventral primary ramus
V
A
Sympathetic trunk

Figure 1.13 The mixed spinal nerve arises from the fusion of axons derived from the primary sensory neurons adjacent to the spinal cord and the motor neurons within the spinal cord. V, developing vertebral column; A, aorta. After Drews.[64]

in the somite mesoderm is also reversed, and axons now traverse the posterior rather than anterior half of each somite (see also Chapter 9).[34]

Postganglionic autonomic neurons arise from a population of crest cells that migrate ventrally beyond the neural tube region to assume a position alongside the aorta, differentiating into the sympathetic (para-aortic) ganglia and sympathetic trunk. Some cells also aggregate in the root of the developing mesentery, forming the sympathetic preaortic ganglia, while others aggregate at the site of the future adrenal medulla (chromaffin cells) or invade the developing gut to generate the enteric nervous system (Fig. 1.14). As discussed in Chapter 5, the phenotypes of crest cells are largely determined by environmental factors. Multipotent crest cells from different levels of the neuraxis encounter different microenvironments, generating regional variations in cell fate. A good example is provided by the enteric nervous system: crest cells from the vagal region (post-otic hindbrain) colonize the entire bowel below the rostral foregut, those from trunk levels colonize only the rostral foregut, while those from sacral levels colonize just the post-umbilical bowel (Fig. 1.15).[35]

Placodal ectoderm

The placodes are epithelial thickenings of the cephalic ectoderm that arise both rostral and lateral to the neural plate.[36] They give rise to the olfactory sensory epithelium, lens, inner ear and anterior pituitary gland, while more caudally the 'neurogenic' placodes also contribute neurons to the sensory ganglia of cranial nerves

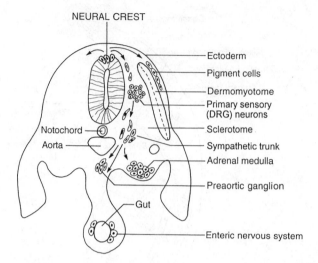

NEURAL CREST

— Ectoderm
— Pigment cells
— Dermomyotome
— Primary sensory (DRG) neurons
Notochord —
Aorta —
— Sclerotome
— Sympathetic trunk
— Adrenal medulla
— Preaortic ganglion
— Gut
— Enteric nervous system

Figure 1.14 The two main pathways of trunk neural crest migration. The dorsolateral pathway, over the dermomyotome, gives rise to pigment cells. The ventral pathway enters the sclerotome (anterior half), and these cells give rise to primary sensory neurons (dorsal root ganglia, DRG) alongside the spinal cord, autonomic (including enteric) neurons, Schwann cells and adrenal medullary cells. After Drews.[64]

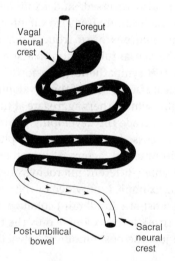

Vagal neural crest
Foregut

Post-umbilical bowel
Sacral neural crest

Figure 1.15 Neural crest origins of the enteric nervous system: cells from the vagal region colonize the entire bowel below the rostral foregut (*arrowheads*), cells from trunk levels colonize only the rostral foregut (*unshaded*), while those from sacral levels ascend to join vagal crest cells to colonize the post-umbilical bowel (*unshaded*). After Gershon.[35]

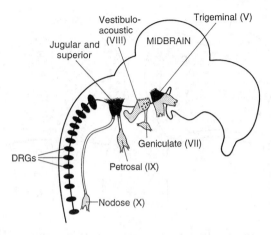

Figure 1.16 Allocation of placode-derived cells (*stippled areas*) to the cranial nerve ganglia in an 8-day chick embryo. The dark regions represent neural-crest-derived cells. Some ganglia (e.g. trigeminal) have a mixed placodal/crest origin. DRGs, dorsal root ganglia. After Le Douarin et al.[36]

V (trigeminal), VII (facial), VIII (vestibulo-acoustic), IX (glossopharyngeal) and X (vagus). Some of these ganglia therefore derive their sensory neurons from both the neural crest and placodes their glia, however, are entirely crest-derived (Fig. 1.16).

Common ground-plans of development in insects and vertebrates

It is traditionally held that patterning of the CNS in insects and vertebrates evolved independently from a more primitive common ancestor, but recent studies have shown that the anatomical ground-plans of early brain development are in fact remarkably similar. This is evident both in the regional expression patterns of homologous pattern-controlling genes and in the arrangement of the first axonal pathways to appear.[1,13,37]

The three main groupings (proto-, deuto- and tritocerebrum) of neuroblasts comprising the most anterior part of the insect brain (future supraoesophageal ganglion) may be equivalent to the vertebrate forebrain/hindbrain region (Fig. 1.17), although the number of further subdivisions in both cases is disputed. Moreover, like the segmental rhombomeres of the vertebrate hindbrain, the paired ganglia of the gnathal segments (which fuse to form the suboesophageal ganglion of the posterior brain) express particular combinations of *Hox* genes and can also be regarded as phylogenetically equivalent. Further similarity is seen in the patterns of expression of orthologous genes in the cells of the CNS midline, such as *Drosophila fork head* and mouse *HNF3β*, and for genes expressed in cells in neighbouring regions (Fig. 1.17; see also Chapter 3). Genes involved in axon guidance at the CNS midline are also highly conserved in the fly and mouse, as discussed in Chapter 9.

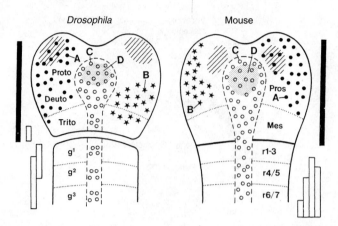

Figure 1.17 Similar patterns of nerve cell groupings and expression of orthologous genes are seen in the anterior region of *Drosophila* neuroectoderm (shortly after gastrulation, *left*) and the mouse neural plate (*right*). For each gene pair (A–D), the expression patterns shown on left or right sides of the embryo are actually symmetrical. A, *tailless/Tlx*; B, *empty spiracles/Emx2*; C, *forkhead/HNF3β*; D, *decapentaplegic/Bmp4*. Open bars, expression domains of *Drosophila HOM-C* and mouse *Hoxa* genes; dark bars, expression domains of *Drosophila orthodenticle* and mouse *Otx2*. Diagonal lines indicate the eye primordia; dashed lines enclose the midline cells of the CNS. Proto, protocerebrum; Deuto, deutocerebrum; Trito, tritocerebrum; Pros, prosencephalon; Mes, mesencephalon; g^1–g^3, suboesophageal ganglia; r1–7, rhombomeres. After Arendt and Nübler-Jung.[1]

The earliest-appearing, 'pioneer' axon growth cones in the developing brain navigate a precise, stereotyped scaffold of axon connectives that shows a strikingly similar overall pattern in insects and vertebrates (Fig. 1.18). In each case, a prominent axonal circle forms in the anterior brain, enclosing the developing foregut in insects[38] and the prospective hypothalamus/infundibulum in the zebrafish,[39] and this is connected laterally in both cases with the developing eye. It seems possible, indeed, that in vertebrates this circle represents the location of the ancestral mouth, before dorsoventral inversion took place during their evolution.[1] More posteriorly, axons in the insect brain navigate segmental commissural axon bundles and two prominent longitudinal bundles that run immediately lateral to the midline cells. An equivalent arrangement is also seen in vertebrate embryos, which have prominent axon tracts alongside the floor plate (medial longitudinal fasciculi) and commissural axons crossing preferentially at rhombomere boundaries.

Differential cell adhesion and morphogenesis

One property of embryonic tissues that is likely to contribute extensively to the morphogenetic processes that occur during early neural development is differential cell adhesion. The role of differential cell adhesion was first demonstrated by classical cell aggregation experiments in which the surface ectoderm and neural tube were

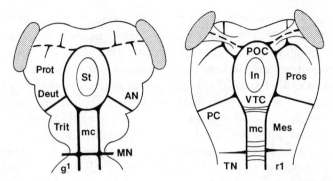

Figure 1.18 Early pattern of axon scaffolds (*bold lines*) in the brains of the developing grasshopper (*left*) and zebrafish (*right*), in the latter case after reopening the neural tube as a flat neural plate. The eye primordia are shown as stippled regions. Axon tracts: POC, post-optic commissure; VTC, ventral tegmental commissure; TN, trochlear (fourth cranial) nerve; AN, antennal nerve; MN, mandibular nerve. Dashed line, optic tract; St, stomodaeum; In, infundibulum; Prot, protocerebrum; Deut, deutocerebrum; Trit, tritocerebrum; Pros, prosencephalon; Mes, mesencephalon; g[1], anterior pair of suboesophageal ganglia; r1, first rhombomere; mc, midline cells. After Arendt and Nübler-Jung.[1]

isolated from early amphibian embryos, dissociated into single cells, and the two populations of cells were mixed together randomly.[40] Over time in culture, the two cell populations segregated from each other, sorting into epidermal and neural regions within the aggregates. Eventually, such aggregates self-organized into the appropriate tissue structure, with the ectodermal cells covering the outside and forming an epidermis with the correct apical–basal polarity, while the neural cells reformed a neural tube with the correct polarity on the inside of the explant. One of the implications of this experiment is that epidermal cells and neural tube cells have molecules on their surface through which they recognize and adhere differentially to each other. Presumably, the differential expression of these adhesion molecules in presumptive neural or epidermal cells during neural induction could contribute to the segregation of ectoderm into neural and epidermal tissues.

The cadherins

One class of cell surface protein that appears to play a role in differential cell adhesion is the cadherin family (see also Chapter 9). The extracellular domain of cadherins contains a homotypic binding site which mediates the interaction of adjacent cells expressing the same cadherin type (homophilic binding). Cells may express multiple cadherin subtypes, so combinatorial cadherin interaction is likely to be important in determining adhesive specificity *in vivo*. Adhesion is dependent on the presence of calcium ions, which link the five successive, repeated subdomains of the extracellular domain, but the molecular basis for the specificity of cadherin interactions is uncertain.[41]

The intracellular cadherin domain binds to members of the catenin family of cytoplasmic proteins, thereby linking the cadherins to the actin-based cytoskeletal network.[42] By binding on both sides of the membrane, the cadherins are thought to provide the transmembrane linkage in the adherens junction, an important means of contact between epithelial cells. Through the formation of adherens junctions, and by interacting with the force-generating, actin-based cytoskeletal network, the cadherins are perfectly placed to regulate cell contacts in epithelial tissues undergoing such morphogenetic processes as cell rearrangement and delamination.

Different members of the cadherin family are expressed in different epithelial tissues, and in different regions of the same tissue. A well-known example of the former is the differential expression of N-cadherin and E-cadherin (also known as L-CAM or uvomorulin) on ectoderm cells that form, respectively, neural tube and epidermis. In vitro aggregation experiments have shown that cells expressing different cadherins will sort out into separate populations.[43] Moreover, disrupting the expression of either cadherin interferes with the segregation and, in vivo, produces neural tube defects.[44] Even variation in levels of expression of a single cadherin can influence cell sorting: when two cell populations expressing different levels of P-cadherin are intermixed, they segregate towards a sphere-within-a-sphere configuration. As predicted on thermodynamic principles,[45] the cell population expressing more P-cadherin forms islands which fuse to become an internal 'medulla'.[46] Thus, the cadherins may provide the molecular basis of the differential adhesion of embryonic cells that was originally observed in cell aggregation assays.

In the early neuroepithelium, the expression of several cadherins is restricted to distinct segmental domains, and within these domains the early neurons differentially express cadherins. Cadherin-6, for example, is expressed in the neural plate with a sharp anterior limit of expression at the future rhombomere 4/5 boundary, and neural tube expression is later confined to rhombomere 6.[47] Cadherins have also been implicated in mediating selective adhesion between successive rhombomeres of the hindbrain, as discussed in Chapter 3, and in segregating the neural crest from the ectoderm (see Chapter 5). In the mantle layer (Fig. 1.11), the sorting of neurons appears to correlate with the cadherins they express, so it has been suggested that differential cadherin expression may influence morphogenetic events in the developing grey matter such as aggregation into brain nuclei and cortical laminae. It is possible, moreover, that grey matter structures expressing particular cadherin combinations become preferentially interconnected to generate functional neuronal circuits.[48]

Several molecular systems besides the cadherins have been implicated in the early morphogenesis of the nervous system and in differential cell–cell adhesion. NCAM, a member of the immunoglobulin superfamily of cell adhesion molecules, is restricted (like N-cadherin) to the neurectoderm rather than presumptive epidermis, and may therefore be involved in mediating their morphogenetic distinction.[49] Its downregulation by migrating neural crest cells, and corresponding upregulation by aggregating cells, may also signify an important role in crest morphogenesis (see Chapter 5),[50] although the early development of the peripheral nervous system in the mouse is unaffected by targeted deletion of the N-CAM gene.[51,52] This class of molecule is further implicated in axon guidance, as discussed in Chapter 9. Extracellular matrix proteins, including collagens, proteoglycans, fibronectin, laminin and the tenascins, and their integrin receptors, may also be involved in the morphogenesis of the neural epithelium. Fibronectin and laminin are prominently expressed, for example, in the basal lamina of the neural tube. However, a full discussion of their roles in epithelial morphogenesis is beyond the scope of this book.

Genetics of neural tube defects

Neural tube defects are the most common neurological malformation encountered in humans at birth; anencephaly and spina bifida each occur in roughly 0.1 per cent of births, the remaining abnormalities taken together being about ten times less frequent. Closure of the neural tube is clearly a complex process, and several relevant mutations and environmental factors have been identified.

Failure of closure of the neural tube at some point along its length is encountered in the mouse mutants *curly tail*, *loop tail*, *splotch* and *exencephaly*. In humans, spina bifida may occur in only one member of a pair of monozygotic twins and is probably usually triggered by environmental factors. Its incidence is reduced significantly by folic acid supplementation during pregnancy, although the mechanism of this protective effect is unknown. Folic acid has also been shown to prevent the neural tube defects seen in *splotch* mutants, providing a model system for understanding its mode of action.[53] The heterozygous form of the *splotch* mutation has a human counterpart, Waardenburg's syndrome, in which there are abnormalities of the ear, eye and hair pigmentation. The *splotch* gene has been identified as the paired-box gene *Pax3*,[54] and the equivalent human gene (*HuP2*) has deletions in Waardenburg's syndrome.[55] There are abnormalities of N-CAM processing in *splotch* mice,[56] so the effect of the *Pax3* mutation may be mediated by abnormal morphogenetic cell movements.

Mutations in another paired-class homeobox gene, *Cart1*, cause acrania and neural tube defects which can be largely overcome with large doses of folic acid.[57] Further examples include the retinoic-acid-inducible transcription factor AP-2, which is necessary for cranial neural tube closure,[58] and *HES1*, the mammalian homologue of *Drosophila enhancer of split* (see Chapter 4), mutations of which cause premature neurogenesis and severe neural tube defects in mice.[59]

General reading

- Drews, U. *Color atlas of embryology* (Thieme Medical Publishers, New York, 1995).
- Gilbert, S. F. *Developmental biology*, 5th edn (Sinauer Associates Inc., Sunderland, Massachusetts, 1998).
- Larsen, W. J. *Human embryology*, 2nd edn (Churchill Livingstone, 1997).
- Gerhart, J. Inversion of the chordate body axis: are there alternatives? *Proc. Natl. Acad. Sci. USA*, **97**, 4445–4448 (2000).

References

1. Arendt, D. and Nübler-Jung, K. Common ground plans in early brain development in mice and flies. *BioEssays* **18**, 255-9 (1996).

2. Thomas, J. B., Bastiani, M. J., Bate, M., and Goodman, C. S. From grasshopper to *Drosophila*: a common plan for neuronal development. *Nature* **310**, 203-7 (1984).

3. Sulston, J. E. and Horvitz, H. R. Post-embryonic cell lineages of the nematode, *Caenorhabditis elegans*. *Dev. Biol.* **56**, 110-56 (1977).

4. Stent, G. S. and Weisblat, D. A. Cell lineage in the development of the leech nervous system. *Trends Neurosci.* **4**, 251-5 (1981).

5. Nardelli-Haefliger, D., Bruce, A. E. and Shankland, M. An axial domain of HOM/Hox gene expression is formed by morphogenetic alignment of independently specified cell lineages in the leech Helobdella. *Development* **120**, 1839-49 (1994).

6. Bode, H. R. Neuron determination in the ever-changing nervous system of *Hydra*. In *Determinants of neuronal identity* (ed. M. Shankland), pp. 323-57 (Academic Press, London, 1992).

7. Karlstrom, R. O., Trowe, T. and Bonhoeffer, F. Genetic analysis of axon guidance and mapping in the zebrafish. *Trends Neurosci.* **20**, 3-8 (1997).

8. Kimmel, C. B. Patterning the brain of the zebrafish embryo. *Annu. Rev. Neurosci.* **16**, 707-32 (1993).

9. Le Douarin, N. M. and Kalcheim, C. *The neural crest* (Cambridge University Press, Cambridge, 1999).

10. Holley, S. A. *et al.* A conserved system for dorsal–ventral patterning in insects and vertebrates involving sog and chordin. *Nature* **376**, 249-53 (1995).

11. Sasai, Y., Lu, B., Steinbeisser, H. and De Robertis, E. M. Regulation of neural induction by the Chd and Bmp-4 antagonistic patterning signals in *Xenopus*. *Nature* **376**, 333-6 (1995). [Published errata appear in *Nature* **377**, 757 (1995) and **378**, 419 (1995).]

12. Arendt, D. and Nübler-Jung, K. Inversion of dorsoventral axis?. *Nature* **371**, 26 (1994).

13. Arendt, D. and Nübler-Jung, K. Comparison of early nerve cord development in insects and vertebrates. *Development* **126**, 2309-25 (1999).

14. Shubin, N., Tabin, C. and Carroll, S. Fossils, genes and the evolution of animal limbs. *Nature* **388**, 639-48 (1997).

15. Copenhaver, P. F. and Taghert, P. H. Origins of the insect enteric nervous system: differentiation of the enteric ganglia from a neurogenic epithelium. *Development* **113**, 1115-32 (1991).

16. Smith, J. L. and Schoenwolf, G. C. Neurulation: coming to closure. *Trends Neurosci.* **20**, 510-17 (1997).

17. Schoenwolf, G. C., Folsom, D. and Moe, A. A reexamination of the role of microfilaments in neurulation in the chick embryo. *Anat. Rec.* **220**, 87-102 (1988).

18. Catala, M., Teillet, M. A., De Robertis, E. M. and Le Douarin, N. M. A spinal cord fate map in the avian embryo: while regressing, Hensen's node lays down the notochord and floor plate thus joining the spinal cord lateral walls. *Development* **122**, 2599-610 (1996).

19. Dale, J. K. *et al.* Cooperation of BMP7 and SHH in the induction of forebrain ventral midline cells by prechordal mesoderm. *Cell* **90**, 257-69 (1997).

20. Adelmann, H. The significance of the prechordal plate: an interpretative study. *Am. J. Anat.* **31**, 55-101 (1922).

21. Alvarez, I. S. and Schoenwolf, G. C. Expansion of surface epithelium provides the major extrinsic force for bending of the neural plate. *J. Exp. Zool.* **261**, 340-8 (1992).

22. Criley, B. B. Analysis of embryonic sources and mechanisms of development of posterior levels of chick neural tubes. *J. Morphol.* **128**, 465-501 (1969).

23. Sarnat, H. B. and Netsky, M. G. *Evolution of the nervous system* (Oxford University Press, Oxford, 1981).

24. Conway Morris, S. *The crucible of creation* (Oxford University Press, New York, 1998).

25. Holland, N. D. and Chen, J. Origin and early evolution of the vertebrates: new insights from advances in molecular in molecular biology, anatomy, and palaeontology. *BioEssays* **23**, 142-51 (2001).

26. Corbo, J. C., Erives, A., Di Gregorio, A., Chang, A. and Levine, M. Dorsoventral patterning of the vertebrate neural tube is conserved in a protochordate. *Development* **124**, 2335-44 (1997).

27. Sauer, F. Mitosis in the neural tube. *J. Comp. Neurol.* **62**, 377-405 (1935).

28. Sauer, F. The interkinetic migration of embryonic epithelial nuclei. *J. Morphol.* **60**, 1-11 (1936).

29. Lunn, E. R., Scourfield, J., Keynes, R. J. and Stern, C. D. The neural tube origin of ventral root sheath cells in the chick embryo. *Development* **101**, 247–54 (1987).

30. Bhattacharyya, A., Brackenbury, R. and Ratner, N. Axons arrest the migration of Schwann cell precursors. *Development* **120**, 1411–20 (1994).

31. Sohal, G. S., Bockman, D. E., Ali, M. M. and Tsai, N. T. DiI labeling and homeobox gene islet-1 expression reveal the contribution of ventral neural tube cells to the formation of the avian trigeminal ganglion. *Int. J. Dev. Neurosci.* **14**, 419–27 (1996).

32. Erickson, C. A. and Weston, J. A. VENT cells: a fresh breeze in a stuffy field? *Trends Neurosci.* **22**, 486–8 (1999).

33. Hörstadius, S. *The neural crest* (Oxford University Press, Oxford, 1950).

34. Keynes, R. J. and Stern, C. D. Segmentation in the vertebrate nervous system. *Nature* **310**, 786–9 (1984).

35. Gershon, M. D. Genes and lineages in the formation of the enteric nervous system. *Curr. Opin. Neurobiol.* **7**, 101–9 (1997).

36. Le Douarin, N. M., Fontaine-Pérus, J. and Couly, G. Cephalic ectodermal placodes and neurogenesis. *Trends Neurosci.* **9**, 175–80 (1986).

37. Reichert, H. and Boyan, G. Building a brain: developmental insights in insects. *Trends Neurosci.* **20**, 258–64 (1997).

38. Therianos, S., Leuzinger, S., Hirth, F., Goodman, C. S. and Reichert, H. Embryonic development of the *Drosophila* brain: formation of commissural and descending pathways. *Development* **121**, 3849–60 (1995).

39. Wilson, S. W., Ross, L. S., Parrett, T. and Easter, S. S., Jr. The development of a simple scaffold of axon tracts in the brain of the embryonic zebrafish, *Brachydanio rerio*. *Development* **108**, 121–45 (1990).

40. Townes, P. L. and Holtfreter, J. Directed movements and selective adhesions of embryonic amphibian cells. *J. Exp. Zool.* **128**, 53–120 (1955).

41. Takeichi, M. Morphogenetic roles of classic cadherins. *Curr. Opin. Cell Biol.* **7**, 619–27 (1995).

42. Ranscht, B. Cadherins and catenins: interactions and functions in embryonic development. *Curr. Opin. Cell Biol.* **6**, 740–6 (1994).

43. Nose, A., Nagafuchi, A. and Takeichi, M. Expressed recombinant cadherins mediate cell sorting in model systems. *Cell* **54**, 993–1001 (1988).

44. Detrick, R. J., Dickey, D. and Kintner, C. R. The effects of N-cadherin misexpression on morphogenesis in *Xenopus* embryos. *Neuron* **4**, 493–506 (1990).

45. Steinberg, M. S. Does differential adhesion govern self-assembly processes in histogenesis? Equilibrium configurations and the emergence of a hierarchy among populations of embryonic cells. *J. Exp. Zool.* **173**, 395–433 (1970).

46. Steinberg, M. and Takeichi, M. Experimental specification of cell sorting, tissue spreading, and specific spatial patterning by quantitative differences in cadherin expression. *Proc. Natl. Acad. Sci. USA* **91**, 206–9 (1994).

47. Inoue, T., Chisaka, O., Matsunami, H. and Takeichi, M. Cadherin-6 expression transiently delineates specific rhombomeres, other neural tube subdivisions, and neural crest subpopulations in mouse embryos. *Dev. Biol.* **183**, 183–94 (1997).

48. Redies, C. and Takeichi, M. Cadherins in the developing central nervous system: an adhesive code for segmental and functional subdivisions. *Dev. Biol.* **180**, 413–23 (1996).

49. Edelman, G. M., Gallin, W. J., Delouvée, A., Cunningham, B. A. and Thiery, J.-P. Early epochal maps of two different cell adhesion molecules. *Proc. Natl. Acad. Sci. USA* **80**, 4384–8 (1983).

50. Thiery, J.-P., Duband, J.-L., Rutishauser, U. and Edelman, G. M. Cell adhesion molecules in early chick embryogenesis. *Proc. Natl. Acad. Sci. USA* **79**, 6737–41 (1982).

51. Cremer, H. *et al.* Inactivation of the N-CAM gene in mice results in size reduction of the olfactory bulb and deficits in spatial learning. *Nature* **367**, 455–9 (1994).

52. Tomasiewicz, H. *et al.* Genetic deletion of a neural cell adhesion molecule variant (N-CAM-180) produces distinct defects in the central nervous system. *Neuron* **11**, 1163–74 (1993).

53. Fleming, A. and Copp, A. J. Embryonic folate metabolism and mouse neural tube defects. *Science* **280**, 2107–9 (1998).

54. Epstein, D. J., Vekemans, M. and Gros, P. Splotch (Sp2H), a mutation affecting development of the mouse neural tube, shows a deletion within the paired homeodomain of Pax-3. *Cell* **67**, 767–74 (1991).

55. Baldwin, C. T., Hoth, C. F., Amos, J. A., da-Silva, E. O. and Milunsky, A. An exonic mutation in the HuP2 paired domain gene causes Waardenburg's syndrome. *Nature* **355**, 637–8 (1992).

56. Moase, C. E. and Trasler, D. G. N-CAM alterations in splotch neural tube defect mouse embryos. *Development* **113**, 1049–58 (1991).

57. Zhao, Q., Behringer, R. R. and de Crombrugghe, B. Prenatal folic acid treatment suppresses acrania and meroanencephaly in mice mutant for the Cart1 homeobox gene. *Nat. Genet.* **13**, 275–83 (1996).

58. Schorle, H., Meier, P., Buchert, M., Jaenisch, R. and Mitchell, P. J. Transcription factor AP-2 essential for cranial closure and craniofacial development. *Nature* **381**, 235–8 (1996).

59. Ishibashi, M. *et al.* Targeted disruption of mammalian hairy and Enhancer of split homolog-1 (HES-1) leads to up-regulation of neural helix–loop–helix factors, premature neurogenesis, and severe neural tube defects. *Genes Dev.* **9**, 3136–48 (1995).

60. Brown, M. C., Hopkins, W. G. and Keynes, R. J. *Essentials of neural development*, p. 176 (Cambridge University Press, Cambridge, 1991).

61. Lacalli, T. Dorsoventral axis inversion: a phylogenetic perspective. *BioEssays* **18**, 251–4 (1996).

62. Campos-Ortega, J. A. and Hartenstein, V. *The embryonic development of Drosophila melanogaster* (Springer-Verlag, Berlin, 1985).

63. Schoenwolf, G. C. and Alvarez, I. S. Role of cell rearrangement in axial morphogenesis. *Curr. Top. Dev. Biol.* **27**, 129–73 (1992).

64. Drews, U. *Color atlas of embryology*, p. 383 (Thieme Medical Publishers, New York, 1995).

65. Romer, A. S. and Parsons, T. S. *The vertebrate body* (W.B. Saunders, Philadelphia, 1977).

2

Origins of the Nervous System: Neural Induction

Early events in vertebrate nervous system development have been most intensively studied in amphibians, particularly the claw-toed frog *Xenopus*. Compared with the embryos of birds and mammals, those of amphibians are very large at early stages and have thereby proved to be ideal subjects for tissue transplantation experiments and, more recently, for genetic manipulation by the direct microinjection of mRNA. By comparison with what is known for amphibian embryos, our understanding of neural induction in amniotes (birds and mammals) is rudimentary. This chapter will be concerned mostly with the details of amphibian development. Although the general principles that emerge can be applied also to the amniote embryo, there are some important differences that will be considered at the end of the chapter.

The nervous system has its origins at the blastula stage of development, when the embryo consists of a ball of cells surrounding a central cavity, or blastocoel. Although nearly spherical in shape, the blastula has recognizable anteroposterior and dorso-ventral axes. The blastocoel lies in the anterior (or animal) hemisphere, surrounded by small cells that will later form the ectoderm and neurectoderm, while the pos-terior (or vegetal) hemisphere consists of large, yolk-laden cells that will contribute to the endoderm (Fig. 2.1). Between the two regions is an equatorial band of cells that will form the mesoderm. The dorsoventral axis is marked by a small surface depression at the prospective dorsal midline, the blastopore, which is the starting point for a series of highly orchestrated cell movements during the subsequent gas-trula stage that result in the internalization of cells from around the equator and posterior half of the embryo. Gastrulation is a complex process of crucial importance in embryogenesis but its details do not directly concern us here (reviewed by Gilbert[1]); suffice it to say that the cell movements of gastrulation transform a ball of cells into a manifestly bilateral embryo with a head end and a tail end and with three distinct structural layers—the ectoderm forms the entire outside surface, enclosing the mesoderm and endoderm internally (Fig. 2.1). These component layers of the gastrula stage embryo are called germ layers because each of them forms a defined subset of structures and organs. The nervous system arises from the ectoderm that forms the dorsal surface of the blastula, whereas the remainder of the ectoderm

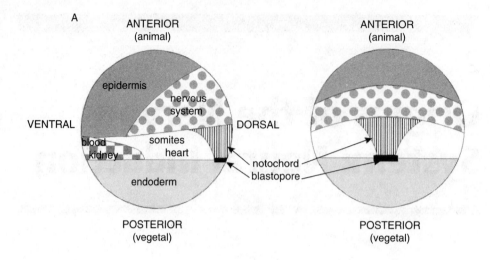

A

ANTERIOR
(animal)

epidermis

nervous
system

VENTRAL

DORSAL

blood
kidney

somites
heart

notochord
blastopore

endoderm

POSTERIOR
(vegetal)

ANTERIOR
(animal)

notochord
blastopore

POSTERIOR
(vegetal)

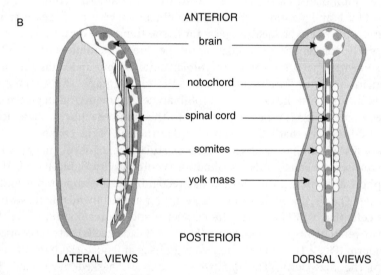

B

ANTERIOR

brain

notochord

spinal cord

somites

yolk mass

POSTERIOR

LATERAL VIEWS

DORSAL VIEWS

Figure 2.1 Fate maps of *Xenopus* embryos at (A) late blastula and (B) neurula stages. Lateral views on the left side and dorsal views on the right. At the blastula stage, the anterior half of the embryo is fated to be ectoderm, the dorsal region of which will become the nervous system and the remainder epidermis. Mesoderm arises from the ring of cells just below the equator of the blastula, known as the marginal zone. Dorsal mesoderm forms the notochord. During gastrulation, the mesoderm and endoderm converge towards the blastopore and move inside the embryo. Further cell rearrangement narrows the mediolateral axis and extends the anteroposterior axis After Gilbert.[1]

largely forms the epidermis. During gastrulation, tissue interactions between the involuting dorsal cells (prospective pharyngeal endoderm and dorsal mesoderm, collectively referred to as mesendoderm) and the overlying ectoderm define the region of the ectoderm that will form the nervous system and establish principal axes, and direct cells within this region towards a neural fate. This process is known as neural induction.

Spemann's organizer

Neural induction was discovered in the 1920s by Spemann and H. Mangold,[2] during the course of grafting experiments on blastula-stage amphibian embryos. They transplanted a small region from around the dorsal rim of the blastopore (the dorsal

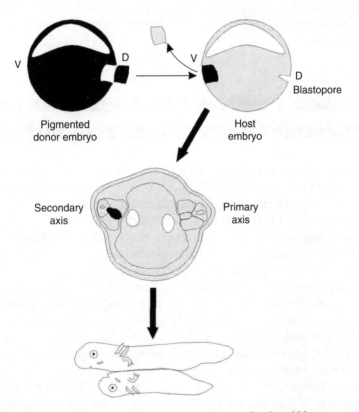

Figure 2.2 Spemann and Mangold's organizer experiment. The dorsal blastopore region is removed from a donor blastula and inserted in place of ventral marginal tissue in a host embryo. The resulting tadpole has two axes, the secondary one being composed of a donor-derived notochord (the normal fate of the grafted tissue) and a host-derived neural tube, induced to form from ventral ectoderm (presumptive epidermis) by the graft. The secondary axis has the same orientation as the primary axis because anteroposterior polarity is already established in the blastula ectoderm. D, dorsal; V, ventral.

blastopore 'lip') to the ventral side of another embryo and found that the host responded by forming an additional embryonic axis (Fig. 2.2) which contained a virtually complete CNS. The only tissues in the supernumerary axis that were contributed by the transplant were those that are normally derived from dorsal mesoderm, such as prechordal mesoderm and notochord; the neural tissue arose from the ventral ectoderm of the host, a region that normally differentiates into epidermis. This experiment heralded a revolutionary advance in our understanding of development because it showed that the nervous system forms in response to inductive signals and that these signals can change the fate of cells. It was later found that the anterior end of the primitive streak in avian embryos, Hensen's node, can also duplicate the dorsal axis, including an induced nervous system, when transplanted to non-neural ectoderm.[3] Thus, vertebrate embryos contain a region, now called the Spemann organizer, that appears to be both necessary and sufficient for inducing dorsal ectoderm to form neural tissue. A more recent experiment in which the Hensen's node of a chick embryo induced neural development in *Xenopus* ectoderm[4] shows that not only the structure itself but also its signals have been conserved through evolution.

The molecular basis of neural induction

The transplantation experiments of the 1920s and 1930s showed that the organizer is the source of a soluble, neural-inducing factor that could neuralize competent ectoderm. The fact that even ventral ectoderm could respond to neural induction implied—incorrectly, as it turns out—that the factor would be a specific molecule capable of dictating the fate of responding cells, that is that it would be an instructive inducer. Identification of the inducer molecule immediately became a high priority and, already in the late 1920s, Holtfreter had devised a simple procedure for testing candidate molecules and substances. When cultured in a salt solution, isolated blastula ectoderm (the so-called animal cap, consisting of uninduced cells, Fig. 2.3) differentiates into epidermis, but it can be induced to form neural tissue if exposed to a source of neural-inducing signals, such as the organizer.[5] However, this assay produced a surprising and for a long time confounding result: isolated ectoderm formed neural tissue when exposed to a wide variety of agents, including heat-treated tissues, tissue extracts, and simple molecules such as turpentine, collectively referred to as artificial inducers.[6,7] Whereas the ability of the organizer to neuralize ventral ectoderm suggested instructive interaction by a specific inducer molecule, the ease with which ectoderm can be neuralized by a wide range of molecules and activities suggested merely permissive interaction—how then could a permissive inducer elicit such a specific response from cells fated to form epidermis? The first clue to resolving this paradox came only recently, after a period of some 60 years of frustrated search for the organizer molecule, from experiments in which animal caps were dissociated

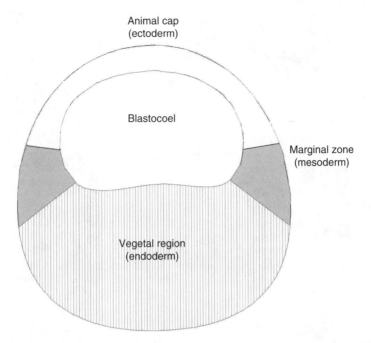

Figure 2.3 Early amphibian blastula sectioned through the middle to show the hollow core (blastocoel) and the extent of the animal cap. All of the ectodermal derivatives in the body arise from the animal cap, but before gastrulation it is not specified to become neural; that is, when explanted as a whole and grown in culture, it produces epidermis but not neurons.

before culture. When tissue organization is disrupted by this means, naive ectoderm cells differentiate into neurons even without the addition of artificial inducers.[8] Thus, because its individual cells can autoneuralize, the ectoderm as a whole would appear to be predisposed to be neural, and intact tissue would be prevented from becoming neural by some inhibitory signal that can be released or diluted out by the process of tissue dissociation. The paradox is therefore resolved by assuming that the uninduced ectoderm, whether it be allocated to nervous system or to epidermis, is already specified as neural. Neural inducers, whether natural or artificial, would work by blocking the inhibitory signal whose continued presence would result in the ectoderm assuming an epidermal fate.

This 'neural default' model derived powerful support from a landmark experiment in which mRNA encoding a modified form of a receptor for transforming growth factor-beta (TGFβ)-like growth factors was injected into early *Xenopus* embryos.[9,10] The TGFβs are a large family of polypeptide growth factors whose various functions include mesoderm induction (activin, Vg-1), induction of chondrogenesis (bone morphogenetic proteins, BMPs), and hormonal regulation of the reproductive system (activin, inhibin). The activities of TGFβs are mediated by a similarly large family of heterodimeric transmembrane receptors, whose type I and type II subunits both have serine/threonine kinase intracellular domains. Ligand binding causes dimerization

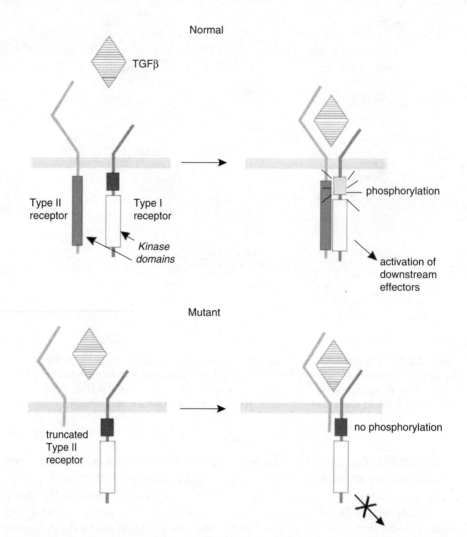

Figure 2.4 Activation of normal activin receptors and the dominant-negative effect of a mutant receptor. Ligand (e.g. TGFβ) binding causes the formation of a heterodimeric complex between type I and type II receptors. A constitutive activity of the type II receptor can then phosphorylate the type I receptor, resulting in downstream signalling. The function of the ligand is to form complexes: when overexpressed at sufficient density, the receptors can signal in the absence of ligand. When a mutant type II receptor that lacks the kinase domain is expressed, it will bind ligand and form complexes with type I receptors but have no activity. If expressed at sufficient density, it will out-compete endogenous type II receptors for ligand, and signalling is blocked. After Harland.[64]

of a type I with a type II subunit, resulting in auto-crossphosphorylation and the activation of a signalling cascade (Fig. 2.4). Lacking an intracellular catalytic domain, the modified, or 'truncated', type II receptor used in this experiment would itself be non-functional and would also form non-functional complexes with native subunits, incapable of crossphosphorylation when binding ligand. Because the truncated receptor would act in a similar fashion to a dominant mutation and interferes with normal signalling, its action is known as 'dominant negative'.

The specific goal of Hemmati-Brivalou and Melton's experiment[9] was to explore the role of TGFβ signalling in the formation of mesoderm. In whole embryos, signal blockade resulted in the absence of mesoderm and consequently of an embryonic axis. But the experiment also had an unexpected outcome: animal caps taken from embryos in which TGFβ-mediated signalling had been disrupted, spontaneously expressed neural markers rather than epidermal markers. This experiment not only mimicked, in intact ectoderm, the autoneuralization of dissociated animal cap cells but also suggested that the endogenous inhibitor would act through a TGFβ receptor. Screening TGFβ-like molecules for their ability to suppress the autoneuralization of dissociated ectoderm revealed that a member of the TGFβ family, BMP4, is particularly potent;[11] BMP4 also effectively epidermalizes the cells—the expectation of an endogenous neural inhibitor. It has since been shown that dominant-negative forms of BMP4 and the related molecule BMP7 neuralize intact animal caps[12] and, crucially, that a number of BMPs, including BMP2, BMP4 and BMP7, are expressed throughout the animal cap during normal development (Fig. 2.5).[13]

The truncated TGFβ receptor experiments, together with the findings for BMPs, suggests that neural induction would involve the inhibition of signalling by these factors. This is indeed the case for three candidate neural inducers that have now been identified: noggin,[14] chordin,[15] and follistatin.[16] All three have direct neuralizing activity and all are expressed exclusively in the organizer at the early gastrula stage. Noggin is a novel protein, whereas chordin is related to the *Drosophila* short gastrulation (sog) protein. Follistatin had previously been characterized as a protein that binds activin (a TGFβ) with high affinity. These three molecules share no obvious sequence homology but each appears to neuralize by blocking BMP signalling, in some cases by direct extracellular binding to the ligand and thereby preventing it from binding to the receptor.[17,18] Presumably, these factors act *in vivo* by titrating out the epidermalizing and neural-inhibitory BMPs from presumptive neural ectoderm and permitting the default state of the ectoderm to be realized.

Why does the embryo have three factors to elicit what appears to be the same response? It may be a case of direct functional redundancy, ensuring that a key event is backed up—much as by wearing both belt and braces. Consistent with this, the individual activity of follistatin or noggin does not appear to be required for neural induction because mice lacking either gene are born and their nervous systems are grossly normal. However, the double knockout of both *chordin* and *noggin* results in severe defects in mouse forebrain development.[19] Could it be that noggin, chordin and the follistatin family have subtly different effects from each other? There are multiple BMPs present in the animal cap that may form heterodimers as well as homodimers, and each of the candidate neural inducers binds preferentially with

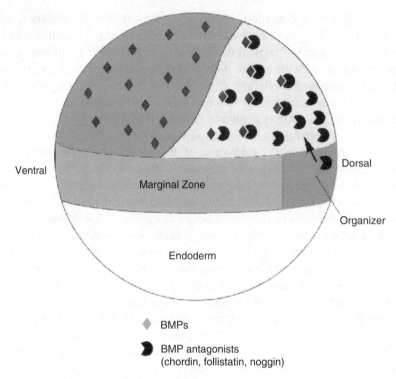

Figure 2.5 The neural default model of induction. Bone morphogenetic proteins (BMPs) are expressed throughout the ectoderm, and their activity promotes epidermal differentiation but suppresses neural differentiation. The organizer produces diffusible factors (e.g. chordin and noggin) that bind to BMPs and prevent them from activating their receptors. In the absence of BMP signalling, the ectoderm can adopt its default state. After Weinstein and Hemmati-Brivanlou.[13]

different BMPs dimers. The fact that none of the three inducers elicits more than primitive neural tissue that, although forebrain-like in terms of early marker expression, lacks the regional characteristics associated with a mature nervous system (considered below) suggests that complex synergy between these factors may be required for normal neural induction. It remains to be seen whether the CNS develops normally when multiple combinations of the neural inducers are inactivated *in vivo*. A further consideration is that the neural tissue induced by BMP inactivation expresses early markers (such as NCAM, Delta and Notch), but it appears that further signals are required to elicit markers of differentiated neurons, such as tubulin.[20]

Another class of neural inhibitors are the WNTs. Related to the *Drosophila* wingless proteins, these are secreted glycoproteins that are required for a number of developmental processes including midbrain and neural crest development (Chapter 3). The inhibition of WNT signalling by soluble WNT antagonists leads to the induction of (anterior) neural markers in animal cap explants.[21,22] One of these antagonists, frzb, is a soluble form of WNT receptor that would defeat WNT signalling by competing with the cell-surface WNT receptor frizzled and is expressed by the organizer;[21] it is not yet clear which WNT family members are specifically expressed in the gastrula ectoderm.

The discovery that *chordin* is the vertebrate homologue of the *sog* gene of *Drosophila* suggests striking parallels in how neural fate is established in the vertebrate and fly embryo, through the action of BMPs and their inhibitors.[23] In *Drosophila*, the early blastoderm is divided into three regions—the hypoderm (the equivalent of epidermis in vertebrate embryos) a ventral neurogenic region equivalent to the neural plate, and the mesoderm. Genetic analysis has shown that the area of the embryo that will form the prospective hypoderm and neurogenic region are specified through the action of the *decapentaplegic* (*dpp*) gene, which encodes a homologue of BMP2 and BMP4[24,25]. In embryos that lack dpp activity, the size of the neurogenic region is increased at the expense of the hypoderm,[26] while increased dpp activity has the opposite effect.[24,27] The size of the hypoderm and neurogenic region in flies is also determined by the activity of *sog*, whose product antagonizes the activity of dpp.[23] Thus, in flies as in vertebrates, the non-neurogenic hypoderm is specified by dpp, and inhibition of dpp by sog specifies the neurogenic region. The conservation of this 'neural default' mechanism in both of the major subgroups of complex animals, the protostomes (e.g. insects) and deuterostomes (e.g. vertebrates), may reflect its acquisition by an ancestral bilateral organism early in metazoan evolution.

Polarity and the establishment of the neuraxis

Initial polarity of the vertebrate CNS is established at about the same time as neural induction, through interactions between the ectoderm and the organizer or its derivatives. Organizer transplantation experiments in amphibian embryos showed that its signals were responsible not only for directing cells towards a neural fate but also for specifying different regions of the CNS.[2] By taking grafts from embryos of different ages, Spemann found that dorsal lip grafts from early gastrulae induced head structures, sometimes even a complete additional embryo, but that grafts from later gastrulae could induce only trunk and tail structures (Fig. 2.6A, C). These experiments suggested that the organizer consists of two components: a 'head' organizer, which induces the anterior part of neuraxis (the forebrain and eyes), and a 'tail' organizer, which induces the caudal part (the rest of the brain and spinal cord). Each component would be the source of signals that induce ectoderm to form neural rather than epidermal tissue and, in addition, signals that determine the region-specific response of the induced ectoderm. Although there is evidence for spatial

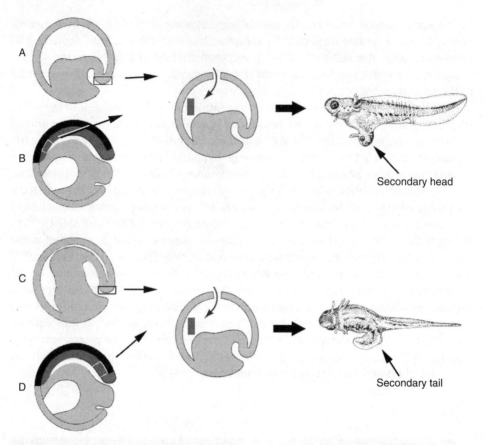

Figure 2.6 Regional specificity of neural induction in relation to the age of the donor tissue. Early blastopore lip tissue induces secondary axial structures with an anterior character when grafted into an equivalent age host gastrula (A), as does the anterior mesoderm formed by the early blastopore lip (B). Later blastopore lip tissue induces posterior secondary axes (C), as does the mesoderm it forms (D). After Gilbert.[1]

segregation of head and tail organizers within the organizer region—small pieces of the early organizer can induce solitary head structures containing only anterior CNS—the spatial readout of the two sets of signals depends more obviously on the temporal progression of gastrulation and the progressive loss of head-inducing activity by cells that remain longer in the organizer region. The mesendoderm that ingresses first through the blastopore moves beneath the prospective neuroectoderm right up to the future anterior pole of the nervous system, where it forms the pre-chordal plate. Later-ingressing cells, which will form the notochord, come to occupy successively more posterior positions relative to the prospective CNS. Thus, future prechordal plate cells invaginate first, come to lie underneath the future forebrain (the prechordal region of the neuraxis) and have forebrain-inducing activity. Future notochord cells invaginate later, come to lie underneath the future midbrain, hind-brain and spinal cord (the epichordal region of the neuraxis), and have the ability to induce progressively more posterior CNS development. It would be expected that head-inducing activity would reside in the prechordal mesendoderm whereas tail-inducing activity would reside in the notochordal mesoderm.

Vertical and planar signalling

The above description assumes that the interactions between organizer cells and ectoderm would occur by a vertical (or radial) route—from underlying mesendoderm to overlying ectoderm. The principal evidence that signalling via this route is important for establishing the polarity of the neuraxis comes from the so-called *einsteck* (pocket) experiments of O. Mangold.[28] Here, pieces of dorsal mesoderm dissected from different anteroposterior (AP) levels of gastrula-stage embryos were inserted into the blastocoel of host embryos, whereupon anterior mesoderm induced ectopic head structures with a brain, while posterior mesoderm induced ectopic tail structures with a spinal cord (Fig. 2.6B, D). These experiments show that qualitatively different inducers are present in different regions of the dorsal mesoderm and that vertical signalling between the mesoderm and overlying ectoderm *could* impose polarity on the neural plate. However, the *einsteck* experiments examined the *potential* of tissue and are, by design, incapable of showing that the vertical signalling route is required, or even used, during normal development.

By contrast, Spemann had originally proposed that polarity of the neuraxis would be imposed by planar signals travelling tangentially through the presumptive neurectoderm—from the organizer lying posteriorly to the ectoderm lying more anteriorly (Fig. 2.7). The existence of such an alternative signalling route was experimentally tested by Holtfreter, who exploited the capacity of amphibian embryos to exogastrulate when treated with hypertonic salt solutions at the start of gastrulation.[29] During exogastrulation, the mesoderm moves outwards rather than inwards and rather than lying beneath the ectoderm remains connected with it at a narrow junction at its posterior pole (Fig. 2.8A). The persistence of contact between the organizer and ectoderm at this junction would presumably have allowed planar signalling, but because the ectoderm of his urodele (*Triturus*) exogastrulae showed no morphological or histological evidence for neural induction, Holtfreter could only conclude that such signalling does not take place. A reasonable assumption would be that vertical signalling alone is required for neural induction and polarization. However, recent re-examinations of *Xenopus*, using molecular markers that were unavailable to Holtfreter, have suggested that planar signalling does operate in anurans. First, in conventional exogastrulae, the morphologically undistinguished sacs of ectoderm that remain attached to the organizer express markers of primitive neural tissue, such as the neural cell adhesion molecule (NCAM), and they also express markers of posterior CNS regions in a correct AP sequence.[30] Second, in an

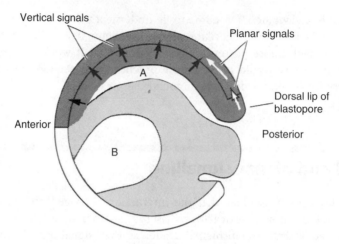

Figure 2.7 Two routes by which signals from the blastopore lip reach the dorsal ectoderm. Planar signals (white arrows), travelling anteriorly within the ectoderm with which the organizer is continuous, could have an effect early on, while the anterior–posterior axis remains short. Vertical signals from the underlying mesoderm (black arrows) are probably the major signalling route to the ectoderm for neural induction, especially as the AP axis lengthens through convergence–extension movements. A, archenteron; B, blastocoel. After Gilbert.[1]

explant culture system in which the dorsal surface of blastula-stage embryos, comprising the presumptive neural ectoderm and organizer mesoderm, is dissected out and cultured as a flat sheet, markers of both neuralization and AP neural pattern are expressed (Fig. 2.8B).[31] Although the gastrulation movements of convergence and extension (see below) seem to occur normally in these so-called 'Keller sandwich' explants,[32] the ectoderm and mesoderm extend away from one another. A prerequisite for molecular differentiation of the ectoderm is that organizer cells remain attached at its posterior end. However, a problem with interpreting both types of experiment is that overt gastrulation in *Xenopus* is preceded by a transient inward movement of organizer cells, which allows the organizer cells to contact the underside of the ectoderm. This cryptic gastrulation would appear to persist under the conditions which produce exogastrulation in *Xenopus* and there would therefore be a period, albeit brief, during which vertical signalling could take place. An explanation for the difference in developmental behaviour of anuran and urodele exogastrulae may lie in the fact that the former have a set of specialized cells in the blastopore (the 'bottle cells') that appear to mediate cryptic gastrulation, whereas these cells do not exist in urodeles.[33] A second complication with these experiments is that mesendoderm cells in the deep layer of the organizer region of *Xenopus*, which form the floor of the blastocoel before gastrulation movements carry them anteriorly, have recently been shown to contribute to head induction in, and to express an inducer molecule (cerberus) already at, the blastula stage.[34] These cerberus-expressing mesendoderm cells may already have initiated neural induction and patterning by vertical signalling

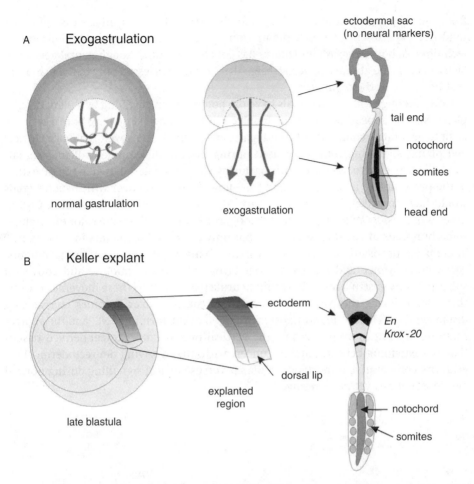

A Exogastrulation

ectodermal sac
(no neural markers)

normal gastrulation

exogastrulation

tail end

notochord

somites

head end

B Keller explant

ectoderm

explanted
region

dorsal lip

En
Krox-20

notochord

somites

late blastula

Figure 2.8 (A) During exogastrulation, the mesoderm fails to invaginate through the dorsal lip of the blastopore and instead extends outwards. The resulting embryo (tadpole stage, right) consists of two sacs connected by a narrow stalk. The ectoderm, which has not been contacted by underlying mesoderm, is not induced and expresses no neural markers. This experiment, conducted with urodele embryos,[29] was taken as evidence that planar signalling is not important in neural induction. (B) The Keller explant consists of the dorsal ectoderm of a blastula-stage *Xenopus* embryo together with the dorsal lip of the blastopore. Two such explants are cultured face to face to prevent the tissues from rolling up ('Keller sandwich') or as single explants under a coverslip ('open-faced Keller sandwich'). As in an exogastrula, the dorsal lip cells do not invaginate beneath the ectoderm but instead extend away from it in the opposite direction. The ectoderm also converges and extends independently of the mesoderm. The later expression of neural markers (e.g. *Engrailed* [En], *Krox-20*) shows that sustained vertical signalling is not required for their induction, but the experiment does not rule out an influence of early vertical contact prior to explantation. After Gilbert.[1]

from the deep layer of the organizer before exogastrulation or, in the case of Keller sandwich experiments, before explantation. A recent study using a modified explant technique in both *Xenopus* and *Triturus* has concluded that although neural genes can be induced in the absence of vertical signals, they are expressed only in the ectoderm that lies close to the organizer.[35]

Thus, although induction signals have the potential for travelling by a planar route, planar signals appear neither to be involved in long-range signalling nor to be suffi-cient to generate a complete AP neural pattern. It is likely, however, that both vertical and planar signalling routes are used during normal development. Planar signals would be expected to have prominence during early gastrulation, when the AP extent of the presumptive neural plate, and therefore the distance over which such signals would have to travel, is extremely short. At this stage (Fig. 2.1), the future CNS of *Xenopus* is considerably wider than it is long; the spinal cord territory, for example, is some hundreds of cell diameters wide but only a few cell diameters in AP extent.[36] These proportions are reversed by cell shape changes and intercalation movements, called convergence and extension, that bring cells to the midline and convert a spherical early gastrula into a long thin neurula (Fig. 2.9).[32] As these movements exert their effect during the course of gastrulation, the organizer becomes increasingly distanced from all but the most posterior region of the forming CNS, and the shorter route for signalling would become the vertical one, from organizer-derived tissues that are extending beneath, and in concert with, the overlying neurectoderm. How-ever, the comparative importance of planar versus vertical signalling during normal development has yet to be resolved.

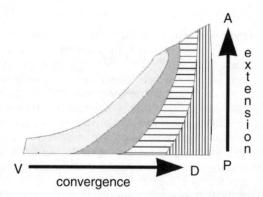

Figure 2.9 Convergence and extension movements, whereby cells converge towards the dorsal midline and then extend away on the AP axis, occur during gastrulation. These movements involve all three germ layers but only the mesodermal regions (dark stipple, lateral plate mesoderm; horizontal hatching, somites; vertical hatching, notochord) are shown here. The shape of embryo is changed by these tissue rearrangements from a sphere into a long thin body with obvious bilateral symmetry. Cell shape and motility drive this morphogenetic change, not cell division or growth.

The two-signal model of neural induction and axis polarization

Two classes of signal are thought to be responsible for inducing and polarizing the neuraxis: the first class, as considered above, would include both the artificial inducers (activators) and the naturally occurring organizer factors noggin, chordin and follistatin. These induce isolated animal cap ectoderm to form neural tissue that is anterior in character, in that it expresses both NCAM and anterior markers such as *Otx2* and *Bf1*. Since the repression of BMP-mediated neural inhibition by these neuralizing factors results in the expression of anterior markers, this could be thought of as the ground state of the CNS as a whole (but see below). A second class of signal, posteriorizing factors would then be required to modify the anterior ground state to a more posterior character.[7,37,38]

These two types of signal could exert spatially distinct effects because, as described above, the mesendoderm ingresses in an anterior (first) to a posterior (later) sequence during gastrulation and moves anteriorly beneath the ectoderm towards the prospective head. Neuralizing signals from early-ingressing mesoderm could induce a default state of anterior neural specification throughout the overlying ectoderm under which the leading mesendoderm passes. Posteriorizing signals from later-ingressing mesoderm would then modify the induced neurectoderm of the more posterior regions, changing its character to a more posterior state. The amount of posteriorizing signal impinging on any one level of the neuraxis might confer its local AP character—the posteriorly increasing response could simply be attributable to the fact that the more posterior the position of the neurectoderm, the longer its exposure to these posteriorizing factors. There could also be an increasing anterior-to-posterior gradient of the signal itself. In this two-signal model, therefore, it is the anterior-to-posterior sequence of mesoderm ingression and its posterior-to-anterior translocation that crucially underlie AP polarity. The organizer lies at the posterior pole of the extending neural plate throughout gastrulation so that, in addition to the vertical signalling route, posteriorizing factors may reach the presumptive neurectoderm by a planar route.

Posteriorizing signals

Candidate posteriorizing signals include retinoic acid (RA), members of the fibroblast growth factor (FGF) and WNT[39] families, and members of the TGFβ superfamily. These molecules are produced by the organizer and its mesodermal derivatives, and they can posteriorize induced neural tissue in animal cap assays and other experimental situations. Posteriorizing signals have also been referred to as transforming signals because they were thought to be incapable of neuralizing ectoderm on their own. A transforming role for RA has been demonstrated in both *Xenopus* and avian embryos. Thus, the misexpression of a constitutively active retinoid receptor (a mutated receptor that is active without binding ligand), which would be expected to increase the effect of retinoid signalling on target gene transcription, results in a posteriorized axis. Conversely, the misexpression of a dominant-negative retinoid receptor, which would be expected to interfere with retinoid-mediated transcription, results in an anteriorized axis.[40] FGFs produce effects that are similar to those of retinoids in *Xenopus* animal cap assays,[41,42] and certain members of the family (especially FGF4) have been shown to both induce and correctly pattern an ectopic neuraxis in chick embryos.[43] Here, when beads coated with FGF4 protein are placed on the extraembryonic epiblast, axes are induced that express a patterned array of posterior markers together with the transcription factor Otx2 (a marker of both midbrain and forebrain). However, they do not express *Bf1* (a rostral forebrain, or telencephalic marker), suggesting that FGF4 is unable to induce the anteriormost elements of neural pattern. In this situation, FGF4 appears to have neuralizing as well as transforming abilities because the ectopic neural induction occurs apparently without the intermediary induction of mesoderm (which could itself possess neuralizing activity). Whereas the ectopic expression of noggin in *Xenopus* animal caps induces *Bf1* but not the posterior marker *Hoxb3*, the combined expression of noggin and FGF can elicit the expression of both anterior and posterior neural markers.[44]

Competence of the ectoderm

Until recently, it has been assumed that the nature of organizer-derived signals alone determines the AP character of neural tissue. However, induction-only models cannot account for the fact that in organizer transplantation experiments, the donor-induced secondary axis consistently has the same polarity and orientation as the host-induced primary axis, irrespective of the orientation and precise position of the graft in the ventral ectoderm. This suggests that AP positional information is present before neural induction in all epiblast cells, regardless of their allocation to neural (dorsal) or non-neural (ventral) structure, and that neural polarity may depend, at least in part, on pre-existing competence in the responding cells. Differential competence on the AP axis has now been shown to be established before gastrulation and involves a posteriorizing influence of the presumptive non-axial mesoderm.[45] The anterior default state of early blastula ectoderm persists in cells at the animal pole, which escape posteriorization by the presumptive mesoderm. Thus, it appears that as well as transforming neural tissue after its neuralization by signals of the organizer, FGFs, WNTs or RA may also act in a graded fashion on the naive ectoderm, producing a posteriorized competence to respond to neuralizing signals.

Specific pathways for head induction

Two lines of evidence suggest that, in addition to the action of the neuralizing factors on ectoderm with pre-specified anterior competence, additional molecular signals are required for complete head induction. First, although noggin-induced animal cap ectoderm has been described as 'forebrain-like' in that it expresses early markers of that region, in reality it is primitive and lacks most of the regional characteristics of forebrain. Second, targeted mutation of either of two homeobox genes, *Lim1* and *Otx2*, expressed by the organizer results in the complete deletion of the anterior head (including forebrain, midbrain and anterior hindbrain, yet the posterior head, trunk and tail develop in apparently normal manner.[46–48] This suggests that the neuralizing/posteriorizing system remains functional but that genetic pathways crucial to anterior head formation have been inactivated by the functional loss of these transcription factors.

Candidate effector molecules in these pathways include the secreted molecules cerberus and dickkopf (dkk1). Cerberus can induce multiple heads without tails when injected as mRNA into early *Xenopus* embryos.[34] Named after the mythological three-headed dog that guarded the infernal regions, cerberus is expressed in the deep cells of the organizer that, during gastrulation, constitute the leading edge of the convergently extending mesendoderm. These cells are thus the first to contact the ectoderm from beneath and move ahead of the prechordal plate. Although they end up in the heart and liver, it is reasonable to suppose that their transient passage beneath the presumptive forebrain region of the ectoderm confers unique properties on that tissue. The heads induced by *Cerberus* overexpression are not complete, however, as they have only a single eye (cyclopia), indicating that Cerberus is not sufficient as a head inducer.

Dickkopf (German for big-head) is a novel protein isolated, like cerberus, by expression cloning from a *Xenopus* cDNA library.[49] It is normally expressed in the presumptive prechordal plate region of the organizer, which has the highest head-inducing potency in organizer transplantation experiments, and its mRNA induces the formation of complete head structures (with two eyes) when coinjected with BMP inhibitors into early embryos. Furthermore, the injection of blocking antibodies to dickkopf leads to microcephaly, showing that this molecule is necessary as well as sufficient (in cooperation with BMP inhibitors) for head induction. Dickkopf is thought to act as an antagonist of WNT signalling in a double inhibitory mechanism reminiscent of that involving noggin and BMPs. WNTs are potent antineuralizing factors that are present, along with BMPs, in gastrula ectoderm. It is not clear whether dickkopf binds WNT proteins themselves or whether they block WNT receptors, or indeed whether they activate signalling pathways that indirectly inhibit WNT signalling. Nor is it clear how transcription factors expressed in the organizer, such as Otx2 and Lim1, regulate the expression of these effector proteins. Notwithstanding these uncertainties, it is clear that there are head-specific induction pathways, and a model for their action proposes the simultaneous suppression of both BMP and WNT signalling. In turn, this implies that 'tail' organizer activity would involve suppression of BMPs (neuralization), without simultaneous WNT suppression. In effect, 'head' organizer activity would involve neuralization and anteriorization, whereas 'tail' organizer activity would involve neuralization and posteriorization.

Recent studies using zebrafish embryos have revealed a further mechanism whereby cell fates may be established in a graded fashion along the AP axis. Overexpression of the TGFβ superfamily factors, activin and nodal-related proteins, converts presumptive forebrain tissue into more posterior neural, or even mesodermal, fates. Conversely, treatment with a specific competitive inhibitor of the activin signalling pathway, antivin, converts posterior CNS into anterior. Increasing antivin dosage results in the progressive anteriorization, such that with a high dose only forebrain and eyes are formed.[50] Both the nodal-related factors and antivin are expressed at the right time and place in the embryo, and, interestingly, both can modulate AP in explants devoid of mesendoderm, suggesting that during normal development these signals may be responsible for planar induction.

The realization that both neural induction and anteriorization involve a double-inhibitory mechanism is, on the one hand, intellectually satisfying and, on the other, puzzling. Satisfying because the formation of nervous system from ectoderm by default, in the absence of instructive BMP signalling, resolves the paradox surrounding artificial inducers and brings to an end the long and frustrating search for the neural inducer. Puzzling because of the implications these mechanisms have for evolution. That head induction involves both the removal of an inhibitor and the absence of posteriorizing signals implies that the default state of the blastula ectoderm is to be forebrain. Yet, we suppose from various lines of evidence that the head is a novel structure acquired in the chordate–vertebrate transition. The early ontogenetic appearance of a phylogenetically later-appearing structure, heterochrony, describes this phenomenon but does not explain how the forebrain-by-default mechanism reached its current ontogenetic pre-eminence during phylogeny.

Neural induction in the amniote embryo

As in amphibians, the primitive ectoderm from which the nervous system arises in chick (the epiblast) acquires a bias towards neural development (i.e. specification) but has to be induced to form a neural plate, presumably through the inactivation of neural inhibitors, by signals from the mesendoderm. Grafts of the avian organizer, Hensen's node, can induce neural differentiation from presumptive non-neural or extraembryonic epiblast, and early nodes induce the expression of anterior neural genes, whereas later nodes induce posterior gene expression.[51] In birds, forebrain induction appears to be a specialized property of the prechordal plate mesendoderm, the first cells to invaginate through the node during gastrulation, as shown by the ability of prechordal tissue to induce forebrain-like differentiation when grafted to the extraembryonic ectoderm.[52] However, in the mouse it appears that the ante-riormost region of the neural axis is induced by signals from presumptive extra-embryonic (visceral) endoderm that already underlies the region before gastrulation commences and are therefore not directly related to the organizer region.[53]

The anterior visceral endoderm (AVE) expresses the transcription factor Otx2, whose loss-of-function by targeted mutation results in deletion of the rostral brain. Otx2 is likely to have two rather separate functions in head development: early expression in the AVE suggests an involvement in either the specification of anterior competence or induction, whereas later expression in the rostral brain itself (anterior to the mid-hindbrain boundary) suggests a subsequent role in the maintenance of the region (Fig. 2.10). Straightforward loss of Otx2 function by targeted mutation in mice deletes the entire head rostral to the middle of the hindbrain; however, two distinct roles for Otx2 have been revealed by ingenious experiments in which Otx2 function has been removed selectively from different regions of the early embryo. First, in mosaics composed of wild-type extraembryonic cells and $Otx2^{-/-}$ embryonic cells (where the anterior visceral endoderm expresses Otx2 but the neurectoderm does not), rostral brain is induced but fails to develop normally.[54] Second, the replacement of *Otx2* by the closely related gene *Otx1* (which is normally expressed late in forebrain development and not in the anterior visceral endoderm) allows the embryo to escape the early gastrulation phenotype of $Otx2^{-/-}$ mutants, showing that *Otx1* can func-tionally substitute for *Otx2* in the visceral endoderm when expressed in the *Otx2* locus under the same spatiotemporal control as *Otx2*.[55] However, for reasons that have yet to become clear, Otx1 protein is not made in early forebrain and midbrain of these knock-in animals despite the fact that the gene is transcribed there in the same manner as *Otx2*. As in the mosaic animals described above, the rostral brain is induced

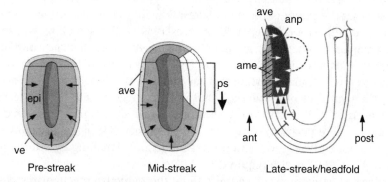

Pre-streak   Mid-streak   Late-streak/headfold

Figure 2.10 At the start of gastrulation in the mouse embryo (pre-streak), visceral endoderm (ve) surrounding the hollow cylindrical epiblast (epi) expresses *Otx2* and also induces widespread *Otx2* expression in the epiblast. As the primitive streak (ps) extends from the posterior pole of the embryo, *Otx2* expression becomes progressively restricted to the anterior of the embryo where, by the late streak stage, it is present in all tissue layers. By this stage, the anterior neural plate (anp) is underlain by mesendoderm (ame) in all but its most rostral region, where it is underlain by the (anterior) visceral endoderm (ave). After Acampora and Simeone.[65] ant, anterior; post, posterior.

but in the absence of early endogenous Otx protein never achieves fore/midbrain status.[56] Instead, the anterior CNS of these animals becomes rapidly transformed into cerebellum and hindbrain—the most anterior region of the neuraxis whose development does not depend on *Otx2*. In addition to dissecting apart two distinct functions of *Otx2* in brain development, this experiment reveals that CNS cells are still labile with respect to AP fate even after they have been neuralized and, in this case, anteriorized by neural induction. Following neuralization (and anteriorization) the rostral brain can have no more than a specification state which, in the absence of appropriate maintenance, can be changed.

Mediolateral extent of the neural plate

In addition to directing competent ectoderm cells towards a neural fate, BMP activity plays a spatial patterning role in defining the area of dorsal ectoderm that will form the neural plate and specifying the neural crest, a distinctive tissue type that forms at the lateral margin of the plate (Chapter 5). This is achieved by a gradient of BMP activity coupled with a dose-dependent response of ectodermal cells (see Chapter 5, Fig. 5.2). Graded BMP activity, high at the epidermal margin of the plate and decreasing medially, has been shown most clearly by the analysis of zebrafish mutants: *chordino*, with a mutation in the chordin gene,[57] has a neural plate that is narrower than normal, whereas *swirl*, with a mutation in Bmp2, has an enlarged neural plate.[58] Analysis of two further mutants, *snailhouse* and *somitabun*, which, together with *swirl*, present a series of progressively more dorsalized phenotypes, has also shown that the extent of the neural crest domain that forms between epidermal ectoderm and neurectoderm depends on thresholds of BMP signalling within a continuous gradient.[59] Where the gradient is shallower, as in *somitabun* mutants, the neural crest domain is wider than normal. This stands in distinction to previous ideas of neural crest induction suggesting that the neural crest formed at the site of contact between the two types of ectoderm,[60] but instead suggests that high, intermediate and low levels of BMP activity are responsible for inducing epidermis, neural crest and neural plate, respectively. However, it is clear that BMP signalling alone, or the lack of it, is not sufficient for neural crest induction; signalling by other pathways such as WNT and FGF is also required.[61-63]

Following the assignment of neural fate by the inductive mechanisms described above, neurectodermal cells enter differentiation pathways leading to a variety of neural fates, a process that is highly patterned such that different neuronal types appear at different positions in the neural plate. The ways in which neural inducers might activate these pathways will be considered in the next two chapters.

Key points

1 The vertebrate nervous system arises from a region of the ectoderm that is induced to form the neural plate rather than epidermis.

2 Classical transplantation studies demonstrated that the inductive signals come from the organizer, at the future posterior end of the neural plate, whose derivatives move beneath the neural plate towards the future head.

3 Organizer signals are also responsible for conferring AP polarity on the neural plate. There are two classes of signal. The first has a neuralizing effect—inhibiting endogenous BMPs, in whose continued presence the ectoderm would differentiate as epidermis. The second either anteriorizes or posteriorizes the neurectoderm, according to its position along the AP axis.

4 Candidate anteriorizing signals include cerberus and dickkopf, expressed by the deep layer cells of the organizer in amphibians, the prechordal mesendoderm in birds, and by the anterior visceral endoderm in mammals.

5 Candidate posteriorizing signals include FGFs, WNTs, retinoids and TGFβs.

6 In combination with the neuralizing activity of BMP antagonists, the anteriorizing and posteriorizing signals would correspond respectively to the 'head' and 'tail' organizers first noted by Spemann in the 1920s.

7 At the close of gastrulation the central nervous system has acquired a coarse-grained AP pattern that will become refined during subsequent stages of development.

8 A gradient of BMP activity across the mediolateral axis of the embryo sets the width of the neural plate and establishes the neural crest at the interface between the epidermis and neural plate.

General reading

■ Acampora, D., Gulisano, M. and Simeone, A. *Otx* genes and the genetic control of brain morphogenesis. *Mol. Cell. Neurosci.* **13**, 1–7 (1999).

■ Harland, R. M. Neural induction in *Xenopus*. In *Molecular and cellular approaches to neural development* (ed. W. M. Cowan *et al.*) (Oxford University Press, 1997).

■ Gilbert, S. F. *Developmental biology*, 6th edn. (Sinauer Associates, Sunderland, MA, 2000).

■ Weinstein, D. C. and Hemmati-Brivanlou, A. Neural induction in *Xenopus laevis*: evidence for the default model. *Curr. Opin. Neurobiol.* **7**, 7–12 (1997).

References

1. Gilbert, S. F. *Developmental biology* (Sinauer Associates Inc., Sunderland, MA, 1998).

2. Spemann, H. *Embryonic development and induction* (Hafner, New York, 1938).

3. Waddington, C. H. Induction by the primitive streak and its derivatives. *J. Exp. Biol.* **10**, 38–46 (1933).

4. Kintner, C. R. and Dodd, J. Hensen's node induces neural tissue in *Xenopus* ectoderm. Implications for the action of the organizer in neural induction. *Development* **113**, 1495–505 (1991).

5. Holtfreter, J. Über die Aufzucht isolierter Teile des Amphibienkeimes. II. *Roux's Arch. Entw. Mech. Org.* **124**, 404–66 (1931).

6. Holtfreter, J. Neural induction in explants which have passed through a sublethal cytolysis. *J. Exp. Zool.* **106**, 197–222 (1947).

7. Saxén, L. Neural induction. *Int. J. Dev. Biol.* **33**, 21–48 (1989).

8. Grunz, H. and Tacke, L. Neural differentiation of *Xenopus laevis* ectoderm takes place after disaggregation and delayed reaggregation without inducer. *Cell Dier. Dev.* **28**, 211–17 (1989).

9. Hemmati-Brivanlou, A. and Melton, D. A. Inhibition of activin receptor signaling promotes neuralization in *Xenopus*. *Cell* **77**, 273–82 (1994).

10. Hemmati-Brivanlou, A. and Melton, D. A. A truncated activin receptor inhibits mesoderm induction and formation of axial structures in *Xenopus* embryos. *Nature* **359**, 609–14 (1992).

11. Wilson, P. A. and Hemmati-Brivanlou, A. Induction of epidermis and inhibition of neural fate by Bmp-4. *Nature* **376**, 331–33 (1995).

12. Hawley, S. H. *et al.* Disruption of BMP signals in embryonic *Xenopus* ectoderm leads to direct neural induction. *Genes Dev.* **9**, 2923–35 (1995).

13. Weinstein, D. C. and Hemmati-Brivanlou, A. Neural induction in *Xenopus laevis*: evidence for the default model. *Curr. Opin. Neurobiol.* **7**, 7–12 (1997).

14. Smith, W. C. and Harland, R. M. Expression cloning of noggin, a new dorsalizing factor localized to the Spemann organizer in *Xenopus* embryos. *Cell* **70**, 829–40 (1992).

15. Sasai, Y. *et al. Xenopus* chordin: a novel dorsalizing factor activated by organizer-specific homeobox genes. *Cell* **79** (1994).

16. Hemmati-Brivanlou, A. and Melton, D. A. Follistatin, an antagonist of activin, is expressed in the Spemann organizer and displays direct neuralizing activity. *Cell* **77**, 283–96 (1994).

17. Zimmerman, L. B., De Jesus-Escobar, J. M. and Harland, R. M. The Spemann organizer signal noggin binds and inactivates bone morphogenetic protein 4. *Cell* **86**, 599–606 (1996).

18. Piccolo, S., Sasai, Y., Lu, B. and De Robertis, E. M. Dorsoventral patterning in *Xenopus*: inhibition of ventral signals by direct binding of chordin to BMP-4. *Cell* **86**, 589–98 (1996).

19. Bachiller, D. *et al.* The organizer factors Chordin and Noggin are required for mouse forebrain development. *Nature* **403**, 658–61 (2000).

20. Messenger, N. J., Rowe, S. J. and Warner, A. E. The neurotransmitter noradrenaline drives noggin expressing ectoderm cells to active *N-tubulin* and become neurons. *Dev. Biol.* **205**, 224–32 (1999).

21. Leyns, L., Bouwmeester, T., Kim, S.-H., Piccolo, S. and De Robertis, E. M. Frzb-1 is a secreted antagonist of wnr-signals expressed in the Spemann organiser. *Cell* **88**, 747–56 (1997).

22. Itoh, K., Tang, T. L., Neel, B. G. and Sokol, S. Y. Specific modulation of ectodermal cell fates in *Xenopus* embryos by glycogen synthase kinase. *Development* **121**, 3979–88 (1995).

23. Holley, S. A., Jackson, P. D., Sasai, Y., Lu, B. and De Robertis, E. M. A conserved system for dorsal–ventral patterning in insects and vertebrates involving sog and chordin. *Nature* **376**, 249–53 (1995).

24. Ferguson, E. A. and Anderson, K. A. *Decapentaplegic* acts as a morphogen to organize dorsal–ventral pattern in the *Drosophila* embryo. *Cell* **71**, 451–61 (1992).

25. Gelbart, W. M. The *decapentaplegic* gene: a TFGβ homologue controlling pattern formation in *Drosophila*. *Development* **122** (Suppl.), 65–74 (1989).

26. Irish, V. F. and Gelbart, W. M. The decapentaplegic gene is required for dorsal–ventral patterning of the *Drosophila* embryo. *Genes Dev.* **1**, 868–79 (1987).

27. Wharton, K. A., Ray, R. P. and Gelbart, W. M. An activity gradient of decapentaplegic is necessary for the specification of dorsal pattern elements in the *Drosophila* embryo. *Development* **117**, 807–22 (1993).

28. Mangold, O. Über die Induktionsfähigkeit der vershiendenen Bezirke der Neurula bon Urodelen. *Naturwissenschaften* **21**, 761–6 (1933).

29. Holtfreter, J. Die totale Exogastrulation, eine Selbstablosung des Ektoderms von Entomesoderm. *Roux's Arch. Entw. Mech. Org.* **129**, 669–793 (1933).

30. Ruiz i Altaba, A. Neural expression of the *Xenopus* homeobox gene Xhox3: evidence for a patterning neural signal that spreads through the ectoderm. *Development* **108**, 595–604 (1990).

31. Doniach, T., Phillips, C. R. and Gerhart, J. C. Planar induction of anteroposterior pattern in the developing central nervous system of *Xenopus laevis. Science* **257**, 542–5 (1992).

32. Keller, R., Shih, J. and Sater, A. The cellular basis for the convergence and extension of the *Xenopus* neural plate. *Dev. Dyn.* 193, 199–217 (1992).

33. Hardin, J. and Keller, R. The behaviour and function of bottle cells during gastrulation in *Xenopus laevis. Development* **103**, 211–30 (1988).

34. Bouwmeester, T., Kim, S., Sasai, Y., Lu, B. and De Robertis, E. M. Cerberus is a head-inducing secreted factor expressed in the anterior endoderm of Spemann's organizer. *Nature* **382**, 595–601 (1996).

35. Chen, Y., Holleman, T., Pieler, T. and Grunz, H. Planar signalling is not sufficient to generate a specific anterior/posterior neural pattern in pseudoexogastrula explants from *Xenopus* and *Triturus. Mech. Dev.* **90**, 53–63 (2000).

36. Keller, R. Vital dye mapping of the gastrula and neurula of *Xenopus* laevis. II. Prospective areas and morphogenetic movements in the deep layer. *Dev. Biol.* **51**, 118–37 (1976).

37. Kelly, O. G. and Melton, D. A. Induction and patterning of the vertebrate nervous system. *Trends Genet.* **11**, 273–8 (1995).

38. Nieuwkoop, P. D. Activation and organization of the central nervous system in amphibians. III. Synthesis of a new working hypothesis. *J. Exp. Zool.* **120**, 83–108 (1952).

39. McGrew, L. L., Lai, C. J. and Moon, R. T. Specification of the anteroposterior neural axis through synergistic interaction of the Wnt signaling cascade with noggin and follistatin. *Dev. Biol.* **172**, 337–42 (1995).

40. Blumberg, B. *et al.* An essential role for retinoid signaling in anteroposterior neural patterning. *Development* **124**, 373–9 (1997).

41. Cox, W. G. and Hemmati-Brivanlou, A. Caudalization of neural fate by tissue recombination and bFGF. *Development* **121**, 4349–58 (1995).

42. Doniach, T. Basic FGF as an inducer of anteroposterior neural pattern. *Cell* **83**, 1067–670 (1995).

43. Alvarez, I. S., Araujo, M. and Nieto, M. A. Neural induction in whole chick embryo culture by FGF. *Dev. Biol.* **199**, 42–54 (1998).

44. Lamb, T. M. and Harland, R. M. Fibroblast growth factor is a direct neural inducer, which combined with noggin generates anterior–posterior neural pattern. *Development* **121**, 3627–36 (1995).

45. Koshida, S., Shinya, M., Mizuno, T., Kuroiwa, A. and Takeda, H. Initial anteroposterior pattern of the zebrafish central nervous system is determined by differential competence of the epiblast. *Development* **125**, 1957–66 (1998).

46. Ang, S.-L. *et al.* A targetted mouse Otx2 mutation leads to severe defects in gastrulation and formation of axial mesoderm and to deletion of the rostral brain. *Development* **122**, 243–52 (1996).

47. Acampora, D. *et al.* Forebrain and midbrain regions are deleted in Otx2$^{-/-}$ mutants due to a defective anterior neuroectoderm specification during gastrulation. *Development* **121**, 3279–90 (1995).

48. Shawlot, W. and Behringer, R. R. Requirement for *Lim-1* in head organizer function. *Nature* **374**, 425–30 (1995).

49. Glinka, A. *et al.* Dickkopf-1 is a member of a new family of secreted proteins and functions in head induction. *Nature* **391**, 357–62 (1998).

50. Thisse, B., Wright, C. V. E. and Thisse, C. Activin- and Nodal-related factors control anteroposterior patterning of the zebrafish embryo. *Nature* **403**, 425–8 (2000).

51. Storey, K. G., Crossley, J. M., De Robertis, E. M., Norris, W. E. and Stern, C. D. Neural induction and regionalisation in the chick embryo. *Development* **114**, 729–41 (1992).

52. Pera, E. and Kessel, M. Patterning of the chick forebrain anlage by the prechordal plate. *Development* **124**, 4153–62 (1997).

53. Thomas, P. and Beddington, R. Anterior primitive endoderm may be responsible for patterning the anterior neural plate in the mouse embryo. *Curr. Biol.* **6**, 1487–96 (1996).

54. Rhinn, M. *et al.* Sequential roles for *Otx2* in visceral endoderm and neuroectoderm for forebrain and midbrain induction and specification. *Development* **125**, 845–56 (1998).

55. Acampora, D. *et al.* Visceral endoderm-restricted translation of Otx1 mediates recovering of Otx2 requirements for specification of anterior neural plate and proper gastrulation. *Development* **125**, 5091–104 (1998).

56. Acampora, D., Gulisano, M. and Simeone, A. Otx genes and the genetic control of brain morphogenesis. *Mol. Cell. Neurosci.* **13**, 1–8 (1999).

57. Schulte-Merker, S., Lee, K. J., McMahon, A. P. and Hammerschmidt, M. The zebrafish organizer requires chordino. *Nature* **387**, 862–3 (1997).

58. Kishimoto, Y., Lee, K. H., Zon, L., Hammerschmidt, M. and Schulte-Merker, S. The molecular nature of zebrafish swirl: BMP2 function is essential during early dorsoventral patterning. *Development* **124**, 2452–61 (1997).

59. Nguyen, V. H. *et al.* Ventral and lateral regions of the zebrafish gastrula, including the neural crest progenitors, are established by a bmp2b/swirl pathway of genes. *Dev. Biol.* **199**, 93–110 (1998).

60. Moury, J. D. and Jacobson, A. G. The origins of neural crest cells in the axolotl. *Dev. Biol.* **141**, 243–53 (1990).

61. Mayor, R., Guerrero, N. and Martinez, C. Role of FGF and noggin in neural crest induction. *Dev. Biol.* **189**, 1–12 (1997).

62. La Bonne, C. and Bronner-Fraser, M. Neural crest induction in *Xenopus*: evidence for a two-signal model. *Development* **125**, 2403–14 (1998).

63. Dorsky, R. I., Moon, R. T. and Raible, D. W. Control of neural crest cell fate by the Wnt signalling pathway. *Nature* **396**, 370–2 (1998).

64. Harland, R. M. Neural induction in *Xenopus*. In *Molecular and cellular approaches to neural development* (ed. W. M. Cowan, T. M. Jessell and S. L. Zipursky), pp. 1–25 (Oxford University Press, New York, 1997).

65. Acampora, D. and Simeone, A. Understanding the roles of Otx1 and Otx2 in the control of brain morphogenesis. *Trends Neurosci.* **22**, 116–22 (1999).

3

Patterning the Central Nervous System

A crude anteroposterior (AP) pattern is set up in the neural plate during, and as a direct result of, neural induction (Chapter 2). At this stage, pattern exists principally at the molecular level, as spatially restricted domains of developmental gene expression; but, as the subsequent process of neural tube morphogenesis (neurulation) begins, so the axis becomes overtly regionalized: the enlarged anterior end of the neural plate continues to expand on closure, but unequally, thereby producing a series of swellings that will eventually form fore-, mid- and hindbrain regions, separated by constrictions in the diameter of the neural tube. The smooth, narrow posterior part of the tube forms the precursor of the spinal cord. Continued morphological subdivision of the neuraxis (most notably in the hindbrain) produces an iterated set of small, segment-like bulges, called neuromeres. These early morphological features of the neuraxis, accompanied by the region-specific neural expression of developmental control genes that begins during gastrulation, dictate the regional plan of the CNS and predict its local specializations. Within each region, a large diversity of neuronal cell types is then generated, with distinct identities in terms of morphology, molecular markers, axonal trajectory, synaptic specificity, neurotransmitter, neurotransmitter receptor, etc. Perhaps most strikingly, individual neurons or groups of similar neurons differentiate at predictable times and positions within the various regions of the neural tube. Some of these subpopulations then undergo an orderly process of migration to specific new and final locations.

Correct specification of this intricate pattern of cell differentiation is crucial to later events in CNS development when the different cell types establish precise arrays of interconnection that assemble functional networks. Activity-dependent processes and regressive events, such as the pruning of axons and cell death, later reinforce and refine initial patterns of connectivity (see Chapters 13 and 14), but an extraordinarily high degree of precision is achieved from the outset, as a direct result of appropriate cell patterning. For the nervous system, as for the entire body, our understanding of patterning processes has advanced rapidly through the discovery of genes that control development, and the elucidation of mechanisms that regulate their spatial and temporal expression. Deciphering the genetic instructions that establish the pattern of neuronal differentiation during development may be the key to understanding the complexities of the adult brain.

It is useful to consider cell pattern in the CNS as if set out on a Cartesian map, whose orthogonal coordinates correspond with the two principal axes of the system, anteroposterior and dorsoventral. The third axis of the CNS, inside–outside (or ventricular–pial), is essentially a maturational gradient of neurogenesis that is rather uniform across the CNS as a whole (with the principal exception of cerebral and cerebellar cortices, see Chapter 7) and will not be considered further here. In previous chapters, we have seen how the AP axis becomes polarized and coarsely regionalized. In this chapter, we will consider the spatial order, or pattern, of neural differentiation. Each of the major brain regions and the spinal cord will be discussed in turn, dealing separately with the AP axis and the dorsoventral (DV) axis. Finally, we will see how patterning information is integrated between the two axes so as to produce correct neuronal specification with respect to position.

Forebrain

In terms of its early development, the forebrain (prosencephalon) is the least studied region of the CNS, especially in mammals where its derivatives include the cerebral cortex, the most prominent and ultimately the most complex region of the brain. Here, later events such as the acquisition of laminar and area (functional) organization are intensively studied (Chapter 7), but a basic and enduring question is how the two major prosencephalic regions, the telencephalon (future cortex and basal ganglia) and diencephalon (future thalamus), and their respective subregions, acquire distinctive identities. A start has been made with the provision of fate maps that can accurately predict the derivation of forebrain structures from the anterior neural plate (Fig. 3.1),[1,2] together with the identification of a number of developmental control genes that are expressed in restricted domains at neural plate and early neural tube stages. Targeted mutation of such genes leads, in some cases, to the disruption of forebrain development and has thereby provided a lead into understanding the genetic pathways involved in patterning the region.

In chick embryos, whose fate map may also reflect the situation in mammals, the telencephalon is seen to arise from the lateral (future dorsal or alar) regions of the anterior neural plate, whereas the medial (later ventral or basal) region gives rise to the diencephalon. During and following neurulation, extensive morphogenetic curvature of the axis (cephalic flexure), accompanied by overfolding of the rapidly expanding areas derived from the lateral/dorsal regions of the neural plate, carry the bilateral telencephalic vesicles forward over the diencephalic vesicle to assume the most rostral position on the neuraxis (Fig. 3.2). The original anterior tip of the neural plate thereby ends up in a ventral and subterminal position, as the pituitary and mammillary region of the hypothalamus. Ventral telencephalic structures (i.e. the

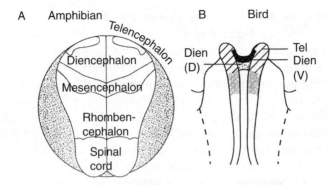

Figure 3.1 Fate maps of an early amphibian (A) and later chick (B) neurula stage. The telencephalon originates from the lateral (future dorsal) region of the neural plate rather than its anterior pole. Neural fold elevation (B) brings the telencephalic (Tel) primordia together in the dorsal midline, and then cephalic flexure carries them forward of the diencephalic (Dien) primordium. A, after Eagleston and Harris;[1] B, after Le Douarin.[2] D, dorsal; V, ventral.

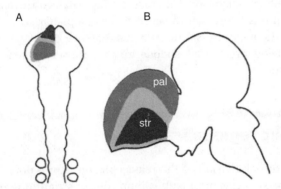

Figure 3.2 Fate map showing the derivation of dorsal (pallium, pal) and ventral (striatum, str) domains of the telencephalon at day 5 of chick development (A) from the prosencephalic vesicle at 1.5 days (B). The pallial region expresses *Emx1* and *Emx2*, whereas the striatal region expresses *Dlx1* and *Dlx2*. After Fernandez *et al.*[124]

striatum and globus pallidus, collectively known as the basal ganglia) thus derive from originally dorsal tissue that moves ventrally during neurulation and anterior neuropore closure. Cephalic flexure also rotates the axis of the diencephalon, such that anterior regions of the diencephalic neural tube assume a ventral position with respect to originally more posterior regions.

The expression of a number of transcription factors supports the notion that the initial subdivision of the forebrain is into telencephalic and diencephalic territories, before each territory is subsequently subdivided. Thus, expression of the winged-helix transcription factor BF-1 demarcates the telencephalon as a single field at the late neural plate stage, before the emergence of a discrete morphological boundary between telencephalon and diencephalon. Loss of *BF-1* function in mice by targeted mutation results in deletion of the ventral telencephalon together with severe reduction of the cerebral hemispheres.[3]

In addition to requiring intrinsic *Otx2* function (Chapter 2), telencephalic specification appears to be under the control of cells at the rostral pole of the neural plate, which constitute one of a number of secondary signalling centres responsible for localized patterning that are set up at various positions in the neural plate during gastrulation. In the zebrafish embryo, a specific transverse row of a dozen ectoderm cells at the anterior neural–non-neural border, the so-called row-1 cells, produce a planar signal required for the expression of telencephalic markers in adjacent cells. Ablation of the row-1 cells results in diencephalic markers expanding into the initially normal-looking telencephalic vesicles. When transplanted heterotopically, row-1 cells can induce expression of forebrain markers by presumptive midbrain neural plate.[4] At a later stage of development, FGF8 emanates from an equivalent region of ectoderm in mouse embryos, the anterior neural ridge (ANR), and appears to influence the expression of *BF-1* in adjoining telencephalic tissues (Fig. 3.3).[5] The signals produced by the ANR of mouse and the row-1 cells of zebrafish cannot be identical because the latter expresses *Fgf8* but the telencephalic territory is specified normally in the *Fgf8*-mutant zebrafish, *ace*.[6] The relationship between the two structures is as yet uncertain, but it is likely that the emergence of a planar signalling centre at the anterior pole of the neuraxis, set up as a consequence of vertical inductive signals from the underlying prechordal endoderm, is a conserved feature of vertebrate neural development.

Telencephalic regionalization

The principal early subdivision of the telencephalon is into dorsal (pallium, future cortex in mammals) and ventral (subpallium, future striatum and globus pallidus) domains, separated by a sharply defined longitudinal boundary. Dorsally expressed genes include the homeobox genes *Emx1* and *Emx2*, the paired box gene *Pax6*, and the T-box gene *Tbr1*. Ventrally expressed genes include homeobox genes of the *Dlx* family, related to *Drosophila distal-less*, and the *Nkx* family. However, these sets of genes do not necessarily have complementary roles: whereas *Emx* genes are expressed in the ventricular neuroepithelium and are therefore candidates for a role in regionalization, *Dlx* genes are expressed in differentiating cells as they leave the ventricular zone, with an implied function in the control of cell differentiation and/or migration.[7] At neural tube and later stages of development, both *Otx* and *Emx* genes are expressed in overlapping domains that encompass the entire rostral extremity of the neuraxis with the exception of the ventral diencephalon (Fig. 3.4). These genes are homologues of the *Drosophila* gap genes *orthodenticle* (*otd*) and *empty spiracles* (*ems*), which function as homeotic selectors in the specification of particular head segments and brain neuromeres. The nested expression of *Emx1* < (within) *Emx2* < *Otx1* < *Otx2* suggests that their proteins may be employed in a combinatorial manner to specify the identity of telencephalic, dorsal diencephalic and mesencephalic regions.[8] In

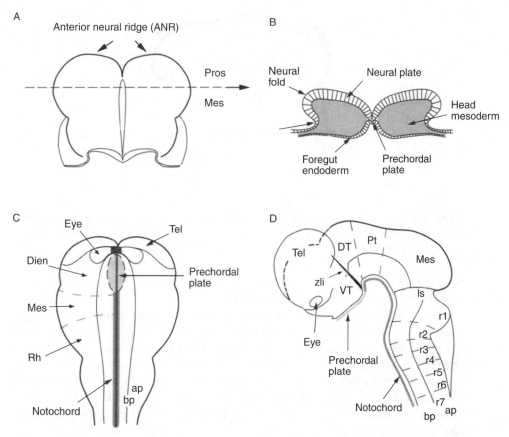

Figure 3.3 Stages in the early morphogenesis of the mouse forebrain. Open neural plate stage (8.5 days post-conception) in dorsal view (A) and section (B) showing the anterior neural ridge, a source of polarizing signals that affect the expression of telencephalic markers. Presumptive brain and eye regions are shown at the later neural plate (C) and closed neural tube (D) stages. ap, alar plate; bp, basal plate; Dien, diencephalon; DT, dorsal thalamus; Is, isthmus; Mes, mesencephalon; Pros, prosencephalon; Pt, pretectum; r, rhombomeres; Rh, rhombencephalon; Tel, telencephalon; VT, ventral thalamus; zli, zona limitans intrathalamica. After Rubenstein and Beachy.[125]

addition, Emx2 protein is expressed in a graded manner in the cortical ventricular zone, such that it is higher in posterior medial cortex, suggesting a role in the specification of functional areas.[9] Loss of *Emx1* and *Emx2* function leads to distinct and restricted structural abnormalities: *Emx1* mutants lose the corpus callosum,[10] whereas *Emx2* mutants lose the hippocampal dentate gyrus[11] and the Cajal–Retzius cells of the neocortex,[12] which are assumed to play a guiding role in the radial migration of cortical neurons (see Chapter 7). Consistent with this, neuronal migration and lamination are severely disrupted in *Emx2* mutants, which have a phenotype similar to the mouse mutant *reeler* in this respect (see Chapter 7). Although an *Emx1; Emx2* double mutant has yet to be described, the null mutant phenotype of Gli3, a zinc-finger transcription factor required for the expression of both *Emx* genes, shows

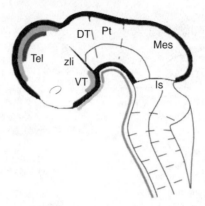

Figure 3.4 Gene expression in the embryonic forebrain. *Otx2* (black) expression encompasses almost the entire forebrain and midbrain, whereas *Emx2* (light grey) and *Emx1* (dark grey) are expressed only in forebrain. For abbreviations, see Fig. 3.3 legend.

disruption of the dorsal telencephalic–diencephalic boundary in addition to the cortical lamination defects seen in the *Emx2* knockout.[13]

Regionalization of the ventral telencephalon into striatal (dorsolateral) and pallidal (ventromedial) areas depends, at least in part, on expression of the homeobox gene *Nkx2.1*, in the latter region. In mice lacking functional Nkx2.1, the striatum is expanded at the expense of pallidal structures. From an analysis of region-specific markers, it appears that the pallidal precursor region (medial ganglionic eminence, MGE) forms initially but rapidly adopts a more dorsal fate, its molecular identity being transformed into that of the striatal precursor (lateral ganglionic eminence, LGE).[14]

The boundary between dorsal and ventral telencephalon, which later forms a prominent junction between cortex and striatum, appears to be established by immiscibility between the cells of the adjoining regions. Tissue culture experiments have shown that when cortical and striatal precursor cells are evenly intermixed in floating aggregates, they can sort out from each other, suggesting a difference in adhesive properties that may relate to the restricted expression of the adhesion molecules R-cadherin and LewisX antigen in the dorsal telencephalon.[15] Expression of these molecules may be regulated by the transcription factor Pax6, whose functional removal by targeted mutation results in the loss of the corticostriatal boundary and the extensive dorsal spread of *Dlx*-expressing cells.[16] Segregation of developmentally distinct domains by differential adhesion, a mechanism that is important in hindbrain patterning, considered below, suggests that ventral and dorsal telencephalic domains are distinct compartments containing committed cells. Transplantation experiments support this view: when tissue pieces or cell aggregates are transposed between prospective cortex and striatum, they continue to express markers characteristic of their original position.[17] At the level of the individual cell, however, this commitment to regional fate appears to be labile: individual cortical precursors grafted to the striatum take on the 'medium spiny' phenotype of striatal neurons, whereas individual striatal precursors can develop into cortical-like pyramidal neurons when surrounded by cortical cells.[18] Thus, a community effect, whereby similar cells enjoy mutual reinforcement of their specification state, seems to be required to maintain their nascent regional identity.

Complicating this simple view of the dorsoventral telencephalic junction as a cell lineage restriction boundary—with its implication that cortical and striatal compartments are segregated into discrete compartments—is the observation that certain classes of *Dlx*-expressing cells originating in the ventral region normally cross this boundary during development.[19–21] Indeed, a large proportion of the small GABAergic inhibitory neurons that populate the cortex are thought to originate not from the expected place, the cortical ventricular zone, but from the striatal and pallidal primordia, the LGE and MGE (see also Chapter 7) (Fig. 3.5). These cortical cells of subcortical origin are depleted in mice that lack functional copies of both *Dlx1* and *Dlx2*, homeobox genes that are normally expressed in the germinative zones of the basal ganglia. In these double-mutant animals (but in neither of the single mutants), the striatum itself is also disrupted by cells failing to migrate out of the germinative layers into the mantle zone.[19] This phenotype suggests that a single functional copy of one of the two *Dlx* genes is required both for normal radial migration of striatal precursors and for their tangential migration across the dorsoventral telencephalic junction into the cortex. A recent study using vital cell marking has confirmed that ventrally derived neurons cross the corticostriatal boundary but that dorsal cells do not cross into ventral territory.[22]

Although it remains unclear how this promiscuity of subcortical cells can be reconciled with the observation of immiscibility between cortical and striatal regions, it may simply be a question of timing. Compartition presupposes the allocation of

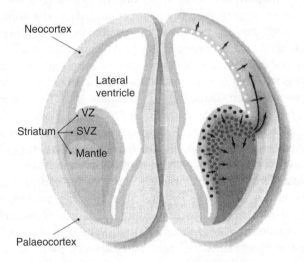

Figure 3.5 Cross-section of the telencephalon of a mouse embryo, showing (left side) the prospective ventral and dorsal regions and (right side) the radial migration of *Dlx*-expressing cells from the germinative zones of the striatal rudiment into the mantle zone and their tangential migration into the neocortex. SVZ, subventricular zone; VZ, ventricular zone. After Lumsden and Gulisano.[21]

defined assemblies of precursor cells whose boundaries are coextensive with the expression domains of genes involved in the acquisition of regional identity. Consistent with this, for as long as the telencephalon consists solely or predominantly of ventricular zone neuroepithelial cells, there is no intermingling between the two regions. Later, the apparent loss of restriction may apply only to specific types of young neuron that have already become specified. Aspects of this specification would include both the downregulation of molecules involved in regional restriction and the gained expression of other (unknown) molecules that would be required for tangential migration.

The major part of the dorsal telencephalon of mammals develops into the neocortex, a region that is characterized by a highly elaborate pattern of functionally (and to some extent structurally) distinct areas. An important influence in neocortical arealization is patterning information imposed by incoming thalamic afferents (see Chapter 7). However, recently described AP countergradients of *Emx2* and *Pax6* expression[23] and the localized expression of signalling molecules in the early dorsal telencephalon tell us that the region must acquire a certain degree of intrinsic pattern before the arrival of these axons. For a further discussion of cortical patterning, see reference 24.

Diencephalic regionalization

The AP axis of the early diencephalon is subdivided by transverse boundaries into two primary regions, the parencephalon (anterior) and synencephalon (posterior), and later into four secondary regions. A prominent boundary, the zona limitans intrathalamica, emerges in the middle of the parencephalon, subdividing it into anterior (future ventral thalamus) and posterior (future dorsal thalamus) regions. The synencephalon is subdivided by growth of the posterior commissure at its border with the midbrain and this posterior region (future pretectum) becomes distinguishable from the anterior synencephalon. Thus, the diencephalon gives the appearance of being subdivided into first two, then three and finally four subregions. Largely on the basis of descriptive histochemical and gene expression studies, it has been proposed that the diencephalon is built piecemeal, like the hindbrain (as we will see below), from a series of metameric units or neuromeres. In the forebrain, these neuromeres have been called 'prosomeres'.[25,26] Experimental evidence for compartition of the diencephalon includes the detection, by vital dye labelling studies, of cell lineage restriction boundaries that align with prominent axon tracts and/or borders of regulatory gene expression that independently define the four regions.[25] However, the existence of cell compartments has been brought into question by an analysis of retrovirally marked clones, which has shown that sibling cells can occupy multiple nuclei throughout the AP extent of the diencephalon.[27] Further cell marking experiments are required to see whether there is a lineage restriction that affects dividing cells but not maturing neurons, as at the dorsoventral telencephalic boundary. Irrespective of the uncertainty surrounding lineage restriction at the boundaries between successive diencephalic prosomeres, there are further concerns about their designation as metameric units or true segments. The essence of segmentation is repetition of a ground pattern and modular organization; although there are examples of developmental control genes that are differentially expressed in different prosomeres, they are not expressed in a repetitive pattern through alternate prosomeres. Given the uncertainty surrounding the designation of diencephalic subregions as true segments (metameres), the term 'prosomere' has similarly infirm status.

The most prominent transverse boundary in the developing diencephalon is that between the future dorsal and ventral thalamus (Fig. 3.3). Known as the zona limitans intrathalamica (zli), it marks the transition from epichordal to prechordal regions of the neuraxis.[28] This is not obvious because the zli develops late by comparison with the morphological boundaries between, for example, forebrain and midbrain or the molecular boundaries that subdivide the hindbrain. By the time the zli does become evident by either morphological or molecular criteria, elongation of the neural tube and cephalic flexure have already resulted in the anterior notochord tip being displaced ventrally and posteriorly away from its original position relative to the neural plate. The zli is colonized by an axon pathway (the mamillothalamic tract), at least in mammals. Furthermore, it not only aligns with the borders of gene expression domains, *Dlx1* and *Dlx2* anteriorly (in the presumptive ventral thalamus) and *Gbx2* and *Wnt3* posteriorly (in the presumptive dorsal thalamus), but itself expresses the important signal molecule Sonic hedgehog (SHH). This property endows the zli with candidacy as a secondary signalling centre, but there is no evidence as yet that it performs such a role. Although speculative, it could be suggested that the zli represents a transverse extension of the midventral floor plate of the neural tube, which overlies the notochord but not the prechordal plate. As we will see below, the floor plate also expresses SHH and has a significant signalling function in regionalization on the dorsoventral axis. Whether or not the zli has a signalling role, it is clear that its position alone witnesses the earliest heterogeneity along the neuraxis, the interface between that part of the nervous system that is induced by notochord and that is induced by prechordal plate.

Another prominent boundary is that between the diencephalon and mesencephalon, marked by the posterior commissure that forms within the caudal (pretectal) region of the diencephalon. At the molecular level, the di/mes boundary appears to form through the repression of mesencephalic *Engrailed* and *Pax2* by diencephalic *Pax6*.[29] Unlike the zli, no signalling function has been attributed to the di/mes boundary.

Midbrain

Like the forebrain, the midbrain (mesencephalon) consists of structurally and functionally distinct dorsal and ventral regions. The ventral midbrain contains the dopaminergic neurons of the substantia nigra and ventral tegmental area, together with motor neurons of the oculomotor (third cranial) nerve. The dorsal midbrain, or tectum, is specialized as a recipient structure for inputs from the eye (retinal ganglion cell axons) and ear. In mammals, the visual and auditory structures are called, respectively, the superior and inferior colliculi. In birds, where much of the experimental work relating to midbrain patterning has been done, the optic tectum dominates the early developing brain as a whole and is elaborately laminated into 16 component layers. The midbrain auditory centre, by contrast, is a small structure at the posterior border of the optic tectum called the torus semicircularis.

The optic tectum has a distinctive AP polarity, manifested by a pronounced variation in cytoarchitecture and the acquisition of different sets of afferent inputs from the retina: the posterior tectum receives axons from the anterior (nasal) retina, whereas the anterior tectum becomes innervated by temporal (posterior) retina (see Chapters 9 and 10). The molecular basis of this topographic discrimination by different sets of retinofugal axons, introduced here because of its relevance to the following discussion, involves ephrin ligands for Eph family receptor tyrosine kinases that are expressed in decreasing posterior-to-anterior gradients in the optic tectum, and may function as growth inhibitors of Eph-receptor-bearing temporal axons.[30] These and other molecular properties of both tectum and retina are crucial to patterning the visual topographic map (see Chapter 10), a process that follows and depends on the acquisition by the tectal primordium of a correctly polarized AP pattern.

The isthmic signalling region

The isthmus is the narrow connection between the midbrain vesicle and hindbrain. Cells in this region have a well-characterized long-range signalling activity that is responsible for generating local AP pattern throughout the midbrain and rostral hindbrain (future cerebellum). The isthmic signalling region is at the midbrain–hindbrain junction, but the latter does not correspond precisely with the morphological constriction that so obviously separates the mesencephalic vesicle from that of rhombomeres 1 and 2. Separating structurally and functionally distinct tectal and isthmo-cerebellar regions of the brain, the junction forms some distance anterior to the constriction and registers with the posterior limit of *Otx2* expression in the early mesencephalic vesicle[31] and the anterior limit of expression of another homeobox gene, *Gbx2*,[32] a vertebrate homologue of *Drosophila unplugged* (Fig. 3.6). The posteriormost, *Otx2*-negative/*Gbx2*-positive region of the vesicle is fated to join rhombomere 1 (r1) in the formation of the cerebellum.[33,34] Thus, it cannot be assumed that obvious morphological features of the neural tube, such as the constrictions between vesicles, necessarily correspond precisely to future subdivisions of the brain.

Isthmic cells are induced to express the secreted signal molecules FGF8 and WNT1 and transcriptional control genes of the *Pax* and *En* families (related to *Drosophila paired* and *engrailed* genes, respectively), which are required for normal development of the region.[35] Although it seems to be the case that *Otx2* represses *Gbx2* and

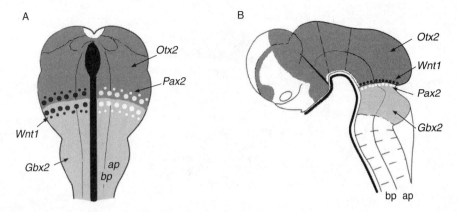

Figure 3.6 Late neural plate (A) and neural tube stage (B) mouse embryos showing the rostral domain of *Otx2* expression meeting the caudal domain of *Gbx2* expression at a sharp interface that becomes the isthmus. *Pax2*, *Wnt1* and *En* (not shown) are expressed in a broad band centred on the isthmus (A). Later, in B, *Wnt1* and *Pax2* expression segregates into two adjacent sharp rings at the *Otx2*–*Gbx2* interface. By this stage, *Gbx2* expression has withdrawn from the posterior rhombencephalon. ap, alar plate, bp, basal plate.

vice versa, it is not clear what mechanism sets the precise position at which their expression domains are juxtaposed. However, several studies have now shown that this interface is directly responsible for establishing the isthmic signalling region. Thus, the depletion of *Otx* function in mice that have only one copy of *Otx2* (and are also null mutant for *Otx1*) moves the isthmus rostrally, to the axial level of the zona limitans.[36] Furthermore, transgenic misexpression experiments in which *Otx2* expression is shifted caudally lead to a corresponding shift of both the *Gbx2* expression boundary and the isthmic signalling region.[37]

Role of the *Engrailed* genes in establishing tectal polarity

Expression of two *En* genes is the earliest known marker for mesencephalic polarity.[35] They are expressed in virtually identical domains, in a gradient that decreases both anteriorly through the mesencephalic vesicle, and posteriorly through the first rhombomere (Fig. 3.7). The main difference between the expression of the two genes is that *En1* is expressed (and its expression is downregulated) earlier than is *En2*. Knockout experiments have shown that *En1* is crucially involved in the early specification of the entire region of its expression,[38] whereas *En2* function is restricted to cerebellar morphogenesis. However, the *En1* mutant phenotype, agenesis of both tectum and cerebellum, is completely rescued by inserting the *En2* cDNA into the *En1* locus, replacing *En1*.[39] This outcome demonstrates that the contrasting phenotypes of

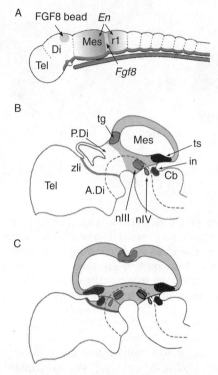

Figure 3.7 Implanting a bead that releases FGF8 protein in the posterior diencephalon (A) of 1.5-day chick embryo results in the transformation of normal posterior diencephalic territory (B) into midbrain (C). In the treated embryo, the ectopic midbrain contains a normal set of midbrain structures laid out in reverse AP polarity to the normal midbrain. This is thought to be due to the induction of Engrailed expression by FGF8 and the formation of a novel anterior-to-posterior gradient of En protein in the diencephalon that is the mirror image of the endogenous En gradient in the midbrain (A). A.Di, anterior diencephalon; Cb, cerebellum; in, isthmic nuclei; Mes, mesencephalon; nIII, oculomotor nucleus; nIV, trochlear nucleus; P.Di, posterior diencephalon; r1, rhombomere 1; Tel, telencephalon; tg, tectal griseum; ts, torus semicircularis. Data from Crossley et al.[45]

En1 and *En2* mutations reflect more the temporal difference in the expression of the two genes than any divergence in the specificity of their protein products.

Transplantation studies in avian embryos have monitored En protein as a marker of tectal polarity and have shown that the En gradient correlates with later-emerging morphology. Thus, when the mesencephalic vesicle is reversed on the AP axis early (on the second day of incubation in the chick embryo), the En gradient readjusts to its original polarity, and both the graded cytoarchitecture and pattern of retinotectal projections develop normally. When reversed on the third day of incubation, however, the En gradient does not adjust, and both cytoarchitecture and retinotectal projection are subsequently inverted.[35] This association has been strengthened by experiments in which *En* is misexpressed using a retroviral vector to drive ectopic expression in the anterior tectum: nasal axons arborize ectopically in the anterior tectum whereas temporal retinal axons fail even to enter the midbrain.[40] Further-more, the altered retinotectal specificity following *En* misexpression in the anterior midbrain is associated with ectopic upregulation of ephrins that are normally expressed only in the posterior tectum, defeating their normal Posterior-to-anterior expression gradient and effectively converting temporal-axon-specific anterior tectum into nasal-axon-specific posterior tectum.[41] Expression of these effector genes, downstream of *En*, suggests that the normal graded expression of *En* may polarize the dorsal mesencephalon.

Regulation of *Engrailed* expression

Graded expression of *En* appears to be regulated by signalling from the isthmus, which forms the posterior border of the mesencephalic field. When grafted to the caudal forebrain, isthmic tissue induces *En* expression and the formation of a com-plete optic tectum from the surrounding tissue.[42] Two secreted signal molecules have been implicated in the isthmic signalling function and the control of *En* expression, WNT1 and FGF8. *Wnt1*, a homologue of the segment polarity gene *wingless* (a regulator of *engrailed* in *Drosophila*) is expressed in the midbrain region of the neural plate and later in a ring of cells at the isthmus. As for their cognates in flies, *Wnt1* and *En* expression appear to be mutually interdependent: in *Wnt1* $^{-/-}$ mice, *En* is expressed normally at first but is then progressively lost, along with the dorsal midbrain.[43] Although WNT1 is required for midbrain and cerebellar development, its ectopic expression fails to mimic the powerful inductive activity of isthmic grafts. Thus, although WNT1 is critically involved in the maintenance of *En* expression, it is not a candidate for inducing *En* expression or for directly setting up midbrain polarity. This has been elegantly shown by a transgenic mouse experiment in which *En* expression driven by the *Wnt1* promoter rescues midbrain development in *Wnt1* $^{-/-}$ mice.[44] However, another secreted factor, FGF8, expressed in a circumferential ring imme-diately posterior to that of *Wnt1*, has been shown to have midbrain-inducing and polarizing abilities. When a bead coated with recombinant FGF8 protein is implanted in the posterior diencephalon of chick embryos, expression of *Fgf8*, *Wnt1* and *En2* is induced in the surrounding tissue.[45] This later displays the character of a complete ectopic midbrain, whose AP polarity is reversed with respect to that of the 'host' midbrain (Fig. 3.7). Thus, neuroectodermal *Fgf8* expression may be sufficient to establish both midbrain pattern and polarity. Significantly, one of the earliest-appearing consequences of FGF8-coated bead implantation in the diencephalon is the downregulation of *Otx2*.

In addition to FGF8, the paired box genes *Pax2*, *Pax5* and *Pax8* are required, singly or together, for specification of the isthmus. The isthmus is deleted in *Pax5* $^{-/-}$ mice,[46] in the *noi* zebrafish mutant (lacking functional *Pax2/5/8*, the only representative of this group of *Pax* genes in fish),[47] and in zebrafish treated with function-blocking antibodies to the Pax2/5/8 protein.[48] In these experiments, the expression of both *Wnt1* and *En2* is also repressed, suggesting their direct positive regulation by Pax proteins. Indeed, consensus Pax binding sites have been identified within an enhancer region of the *En2* gene: when these sites are mutated, the midbrain–hindbrain domain of reporter expression is lost.[49] Extensive interaction and cross-regulation between En, Pax and FGF8 appears to be required to maintain isthmic identity (Fig. 3.8). Ectopic isthmus formation following the misexpression of *Otx2* in rhombomere 1[37] may be explained as follows. *Otx2* represses *Gbx2*, which is required for rostral hindbrain differentiation,[32] but induces the expression of *Pax2*. This, in turn, activates the feedback loop with *En* and *Fgf8* and leads to conversion of cerebellar territory into tectal territory and the establishment of an ectopic isthmus at its posterior border.

Whereas isthmic grafts induce tectal development in the caudal diencephalon, the same grafts to the dorsal hindbrain induce cerebellar development,[50] demonstrating that the competence of rhombencephalic tissue to respond to isthmic signals differs from that of mesencephalic and caudal diencephalic regions. However, FGF8 alone appears insufficient for inducing ectopic *En2* expression or cerebellar development in the hindbrain, implicating additional signalling molecules at the isthmus.[45]

In the midbrain, the alar plate forms the tectum and the basal plate forms the tegmentum, the oculomotor nucleus and the dopaminergic neurons of the substantia nigra. Patterning of the mesencephalic vesicle into these sharply distinct dorsoventral domains appears to be under the control of Sonic hedgehog, expressed by the floor plate. Misexpression of *Shh* results in expansion of the tegmentum at the expense of the tectum.[51] In the course of this transformation, SHH mediates the repression of genes associated with isthmic signalling and tectal polarity, including *En1/2*, *Pax2*, *Pax5* and *Fgf8*, while inducing the expression of ventral genes such as *Isl1* and *Lim1/2*.

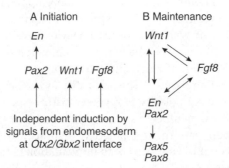

Figure 3.8 Regulatory pathways involving *Pax*, *Wnt1*, *Fgf8* and *En* genes. Following the independent induction of these genes (A), they become mutually interdependent for their expression (B). Ectopic expression of one of the genes will activate the others in a positive feedback loop. Although FGF8 does not normally induce *En*, it can do so. When misexpressed in tissue that is competent to express all four genes, a new isthmus is formed. The *Otx2–Gbx2* interface is probably required during normal development for locating and sharpening the initial expression domains of these four genes.

Hindbrain

The hindbrain (rhombencephalon) is characterized by a comparatively small number of cell types belonging to well-defined categories and disposed in an arrangement that is broadly similar to that of the spinal cord. Dorsal regions, developing from the alar, or lateral region of the neural plate, contain second-order sensory interneurons and relay neurons whereas ventral regions, developing from the basal, or medial region of the neural plate, contain motor neurons. Alongside the hindbrain (Fig. 3.9)

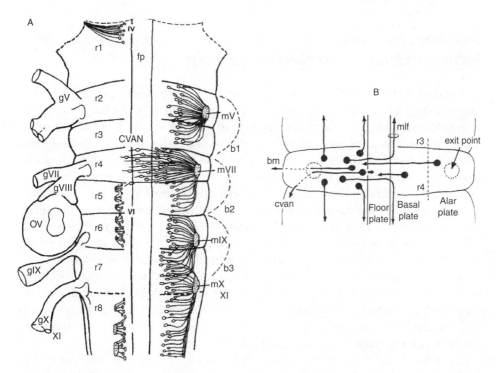

Figure 3.9 (A) Rhombomeric organization of the hindbrain in a 4-day chick embryo. The left side shows the cranial sensory ganglia (gV–gX), otic vesicle (ov) and somatic motor nerve nuclei (IV–XII) in relation to the rhombomeres (r1–r8). The right side shows the organization of the branchiomotor nerve nuclei (mV–mXI) in relation to both their rhombomeres of origin and their branchial arch target regions (b1–b3). The contralaterally migrating efferent neurons of the vestibuloacoustic nerve (cvan), which share an exit point with VIIth nerve neurons, are shown crossing the floor plate (fp) in rhombomere 4. After Lumsden and Keynes.[53]
(B) Typical organization of projection interneurons in an avian rhombomere. Neurons are defined by their cell body position (lateral, medial) and their axonal trajectory (crossed or uncrossed, ascending or descending, lateral or medial pathway). Rhombomere 4, as shown, is distinct from other rhombomeres in forming contralaterally migrating efferent neurons (cvan). mlf, medial longitudinal fascicle.

is a series of cranial sensory ganglia, of combined neural crest and placodal origin. These are associated with motor nerves that innervate the subjacent branchial arches—trigeminal (cranial nerve V), facial (c.n. VII), glossopharyngeal (c.n. IX) and vagal/accessory (c.n. X/XI)—or with the vestibuloacoustic efferent nerve (c.n. VIII). The motor nuclei of these cranial nerves develop in the basal plate but their axons leave the hindbrain through specialized conduits in the alar plate that also serve as entry points for axons from the ganglia. The remaining cranial nerves of hindbrain origin—trochlear (c.n. IV), abducens (c.n. VI) and hypoglossal (c.n. XII)—are somatic motor and are not associated with peripheral ganglia. In addition to the sensory and motor elements, the hindbrain contains numerous types of projection interneuron. The cerebellum is a specialization of the anterior end of the hindbrain.

Segmentation and neuronal pattern

Regional diversity in the hindbrain is acquired through a process of segmentation,[52] whereby the parent neuroepithelium becomes subdivided on its AP axis into a series of discrete domains, rhombomeres. Segmentation suggests the early allocation of defined sets of precursor cells and the existence of precise boundaries to both cellular assemblies and realms of gene action, and is therefore presumed to allow each successive segment to adopt a specific identity, distinct from its neighbours.

In the avian embryo, the segmented pattern of the hindbrain begins to emerge immediately following neural tube closure as a series of constrictions, the inter-rhombomere boundaries, progressively subdivide the length of the hindbrain neural tube. The pattern of eight rhombomeres is complete at the onset of neurogenesis (Fig. 3.10). Inter-rhombomere boundaries later become colonized by axons, perhaps on account of both the local expression of growth-promoting molecules[53] and the availability of extracellular space.[54] Segmentation of the vertebrate hindbrain bears a superficial resemblance to segmentation of the *Drosophila* embryo: rhombomeres form by subdivision rather than by budding from a growth zone (as do vertebrate somites), and they have a pairwise organization.

Two patterns of metameric cellular organization can be distinguished in the embryonic hindbrain. The first is a repeat pattern through every segment involving eight identified types of reticular neuron (Figs 3.9 and 3.11), the formation of which endows each sequential rhombomere with a more or less complete set.[55] The second is a two-segment repeat pattern involving the branchial motor neurons. These first appear in the even-numbered rhombomeres, r2 (trigeminal), r4 (facial) and r6 (glossopharyngeal), the same rhombomeres that contain their respective exit points in the alar plate. Thereafter, further neurons are formed in the intervening odd-numbered rhombomeres, each in association with the cluster of motor neurons in the anteriorly adjacent rhombomere.[53] Later in development, the segmental origins of these cells become obscured as certain interneurons become more numerous in particular rhombomeres and the motor nuclei condense and migrate to new positions. In

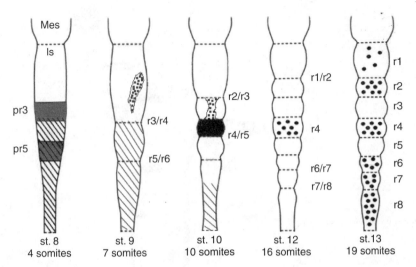

Figure 3.10 Stages in hindbrain morphogenesis in the chick embryo. At stage 8, territories corresponding with presumptive rhombomeres 3 and 5 (pr3, pr5) are marked by *Krox20* expression, while *Hoxb1* is expressed at low level in the caudal hindbrain (hatch). The first rhombomere boundaries are evident morphologically at stage 9. By stage 10, low-level *Hoxb1* has retreated and high-level expression is restricted to r4, now delineated by both of its boundaries. Clones marked after boundary formation do not spread into adjacent rhombomeres, although they may do if marked before boundary formation (stippled areas). Dierentiating neurons appear first in r4 (stage 12) and last in r3 and r5.

addition, the neural crest cells that populate the branchial arches emigrate from the dorsal margin of the hindbrain in segmental fashion, migrating from r2, r4 and r6 into the first, second and third arches, respectively.[56] These cells (which are discussed in more detail in Chapter 5) contribute to the cranial ganglia, form the cartilage and bone of the arches, and confer motor axon targeting specificity on the branchial musculature. The two-segment repeat pattern of the early hindbrain thus generates a close anatomical[53] and functional[57] correspondence between motor neuronal populations within the brain and their target structures in the segmented series of branchial arches that lies directly ventral to it.

Each rhombomere can also be considered to have an individual identity as, among other unique characteristics, its component neurons display rhombomere-specific axon navigation behaviour with respect to the specific synaptic targets. Notable rhombomere-specific cell populations include the Mauthner cells of lower verte-brates and a group of contralaterally migrating efferent neurons that innervate the hair cells of the inner ear, both of which develop exclusively in r4 (Figs 3.9B and 3.11). Rhombomere 1 is distinct in respect of its lack of branchial motor neurons and its being the precursor region of the cerebellum. The dorsolateral margins of r1 (the rhombic lips) contribute a very large migratory cell population that forms the

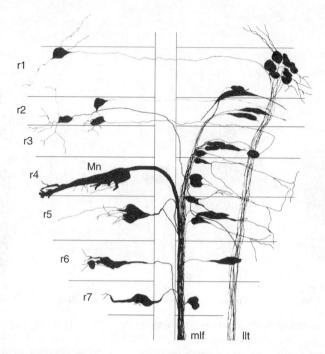

Figure 3.11 Reticulospinal neurons in a 5-day zebrafish embryo in relation to diagrammatic rhombomeres. Ipsilaterally projecting cells are shown on the right side and contralaterals on the left; both sets of axons project down one of two major longitudinal pathway, the medial longitudinal fascicle (mlf) and the lateral longitudinal tract (llt). All of these cells are individually identifiable by position and pathway choice. The Mauthner neuron (Mn) is a single large cell in r4. After Kimmel *et al.*[126]

external germinal layer and later the internal granule cell layer of the cerebellum (see also Chapter 7).[33]

Thus, although not obvious from the adult structures, segmentation is crucially involved in specifying the pattern of developing structures in the hindbrain region. It is therefore of considerable importance to understand how rhombomeres are formed, how they acquire their early even/odd alternation and how their individual identity is finally conferred.

Compartment-like properties of rhombomeres

Developmental compartments provide a way of allocating blocks of cells with distinct properties. The containment of polyclonal assemblages of neuroepithelial cells within rhombomeres has been shown by lineage tracing studies in chick.[58] Although able to mingle freely within a particular rhombomere, neuroepithelial cells do not move from one rhombomere to another (Fig. 3.12). Compartmental restriction of cell

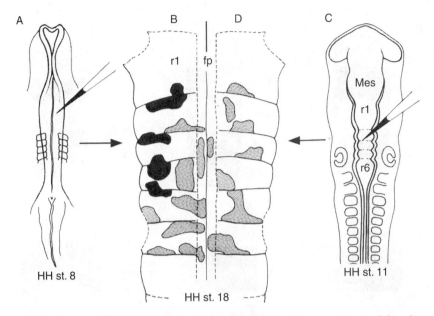

Figure 3.12 Cell dispersal in the chick hindbrain in relation to the emergence of rhombomere boundaries. Single cells labelled with an intracellular fluorescent tracer in the neural plate or tube (A, C) divide several times over 2 days to form clones that are detectable in a flat-mounted 3.5-day hindbrain (B, D). Clones marked before boundary formation (A) may be found straddling a boundary (black patches in B). Clones marked near an already-formed boundary (C) are always restricted from spreading into an adjacent rhombomere (D). After Fraser *et al.*[58]

mingling begins at the time rhombomeres become delineated by their boundaries and persists while the epithelium is predominantly germinative; later, young neurons may escape the restriction once they have acquired their ultimate positional specification. Rhombomeric domains of the germinative (ventricular) zone remain lineage-restricted up to late stages, when neurogenesis is nearing completion.[59]

Rhombomeres partition from one another according to an adhesion differential that displays a two-segment repeat pattern.[60,61] Consistent with an expected tendency of neighbouring cell groups to separate from one another, enlarged intercellular space is the earliest manifestation of rhombomere boundaries.[54] Complementing this adhesive differential is an alternating periodicity to the expression domains of the Eph-like receptor tyrosine kinases and their ephrin ligands:[30,62] three receptors (EphA4, EphB2, EphB3) are expressed in odd-numbered rhombomeres (r3, r5), whereas their ephrin-B (transmembrane class) ligands are expressed in the even-numbered rhombomeres, r2, r4 and r6. Interaction between these ligand–receptor partners has been shown to mediate repulsive interactions that serve to sharpen rhombomere borders and prevent cell mixing between adjacent rhombomeres (Fig. 3.13).[63,64] Eph–ephrin interaction may also provide a potential mechanism by which cells in adjacent rhombomeres interact with each other to establish additional cell states at the inter-rhombomere boundaries. Upstream control of Eph and ephrin expression is expected to be exerted by transcription factors that may share their

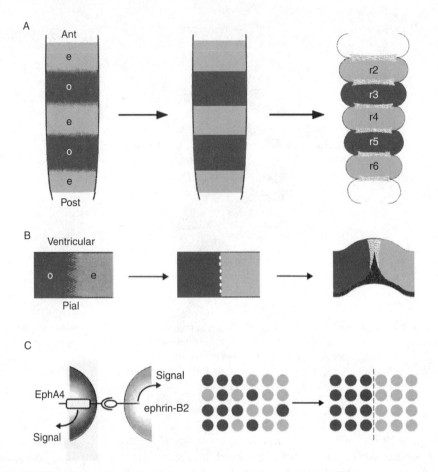

Figure 3.13 Interaction between Ephs expressed on odd rhombomere cells (o) and ephrins expressed on even rhombomere cells (e) may function in segregating cells into like groups, thereby sharpening an initially fuzzy boundary between adjacent rhombomeres. The sequence of steps in boundary formation is shown in dorsal view in A, and in parasagittal section in B. The first morphological evidence of boundary formation is the appearance of intercellular space (middle figure in B), suggesting partial de-adhesion of odd and even cells, an event which is followed by elevation of a ventricular ridge below which axons of the marginal zone collect preferentially. Interaction between Ephs and ephrins (C) results in bidirectional signalling and cell-sorting behaviour. Data from Xu et al.,[63] after Lumsden.[64]

two-segment repeat expression pattern. The zinc-finger gene *Krox20* is expressed in two stripes in the neural plate that become r3 and r5,[65] and its product directly regulates expression of *EphA4*.[66] In *Krox20* null mutant animals, r3 and r5 are deleted and a partially fused r2/r4/r6 territory develops—a phenotype consistent with *Krox20* being responsible for generating single-compartment periodicity from cues established by upstream genes.[67] Candidates in the latter category include *kreisler* and its zebrafish homologue, *valentino*, a leucine zipper gene of the *b-zip Maf* proto-oncogene family that is expressed in r5 and r6.[68,69] Although direct interaction has yet to be demonstrated, the r5 stripe of *Krox20* is missing in *kreisler* null mutant mouse embryos, whose neural tube is unsegmented posterior to the r3–r4 boundary, suggesting the loss of r5 and r6 as identifiable territories.[70] In the *valentino* mutant, prospective r5 and r6 lack their specific segmental identity.

The small number of known or candidate segmentation genes remains a major gap in our understanding of hindbrain segmentation. Despite the conserved role of Hox genes in specifying segmental identity (see below), the upstream pathway of segment formation appears not to be conserved between flies and vertebrates. However, segmentation is a generic property of metazoan organization that has evolved many times, making it likely that *Hox* genes have been coupled independently to segmentation—in flies, the coupling is via pair rule and segment polarity genes whereas in vertebrates, the mechanism of coupling is not understood, although *kreisler* and *Krox20* are both clearly involved.

Hox genes and rhombomere identity

The emergence of regional pattern along the AP axis depends on the expression of position-specifying genes. The hindbrain provides us with the best example of how positional values are set up in the neuroepithelium, through the use of a set of genes whose close relatives have long been known to specify positional values along the main body axis of the fly embryo. These homeotic selector (*HOM-C*) genes are the master control genes that coordinate the regulators of all processes involved in the development of structures appropriate to axial position in the epidermal segments of the fly. Consistent with their serving a similar function in vertebrates, the homologues of these genes, the *Hox* family of homeobox genes, retain a clustered chromosomal organization in which the relative position of a gene in the cluster reflects its boundary of expression along the AP axis (the principle of colinearity). Duplications during evolution of the vertebrate genome have increased the number of *Hox* genes such that mammals may possess up to four copies of genes that are represented singly in *Drosophila*. Divergence of these paralogous genes, together with cross-regulation between them, would be expected to increase the resolution of pattern control.

Rhombomeres are thought to acquire their positional values (and hence their individual identities) under the influence of the *Hox* genes. These are expressed in overlapping, or nested, domains along the axis of the early vertebrate embryo, those at the 3′ ends of the clusters being expressed most anteriorly, in the hindbrain, where there is a striking correspondence between their rostral expression boundaries and the interfaces between rhombomeres.[71] *Hox* gene expression precedes rhombomere formation but becomes progressively sharpened such that the borders of their expression domains coincide with the emerging rhombomere boundaries. In the fully segmented hindbrain, genes situated 3′ in the genomic *Hox* clusters are expressed in an ordered and nested set of domains along the AP axis of the hindbrain, with a two-rhombomere periodicity. Superimposed on this pattern are rhombomere-specific

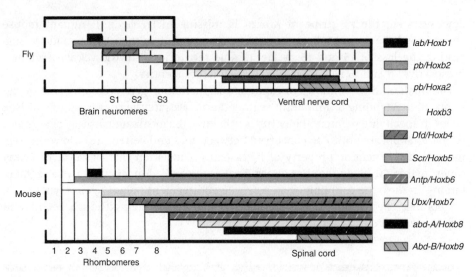

Figure 3.14 Nested expression domains of *Hox* genes in fly and mouse. The nine homeotic genes of *Drosophila* are shown on the left, together with their homologues in the vertebrate HoxB cluster. In flies, the homeotic genes are grouped in two complexes, the Antennapedia complex contains six genes (*labial* to *Antennapedia*, in 3′ to 5′ sequence) while the Bithorax complex contains the remaining three genes (*Ultrabithorax* to *Abdominal-B*). The sequence of genes within these chromosomal groups is reflected by their temporal and spatial order of expression along the anteroposterior axis of the body in both flies and vertebrates. After Hirth *et al.*[72]

variations in expression levels. In addition to the conservation of individual sequence and chromosomal organization between the *Hox* clusters of fly and vertebrate, there is a striking correspondence of the expression domains of the homologous genes between their respective central nervous systems (Fig. 3.14).[72]

Considering the distribution of transcripts and the general synergy between *Hox* genes detected in mouse null mutants, it is possible that the identity of individual rhombomeres could be defined by the cooperative action of Hox proteins.[73] They may also have singular influences on rhombomere phenotype, as has been well documented for *Hoxb1*, a gene which is uniquely expressed at high level in r4. Targeted mutation of *Hoxb1* in mice leads to the transformation of r4 to an r2-like identity[74] whereas ectopic overexpression of *Hoxb1* in chick embryos, by means of a retroviral vector, leads to the opposite transformation.[75] These transformations have been documented in most detail for the behaviour of motor neurons (Fig. 3.15): in the absence of functional Hoxb1 protein, facial motor neurons fail to undertake their normal caudal migration from r4 into r6 and the contralateral migration of vestibuloacoustic efferent neurons developing in r4 also fails. Instead, both types of motor neuron migrate dorsolaterally, in the manner of trigeminal motor neurons. The misexpression of *Hoxb1* in r2 causes the motor axons leaving the hindbrain by way of the r2 exit point to ignore their normal target, the first branchial arch, and instead turn sharply caudal and grow into the second branchial arch. Both gain and loss of *Hoxb1* function result in transformations that can be properly described as homeotic,

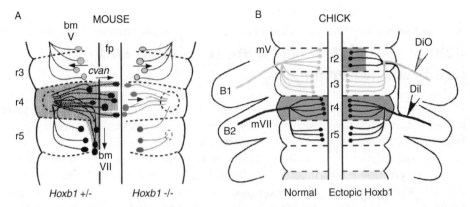

Figure 3.15 Effects of loss (A) and gain (B) of *Hoxb1* function on the identity of motor neurons developing in r4, the normal domain of *Hoxb1* expression (shaded). In the null mutant mouse (right side of A) motor neurons differentiate and extend axons but then fail to undergo their normal migrations across the floor plate (in the case of the contralateral vestibuloacoustic neurons, cvan) and caudally into r6 (in the case of facial branchiomotor neurons, bm VII). When Hoxb1 is overexpressed in basal r2, motor neurons extend their axons via a novel pathway to the second arch, suggesting that their identity has changed from trigeminal (mV) to facial (mVII), although this is only seen in their pathfinding specificity. Axons traced by retrograde labelling after injection of fluorescent dyes (DiI and DiO). A, data from Studer *et al.*;[74] B, data from Bell *et al.*[75]

in that one member of the meristic series adopts the likeness of another member of the series.[76] However, it should be noted that, through the dearth of markers for specific cell types and their regional variants, we are as yet unable to characterize completely the properties and peculiarities of individual rhombomeres and therefore cannot assess how complete the transformations are. However, it is clear that *Hoxb1* is responsible for regulating, directly or indirectly, eector molecules involved in neuronal migration and axon guidance that are restricted to, or dierentially expressed in, r4. The results of losing the function of other *Hox* genes on hindbrain development are less clear-cut. Loss of *Hoxa1* function, for example, results in the deletion of r5, reduction of r4 and loss of specific neuronal nuclei,[77] abnormalities that are not obviously consistent with the gene being responsible for conferring specific identity on an existing repetitive ground-plan; but it remains possible that *Hox* genes could have dual roles, both in segmentation and segment identification.[78]

Although it is most likely that positional value is conferred on rhombomeres by *Hox* gene expression, it is unclear how the *Hox* genes themselves become activated at appropriate levels of the neuraxis. Extensive cross-regulation between the various *Hox* genes is certainly involved[79] and regulators upstream of the *Hox* genes include *kreisler* and *Krox20* which, in addition to controlling segmentation of the neuroepithelium, act in a parallel but clearly related process directly to regulate the *Hox* genes. Thus, *kreisler* directly modulates expression of paralogue group 3 *Hox* genes in r5[80] and *Krox20* is a direct modulator of the r3/r5 activity of both *Hoxa2* and *Hoxb2*.

Role of retinoids in *Hox* gene regulation and hindbrain patterning

In addition to these candidate genetic regulators of specific subsets of *Hox* gene expression, there is also evidence that retinoids (e.g. retinoic acid, RA) act as overall regulators of nested *Hox* expression, consistent with their global posteriorizing effect on CNS regionalization (see Chapter 2). In this context, RA may act as a morphogen conferring positional information on cells at different AP levels of the hindbrain by differentially regulating *Hox* gene expression. The evidence for this is as follows. First, RA is an active derivative of vitamin A, whose deficiency leads to dysmorphogenesis, as does an excess of vitamin A. In both cases, the defects are particularly severe in the hindbrain and branchial arch region. Excess RA causes a concomitant dose-dependent anterior-to-posterior transformation of cell fate, in which the hindbrain is expanded at the expense of the mid- and forebrain. Second, this change in regional fate is associated with changes of *Hox* gene expression patterns in a manner consistent with the principle of colinearity; there is a direct correspondence between the location of a *Hox* gene in the cluster and its responsiveness to RA in which 3' genes respond more rapidly and at a lower RA concentration than more 5' genes. The changes of expression are followed by stable changes in morphology, including the ordered transformation of anterior rhombomere cell types to those of a more posterior type, suggesting that a retinoid signal normally regulates the pattern of *Hox* expression.[81] Third, RA is lipophilic and can diffuse directly across cell membranes and exerts its effects on development by controlling target gene transcription via multiple types of RA receptors (RARs and RXRs), members of the nuclear receptor superfamily. RA-bound receptors act as transcription factors that bind as homodimers (RXR–RXR) or heterodimers (RAR–RXR) to RA response elements (RXREs and RAREs) in the promoters of target genes.[82] The promoters of at least some of the *Hox*genes contain RAREs, which have been shown to be required for gene activation.[83] Fourth, targeted disruption of the retinaldehyde dehydrogenase gene (*Raldh2*), essential for the synthesis of active RA, leads to major alterations in *Hox* expression and impairment of segmentation throughout the hindbrain.[84] Significantly, at the neural plate and early tube stages during which patterned *Hox* gene expression commences, Raldh2 is not present in the neuroepithelium itself, but in the presomitic mesoderm that underlies the neurectoderm of the future spinal cord. The forebrain and midbrain, by contrast, express an enzyme (Cyp26) which inactivates retinoids. Thus, these two regions could conceivably act as source and sink in a concentration gradient that spans the intervening hindbrain.[85] The patterning effect of RA, mediated via the nested expression of *Hox* genes along the anteroposterior axis, can be considered both as a local patterning influence on the hindbrain and, more generally, as a posteriorizing element of neural induction (Chapter 2).

While retinoids may be responsible for the posterior-to-anterior display of *Hox* gene expression, it appears that the anterior limit of *Hox* expression, at the r1–r2 boundary, is set by isthmic signals, in particular FGF8.[86] Inhibition of FGF8 *in vivo* allows r1 to express *Hox* genes, whereas ectopic FGF8 represses *Hox* expression elsewhere in the hindbrain. Thus, opposing gradients of diffusible molecules may act to confer coarse pattern on the AP axis of the hindbrain, prominent features of which are a *Hox* negative region, which ultimately forms the cerebellum, and successive domains of nested *Hox* expression which later form an iterated set of pontine and medullary nuclei.

Spinal cord

The spinal nerves comprise a ladder-like array of dorsal root ganglia (DRG) and ventral motor roots along the length of the spinal cord, an obvious manifestation of segmentation. However, in contrast to the intrinsic segmentation that operates in the hindbrain, no evidence of segmental patterns of neuronal differentiation or clear evidence of cell lineage restriction along the AP axis of the spinal neural tube have been found in higher vertebrates. Rather, the spinal nerves are segmented by an extrinsic mechanism, pattern being imposed on the unsegmented neural crest cells and motor axons by a serially-reiterated asymmetry in the sclerotomal component of the mesoderm that lies directly alongside the spinal neural tube.[87] Neural crest cells collect to form DRG preferentially within the rostral half sclerotome of each somite, which is also permissive for axon growth, whereas the caudal half sclerotome of each somite excludes both neural crest cells and motor axons through expression of proteins that inhibit cell migration and cause the collapse of growth cones.[88] Subdivision of the paraxial mesoderm into AP-polarized somites thus ensures a positional correspondence between the segmented dermomyotome on the one hand and its sensorimotor innervation on the other (Fig. 5.3).

Dorsoventral pattern in the spinal cord

The spinal cord has a characteristic dorsoventral (DV) distribution of cell types throughout its AP extent. Specialized non-neurogenic cells form the floor plate, a narrow strip at the ventral midline, which segregates the bilateral halves of the tube; on each side, motor neurons differentiate in the ventral third, relay neurons in the middle third, and smaller interneurons in the dorsal third. The most dorsal region, represented early on by the neural folds that mark the transition between cells with neural and epidermal fates, produces the migratory neural crest cells that give rise to the glia and the majority of neurons in the peripheral nervous system. Later, after the neural crest cells have departed, the dorsal midline is formed by a non-neurogenic roof plate. A similar pattern prevails in the hindbrain and parts of the midbrain.

A number of developmental control genes containing the *Drosophila paired*-type box (*Pax* genes) are expressed in sharply defined dorsoventral domains in the neural tube. *Pax3*, for example, is expressed in the dorsal (alar) half of the neural tube, whereas *Pax6*, is expressed in the dorsal two-thirds of the tube, excluding the most dorsal cells.[89] Homozygous *Pax3* null mutants (the *Splotch* mouse mutant) have spina bifida and lack dorsal root ganglia and other neural crest derivatives. *Pax6* null mutants (the *small eye* mutant) lack eyes and olfactory epithelium. Both genes are expressed during the period when the dorsoventral axis of the neural tube is being patterned. The possibility exists, therefore, that *Pax* genes may encode positional value on the DV axis in much the same way as *Hox* genes do on the AP axis.

A wealth of data from both genetic experiments, tissue recombinations and transplantations has demonstrated that the notochord, the mesodermal skeletal structure that directly underlies the midline of the neural plate and tube, is an important signalling centre in the control of cell pattern in the ventral region of the overlying neuroectoderm. The notochord derives from the chordamesoderm that has an earlier, more general role in initial neuralization of the ectoderm, discussed in Chapter 2. As the notochord condenses, it takes on the more specific role of local signalling centre, controlling the patterning of both floor plate and motor neurons. Thus, surgical removal of the notochord at the late neural plate stage results in a near-normal-sized neural tube in which dorsal markers, such as *Pax3*, appear down the entire DV axis and in which both floor plate and motor neurons fail to appear.[90] Similarly, ventral cell types are absent from the spinal cords of mouse and zebrafish mutants in which notochord formation is genetically perturbed. These findings suggest that the ventral tube takes on dorsal character and that multipotent precursors in the ventral region switch fate in the absence of signals from the notochord. Similarly, implanting a supernumerary notochord alongside the lateral region of the neural plate causes *Pax3* and *Pax6* expression to retreat dorsally and later results in the formation of an additional group of floor plate cells, with flanking columns of ectopic motor neurons, along the line of contact with the grafted notochord (Fig. 3.16).[91,92] Again, it appears that the fate of cells has changed in response to the notochord: cells originally fated to form mid/dorsal interneurons switch fates to become ventral cell types in the presence of notochord, a transformation that is presaged by altered domains of *Pax* gene expression. Furthermore, the notochord (or notochord-conditioned medium) can induce both floor plate and motor neuron development in lateral neural plate tissue cultured in isolation from the rest of the embryo, demonstrating that an inductive signal from the notochord is sufficient to initiate the development of these two ventral cell types, even in heterotypic tissue.[93,94] These experiments show not only the power of the midline axial signal to influence the choice of cell fate, but also the multipotential competence of responding neural tube cells. Whereas floor plate induction seems to require intimate contact with notochord, motor neuron induction occurs at a small distance—suggesting that a diffusible molecule is involved. At a slightly later stage, the floor plate itself acquires the same inductive capabilities as the notochord: it can induce motor neurons in competent neural plate and it can homeogenetically induce itself.

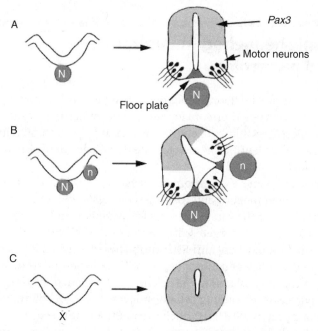

Figure 3.16 Cross-sections of the developing axis showing (A) the normal relationship between notochord (N), floor plate, and motor neurons. When a supplementary notochord (n) is grafted alongside the neural plate (B), an additional floor plate and motor neuron column is induced and *Pax3* expression, normally extending through the dorsal half of the spinal cord, retreats on the operated side. Conversely, when the notochord is extirpated early in development (C), both floor plate and motor neurons fail to develop and *Pax3* is expressed throughout the dorsoventral extent of the cord. Data from Yamada *et al.*[92] and Goulding *et al.*[91]

While these and other experiments clearly show that the notochord is sufficient for floor plate induction, it is less clear that it is necessary for this function. That it is necessary has been presumed primarily on the results of notochord removal experiments in chick, as described above. This view is widely accepted but it has not gone unchallenged. The alternative possibility is that the floor plate acquires its signalling and patterning properties in parallel with but independently from the notochord, as a result of their common origin from the node. In this view, it has been proposed that the absence of floor plate and motor neurons following notochord removal is due not to the elimination of an inducer tissue but to the mechanical ablation of the floor plate itself. Because the midventral cells of the neural tube and the underlying chordal mesoderm are confluent or at least tightly adherent at the site of these operations, inadvertent removal of the floor plate precursors is at least a possibility. For a detailed exposition of these divergent views on the origin of floor plate inductive properties the reader is referred to two recent reviews.[95,96]

Role of Sonic hedgehog in ventral spinal cord patterning

Although motor neuron and floor plate induction appear to require different signals, the one diffusible and the other contact-dependent, molecular studies have shown that a single molecule, Sonic hedgehog, can account for both activities.[97,98] *Sonic hedgehog* was originally identified as a vertebrate homologue of the *Drosophila* segment polarity gene *hedgehog*.

Sonic hedgehog (*Shh*) gene expression displays the appropriate dynamics, being expressed first in the notochord and then the floor plate and when misexpressed in the dorsal neural tube, SHH can elicit ectopic floor plate and motor neuron development,[98-100]. Furthermore, targeted disruption of the *Shh* gene in mice[101] and the application of function-blocking anti-SHH antibodies to avian embryos[102] both result in the absence of floor plate and motor neurons. These experiments demonstrate that SHH protein is necessary as well as sufficient for the induction of these cell types. Moreover, the choice of responding cell fate appears to depend on the concentration of Sonic hedgehog protein (SHH) to which the multipotent precursor is exposed: the concentration threshold for motor neuron induction is about five times lower than that required for floor plate induction.[103] Biochemical studies have revealed a mechanism whereby cells at different DV positions in the naive neural tube could be exposed to different concentrations. The SHH precursor protein synthesized by notochord is autoproteolytically cleaved to generate an inductively active N-terminal product (SHH-N), the majority of which is retained on the secreting cell surface, and an inductively inactive C-terminal product, which plays a role in the cleavage process and in coupling the SHH-N peptide to the cell surface.[104-106] Midventral neural tube cells, which are in contact with the notochord, are thus likely to be exposed to a high local concentration of SHH-N, exceeding the threshold for floor plate induction, whereas the small amount of SHH-N that can diffuse freely from the notochord is sufficient to induce motor neuron development by more distant cells (Fig. 3.17). A remaining question, how cells interpret their local concentration of SHH into a positionally appropriate choice of fate, is considered in Chapter 4.

Target genes induced in neural plate tissue by SHH-N signalling include the winged-helix transcriptional control gene *HNF3β*, a marker of floor plate cells,[100] the LIM-homeobox gene *Isl1*, a marker of motor neurons,[107,108] and the homeobox genes *Nkx2.1* and *Nkx2.2*, markers of ventrolateral neural tube cells.[109,110] SHH signalling also represses the homeobox gene *Msx1* and the *paired* box genes *Pax3* and *Pax6*, suggesting that inactivation of certain transcription factors is a required step in the specification of ventral fate.[91,111] Indeed, the misexpression of *Pax3* in the ventral neural tube of transgenic mice inhibits floor plate and motor neuron differentiation.[112] Although Isl1 is used as a molecular marker for postmitotic motor neurons, it is now becoming clear that Isl1 functions in the developmental progression of both motor neurons and other ventral cell types, most notably those of the forebrain (see

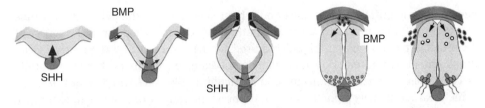

Figure 3.17 Series of stages in development of the dorsal axial organs showing the early action of Sonic hedgehog (SHH) from the notochord in floor plate induction, the ensuing expression of SHH within the floor plate itself and the SHH-dependent induction of motor neurons in the ventrolateral neural tube. Bone morphogenetic proteins (BMPs) expressed in dorsal ectoderm induce the differentiation of neural crest cells (black) at the margins of the approaching neural folds. These cells are subsequently released into the interior of the embryo following neural tube closure. With detachment of the neural tube from overlying ectoderm, BMPs also become expressed in the roof plate of the neural tube (white) where they influence the differentiation of dorsal cell types.

below). That Isl1 is required for motor neuron survival and maturation has been shown by targeted mutation in mice and antisense oligonucleotide treatment of chick neural tube explants.[107] In both cases, motor neurons are formed but die soon afterwards and a small population of ventral interneurons that are distinguished by their expression of *En1* fails to appear. Because these cells do not themselves express *Isl1*, it can be presumed that their differentiation normally depends on an interaction with young motor neurons. This raises the possibility that a series of inductive interactions could extend up the DV axis of the tube, providing a reliable and precise mechanism for generating the large number of different interneuron cell types that it finally produces.

Recently, a study of the requirements for induction of subtypes of interneuron in the ventral half of the spinal cord has revealed the existence of an additional, SHH-independent signalling pathway. This is mediated by retinoids that are probably provided by the newly formed mesoderm lying alongside the neural tube.[113]

Patterning influence of the dorsal ectoderm and roof plate

Cell pattern in the dorsal half of the spinal cord is unaffected by early notochord removal; rather, dorsal marker gene and antigen expression spreads into the ventral neural tube, suggesting that 'dorsal' may be the default state of the neural plate and early tube. Dorsal cell types are marked by the expression of transcription factors, such as Slug (neural crest),[114] and the LIM homeodomain proteins Lmx1 (roof plate)[115] and LH2 (dorsal interneurons).[116] However, these markers are not expressed by default but require inductive signals from the epidermal ectoderm with which the neural plate is initially continuous and which later overlies the closed neural tube (Fig. 3.17). At the neural plate stage, the flanking epidermal ectoderm is the source of a contact-dependent planar signal required for neural crest and (later) roof plate development. This interaction appears to be mediated by members of the BMP family of TGFβ-related signalling molecules, in particular BMP4 and BMP7.[111] Both proteins (which earlier in development act to suppress neuralization; see Chapter 2) are expressed in the dorsal non-neural ectoderm and both recombinant proteins can induce neural crest, interneuron and roof plate cell phenotypes. At the neural tube stage, these dorsal signals are expressed in the roof plate.

The above studies have shown that BMPs produced by the epidermal ectoderm and roof plate are involved in neuronal induction in the dorsal neural tube but have not resolved the comparative importance of the two sources with regard to the induction of specific subtypes of interneuron. It has since been shown that signalling from the roof plate plays a crucial role in the generation of distinct classes of dorsal inter-neuron, as defined by LIM gene expression.[117] Genetic ablation of the roof plate, brought about by expressing a cell toxin under the control of a roof plate-specific gene (*Gdf7*), results in the absence of three interneuron subtypes normally found in the dorsal third of the neural tube and their replacement by a normally midlateral population of interneurons. Cell lineage analysis shows that failure of the dorsal interneurons to appear is due to the elimination of non-autonomous signals ema-nating from the roof plate. The loss of roof plate cells and attendant mis-specifica-tion of interneurons in the dorsal neural tube have also been described in *dreher* mouse mutants, which have a loss-of-function mutation in the *Lmx1a* LIM homeobox gene.[118]

The acquisition by roof plate cells of signalling properties expressed earlier by the epidermal ectoderm suggests the operation of a homeogenetic induction analogous to the transfer of *Shh* expression from notochord to floor plate. In both cases, the transfer of inducing ability attends the physical separation of the initial signalling centre from the neurectoderm and may thus serve to control the levels of signal molecule within tight limits. However, unlike the ventral neural tube, where differ-ent levels of SHH-N induce different cell types, the patterning of dorsal neural tube interneurons does not appear to depend on differing levels of BMP protein. Rather, the same concentration produces a number of different cell types.[116] Although the question of how these distinct cell types is produced is unresolved, their sequential appearance during normal development suggests that the time at which multipotent precursors are exposed to BMPs may be a determinant of their fate.

Role of Sonic hedgehog in dorsoventral patterning of the anterior CNS

Motor neuron differentiation is coextensive with the notochord/floor plate along the AP axis; both have an anterior limit close to the midbrain–forebrain junction. Thus, the forebrain (telencephalon and diencephalon) is devoid of motor neurons and, anterior to the zona limitans (see above), has no floor plate nor is it underlain by notochord. The absence of these midline structures therefore raises the issue of how the bilateral organization of the forebrain and the differentiation of its ventral cell types are controlled. It appears that even in this terminal expansion of the CNS, a common mechanism is used for ventral patterning. As a result of signalling from the underlying prechordal mesoderm, *Shh* is expressed in mid-ventral cells of the forebrain, and tissue culture experiments have shown that SHH-N can induce lateral or dorsal forebrain cells to express the LIM-homeobox gene *Isl1*, an early marker of ventral (motor neuron) specification in the more caudal regions of the CNS.[109,119] However, the normal expression of *Isl1* in the forebrain shows that, rather than being specific to motor neurons, it is a general marker of ventral character: the Isl1-positive cells induced by SHH are forebrain-specific, in that they express the homeobox genes *Nkx2.1* and *Nkx2.2* and do not express any of the markers characteristic of motor neurons. SHH emanating from the ventral midline of the forebrain is responsible for differentiation of the basal ganglia, which are major ventral regions of the telencephalon, in a concentration-dependent manner (Fig. 3.18). High levels of SHH induce the medial ganglionic eminence (future globus pallidus), whereas lower levels induce lateral ganglionic eminence (future striatum/caudate-putamen).[120]

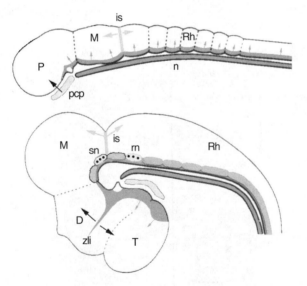

Figure 3.18 Responses of cells in the ventral neural tube to Sonic hedgehog signalling differ with position along the AP axis. Motor neurons form at most AP positions in the hindbrain except caudal r1, where serotonergic neurons of the raphé nucleus (rn) develop in their place. Similarly, motor neurons and dopaminergic neurons (substantia nigra, sn) develop at the same DV position but different AP positions in the midbrain. *Shh* expression later extends into the ventral telencephalon where it influences the development of the basal ganglia. D, diencephalon; is, isthmus; M, mesencephalon; n, notochord; P, Prosencephalon; pcp, prechordal plate; Rh, rhombencephalon; T, telencephalon; zli, zona limitans intrathalamica.

Coordination of AP and DV patterning mechanisms

There is marked variation in the neural cell types that differentiate at the same DV position but different AP positions of the axis. Besides inducing motor neurons and floor plate at mid- and hindbrain levels of the neuraxis, SHH signalling is also involved in the development of region-specific neuronal subpopulations in those brain regions that, like motor neurons, develop alongside the floor plate.[121] Thus, dopaminergic neurons that form the substantia nigra appear in a region of the posterior ventral midbrain where there are no motor neurons—in the gap between oculomotor and trochlear nuclei. Serotonergic neurons that form the raphé nucleus of the hindbrain develop both in regions where there are no motor neurons (such as posterior rhombomere 1), and in more posterior regions which also contain motor neurons (Fig. 3.19). In the latter case, it appears that serotonergic neurons are induced during a second phase of SHH-mediated signalling after motor neuron induction has been completed. These observations suggest that a single signalling system, SHH, can

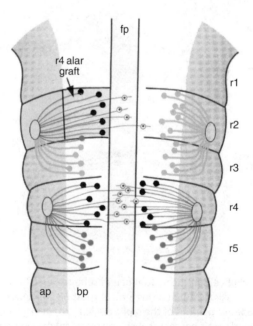

Figure 3.19 Alar plate cells have the potential to become motor neurons when grafted near to the floor plate but the subtype of motor neuron is dictated by the AP origin of the cells. Here, a graft of r4 alar plate in place of r2 basal plate has formed both r4 (facial)-type branchiomotor neurons and r4-specific cva neurons. Data from Simon et al.[123]

induce the formation of different cell types at different positions along the AP axis, or at different times in development. This implies that SHH is permissive rather than instructive, that the choice of induced cell fate would depend on some pre-existing competence in the neuroepithelium, and that this competence would vary with AP position in terms of the local repertoire of possible responses to SHH signalling. That the response to SHH induction is AP position-specific is well illustrated by the dopaminergic neurons of the posterior midbrain: these can be induced to form in lateral regions of the neural plate either by contact with notochord or floor plate or by treatment with SHH protein, but only when the responding tissue is explanted from the midbrain level of the neural tube.

Thus, the patterning activities of SHH operate within the context of previously established AP positional cues and previously specified AP regional identity. Before SHH acts on the tissue, however, the AP regional identity of any particular cell is not manifested as any definitive cell phenotype, rather it would take the form of a repertoire of possible phenotypes, restricted to those fates that are appropriate to the cell's precise AP position. The ultimate choice of cell-type fate would await the permissive midline signal, whose influence in selecting which of the number of possible fates should be adopted would be its concentration. This has been most clearly demonstrated *in vivo* for cell type determination in the avian hindbrain, where (as described above) each rhombomere has a unique identity. Rhombomere 4, for example, expresses *Hoxb1* at high level and later develops a population of cholinergic motor-like neurons alongside the floor plate, the contralateral vestibuloacoustic efferent neurons (CVAN) whose target specificity (the inner ear) and contralateral cell body migration endow them with a prominent and unique phenotype.[122] When the ventral (basal) plate of r4 (the normal source of CVAN) is transplanted in place of the basal plate of r2 (where the motor neurons normally project exclusively ipsilaterally), *Hoxb1* expression is sustained and CVAN develop in the graft, demonstrating that at the time of grafting AP positional value has already been determined and is no longer labile. However, the CVAN also differentiate in grafts of the dorsal (alar) plate of r4 when it is grafted in place of basal r2, provided that the graft comes into proximity with the notochord/floor plate (Fig. 3.19).[123] Thus, an r4-specific basal plate cell type is formed in response to ventral midline signalling, irrespective of the original dorso-ventral position of the precursors. This shows that DV fate is still labile at a time when AP fate is already fixed and, therefore, that the graft tissue must contain cells which are multipotent (alar plate never normally form motor neurons). Although multipotent, however, their range of potentials is already restricted to those that are appropriate to r4; midline signals then determine which specific cell type should develop at a particular DV position.

An interesting but as yet hardly explored question is whether the coordination between AP and DV patterning seen for the ventral neural tube also pertains to midline signalling in the dorsal tube. Marked differences exist between the dorsal cell content of spinal cord, hindbrain (cerebellum) and midbrain (optic tectum) as well as between the cephalic and spinal neural crest.

Key points

1 Pattern formation is the spatial ordering of cell differentiation. An early phase during which regions and subregions are specified is followed by the acquisition of individual cell identity

2 The CNS has two principal axes, anteroposterior and dorsoventral, along which both regional and cell pattern is established. The third axis, inside–outside, is largely a maturational gradient, with neurons being born next to the ventricle and then migrating to outer regions. The anteroposterior axis is known as the neuraxis.

3 Each of the principal brain regions—forebrain, midbrain, and hindbrain—is morphologically distinct as an individual swelling (vesicle) of the neural tube before any neurons are born, and each is characterized by the expression of region-specific transcription factors.

4 Subdivision of the forebrain (prosencephalon) into telencephalic and diencephalic regions involves planar signalling from the anterior pole of the neuraxis.

5 The telencephalon is subdivided by a major longitudinal boundary into dorsal (pallial) and ventral (subpallial) regions which express different transcription factors and have distinct regional fates. In mammals, the pallium forms the cerebral cortex whereas the subpallium forms the basal ganglia.

6 The diencephalon is subdivided by a major transverse boundary, the zona limitans intrathalamica, into anterior (later ventral thalamus) posterior (later dorsal thalamus) regions. A third territory, the pretectum, forms at its border with the midbrain.

7 A prominent signalling centre at the narrow region of the tube between midbrain and hindbrain vesicles (the isthmus) is responsible for specifying midbrain and cerebellar fate and for establishing the anteroposterior polarity of the dorsal midbrain, the optic tectum.

8 Hindbrain development is characterized by the process of segmentation. A modular organization of neuronal subtypes and nuclei is set up by the early transverse subdivision of the hindbrain into a set of eight rhombomeres. Rhombomere identity is controlled by transcription factors of the Hox family.

9 Cell pattern is rather uniform along the anteroposterior axis of the spinal cord but has distinct variation down the dorsoventral axis, where motor neurons form ventrally, relay neurons in the middle third and small interneurons form dorsally.

10 Dorsoventral polarity of the spinal cord is established by signalling centres at ventral and dorsal poles—the floor plate and the roof plate. Both of these are non-neurogenic structures that join the left and right halves of the spinal cord together at the midline.

11 The ventral signalling centre is induced by signals from the underlying notochord. The best known of its signals is Sonic hedgehog, which influences cell pattern in the ventral third of the spinal cord.

12 The dorsal signalling centre, along with the overlying epidermal ectoderm, releases bone morphogenetic proteins which influence cell pattern in the dorsal third of the cord.

General reading

- Fraser, S. E. and Harland, R. M. The molecular metamorphosis of experimental embryology. *Cell* **100**, 41–55, 2000.

- Jessell, T. M. and Lumsden, A. Inductive signals and the assignment of cell fate in the spinal cord and hindbrain. In *Molecular and cellular approaches to neural development* (ed. W. M. Cowan, T. M. Jessell and S. L. Zipursky), pp. 290–333 (Oxford University Press, New York, 1997).

- Lumsden, A. and Krumlauf, R. Patterning the vertebrate neuraxis. *Science* **274**, 1109–15, 1996.

- Rubenstein, J. L. R. and Beachy, P. A. Patterning of the embryonic forebrain. *Curr. Opin. Neurobiol.* **8**, 18–26, 1998.

- Ragsdale, C. W. and Grove, E. A. Patterning the mammalian cerebral cortex. *Curr. Opin. Neurobiol.* **11**, 50–8, 2001.

References

1. Eagleston, G. W. and Harris, W. A. Mapping of the presumptive brain region in the neural plate of *Xenopus laevis*. *J. Neurobiol.* **21**, 427–40 (1990).

2. Le Douarin, N. Cephalic placodes and neurogenesis. *Trends Neurosci.* **9**, 175–80 (1986).

3. Xuan, S. *et al.* Winged helix factor BF-1 is essential for the development of the cerebral hemispheres. *Neuron* **14**, 1141–52 (1995).

4. Houart, C., Westerfield, M. and Wilson, S. A small population of anterior cells patterns the forebrain during zebrafish gastrulation. *Nature* **391**, 788–92 (1998).

5. Shimamura, K. and Rubenstein, J. L. R. Inductive interactions direct early regionalisation of the mouse forebrain. *Development* **124**, 2709–18 (1997).

6. Shanmugalingam, S. *et al.* Ace/Fgf8 is required for forebrain commissure formation and patterning of the telencephalon. *Development* **127**, 2549–61 (2000).

7. Bang, A. and Goulding, M. Regulation of vertebrate neural cell fate by transcription factors. *Curr. Opin. Neurobiol.* **6**, 25–32 (1996).

8. Boncinelli, E., Gulisano, M. and Broccoli, V. *Emx* and *Otx* homeobox genes in the developing mouse brain. *J. Neurobiol.* **24**, 1356–66 (1993).

9. Mallamaci, A. *et al.* EMX2 protein in the developing mouse brain and olfactory area. *Mech. Dev.* **77**, 165–72 (1998).

10. Qiu, M. *et al.* Mutation of the *Emx-1* homeobox gene disrupts the corpus callosum. *Dev. Biol.* **178**, 174–8 (1996).

11. Pellegrini, M., Mansouri, A., Simeone, A., Boncinelli, E. and Gruss, P. Dentate gyrus formation requires *Emx2*. *Development* **122**, 3893–8 (1996).

12. Mallamaci, A. *et al.* The lack of *Emx2* causes impairment of Reelin signaling and defects of neuronal migration in the developing cerebral cortex. *J. Neurosci.* **20**, 1096–118 (2000).

13. Theil, T., Alvarez-Bolado, G., Walter, A. and Ruther, U. *Gli3* is required for *Emx* gene expression during dorsal telencephalon development. *Development* **126**, 3561–71 (1999).

14. Sussel, L., Marin, O., Kimura, S. and Rubenstein, J. L. R. Loss of *Nkx2.1* homeobox gene function results in a ventral to dorsal molecular

respecification within the basal telencephalon: evidence for a transformation of the pallidum into the striatum. *Development* **126**, 3359–70 (1999).

15. Götz, M., Wizenmann, A., Reinhardt, S., Lumsden, A. and Price, J. Selective adhesion of cells from different telencephalic regions. *Neuron* **16**, 551–64 (1996).

16. Stoykova, A., Fritsch, R., Walther, C. and Gruss, P. Forebrain patterning defects in small eye mutant mice. *Development* **122**, 3453–65 (1996).

17. Magrassi, L. *et al*. Basal ganglia precursors found in aggregates following embryonic transplantation adopt a striatal phenotype in heterotopic locations. *Development* **125**, 2847–55 (1998).

18. Fishell, G. Striatal precursors adopt cortical identities in response to local cues. *Development* **121**, 803–12 (1995).

19. Anderson, S. A., Eisenstat, D. D., Shi, L. and Rubenstein, J. L. R. Interneuron migration from basal forebrain to neocortex: dependence on *Dlx* genes. *Science* **278**, 474–6 (1997).

20. Lavdas, A. A., Grigoriou, M., Pachnis, V. and Parnavelas, J. G. The medial ganglionic eminence gives rise to a population of early neurons in the developing cerebral cortex. *J. Neurosci.* **99**, 7881–8 (1999).

21. Lumsden, A. and Gulisano, M. Neocortical neurons: where do they come from? *Science* **278**, 402–3 (1997).

22. Chapouton, P., Gartner, A. and Gotz, M. The role of Pax6 in restricting cell migration between developing cortex and basal ganglia. *Development* **126**, 5569–79 (1999).

23. Bishop, K. M., Goudreau, G. and O'Leary, D. D. M. Regulation of area identity in the mammalian neocortex by Emx2 and Pax6. *Science* **288**, 344–9 (2000).

24. Ragsdale, C. W. and Grove, E. A. Patterning the mammalian cerebral cortex. *Curr. Opin. Neurobiol.* **11**, 50–8 (2001).

25. Figdor, M. C. and Stern, C. D. Segmental organisation of embryonic diencephalon. *Nature* **363**, 630–4 (1993).

26. Rubenstein, J. L. R., Martinez, S., Shimamura, K. and Puelles, L. The embryonic vertebrate forebrain: the prosomeric model. *Science* **266**, 578–80 (1994).

27. Cepko, C. L., Golden, J. A., Szele, F. G. and Lin, J. C. Lineage analysis in the vertebrate central nervous system. In *Molecular and cellular approaches to neural development* (ed. W. M. Cowan, T. M. Jessell and S. L. Zipursky), pp. 391–439 (Oxford University Press, New York, 1997).

28. Zeltser, L., Larsen, C. and Lumsden, A. Molecular events leading to formation of the zona

limitans intrathalamica, the major divisional boundary of the vertebrate forebrain. Unpublished data (2001).

29. Matsunaga, E., Araki, I. and Nakamura, H. *Pax6* defines the di-mesencephalic boundary by repressing *En1* and *Pax2*. *Development* **127**, 2357–65 (2000).

30. O'Leary, D. D. M. and Wilkinson, D. G. Eph receptors and ephrins in neural development. *Curr. Opin. Neurobiol.* **9**, 65–73 (1999).

31. Millet, S., Bloch-Gallego, E., Simeone, A. and Alvarado-Mallart, R.-M. The caudal limit of *Otx2* gene expression as a marker of the midbrain/hindbrain boundary: a study using a chick *Otx2* riboprobe and chick/quail homotopic grafts. *Development* **122**, 3785–97 (1996).

32. Wassarman, K. M. *et al*. Specification of the anterior hindbrain and establishment of a normal mid/hindbrain organizer is dependent on *Gbx2* gene function. *Development* **124**, 2923–34 (1997).

33. Wingate, R. J. T. and Hatten, M. E. Cerebellar rhombic lip derivatives. *Development* **126**, 4395–404 (1999).

34. Hallonet, M. E., Teillet, M.-A. and Le Douarin, N. A new approach to the development of the cerebellum provided by the quail-chick marker system. *Development* **108**, 19–31 (1990).

35. Joyner, A. L. *Engrailed*, *wnt* and *pax* genes regulate midbrain–hindbrain development. *Trends Genet.* **12**, 15–20 (1996).

36. Acampora, D., Avantaggiato, V., Tuorto, F. and Simeone, A. Genetic control of brain morphogenesis through *Otx* gene dosage. *Development* **124**, 3639–50 (1997).

37. Broccoli, V., Boncinelli, E. and Wurst, W. The caudal limit of *Otx2* expression positions the isthmic organizer. *Nature* **401**, 164–8 (1999).

38. Wurst, W., Auerbach, A. B. and Joyner, A. L. Multiple developmental defects in *Engrailed-1* mutant mice: an early mid-hindbrain deletion and patterning defects in forelimbs and sternum. *Development* **120**, 2065–75 (1994).

39. Hanks, M., Wurst, W., Anson-Cartwright, L., Auerbach, A. B. and Joyner, A. L. Rescue of the *En-1* mutant phenotype by replacement of *En-1* with *En2*. *Science* **269**, 679–82 (1995).

40. Itasaki, N. and Nakamura, H. A role for gradient en expression in positional specification of the optic tectum. *Neuron* **16**, 55–62 (1996).

41. Logan, C. *et al*. Rostral optic tectum adopts a caudal phenotype following ectopic engrailed expression. *Curr. Biol.* **6**, 1006–104 (1996).

42. Itasaki, N., Ichijo, H., Hama, C., Matsuno, T. and Nakamura, H. Establishment of rostrocaudal polarity in tectal primordium: engrailed expression and subsequent tectal polarity. *Development* **113**, 1133–44 (1991).

43. McMahon, A. P., Joyner, A. L., Bradley, A. and McMahon, J. A. The midbrain-hindbrain phenotype of *Wnt-1⁻/Wnt-1⁻* mice results from stepwise deletion of *Engrailed*-expressing cells by 9.5 days postcoitum. *Cell* **69**, 581–95 (1992).

44. Danielian, P. S. and McMahon, A. P. Engrailed-1 as a target of the Wnt-1 signalling in vertebrate midbrain development. *Nature* **383**, 332–4 (1996).

45. Crossley, P. H., Martinez, S. and Martin, G. R. Midbrain development induced by FGF8 in the chick embryo. *Nature* **380**, 66–8 (1996).

46. Urbanek, P., Wang, Z. Q., Fetka, I., Wagner, E. F. and Busslinger, M. Complete block of early B cell differentiation and altered patterning of the posterior midbrain in mice lacking Pax5/BSAP. *Cell* **79**, 901–12 (1994).

47. Lun, K. and Brand, M. A series of zebrafish *no isthmus* alleles of the *Pax2.1* gene reveals multiple signalling events in development of the midbrain-hindbrain primordium. *Development* **125**, 3049–62 (1998).

48. Krauss, S., Maden, M., Holder, N. and Wilson, S. W. Zebrafish *pax[b]* is involved in the formation of the midbrain–hindbrain boundary. *Nature* **360**, 87–9 (1992).

49. Song, D.-L., Chalepakis, G., Gruss, P. and Joyner, A. L. Two Pax-binding sites are required for early embryonic brain expression of an *Engrailed-2* transgene. *Development* **122**, 627–35 (1996).

50. Martinez, S., Marin, F., Nieto, M. A. and Puelles, L. Induction of ectopic engrailed expression and fate change in avian rhombomeres: intersegmental boundaries as barriers. *Mech. Dev.* **51**, 289–303 (1995).

51. Watanabe, Y. and Nakamura, H. Control of chick tectum territory along the dorsoventral axis by Sonic hedgehog. *Development* **127**, 1131–40 (2000).

52. Lumsden, A. The cellular basis of segmentation in the developing hindbrain. *Trends Neurosci.* **13**, 329–35 (1990).

53. Lumsden, A. and Keynes, R. Segmental patterns of neuronal development in the chick hindbrain. *Nature* **337**, 424–8 (1989).

54. Heyman, I., Kent, A. and Lumsden, A. Cellular morphology and extracellular space at rhombomere boundaries in the chick embryo hindbrain. *Dev. Dyn.* **198**, 241–53 (1993).

55. Clarke, J. D. and Lumsden, A. Segmental repetition of neuronal phenotype sets in the chick embryo hindbrain. *Development* **118**, 151–62 (1993).

56. Lumsden, A., Sprawson, N. and Graham, A. Segmental origin and migration of neural crest cells in the hindbrain region of the chick embryo. *Development* **113**, 1281–91 (1991).

57. Fortin, G., Jungbluth, S., Lumsden, A. and Champagnat, J. Segmental specification of GABAergic inhibition during development of hindbrain neural networks. *Nat. Neurosci.* **2**, 873–7 (1999).

58. Fraser, S., Keynes, R. and Lumsden, A. Segmentation in the chick embryo hindbrain is defined by cell lineage restrictions. *Nature* **344**, 431–5 (1990).

59. Wingate, R. and Lumsden, A. Persistence of rhombomeric organisation in the postsegmental avian hindbrain. *Development* **122**, 2143–52 (1996).

60. Guthrie, S. and Lumsden, A. Formation and regeneration of rhombomere boundaries in the developing chick hindbrain. *Development* **112**, 221–9 (1991).

61. Wizenmann, A. and Lumsden, A. Segregation of rhombomeres by differential chemoaffinity. *Mol. Cell. Neurosci.* **9**, 448–59 (1997).

62. Nieto, M. A., Gilardi, H. P., Charnay, P. and Wilkinson, D. G. A receptor protein tyrosine kinase implicated in the segmental patterning of the hindbrain and mesoderm. *Development* **116**, 1137–50 (1992).

63. Xu, Q., Mellitzer, G., Robinson, V. and Wilkinson, D. G. *In vivo* cell sorting in complementary segmental domains mediated by Eph receptors and ephrins. *Nature* **400**, 267–71 (1999).

64. Lumsden, A. Closing in on rhombomere boundaries. *Nat. Cell Biol.* **1**, E83–5 (1999).

65. Wilkinson, D. G., Bhatt, S., Chavrier, P., Bravo, R. and Charnay, P. Segment-specific expression of a zinc-finger gene in the developing nervous system of the mouse. *Nature* **337**, 461–5 (1989).

66. Theil, T. *et al.* Segmental expression of the *EphA4* (*Sek-1*) receptor tyrosine kinase in the hindbrain is under direct transcriptional control of Krox-20. *Development* **125**, 443–52 (1998).

67. Schneider-Maunoury, S., Seitanidou, T., Charnay, P. and Lumsden, A. Segmental and neuronal architecture of the hindbrain of *Krox-20* mouse mutants. *Development* **124**, 1215–26 (1997).

68. Moens, C. B., Cordes, S. P., Giorgianni, M. W., Barsh, G. S. and Kimmel, C. B. Equivalence in the genetic control of hindbrain segmentation in fish and mouse. *Development* **125**, 381–91 (1998).

69. Manzanares, M. *et al.* The role of *kreisler* in segmentation during hindbrain development. *Dev. Biol.* **211**, 220–37 (1999).

70. McKay, I. J. *et al.* The *kreisler* mouse: a hindbrain segmentation mutant that lacks two rhombomeres. *Development* **120**, 2199–211 (1994).

71. Wilkinson, D. G., Bhatt, S., Cook, M., Boncinelli, E. and Krumlauf, R. Segmental

expression of Hox-2 homeobox-containing genes in the developing mouse hindbrain. *Nature* **341**, 405–9 (1989).

72. Hirth, F., Hartmann, B. and Reichert, H. Homeotic gene action in embryonic brain development of *Drosophila*. *Development* **125**, 1579–89 (1998).

73. Krumlauf, R. *Hox* genes in vertebrate development. *Cell* **78**, 191–201 (1994).

74. Studer, M., Lumsden, A., Ariza-McNaughton, L., Bradley, A. and Krumlauf, R. Altered segmental identity and abnormal migration of motor neurons in mice lacking *Hoxb1*. *Nature* **384**, 630–4 (1996).

75. Bell, E., Wingate, R. J. T. and Lumsden, A. Homeotic transformation of rhombomere identity after localized *Hoxb1* misexpression. *Science* **284**, 2168–71 (1999).

76. Bateson, W. *Materials for the study of variation* (Cambridge University Press, Cambridge, 1894).

77. Mark, M. *et al.* Two rhombomeres are altered in *Hoxa1* mutant mice. *Development* **119**, 319–38 (1993).

78. Gavalas, A. *et al. Hoxa1* and *Hoxb1* synergise in patterning the hindbrain cranial nerves and second pharyngeal arch. *Development* **125**, 1123–36 (1998).

79. Sharpe, J., Nonchev, S., Gould, A., Whiting, J. and Krumlauf, R. Selectivity, sharing and competitive interactions in the regulation of *Hoxb* genes. *EMBO J.* **17**, 1788–98 (1998).

80. Manzanares, M. *et al.* Conserved and distinct roles of kreisler in regulation of the paralogous *Hoxa3* and *Hoxb3* genes. *Development* **126**, 759–69 (1999).

81. Marshall, H. *et al.* Retinoic acid alters hindbrain Hox code and induces transformation of rhombomeres 2/3 into a 4/5 identity. *Nature* **360**, 737–41 (1992).

82. Mangelsdorf, D. J. and Evans, R. M. The RXR heterodimers and ophan receptors. *Cell* **83**, 841–50 (1995).

83. Marshall, H., Morrison, A., Studer, M., Popperl, H. and Krumlauf, R. Retinoids and *Hox* genes. *FASEB J.* **10**, 969–78 (1996).

84. Niederreither, K., Vermot, J., Schuhbaur, B., Chambon, P. and Dollé, P. Retinoic acid synthesis and hindbrain patterning in the mouse embryo. *Development* **127**, 75–85 (2000).

85. Maden, M. Unpublished data (2000).

86. Irving, C. and Mason, I. Signalling by FGF8 from the isthmus patterns anterior hindbrain and establishes the anterior limit of *Hox* gene expression. *Development* **127**, 177–86 (2000).

87. Keynes, R. and Stern, C. Segmentation in the vertebrate nervous system. *Nature* **310**, 786–9 (1984).

88. Davies, J., Cook, M., Stern, C. D. and Keynes, R. J. Isolation from chick somites of a glycoprotein that causes collapse of dorsal root ganglion growth cones. *Neuron* **4**, 11–20 (1990).

89. Chalepakis, G., Stoykova, A., Wijnholds, J., Tremblay, P. and Gruss, P. Pax gene regulators in the developing nervous system. *J. Neurobiol.* **24**, 1367–84 (1993).

90. Tanabe, Y. and Jessell, T. M. Diversity and pattern in the developing spinal cord. *Science* **274**, 1115–23 (1996).

91. Goulding, M. D., Lumsden, A. and Gruss, P. Signals from the notochord and floor plate regulate the region-specific expression of two *Pax* genes in the developing spinal cord. *Development* **117**, 1011–16 (1993).

92. Yamada, T., Placzek, M., Tanaka, H., Dodd, J. and Jessell, T. M. Control of cell pattern in the developing nervous system: polarizing activity of the floor plate and notochord. *Cell* **64**, 635–47 (1991).

93. Yamada, T., Pfaff, S., Edlund, T. and Jessell, T. M. Control of cell pattern in the neural tube: motor neuron induction by diffusible factors from notochord and floor plate. *Cell* **73**, 673–86 (1993).

94. Placzek, M., Jessell, T. M. and Dodd, J. Induction of floor plate differentiation by contact-dependent, homeogenetic signals. *Development* **117**, 205–18 (1993).

95. Placzek, M., Dodd, J. and Jessell, T. M. The case for floor plate induction by the notochord. *Curr. Opin. Neurobiol.* **10**, 15–22 (2000).

96. Le Douarin, N. M. and Halpern, M. E. Origin and specification of the neural tube floor plate: insights from the chick and zebrafish. *Curr. Opin. Neurobiol.* **10**, 23–30 (2000).

97. Krauss, S., Concordet, J. P. and Ingham, P. W. A functionally conserved homolog of the *Drosophila* segment polarity gene hh is expressed in tissues with polarizing activity in zebrafish embryos. *Cell* **75**, 1431–44 (1993).

98. Roelink, H. *et al.* Floor plate and motor neuron induction by vhh-1, a vertebrate homolog of hedgehog expressed by the notochord. *Cell* **76**, 761–75 (1994).

99. Tanabe, Y., Roelink, H. and Jessell, T. M. Induction of motor neurons by Sonic hedgehog is independent of floor plate differentiation. *Curr. Biol.* **5**, 651–8 (1995).

100. Ruiz i Altaba, A., Placzek, M., Baldassare, M., Dodd, J. and Jessell, T. M. Early stages of notochord and floor plate development in the chick embryo defined by normal and induced expression of HNF3β. *Dev. Biol.* **170**, 299–313 (1995).

101. Chiang, C. *et al.* Cyclopia and defective axial patterning in mice lacking Sonic hedgehog gene function. *Nature* **383**, 407–13 (1996).

102. Marti, E., Bumcrot, D. A., Takada, R. and McMahon, A. P. Requirement of 19K form of Sonic hedgehog for induction of distinct ventral cell types in CNS explants. *Nature* **375**, 322–5 (1995).

103. Roelink, H. *et al.* Floor plate and motor neuron induction by different concentrations of the amino-terminal cleavage product of sonic hedgehog autoproteolysis. *Cell* **81**, 445–55 (1995).

104. Bumcrot, D. A., Takada, R. and McMahon, A. P. Proteolytic processing yields two secreted forms of Sonic hedgehog. *Mol. Cell. Biol.* **15**, 2294–303 (1995).

105. Lee, J. J. *et al.* Autoproteolysis in hedgehog protein biogenesis. *Science* **266**, 1528–37 (1994).

106. Porter, J. A. *et al.* The product of hedgehog autoproteolytic cleavage active in local and long-range signalling. *Nature* **374**, 363–6 (1995).

107. Pfaff, S. L., Mendelsohn, M., Stewart, C. L., Edlund, T. and Jessell, T. M. Requirement for LIM homeobox gene *Is11* in motor neuron generation reveals a motor neuron-dependent step in interneuron differentiation. *Cell* **84**, 1–20 (1996).

108. Ericson, J., Thor, S., Edlund, T., Jessell, T. M. and Yamada, T. Early stages of motor neuron differentiation revealed by expression of homeobox gene Islet-1. *Science* **256**, 1555–60 (1992).

109. Ericson, J. *et al.* Sonic hedgehog induces the differentiation of ventral forebrain neurons: a common signal for ventral patterning within the neural tube. *Cell* **81**, 747–56 (1995).

110. Briscoe, J. *et al.* Homeobox gene *Nkx2.2* and specification of neuronal identity by graded Sonic hedgehog signalling. *Nature* **398**, 622–7 (1999).

111. Liem, K. F., Tremml, G., Roelink, H. and Jessell, T. M. Dorsal differentiation of neural plate cells induced by BMP-mediated signals from epidermal ectoderm. *Cell* **82**, 969–79 (1995).

112. Tremblay, P., Pituello, F. and Gruss, P. Inhibition of floor plate differentiation by Pax3: evidence from ectopic expression in transgenic mice. *Development* **122**, 2555–67 (1996).

113. Pierani, A., Brenner-Morton, S., Chiang, C. and Jessell, T. M. A Sonic hedgehog-independent, retinoid-activated pathway of neurogenesis in the ventral spinal cord. *Cell* **97**, 903–15 (1999).

114. Nieto, M. A., Sargent, M. G., Wilkinson, D. G. and Cooke, J. Control of cell behavior during vertebrate development by *Slug*, a zinc finger gene. *Science* **264**, 835–9 (1994).

115. Riddle, R. D. *et al.* Induction of the LIM-homeobox gene *Lmx1* by WNT7a establishes dorsoventral pattern in the vertebrate limb. *Cell* **83**, 631–40 (1995).

116. Liem, K., Tremml, G. and Jessell, T. M. A role for the roof plate and its resident TGFβ-related proteins in neuronal patterning in the dorsal spinal cord. *Cell* **91**, 127–38 (1997).

117. Lee, K. J., Dietrich, P. and Jessell, T. M. Genetic ablation reveals that the roof plate is essential for dorsal interneuron specification. *Nature* **403**, 734–40 (2000).

118. Millonig, J. H., Millen, K. J. and Hatten, M. E. The mouse Dreher gene *Lmx1a* controls formation of the roof plate in the vertebrate CNS. *Nature* **403**, 764–9 (2000).

119. Barth, K. A. and Wilson, S. W. Zebrafish *Nkx2.2* is influenced by Sonic hedgehog/vertebrate hedgehog-1 and demarcates neuronal differentiation in the embryonic forebrain. *Development* **121**, 1755–68 (1995).

120. Kohtz, J. D., Baker, D. P., Corte, G. and Fishell, G. Regionalization within the mammalian telencephalon is mediated by changes in responsiveness to Sonic hedgehog. *Development* **125**, 5079–89 (1998).

121. Hynes, M. and Rosenthal, A. Specification of dopaminergic and serotonergic neurons in the vertebrate CNS. *Curr. Opin. Neurobiol.* **9**, 26–36 (1999).

122. Simon, H. and Lumsden, A. Rhombomere-specific origin of the contralateral vestibulo-acoustic efferent neurons and their migration across the embryonic midline. *Neuron* **11**, 209–20 (1993).

123. Simon, H., Hornbruch, A. and Lumsden, A. Independent assignment of antero-posterior and dorso-ventral positional values in the developing chick hindbrain. *Curr. Biol.* **5**, 205–14 (1995).

124. Fernandez, A. S., Pieau, C., Reperant, J., Boncinelli, E. and Wassef, M. Expression of the *Emx-1* and *Dlx-1* homeobox genes define three molecularly distinct domains in the telencephalon of mouse, chick, turtle and frog embryos: implications for the evolution of telencephalic subdivisions in amniotes. *Development* **125**, 2099–111 (1998).

125. Rubenstein, J. L. R. and Beachy, P. A. Patterning of the embryonic forebrain. *Curr. Opin. Neurobiol.* **8**, 18–26 (1998).

126. Kimmel, C. B., Sepich, D. S. and Trevarrow, B. Development of segmentation in zebrafish. *Development* **104** (Suppl.), 197–207 (1988).

4

The Emergence of Neural Fate

In this chapter we will describe the general processes whereby a neuron differentiates from a progenitor cell. Having surveyed the mechanisms involved in this process of neurogenesis, in both *Drosophila* and vertebrates, we will consider how neurogenic programmes may be integrated with the mechanisms of neural induction and patterning, such that distinct neuronal cell types develop at different positions in the neural epithelium.

The common ancestor of vertebrates and invertebrates possessed a nervous system, so it is perhaps not surprising that the study of nerve cell origins and differentiation in invertebrate systems, and particularly its molecular genetic dissection in *Drosophila*, has provided important insights into the mechanisms of neurogenesis more generally. A recurring theme in the analysis of cell fate in any organism concerns the degree to which that fate is determined by the cell's environment, being 'induced' by instructive interactions with molecules derived from neighbouring cells, and to what extent fate is dictated by the cell's lineage—the particular parcellation of cytoplasmic determinants that it receives from its parent cell. In *Drosophila*, where the major advances in understanding have been made, single neuroblasts are selected from an initially homogeneous population of ectoderm cells (the neurogenic region, or neurectoderm) as a result of a series of cell interactions that act progressively to restrict cell fates. Initially, all of the cells form an 'equivalence group', in which the individual cells can substitute for each other during the acquisition of specific cell fate. Equivalence is progressively lost through a process of cell–cell interaction characterized by lateral inhibition with feedback, the principle of which is that the more inhibition a cell receives the less it is able to deliver. The importance of cell–cell signalling in these decisions is indicated by the finding that a cell that would normally differentiate as an epidermoblast can adopt a neural fate when a neighbouring neuroblast is ablated. Later, once neuroblasts have formed, a second mechanism involving the asymmetric distribution of cytoplasmic determinants comes into play during the subsequent divisions of the neuroblast. Although the process of neural fate selection is ultimately complex, with more than 30 genes being known to be involved in the process in the fly, it is essentially a series of simpler binary choices.

Neural cell fate determination in *Drosophila*

The first step is the specification of discrete regions of the ectoderm, within which each cell has the potential to produce neural precursor cells (Fig. 4.1). These proneural clusters are characterized by the cell autonomous expression of the *proneural genes*, which encode a group of transcription factors of the basic helix–loop–helix class (bHLH proteins), and are set up as a prepattern in the ectoderm as a component of the positional information system operating during early embryogenesis, such that the pattern of proneural clusters is registered with the segmented body plan. Proneural gene expression endows the potential to become neural. Later, cells within the cluster compete with each other such that the ability to form a neural precursor is restricted to one cell in the cluster. Which particular cell is singled out is determined by signalling between adjacent cells in a process known as lateral specification. This is one use of a mechanism that is widely used during development to impose differences between groups of cells that are otherwise equivalent. Lateral specification involves the *neurogenic genes*, which encode the transmembrane proteins Notch and Delta. Expression of Delta is controlled by the proneural genes, and the protein is a ligand that activates the Notch receptor. In turn, activated Notch generates intracellular signals leading to the repression of proneural gene expression and the down-regulation of Delta. Once singled out, the neural precursor starts to express neural precursor genes, which are common to all precursors and may direct general neural differentiation, and neuronal-type selector genes, whose expression is restricted to specific subsets of precursors.

The system has an essentially stochastic character. Fluctuation in the level of expression of proneural genes between the cells of cluster leads to variation in Delta expression which leads, through intercellular signalling, to variation in Notch expression. Such initial variation in the levels of Notch expressed by two neighbouring cells is amplified by a local feedback loop, since the cell with more Notch will express less Delta and so activate less Notch in its neighbour; cells that are relatively weak in Notch signalling become neurons, while those with relatively strong Notch signalling become epidermoblasts, the progenitor cells of the epidermis.[1] The newly determined neuroblasts move deeper into the embryo to develop the CNS, while the PNS develops from remaining epidermoblasts that undergo a further decision between neural and non-neural fates, some becoming sensory organ precursor cells and the rest differentiating as epidermal cells. In both CNS and PNS the course of neural precursor differentiation follows a precise series of asymmetrical cell divisions. In the CNS,[2] the neuroblasts that delaminate from the ventral neurectoderm undergo a stereotyped series of asymmetric divisions, at each one producing a smaller ganglion mother cell from the inner (basal) surface; each ganglion mother cell then divides equally to produce two postmitotic neurons or glia (Fig. 4.1). Each neuroblast

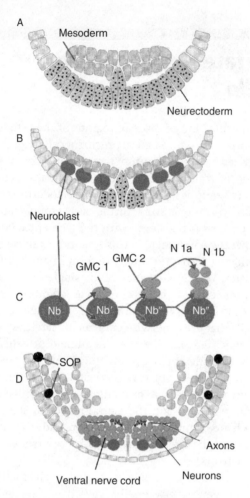

Figure 4.1 Cross-sections of an insect embryo showing early stages in the formation of the ventral nerve cord. Progenitors in the neurectoderm (A) delaminate to give rise to neuroblasts (B), which go through a series of asymmetric divisions (C) to produce a stack of ganglion mother cells (GMCs). Each GMC then divides to produce two neurons (e.g. N1a, N1b). Neurons form the outer layer of the nerve cord, surrounding their axons (D). Individual sense organ precursor (SOP) cells delaminate from the epidermis at various positions. After Harris and Hartenstein.[118]

generates an invariant lineage. In the PNS, the selected sense organ precursor (SOP) cell divides twice to produce the four cells of which the external sensory (ES) organ is composed—bristle cell, socket cell, sheath (glial) cell and neuron. A similar pattern of precursor cell division is involved in the production of the second main component of the PNS, the internal stretch receptors (chordotonal organs). The developing ES organ of the adult fly has proved to be a highly approachable system for understanding the controls of neurogenesis (Fig. 4.2).

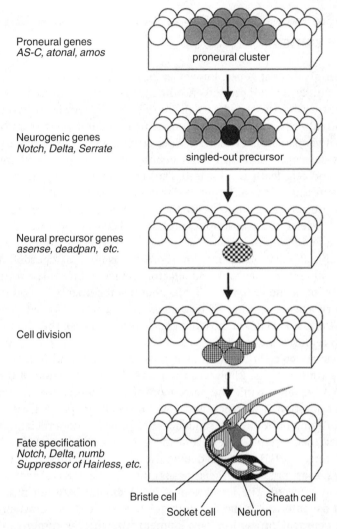

Proneural genes
AS-C, atonal, amos

proneural cluster

Neurogenic genes
Notch, Delta, Serrate

singled-out precursor

Neural precursor genes
asense, deadpan, etc.

Cell division

Fate specification
Notch, Delta, numb
Suppressor of Hairless, etc.

Bristle cell   Sheath cell
Socket cell   Neuron

Figure 4.2 Progressive specification of external sensory organ fate in *Drosophila*. Proneural gene expression in the ectoderm defines a cluster of cells with the potential to form a sense organ. Individual cells within the cluster compete with each other through Delta–Notch interaction such that one cell is singled out to express proneural genes at high level, while the others become epidermal. The singled-out precursor expresses genes involved in differentiation and identity before going through two rounds of asymmetric division to produce the four component cells of the sense organ. After Anderson and Jan.[1]

Proneural genes

A small cluster of adjacent genes, known as the *Achaete–Scute* complex (*AS-C*) are key members of a family of bHLH protein-encoding genes that are referred to as proneural genes because they are associated with the initial steps in neurogenesis during which naive ectodermal cells acquire the potential to be neural precursors.[3,4] They are generally positive regulators of cell fate. Flies lacking AS-C lack ES organs. They also have a poorly developed CNS with fewer neuroblasts; these proliferate more slowly than normal and cell death is increased. During normal development the regional domains of expression of the different *AS-C* transcripts overlap, and the *AS-C* genes are suggested to provide neuroblasts with their specific identities on the basis of a combinatorial code of *AS-C* transcript expression. *AS-C* genes operate in concert with two other proneural genes, *atonal*[5,6] and *amos*,[7,8] to specify the entire peripheral nervous system. *atonal* is necessary for the development of chordotonal organs, whereas *amos* (absent md neurons and olfactory sensilla) directs the formation of a minor component of the PNS, the solo-MD neurons, together with two specific sub-sets of olfactory sensilla (specialized ES organs). Loss of both *AS-C* and *atonal* function removes most of the PNS (ES organs and chordotonal organs); the additional loss of *amos* function removes the rest.

Proneural genes typically function as heterodimers and bind to a common DNA sequence of six nucleotides, known as the E-box. The basic region of the molecule binds this DNA sequence while the helix–loop–helix region is involved in dimerization.[9] A major question is whether, and how, they deliver specificity in target gene regulation. Differing DNA binding sequences are probably not crucial; rather, it has been suggested that specific protein cofactors are involved. One of these is the ubiquitously expressed bHLH protein, daughterless, which is required for the development of all sensory organs;[10] in *daughterless* mutants, the PNS is absent, and the CNS is also partially affected. The formation of heterodimers between proneural gene products and daughterless is thought to regulate specific target downstream genes that initiate neuronal progenitor development,[9,11] whereas dimerization of proneural gene products with negative regulatory HLH proteins, such as extra-macrochaetae and hairy,[12] prevents their binding to DNA.

The expression of proneural genes in discrete domains of the ectoderm appears to be directed by a large number of regulatory elements in the complex, which are assumed to respond to the products of prepatterning genes that are expressed either alone or in combination in different regions of the embryo. Prepatterning genes for the CNS expression of proneural genes include the pair rule and segment polarity genes that set up a general system of positional information in the embryo.[13] Prepatterning genes that direct the expression of proneural genes in the peripheral sensory system include *lozenge* (which prepatterns *amos* expression),[8] the segment polarity gene *wingless* (*wg*)[14] and genes of the *iroquois* complex (*IRO-C*),[15,16] which are themselves expressed in response to more global signals such as *decapentaplegic*. The activity of *wg* and *IRO-C* genes is required for different subsets of bristles on the back of the fly.

The establishment of a number of proneural regions, each in the position of a presumptive sense organ and each containing a cluster of cells that have the potential for neurogenesis, is followed by a competitive process within each cluster that results in the emergence of only one of these cells as the SOP cell responsible for producing all cells of the ES organ. This competition involves the neurogenic genes, whose action enhances the expression of proneural genes in one cell and suppresses their action in the others.

Neurogenic genes

The hallmark of the *Drosophila* neurogenic genes is that their loss-of-function causes presumptive epidermoblasts in the neuroectoderm to become neuroblasts instead. As a consequence, some four times as many neuroectoderm cells initiate neurogenesis, causing massive hyperplasia of the CNS, increased numbers of sensory neurons, deficient epidermis and embryo lethality. The first neurogenic locus (*Notch*) was discovered in the 1930s, since when several more have been identified, in particular *master mind* (*mam*), *big brain* (*bib*), *neuralized* (*neu*), *Delta* (*Dl*), *Serrate* (*Ser*) and *Enhancer of split* (*E(spl)*).[17-19] It is now recognized that Notch signalling is also involved in mediating cell fate decisions outside the nervous system.[20] Transplanting single neuro-ectodermal cells from the neurogenic mutants into the neuroectoderm of wild-type flies has addressed whether or not the mutations are cell-autonomous, and result in abnormal reception by the mutant cell of epidermalizing environmental signals.[21] It turns out that *Notch*, *mam*, *bib*, *neu* and *Dl* are not cell-autonomous, for mutant cells develop normally when surrounded by wild-type cells, and the interpretation is therefore that the mutant cells have normal receptor mechanisms but transmit abnormal signals to their neighbours. In contrast, *E(Spl)* is cell-autonomous; mutant cells develop only neural clones after transplantation into a wild-type background, suggesting that here the mutant cells cannot read the epidermalizing signal.

Since the phenotypes caused by the mutant neurogenic genes are similar, it can be anticipated that their products interact functionally in the specification of neural versus epidermal phenotype, and this is indeed the case. With the exception of *bib*, all the neurogenic loci operate within the same developmental pathway, with *E(Spl)* forming the last link in the chain, although less is known about how their products interact at the molecular level. The *Notch* product is a large transmembrane protein containing 36 extracellular EGF-like repeats, consistent with a role in the direct mediation of cell–cell interactions, and it is homologous to the product of the *lin-12* gene of *C. elegans* which controls several cell fate decisions during nematode development.[22,23] Its extracellular domain acts as a receptor for Delta or Serrate on neighbouring cells, while proteolytic cleavage[24,25] of its intracellular domain (known as NICD) allows the latter to bind and translocate a cytoplasmic DNA-binding protein,

A

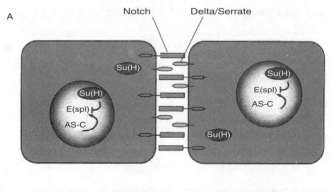

Notch   Delta/Serrate

B

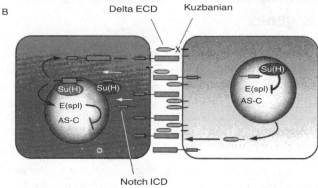

Delta ECD   Kuzbanian

Notch ICD

C

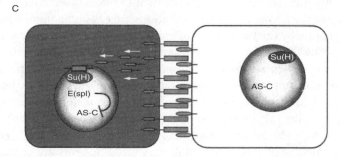

Figure 4.3 Lateral inhibition in the specification of a neuronal precursor (*right*) and an epidermal precursor (*left*) from two cells which are equivalent, other than a slight imbalance between them of *Delta* (or *Serrate*) expression. *Delta* expression is positively regulated by *Achaete–Scute* complex (*AS-C*) genes. Notch activation induces *Notch* and represses *AS-C* and *Delta* whereas lack of Notch activation allows *AS-C* and *Delta* expression to continue. This feedback amplifies the initial imbalance until the right cell expresses *AS-C* and *Delta* at high level while the left cell expresses *Notch* at high level and *AS-C* is repressed. Repression is mediated by the intracellular domain (ICD) of Notch which is released upon activation by Delta and transports Suppressor of Hairless (Su(H)) to the nucleus. Activation of negative regulators of fate (e.g. *Enhancer of Split, E(spl)*) by Su(H) leads to the repression of *AS-C*. Delta acts either as a membrane-inserted ligand or as a freely diffusible extracellular domain (ECD) released by the action of an enzyme, Kuzbanian. After Kopan and Turner.[23]

Suppressor of Hairless (Su(H)), to the nucleus.[26] Su(H) transduces the Delta–Notch signal by direct transcriptional activation of the *E(Spl)* complex and other genes that have promoters containing Su(H) binding sites (Fig. 4.3).[27] Proteins encoded by the *E(Spl)* complex, together with the products of *Hairy* and *Extramacrochaetae*, are negative regulators of neurogenesis that, in some cases, function by heterodimerizing with AS-C proteins and prevent their binding DNA.

The *Delta* locus is complex, and the transcript sequences indicate another trans-membrane protein with extracellular EGF repeats. *Delta* is initially expressed throughout the neurogenic regions of the embryo, but then becomes restricted to the cells that proceed to a neural fate. The *E(Spl)* locus (so-called because the mutation enhances the phenotype of the *Notch* allele *split*) is a member of a larger complex, and encodes at least 11 major transcripts that are all expressed during neurogenesis; some of these become restricted to the epidermal lineage in a manner complementary to the neurally-fated expression of *Delta*, and several of the encoded proteins probably act as transcriptional regulators within the cell.[19]

The neurogenic gene *kuzbanian* encodes a transmembrane metalloprotease which is thought to cleave Delta from the cell surface, which may be necessary for Notch activation (the phenotype of *Kuz* mutants is similar to those associated with loss of Notch signalling).[28] The production of soluble Delta may also allow Notch signalling to occur independently of cell contact. Other extracellular modulators of Notch signalling include Fringe,[29] whose activity enhances Notch activation by Delta but inhibits its activation by Serrate, a process that has been implicated in the formation of regional boundaries.

Sensory cell lineages

Once they have been determined by the sequential action of proneural and neurogenic genes, neural precursor cells adopt a distinctive mitotic behaviour and give rise to stereotyped lineages whose nature and specific cell progeny depend on position in the embryo. At least eight different types of lineage have been described in the nervous system of the fly, the simplest and best understood of which is that of the SOP cell of the ES organ (Fig. 4.4).[1,30] The first division of the SOP generates two secondary precursor cells (pIIa and pIIb), each of which divides again to produce four terminally differentiated cells: pIIa produces two non-neural cells, the bristle and its socket cell, whereas pIIb produces two neural cells, a sensory neuron and its sheath (glial) cell. Because all four daughter cells have a different fate, these divisions are known as asymmetric. SOP cells, as well as the neuroblasts of the presumptive CNS, are selected from the proneural region through expression of the proneural genes, and are then singled out from their neighbours by Notch signalling. The study of temperature-sensitive mutants of *Notch* and *Delta* has shown that *Notch–Delta* signalling continues to be important for generating the asymmetric divisions of the SOP cell.[31,32] Reducing *Notch* function after the period of neuroblast segregation, for example, affects the first SOP cell division, transforming pIIa to pIIb and generating two neurons and

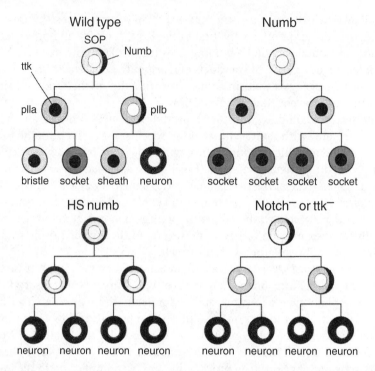

Figure 4.4 Cell fate in the external sensory organ precursor lineage of wild-type and various mutant flies. In wild-type animals, the neuronal determinant Numb is segregated to one pole of the dividing SOP cell such that it is inherited by one daughter of the asymmetric division (pIIb) but not the other (pIIa). Numb is later re-expressed in pIIb and again segregated to one daughter of the second asymmetric division, which becomes the neuron. The other three cells become supporting cells. Numb is required to suppress Notch so that in *numb* mutants all four grand-daughters become socket cells, whereas the overexpression of numb using a heat shock promoter (HS numb) allows all of them to become neurons. The same happens in *Notch* mutants and mutants for *tramtrack*, a neuronal fate-suppressing zinc-finger gene positively regulated by Notch. The presence of tramtrack in the nucleus is shown in black in the wild-type and *numb*⁻ situations.

two sheath cells; if the temperature shift also affects the pIIb progeny, the result is a further transformation of sheath cell to neuron, with the net outcome of four neurons.

It is clear that the asymmetry between sibling cells in the SOP lineage involves the asymmetric distribution of cytoplasmic determinants, rather than an inductive interaction with neighbouring cells. During most of the cell divisions in the *Drosophila* ectoderm prior to neurogenesis, the mitotic spindles are oriented parallel to the surface, but in the precursor cells of the CNS and PNS the spindles are oriented perpendicular to the surface, a reorientation that correlates with the asymmetric segregation of the product of the *numb* gene.[33] Immunocytochemical experiments have shown that Numb protein is associated with the cytoplasmic side of the cell membrane and is localized in a crescent in the SOP cell.[33,34] During the first division of the SOP cell, the numb crescent is preferentially distributed to pIIb, where its presence is likely to confer a pIIb fate. Indeed, in *numb* loss-of-function mutants, the SOP cell divides into two pIIa cells, transforming the neuron and sheath cell into a bristle cell and socket cell, giving a PNS phenotype that is a mirror image of the *Notch* phenotype (Fig. 4.4). Following the first division, Numb is re-expressed in the pIIb cell and becomes asymmetrically localized such that it is preferentially distributed to the prospective neuron. Consistent with Numb function being to assign neural fate, forced expression of *numb* in the pIIa cell transforms it to a pIIb fate,[33] with the ultimate production of four neurons. Although the mechanism whereby Numb protein becomes localized is unclear, it appears to determine the fate of the cell in which it becomes localized.

With the exception of the eye (see Chapter 8), the asymmetric segregation of Numb appears to be an important feature of cell fate determination throughout the developing PNS and CNS, and its deployment must interact in some way with the *Notch–Delta* signalling pathway. In a determinate lineage such as that of the ES organ, where a cell's parentage plays an important role in specifying its fate, it is possible that the inheritance of Numb protein is used to bias the lateral-inhibitory competition towards a predictable rather than a stochastic outcome. For example, if Numb suppresses the function of Notch, the cell that receives Numb from the parent will produce more Delta, so increasing its ability to inhibit its sibling. Consistent with this, *Notch* has been shown to act downstream of *numb*; in *Notch–numb* double mutants, the phenotype resembles the *Notch* mutant phenotype, and there is also evidence for a direct interaction between Notch and Numb protein, suggesting that Numb binds to and inactivates the intracellular domain of the Notch protein, precluding the nuclear translocation of the *Su(H)* product.[35-37] Notch signalling, due to absence of Numb, results in expression of the *tramtrack* gene (*ttk*) in pIIa but not pIIb and, at the second division of pIIb, in the sheath cell but not the neuron (Fig. 4.5). The *ttk* product is thus assumed to be an effector of the asymmetry produced by the Notch–Numb system in terms of realizing the four different cell fates.[38]

The SOP lineage is apparently neuronal by default: in both of the successive divisions of the SOP cell, one daughter of each pair adopts the default state, whereas the other is driven by Notch signalling and ttk activity to a new fate. The default state of

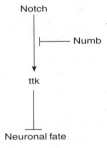

Figure 4.5 The inheritance of Numb by the daughter cell of a division assigns neuronal fate by blocking the Notch pathway. Notch is prevented from activating its downstream targets, such as *tramtrack* (*ttk*), which act as suppressers of neuronal fate.

the first division is the pIIb cell, which retains neuronal potential, whereas the pIIa cell is driven by ttk and proneural repression to an alternate, non-neural fate. In the subsequent pIIb division, the neuron is the default fate and the sheath cell is the alternate fate. This neuronal-by-default view is supported by the observation that the SOP turns directly into a neuron when it is prevented from dividing.[39]

Asymmetric divisions and cell polarity during CNS neurogenesis

A similar interaction between *Notch* and *numb* has been identified in one of the smaller lineages in the developing fly CNS, where one neuroblast (e.g. MP2) divides asymmetrically to produce two daughter neurons (vMP2 and dMP2), without an intermediate ganglion mother cell (GMC) stage.[37] During this cell division, Numb protein is selectively distributed to the dMP2 cell, where it suppresses Notch and leads to the dMP2 phenotype. In *numb* mutants, dMP2 is transformed into a second vMP2 whereas when numb is driven ectopically in vMP2 it is transformed into a second dMP2. In this example it also appears that the Delta-mediated signalling generating the vMP2 phenotype is derived not from vMP2 and dMP2 themselves, as in the SOP model outlined above, but from neighbouring cells in the mesoderm and neuroectoderm (Fig. 4.6). Although all neuroblasts in the fly CNS partition Numb asymmetrically into their progeny GMC, it is not clear whether an asymmetric segregation of Numb contributes to the difference between neuroblasts and their GMCs.

Neurogenesis is of course likely to involve multiple molecular interactions, and a variety of other contributing genes have been identified in *Drosophila*. A further example of an intrinsic factor that is distributed asymmetrically during lineage divisions in the CNS is Prospero, a homeodomain protein required for normal ganglion mother cell development.[40] Neuroblasts synthesize Prospero protein but retain it cytoplasmically before partitioning it into their daughter GMCs, where it enters the nucleus and functions as a transcription factor. The asymmetric distribution of both Numb and Prospero into GMCs is preceded by their asymmetric localization to a crescent-shaped domain of the basal cortex of the neuroblast where the GMC will bud off (Fig. 4.7). Localization of Prospero to the basal side of the neuroblast requires an anchoring protein, Miranda, which also functions to release Prospero for nuclear entry once segregated to a GMC.[41,42] Localization of Numb in both neuroblasts and SOPs involves its binding with another protein, Partner of Numb (Pon).[43]

Operating upstream of *numb* and *prospero* is the product of *inscuteable*, which is involved in the elaboration of a perpendicularly oriented mitotic spindle in neuroblasts, and which is therefore necessary for normal asymmetric cytoplasmic localization of both Numb and Prospero.[44] Inscuteable is responsible for coordinating the axis of asymmetric localization of cytoplasmic determinants with the axis of segregation of these determinants to the GMC (Fig. 4.7). In the absence of Inscuteable, mitotic spindles and basal crescents are randomly oriented both to the apical–basal axis of the epithelium and with respect to each other. The localization of Inscuteable

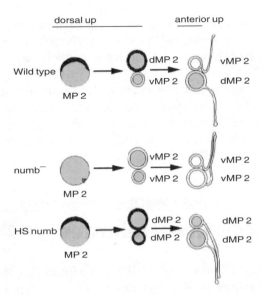

Figure 4.6 Numb and Notch involvement in specifying the fate of sibling neurons in the CNS of *Drosophila*. In wild-type flies, the MP2 neuroblast produces two neurons directly, without an intervening ganglion mother cell stage. Numb is distributed asymmetrically to the dorsal daughter (dMP2) where it antagonizes the Notch signal but allows the ventral daughter (vMP2) to receive it. The bias in Notch signalling leads to distinct cell fates characterized by axonal trajectory—posterior in dMP2 and anterior in vMP2. In *numb⁻* mutants both cells adopt the vMP2 phenotype whereas both adopt the dMP2 phenotype when *numb* is overexpressed by heat shock. After Spana and Doe.[37]

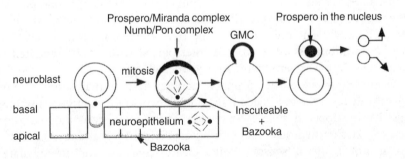

Figure 4.7 Asymmetric localization of cell fate determinants in fly CNS development. Bazooka is localized to the apical cortex of epithelial cells and during neuroblast delamination recruits newly expressed Inscuteable apically. Inscuteable then coordinates the change of spindle orientation with the localization of Prospero and Numb, together with their anchoring proteins, Miranda and Pon, to the basal cortex where they segregate into the daughter ganglion mother cell (GMC). Soon after division, Prospero moves in the nucleus where it acts as a transcription factor influencing cell fate selection by the daughter neurons. After Matsuzaki.[119]

to the apical pole of delaminating neuroblasts has been found to depend not only on specific domains of the protein, which also confer the ability to orient the spindle,[45] but also on the presence at the apical pole (of all epithelial cells) of the PDZ domain protein, Bazooka.[46,47]

bHLH gene expression, a crucial event in initiating neurogenesis, is not confined to the early stages when the proneural genes are activated; rather, a cascade of bHLH proteins ensues during lineage divisions, with genes such as *asense* and *deadpan* becoming expressed in cells as they realize their neural potential and finally differentiate into neurons.[48,49]

Neurogenesis in vertebrates

Neurogenesis in vertebrates bears interesting comparison with the process in the fly. In both cases the neurectodermal cells appear to express a primary neural fate. In vertebrates, this tendency is reinforced by further neuralizing signals (e.g. noggin, chordin, follistatin, see Chapter 2) that antagonize signals that would otherwise direct the cells away from a neural fate. In flies, neuralization is primarily determined by the strength of a cell's ability to epidermalize its neighbours and so reinforce its own neuralization. The identification of vertebrate homologues of *AS-C* and other proneural genes, *Notch*, *Delta* and *numb*, also suggests that the details of phenotype determination in the vertebrate CNS may turn out to be fundamentally similar, despite superficial differences.

In vertebrates, sensory and autonomic neurons arise in the periphery from the migratory neural crest or, in the specific cases of cranial sensory neurons, olfactory neurons, and the sensory epithelia of the inner ear, from ectodermal placodes (see Chapter 5). The principal location of neurogenesis in vertebrate embryos, however, is the epithelium of the neural plate and tube. Here, the first neurons arise in a number of distinct locations as scattered cells interspersed with undifferentiated neuroepithelial cells. In lower vertebrates such as the zebrafish and *Xenopus*, the first neurons form part of an entire 'primary' nervous system that forms rapidly with comparatively few cells to provide functional networks for the free-swimming larva, a stage that is skipped in higher vertebrates. In the spinal cord region of the neural plate/tube, the first neurons develop in three distinct longitudinal domains, medial (motor neurons), lateral (sensory (Rohon–Beard) neurons), and intermediate (interneurons) (Fig. 4.8). Although an analogy can be drawn between each of the three domains of initial neurogenesis in lower vertebrates and a *Drosophila* proneural cluster, there is a significant difference: in vertebrate embryos all cells of the neural plate are allocated to a solely neural fate. The subsequent singling-out of cells may involve decisions such as to become neuronal versus glial (or neuronal now versus neuronal later) but becoming epidermal is no longer an option. Thus, in vertebrates, proneural and neurogenic genes act within a context of already established neural (but not necessarily neuronal) fate. An attendant difference is that whereas flies form

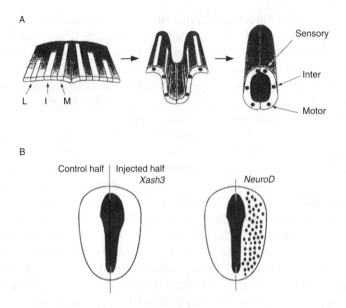

Figure 4.8 (A) Three longitudinal stripes of *Xash3* neural determination gene expression in the *Xenopus* neural plate presage zones of primary neurogenesis (M, medial; I, intermediate; L, lateral) where columns of motor neurons, interneurons and sensory neurons, respectively, develop in the neural tube. The repressor *Zic2* is expressed in between the three zones of neurons. (B) Ectopic overexpression of *Xash3* results in expansion of the neural plate at the expense of epidermis, whereas overexpression of neuronal differentiation gene *NeuroD* results in the ectopic differentiation of neurons from epidermal precursors. After Anderson and Jan.[1]

their CNS by polyinvagination of single neuroblasts from the surface epidermis, the vertebrate neural plate invaginates as a whole, segregating from flanking epidermis by molecular interactions (see below) and the morphogenetic movements of neurulation.

bHLH genes

In addition to their crucial role in development of the *Drosophila* nervous system, bHLH transcription factors have been shown to be important regulators of the vertebrate myogenic lineage. Subsequently, several vertebrate homologues of both *AS-C* and *atonal* have been cloned, and some of these have been shown to have proneural characteristics, as determination factors in neurogenesis.[1,50] These include *Xash* and *Mash* (*Xenopus* and mouse *Achaete–Scute* homologues), *Math* (mouse *atonal* homologue), and the *neurogenin* family (relatives of *atonal*). Later expressed bHLH genes include *NeuroD* (a more distant relative of *atonal*) which has the characteristics of a differentiation factor. Negative regulators include *Hes* (a homologue of *Hairy*) and *Id* (a homologue of *Extramacrochaetae*). Although the large size and complexity of the vertebrate nervous system has meant that functional data are difficult to interpret, it appears that cascades of bHLH factors may operate during all stages of neurogenesis, from the commitment of neural precursors through proliferation and migration to terminal differentiation. At each stage, it is presumed that specific bHLH proteins may regulate target genes that are instrumental in reaching the next step. As in the fly, the progression towards a particular fate is expected to be regulated by a balance between positive and negative bHLH and HLH proteins.

Mash1, originally cloned from a neural crest cell line, is expressed in the CNS and PNS and may be involved in both the determination of neural fate and subsequent steps of precursor differentiation. Knockout studies have shown that *Mash1* is required for the early development of olfactory, autonomic and telencephalic neurons.[51,52] Overexpression of its homologue in *Xenopus*, *Xash3*, causes expansion of the neural plate at the expense of epidermis, overproliferation of neural precursor cells and ectopic neuronal differentiation (Fig. 4.8).[53] *Math1* is expressed in the cranial sensory ganglia and the ventricular zone of the dorsal neural tube. Later, it is strongly expressed in the rhombic lip of the hindbrain whose principal derivative is the granule cells that form the external germinal layer (EGL) of the cerebellum. Loss of *Math1* function removes these cells, suggesting that *Math1* is required for production and/or migration of granule cell precursors from the rhombic lips.[54]

The *neurogenins* may have a more general role in vertebrate neurogenesis, in both the CNS and the PNS. Indeed, a number of lines of evidence suggest that neurogenins lie at the start of a core programme of neurogenesis, activating a pathway that leads to the activation of other bHLH factors that are either determinants of neural fate or that promote specialized aspects of neuronal differentiation. In *Xenopus* embryos, expression of the *neurogenin*-related gene *XNGNR1* begins at late gastrulation, ahead of *Delta* expression, and defines the three prospective territories of primary neurogenesis in the neural plate.[55] Overexpression of *XNGNR1* leads to expansion of the domain in which *Delta* is subsequently expressed and the overproduction of primary neurons, which are no longer confined to the three territories.[55]

The final common pathway for many neuronal lineages is the direct regulation by the different *neurogenins* of the later-expressed differentiation regulator *NeuroD*.[50] This is expressed transiently in developing neurons in many regions of the nervous system and expression in the CNS is maintained in fully differentiated neurons. When overexpressed in *Xenopus* embryos, NeuroD is sufficient to convert non-neural ectodermal cells into neurons and to cause premature differentiation of neural precursor cells.[56] Opposing the function of NeuroD and related positive regulators are negative regulators of cell fate, the serine threonine protein kinase $GSK3\beta$[57] and Hes1 and Hes5, which are structurally related to hairy and E(spl). *Hes1* null mutation results in premature neuronal differentiation,[58] a phenotype similar to that produced by *NeuroD* overexpression, whereas the opposite result, failure of neural differentiation, is obtained when *Hes1* expression is maintained in CNS precursors.[59] As expected by analogy with neurogenesis in *Drosophila*, these effects are correlated with changes in the expression of *AS-C* homologues.

NEUROGENESIS IN VERTEBRATES **107**

Neurogenic genes

Homologues of *Notch* and its ligands, *Delta* and *Serrate*, have been cloned from several vertebrate species, together with a third ligand, *Jagged*, which is closely related to *Serrate*. As with the bHLH genes so with the neurogenic genes, our understanding of function in vertebrates is at present rudimentary in comparison with what is known for *Drosophila*. Progress is rapid, however, primarily through overexpression studies by direct injection of mRNA into the two-cell stage *Xenopus* embryo and also through null mutation in mice. Using the former strategy, a conserved function in neurogenesis for Delta and Notch homologues has been shown whereby Delta binds and activates Notch on neighbouring cells, causing the suppression of both proneural gene activity and *Delta* expression. Thus, overexpression of either *Delta1* or a constitutively active form of *Notch1* reduces the number of primary neurons that form at the neural plate stage.[60] Presumably, when all cells are forced to express *Delta1*, they each inhibit each other. Furthermore, feedback to the lateral inhibition system has been shown by the injection of mRNA encoding a form of Notch1 with a truncated extracellular domain, or just the intracellular domain alone.[60] Both of these proteins have a dominant active function and not only block the production of neurons but inhibit the expression of *Delta*. By contrast, the injection of mRNA encoding a mutant form of Delta1 with a truncated intracellular domain results in the overproduction of primary neurons. Truncated Delta presumably acts as a dominant negative protein that would interfere with the normal delivery of lateral inhibition through the resident full-length Delta. The additional neurons formed in this situation are confined to the three zones of the spinal neural plate (medial, lateral and intermediate) where Delta is normally expressed and primary neurons normally formed. This indicates that the regulation of neurogenesis by Delta–Notch signalling operates within the context of pre-existing proneural gene expression, particular that of *neurogenin*.

Control of neurogenesis by Delta–Notch signalling operates not only during primary neurogenesis in frogs but also during the main period of neurogenesis in both lower and higher vertebrates. In the chick embryo spinal cord, for example, *Notch* is expressed by all mitotic cells in the ventricular zone whereas *Delta* expression is confined to a subset of non-dividing cells, presumably young neurons. In the retina of both *Xenopus* and chick embryos, activated forms of Notch inhibit neurogenesis just as with *Xenopus* primary neurons.[61,62] Furthermore, blocking Notch expression in the chick retina with antisense oligonucleotides increases neuron production.[61] A further conserved component in the control of neurogenesis between fly and vertebrate is the downstream targets of Notch signalling, involving the hairy-E(spl) homologues mentioned above.

Regional variation in bHLH gene expression

While the existence of proneural and neurogenic genes in vertebrates and their role in neurogenesis has been well documented, their role in determining cell type selection remains poorly understood. That they might have such a role is suggested by the fact that the bHLH genes and the Notch ligands cloned from vertebrates are expressed in only a subset of regions or lineages of the CNS or PNS, showing that the progress of neurogenesis in any one region or lineage involves patterning decisions made at an earlier stage. As we will see with this brief survey of regional diversity in their expression, the use of diverse 'proneural' and 'neurogenic' genes does also contribute to regional or cell type differentiation, suggesting that neurogenesis be considered as a patterning process in its own right and not simply as a generic programme for making a neuron.

In the PNS, two neurogenin family members have nearly complementary expression between the two principal cell groups contributing the neurons of sensory ganglia: *Ngn1* is expressed in the neural crest-derived proximal cranial ganglia, whereas *Ngn2* is expressed by the ectodermal placode-derived distal cranial ganglia. In both cases, these bHLH genes are required for neurogenesis.[63,64] In the spinal cord, *neurogenin*, *Mash1* and *Math1*, are expressed in complementary and non-overlapping dorsoventral domains of the ventricular zone, as are *Delta* and *Serrate/Jagged*. In the forebrain, dorsal telencephalic cells express *Ngn2* whereas ventral cells express *Mash1*. Loss of Ngn function in the cortex of *Ngn2* mutants and *Ngn1;Ngn2* double mutants allows *Mash1* expression to spread dorsally, showing that *Ngns* are required to repress *Mash1* in the cortex. Furthermore, in both these *Ngn* knockout animals and knock-in mutants carrying *Mash1* in the *Ngn2* locus, cortical cells express ventral markers such as *Dlx*.[65] This demonstrates that genes with an ascribed function in neuronal determination can act in the acquisition of neuronal identity, transferring patterning information from upstream regionalization genes. Potential regulators of *Ngn2* and *Mash1* expression are *Pax6* and *Gsh2*,[66] which are expressed in dorsal and ventral regions of the early telencephalon, respectively.

Activation of neurogenic programmes by neural induction

The suppression of BMP signalling in *Xenopus* embryos by antagonists such as noggin and chordin leads to the upregulation of genes that drive cells towards a neural fate; in some cases such genes form a molecular link between neural induction and proneural gene expression and are instrumental in the acquisition of neural (as compared with epidermal) fate. Differential screens designed to detect genes that are upregulated by chordin or noggin in *Xenopus* animal caps have isolated a number of candidates. These include members of the *Sox* family of HMG box transcriptional regulators, whose products are thought to endow competence by bending the DNA on which they bind, thereby opening specific regions for transcription. *SoxD* is the earliest of these genes to be expressed in *Xenopus*, with transcripts being already widely distributed at the blastula stage. This early, widespread expression suggests a role in conferring the neural-default state of the uninduced dorsal ectoderm.[67] *SoxD* expression increases and becomes progressively restricted as the events of gastrulation define the neural plate. Forced expression of *SoxD* in animal cap ectoderm promotes the expression of *neurogenin* and neural differentiation of anterior character, whereas expression of a dominant negative form, lacking the HMG box, blocks neuralization and suppresses the differentiation of anterior neural tissue in injected embryos. Another competence-endowing gene, *Sox2*, is expressed later in the neural plate but does not have the independent neuralizing activity seen for *SoxD*.

The anteriorly expressed winged helix transcription factor BF-1, one of the earliest markers of telencephalic development whose ablation in mice leads to the specific loss of telencephalic tissue,[68] appears to play a dual role in positioning rostral neurogenesis in *Xenopus* embryos. Misexpression at high levels suppresses neuronal differentiation in the expressing cells but induces neurogenesis in adjacent cells, whereas lower level expression causes expansion of the neural domain.[69]

Also activated by neural inducers and playing a role in neural specification are members of the *Iroquois* and *Zic* gene families. The *Drosophila iroquois* relative, *Xiro3*, promotes the expression of the proneural gene *Xash-3* in *Xenopus* embryos[70] and may function in defining the neural plate as distinct from the neural crest,[71] with whose differentiation several of the *Zic* family of zinc-finger genes are also associated.[72,73] While some of the *Zic* genes positively regulate neurogenins, the effect of *Zic2* appears to be the opposite. It is expressed in longitudinal domains of the neural plate that are complementary to the three stripes where neurogenesis is initiated.[73] Since Zic2 is thought to have a repressor activity on more widely expressed neuralizing genes, its expression is consistent with restricting neurogenesis to these three stripes.

Integration of neurogenic programmes with patterning mechanisms

A major, but comparatively little understood, issue is how neurogenic programmes might be integrated with patterning mechanisms such that distinct neuronal cell types develop at different positions in the neural epithelium. The generation of three neurogenic domains in the lower vertebrate spinal cord, referred to above, provides a promising system for the analysis of how dorsoventral patterning mechanisms lead to the expression of positive and negative neurogenic regulators. Here again, studies on *Drosophila* have provided clues. In the fly CNS, the early production of neuroblasts is also in three longitudinal columns, whose positioning depends on the expression of three homeobox genes, *vnd* (*ventral neural defective*), *ind* (*intermediate neural defective*), and *msh* (*muscle segment homeobox*).[74,75] Expression of these genes in parallel stripes in the neurectoderm (Fig. 4.9) depends on *vnd* repressing *ind* in the ventral column, and *ind* repressing *msh* in the intermediate column. In vertebrate neural plate, the homologues of these genes (*Nkx2.2*, *Gsh1* and *Msx*, respectively) are also expressed in three discrete parallel stripes, corresponding with later neurogenin expression.[76] At this point, we have only the intriguing parallel in the positioning of these genes, and know little about their precise role and regulation in vertebrates, although it is clear that expression of the most dorsal gene, *Nkx2.2*, is positionally regulated by SHH.[77] At

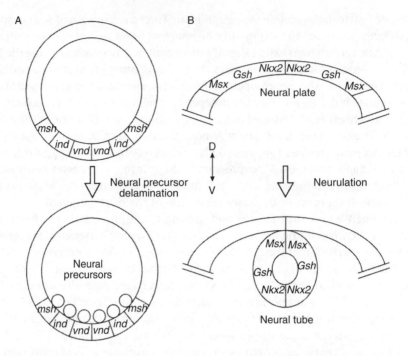

Figure 4.9 Comparison of neurogenic domains in the embryo of *Drosophila* (A) and the spinal cord region of lower vertebrate embryos (B). In both organisms neurons are produced in three longitudinal columns that are marked by the expression of homologous genes. In *Drosophila*, neuroblasts delaminate directly from the neurectoderm, whereas in vertebrates the entire neural plate invaginates before or during initial neurogenesis, thereby inverting the original ventral–dorsal polarity of the neurectoderm. After Chan and Jan,[120], from Weiss *et al.*[75]

this point, it should be recalled that the ventralmost region of the neural tube starts out as the dorsalmost region of the neural plate (Fig. 4.9) and that the vertebrate body axis as a whole is dorsoventrally inverted relative to that of the fly (see Chapter 1).

Role of cell proliferation in the determination of fate

Studies of cell proliferation in the neural tube, using labelling of S-phase cells by tritiated thymidine labelling or BrdU, have allowed a number of broad conclusions to be drawn about the patterns of cell proliferation, migration and assembly in the developing nervous system. First, phylogenetically older neurons, and brain regions, tend to appear early in development, as do the largest neurons in any particular region. The pyramidal neurons for example, are among the first cerebral cortical neurons to become postmitotic, and this could be related to the need for their growth cones to navigate to remote target sites while the distances in the embryo are still small. Second, in regions of grey matter where cells are stacked in superimposed layers, such as the cortex and the optic tectum, these layers are usually laid down by a continuous, ordered migration of postmitotic cells in a ventricular-to-pial ('inside-out') direction; the granular layers of the hippocampal dentate gyrus and cerebellar cortex do, however, provide exceptions to this rule (see Chapter 7). In non-laminated regions, by contrast, such as the aggregated nuclei of the thalamus and hypothalamus, cells assemble in an 'outside-in' sequence. For any particular region of the nervous system, whether developing inside-out or outside-in, mechanisms must exist that determine the size of its mature cell population, and these are likely to involve controls on the extent of precursor cell proliferation and differentiation, as well as the regulation of cell death. The control and function of cell death is discussed in Chapter 13, while the control of cell proliferation will be considered here.

The cell cycle

Cell division is controlled by an elaborate network of molecular interactions that regulate particular phases of the cell cycle, and the cycle shows both an intrinsic, autonomous drive and a susceptibility to external molecular signals derived from the local cell environment. Many of the details have been worked out in recent years from studies of yeast genetics and tumour biology, and a full discussion is beyond the scope of this book. Overall, the cycle is regulated by the timed modification of protein structure resulting from phosphorylation/dephosphorylation and ubiquitin-mediated protein degradation. The key regulatory interactions of the cycle are, of course, likely to hold for all cells, including the progenitors of differentiated neurons and glia, but the individual molecular components operating at particular regions and times during vertebrate CNS development remain largely unresolved.

It is likely that there are stage- and region-specific variations in cell-cycle control during neural development. Cell-cycle regulation may be important in shaping early CNS morphogenesis, as suggested by the study of single neural lineages in the zebrafish. During gastrulation, cells in single clones tend to divide synchronously, orienting their divisions, intercalations and movements in the same way at particular cell cycles. As a result, an individual neural lineage becomes aligned into a single discontinuous string of cells along the early neural tube.[78] A further division then converts this clonal string into a bilateral pair of strings straddling the midline, each contributing a part of the wall of the neural tube. Whether such cell cycle-specific morphogenesis involves cell-autonomous mechanisms, such as counting cell cycles, is at present uncertain. Regional differences in proliferation rate probably contribute to the complex folding of the neural tube as development proceeds (see Chapter 1) and could also influence the relative sizes of different populations of cells in the developing CNS, for example generating more neurons in striate versus extrastriate cerebral cortex.[79] For any particular area, however, the final cell numbers are determined by the interplay between cell proliferation and cell death (see Chapter 13).

A number of cell cycle components that may be involved in the regulation of region-specific CNS development have been identified. These include the retinoblastoma protein, pRb, which inhibits progression of the cycle through G1–S; pRb knockout mice show regional defects in neurogenesis, particularly in the hindbrain.[80] As a further example, the D2-cyclin, also involved in regulating the G1–S transition, is expressed in cells of the proliferating external granular layer of the cerebellum after migration of their precursors from the rhombic lip (Chapter 7) but not at earlier stages, suggesting that this particular cyclin participates in the final stages of granule cell differentiation.[81] For the vertebrate nervous system it seems generally to be the case that cell fates are determined around the stage of the final mitosis, as will be seen below for motor neurons (see also Chapter 7 for cortex). An interesting exception is the chick hindbrain, where neuronal fate appears to be decided in precursors, several rounds of division before the last.[82] As a consequence, a single precursor produces a clone of, for example, eight identical neurons.

Precisely how cell-cycle regulators interact with those of cell fate remains unclear.[83] Examples have been identified in *C. elegans* where exit from the uncommitted stem cell state and initiation of differentiation are controlled independently, both by loss of repression of differentiation-inducing genes and by activation of transcriptional regulators that promote differentiation along particular lineage pathways, but it is unclear whether this is also the case in mammals.[84] The study of genes such as the vertebrate homologues of *notch* and *delta*, which may maintain presumptive neural cells in an undifferentiated state, and those such as *NeuroD* and *neurogenin*, that read out that differentiation, will be important areas for future research.

As might be predicted, both cell-autonomous and environmental factors appear to influence the decision of neural cells to divide or to exit the cell cycle and differentiate, and a variety of studies have revealed the importance of cell interactions in the control of cell proliferation. For example, addition of glial membrane fractions to cultured mouse cerebellar granule progenitor cells blocks their proliferation and the glia-derived *anachronism* product inhibits proliferation[85] of neighbouring neuroblasts in *Drosophila*.[86] The neurotransmitters GABA and glutamate have also been implicated as anti-mitogens in the control of cortical neurogenesis.[87] Many different mitogenic factors have been identified that may drive division of neural progenitor cells during development, including a variety of growth factors such as FGFs,[88] PDGF and insulin-related growth factors,[89] as well as WNT1, whose ectopic expression in the mouse spinal cord substantially increases the number of proliferating cells in the ventricular zone,[90] and SHH.[91] In some cases the ability to manipulate the expression of these molecules in transgenic mice has been critical in defining their functions *in vivo* (see Chapter 6), while the *in vitro* approach has also been useful for examining their role in the parallel process of cell differentiation. For further discussion of the relationship between cell cycle and cell fate, the reader is referred to a recent review by Ohnuma *et al.* (see General Reading at the end of this chapter).

Asymmetrical cell division

An asymmetric division is one where those constituents of the mother cell that are able to affect cell fate are unequally distributed between the two daughter cells. There is substantial descriptive evidence for asymmetrical division in the vertebrate neuro-epithelium, where a mother cell produces one daughter that immediately differentiates as a neuron and one that goes on to divide again (Fig. 4.10). Where this pattern occurs repeatedly the dividing cell can be described as a self-renewing stem cell.

The mammalian cerebral cortex provides the best-known example of asymmetrical cell division in the vertebrate CNS. Here, early cell divisions are symmetrical and multiplicative, resulting in an increased number of cells in the ventricular zone. As neurogenesis commences, there is a gradual shift towards asymmetrical, stem cell-like divisions, in which one of the daughters stays in the ventricular zone and the other leaves. The change in mode of division is thought to involve a change in cleavage plane orientation from vertical (perpendicular to the plane of the ventricular cell layer) in symmetrical division to horizontal (parallel to the cell plane) in asymmetrical division, as for fly neuroblasts. Although stereotyped lineages have been described for mouse cortical ventricular zone cells *in vitro*[92] there is little evidence to

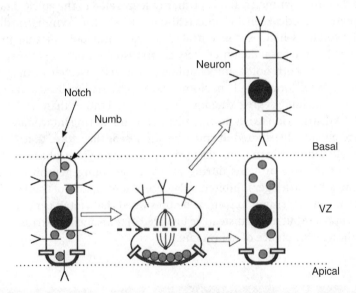

Figure 4.10 Numb and Notch involvement in asymmetric divisions during mammalian cortical neurogenesis. Both proteins are distributed during interphase but become localized to opposite poles as a ventricular zone (VZ) precursor enters division. If the cleavage plane is perpendicular to the apical surface and the division symmetrical, both daughters inherit both proteins (not shown). When the cleavage plane is parallel, as shown here, and the division asymmetrical, the basal daughter which migrates radially and becomes a neuron appears to inherit Notch whereas the apical daughter, which stays in the VZ and may divide again, inherits Numb. After Huttner and Brand.[93]

suggest that the successive divisions within such lineages generate different kinds of neuron in any predictable way. Stereotyped programmes of cell division suggest, but are not themselves evidence for, intrinsic determination of daughter cell fate. It is equally possible that the succession of postmitotic daughters thrown off in a stem cell lineage share a generic neuronal identity and that their ultimate choice of fate awaits a variety of extrinsic cell fate determinants encountered during or after migration out of the ventricular zone.

The change in cleavage plane orientation would presumably result in a corresponding change from equal to unequal subdivision of any cytoplasmic fate determinants whose distribution in the mother cell has an apical–basal polarity.[93] Indeed, mammals have homologues of some of the cytoplasmic determinants of asymmetrical division found in the fly, and these show a polarized distribution in cortical neuro-epithelial cells. These include Notch1 and a mouse homologue of Numb, m-Numb,[94] which is more than 50 per cent homologous to its fly counterpart and can be used to rescue *numb* mutations in *Drosophila*. Also as in fly, m-Numb binds to the cytoplasmic tail of Notch1. A further gene is *numblike*, which is expressed in postmitotic neurons in the cortical plate but not in progenitors in ventricular zone.[95] *m-numb* is expressed by dividing ventricular cells, and its product becomes asymmetrically localized in the apical half of the cell regardless of the orientation of cell cleavage planes. Where cell divisions are symmetrical, m-Numb protein is evenly distributed to the daughter cells, but where they are asymmetrical it is primarily segregated to the apical daughter cell. The asymmetry of cortical cell divisions is also marked by the asymmetric distribution of Notch1 protein, which is concentrated at the basal pole of the dividing cell and segregated to the basal daughter.[96] By comparison with their counterparts in fly neuroblasts, where both notch and Numb are localized together in the prospective ganglion mother cell (or pIIb cell), m-Numb and Notch1 are localized at opposite poles of the cell with m-Numb segregating into the apical cell rather than the basal neuron. However, this distribution exists during mitosis and not during interphase, when both proteins are equally distributed. It must be supposed, therefore, that Notch–Numb binding would inhibit Notch signalling principally during interphase. Following the segregation of the two proteins during mitosis, the young neuron inherits Notch which, because it is no longer inhibited by Numb, is now capable of transducing signals to the nucleus. In this situation it must be presumed that Notch is no longer able to suppress neural fate but might instead be involved in transducing extrinsic signals that influence the specific choice of neural fate.

Development of specific neuronal types in vertebrates

Following neural induction and the expression of genes involved in regionalization and neurogenesis, neural progenitors remain capable of adopting a wide range of specific cell fates. Though multipotent, they are presumably primed to respond to positional signals that regulate specific neural identity genes. The latter would include transcriptional control genes that are involved in the acquisition of a mature neuronal phenotype, including such aspects as choice of neurotransmitter, axonal pathway selection and target connectivity. Our understanding of the mechanisms whereby diverse neuronal types acquire their specific identities is rudimentary. However, substantial progress has been made in respect of developing motor and sympathetic neurons.

The motor neuron

All types of motor neuron share features such as large size of the cell body and its ventral position in the neural tube, cholinergic neurotransmission, and the ability of the growth cone to penetrate the outer limiting membrane of the tube. This peculiarity of their growth behaviour allows motor neuron cell bodies to be cleanly and reliably identified by applying retrograde tracers to their axons in the periphery and has contributed to the intensive study of this neuronal type. Although there is an enormous diversity of motor neuron types, most obviously in terms of their target specificity, three classes are generally recognized: somatic motor neurons, which innervate skeletal muscles; branchiomotor neurons, which innervate muscles developing in the branchial arches; and visceromotor neurons, which innervate postganglionic neurons in the sympathetic chains and parasympathetic ganglia. In all cases, and regardless of peculiarities of their later migration behaviour, motor neurons first appear during development very close to the floor plate, a narrow strip of non-neuronal cells at the ventral midline of the neural tube.

Motor neuron differentiation depends on signals emanating from the floor plate, especially the secreted morphogen Sonic hedgehog (SHH; described in more detail in Chapter 3). As shown by *in vitro* studies of explanted pieces of naive neural tissue, different defined thresholds of concentration of SHH induce multipotent neural progenitors to enter different pathways of differentiation, including that leading to the motor neuron phenotype.[97] *In vivo*, this translates into different responses to a presumed gradient of SHH according to different positions on the dorsoventral axis of the neural tube. In the ventral half of the plate/tube SHH represses *Pax3*, which itself antagonizes the differentiation of motor neurons,[98,99] and induces both *Pax6* and *Nkx2.2* homeobox gene expression.[100] At a precise DV position within this ventral (Pax6[+], neurogenin[+]) domain, proliferating progenitor cells respond to floor plate-derived SHH by expression of the homeobox gene *MNR2* (Fig. 4.11). (The threshold for this response *in vitro* is 2 nM.)[97] Then, as they become postmitotic young neurons, MNR2[+] cells express the LIM-homeobox genes *Isl1* and *Isl2*. MNR2 is seen as a candidate determinant of motor neuronal fate because, when overexpressed in the dorsal neural tube, cells normally fated to become interneurons instead express motor neuron markers such as Isl1, Isl2 and choline acetyl transferase (ChAT, a early expressed marker of cholinergic differentiation) and go on to acquire phenotypic

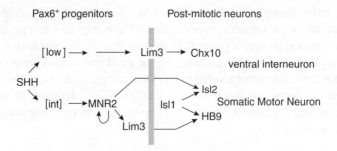

Figure 4.11 Involvement of transcription factors in determining neuronal fate in the higher vertebrate spinal cord. The motor neuron lineage arises from precursors that are induced by relatively high levels of Sonic hedgehog (SHH, int) and express the homeodomain protein MNR2. As they become postmitotic (grey bar) the LIM-homeodomain proteins Isl1 and Lim3 are required for expression of the motor neuron-specific markers, HB9 and Isl2. In the absence of MNR2, at relatively low levels of SHH signalling, Lim3 is sufficient to induce the interneuron marker Chx10. After Tanabe et al.[101]

traits characteristic of differentiated motor neurons, including the extension of axons into the periphery.[101] In addition to positively regulating the expression of Isl1, MNR2 positively regulates its own expression, thereby allowing motor neuron differentiation to proceed independently of SHH availability. The two homeodomain transcription factors appear to work synergistically to promote motor neuron differentiation, as their coexpression in the dorsal neural tube increases the number of ectopic motor neurons over that produced by MNR2 misexpression alone. An essential role for Isl1 is shown by targeted disruption of the *Isl* gene, which results in the early loss of motor neuron precursors through apoptosis.[102] Thus, ventral neural tube cells that have already been committed to a general neural fate by *neurogenin* expression are exposed to an appropriate level of SHH protein by virtue of their precise position relative to the floor plate. They respond to SHH signalling by expressing MNR2 and enter an initial phase of motor neuron development. They then express Isl1, which commits them to motor neuron differentiation or, if they are unable to express Isl1 (as in the case of the Isl1 mutant mouse), they adopt the alternative fate of death.

MNR2 has the ability to override the normal differentiation programme of dorsal neural tube cells, where BMP signalling is thought to influence a variety of interneuron fates, and to suppress the expression of dorsal transcription factors such as Lhx2 and Brn3.0. MNR2 is thus implicated in the choice between interneuron and motor neuron fates. Less clear is whether MNR2 also directs cells into a specific somatic motor neuron pathway, as some evidence suggests, or whether it functions as a more general motor neuron determinant of cells that only later decide whether they are somatic or visceral motor in subtype. An important aspect of neuronal phenotype is the type of transmitter that the cell releases. MNR2 provides an example of an upstream regulator of cholinergic differentiation but whether or not it is a direct regulator of the *ChAT* gene remains unclear.

Although the spinal cord has a superficial uniformity of pattern along the AP axis, with no clear evidence for intrinsic segmentation (as discussed in Chapter 3), distinct

AP variation in cellular composition exists. This is particularly the case for the motor neurons. Those motor neurons that innervate the limbs form expanded populations in the lateral motor columns of the brachial and lumbar cord and are distinct from motor neurons of cervical and thoracic levels—both in their obvious choice of peripheral target and in the expression of different combinations of LIM-homeobox genes.[103] The expression of a specific set of LIM-homeobox genes, a 'LIM code', is believed to confer motor neuron subtype identity, pathfinding behaviour and target specificity (Fig. 4.12). Functional evidence in support of this idea has come from a comparison between motor neurons that have ventral exit points and those (at hindbrain level) that have dorsal exit points.[104] The former express the LIM genes *Lhx3* and *Lhx4* during their final progenitor division, whereas the latter do not. Mice with double knockouts of these genes lack ventrally exiting motor neurons, which appear to be transformed into dorsally exiting types. *Lhx3* ectopically expressed in the caudal hindbrain leads to the formation of ectopic ventrally exiting motor neurons and the absence of dorsally exiting ones, with no change in overall motor neuron number.

At a finer level of pattern, the columnar organization of motor neurons is subdivided into functionally distinct pools of cells, each of which innervates a single muscle in trunk or limb. Individual pools of motor neurons are uniquely marked by the expression of ETS domain transcription factors, as are the sensory neurons that transmit proprioceptive information, in monosynaptic reflex pathways, from the muscle to the motor neurons. The motor and sensory neurons that innervate the same muscle express the same combination of ETS genes. These may thus play a role in specifying neuronal identity at the level of the single unit, and may be instrumental in setting up the precise matching of connectivity within the spinal cord.[105,106]

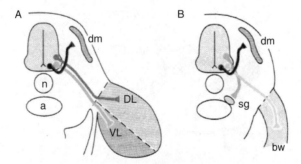

Figure 4.12 Motor neurons that innervate different peripheral targets express different combinations of LIM-homeodomain proteins. At limb levels (A), a specialized lateral motor column differentiates, whose more medially sited neurons express Isl1 and Isl2 and innervate muscles in the ventral limb (VL); more laterally sited neurons in the lateral motor column express Isl2 and Lim1 and innervate muscles in the dorsal limb (DL). At trunk levels (B), where the sympathetic chain (sg) is present, preganglionic motor neurons in the Column of Terni express Isl1, whereas the body wall (bw) is innervated by medial motor column neurons that express Isl1 and Isl2. At all levels of the axis, epaxial muscle derived from the dermomyotome (dm) is innervated by medial motor column neurons that express Isl1, Isl2, Lim3 and Gsh4. n, notochord; a, aorta. After Tsuchida *et al.*[103]

In zebrafish, which form a much smaller number of neurons by comparison with that of amniotes, and in which individual neurons are identifiable, the spinal motor neurons form a continuous column along the AP axis but acquire a consistent segmental arrangement in register with successive myotomes (Fig. 4.13). In each segment, there are three neurons (in rostral, mid and caudal positions relative to the somite) that are identifiable by their axonal trajectory and connectivity with specific regions of the myotome, together with one variable motor neuron that can adopt a different fate in different segments.[107] Single neuron transplantation has shown that the individual identity of these cells remains labile up to a late postmitotic stage in their differentiation and appears to be determined by their position relative to one another and to the paraxial mesoderm. Thus, a prospective middle (MiP) cell transplanted to the caudal (CaP) position 2–3 hours before axonogenesis acquires Cap identity, in respect of LIM homeobox gene expression, trajectory and target domain, but retains MiP identity if transplanted later.[108,109]

Candidate for upstream control of AP variation in motor neuron subtype are the *Hox* genes. Those lying progressively more 5′ in the *Hox* clusters are expressed in progressively more posterior regions of the spinal cord and may confer regional identity on, for example, brachial versus thoracic domains.[110] Transposition of prospective brachial and thoracic regions in chick leads to a change in *Hox* gene coding, a change in LIM-homeobox gene coding, respecification of motor neuron identity, and adoption of columnar organization appropriate to their new positions.[111] A likely source of molecular signal that might confer this positional information is the paraxial mesoderm that flanks the neural tube, known to be a rich source of retinoic acid (RA) and other, yet unidentified, signals. The paraxial mesoderm is also

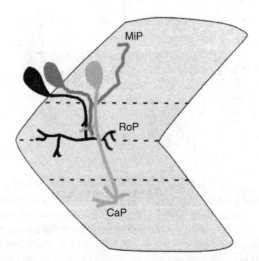

Figure 4.13 Parts of a single spinal segment of a young zebrafish embryo in lateral view. The myotome (*shaded*) is innervated by three primary motor neurons, which have rostral (RoP), mid (MiP) and caudal (CaP) positions in relation to each other. Each of these neurons innervates a distinct territory of a myotome. After Eisen.[107]

implicated in the specification of primary motor neurons in the zebrafish embryo, although the signals that operate in this system are unknown.

Developmental control of neurotransmitter phenotype

Acquiring a specific neuronal phenotype involves the coordinated regulation of a extensive range of molecules, including the axon guidance receptors, recognition molecules and synaptic proteins required for the insertion of a neuron into a functional network, the enzymes responsible for transmitter synthesis, the specific constituents of storage and release vesicles, and the transporter proteins required for reuptake of the transmitter after its release from terminals. An unresolved issue is how differentiating neurons coordinate the expression of the relevant genes, although it appears that cholinergic neurons (including motor neurons) achieve at least a part of this coordination by expressing the synthetic enzyme ChAT and the vesicular acetyl choline transporter under the same *cis*-regulatory elements.[112] On a wider scale, since neurotransmitters and their receptors are expressed before synaptic connections are made, there must also be regulatory mechanisms that coordinate neurotransmitter phenotype with the expression of axon guidance receptors, recognition molecules and synaptic proteins. Beyond this, another requirement is that the neuronal or non-neuronal target cells express receptors that are appropriate for the transmitters expressed by their future synaptic partners.

There are also candidate determinants for other transmitter phenotypes, such as dopaminergic and noradrenergic neurons. For example, the transcription factor Nurr1 is an orphan nuclear receptor protein whose loss through targeted mutation in mice results in the absence of dopamine (DA) synthesis in the substantia nigra and tegmental area of the midbrain, the principal DA expressing regions of the brain.[113,114] However, Nurr1 is neither a necessary nor a sufficient determinant of the entire dopaminergic phenotype because other groups of DA cells survive and express normally in the *Nurr1* mutant mouse and the gene is also expressed in other types of neuron. Similarly, the proneural gene *Mash1* seems to be a major, but not exclusive, determinant of the noradrenergic (NA) phenotype.[115] All central and nearly all peripheral NA neurons of the *Mash1*$^{-/-}$ mouse fail to express the NA-synthesizing enzyme dopamine β-hydroxylase (DBH). Downstream targets regulated by Mash1 include the homeobox genes of the *Phox2* family,[116] which are expressed in all NA neurons at the time of their differentiation and whose protein products bind directly to the regulatory elements in the *DBH* promoter. The principal noradrenergic nucleus of the brain, the locus coeruleus, is absent in *Phox2a*$^{-/-}$ mice.[117] A further example of the control of neurotransmitter phenotype is provided by the switch between noradrenergic and cholinergic transmission that occurs for certain neurons of the sympathetic nervous system; this topic is considered in Chapter 5.

Key points

1 The production of a specific neuronal type in a particular region of the nervous system can be resolved into three major phases, which overlap to a considerable extent—induction (neural vs. non-neural), pattern formation (which type of cell at what position) and neurogenesis (differentiation of the cell). The last phase, production of a neuron which is identifiable by both general type (e.g. motor neuron vs. interneuron) and local subtype (e.g. facial vs. trigeminal motor neuron), is reached by a process in which the potentials of the neuron's antecedents are progressively restricted.

2 Studies of neurogenesis in *Drosophila*, in particular during the development of the external sensory (ES) organ of the PNS, have identified genes and revealed developmental mechanisms that are also used in vertebrate neurogenesis.

3 Prepattern genes establish patches of cells with neural potential by regulating proneural genes, e.g. those of the *Achaete–Scute* complex. Cells in the patch (a proneural cluster) are equivalent to each other but only one will go on to form an ES organ.

4 Selection of the precursor cell involves signalling between adjacent cells, in a process of lateral inhibition. This involves the neurogenic genes, *Delta* and *Notch*.

5 Once singled out, an ES organ precursor expresses genes which direct neural differentiation and undergoes a series of asymmetrical divisions that produce all the cells of the ES organ. The default state of the lineage is neuronal but this fate is suppressed in the non-neural siblings by Notch signalling.

6 Vertebrate homologues of *Drosophila* proneural genes have been shown to play similar roles, as determination factors in neurogenesis, in both the CNS and PNS. Similarly, vertebrate homologues of Notch and its ligands function in lateral inhibitory specification.

7 Neural induction in vertebrates activates neurogenic programmes via, for example, *Sox* and *Zic* genes.

8 Motor neurons provide the best worked-out example of how induction, patterning and neurogenic programmes are integrated to produce an appropriate neuronal type at the appropriate position in the neural tube.

9 Remaining questions include how neuronal migration and axonal navigation behaviours, crucial aspects of a neuron's phenotype, are determined during the acquisition of cell fate.

General reading

■ Anderson, D. J. and Jan, Y. N. The determination of the neuronal phenotype. In *Molecular and cellular approaches to neural development* (ed. W. M. Cowan, T. M. Jessell and S. L. Zipursky), pp. 26–63 (Oxford University Press, New York, 1997).

■ Goridis, C. and Brunet, J.-F. Transcriptional control of neurotransmitter phenotype. *Curr. Opin. Neurobiol.* **9**, 47–53, 1999.

■ Ohnuma, S., Philpott, A. and Harris, W. A. Cell cycle and cell fate in the nervous system. *Curr. Opin. Neurobiol.* **11**, 66–73, 2001.

■ Pfaff, S. and Kintner, C. Neuronal diversification: development of motor neuron subtypes. *Curr. Opin. Neurobiol.* **8**, 27–36, 1998.

■ Tanabe, Y. and Jessell, T. M. Diversity and pattern in the developing spinal cord. *Science* **274**, 1115–23, 1996.

■ Vervoort, M., Dambly-Chaudiere, C. and Ghysen, A. Cell fate determination in *Drosophila. Curr. Opin. Neurobiol.* **7**, 7–12, 1997.

References

1. Anderson, D. J. and Jan, Y. N. The determination of the neuronal phenotype. In *Molecular and cellular approaches to neural development* (ed. W. M. Cowan, T. M. Jessell and S. L. Zipursky), pp. 26–63 (Oxford University Press, New York, 1997).

2. Doe, C. Q. and Skeath, J. B. Neurogenesis in the insect central nervous system. *Curr. Opin. Neurobiol.* **6**, 18–24 (1996).

3. Ghysen, A. and Dambly-Chaudiere, C. From DNA to form: the *achaete–scute* complex. *Genes Dev.* **7**, 723–33 (1988).

4. Campuzano, S. and Modolell, J. Patterning of the *Drosophila* nervous system: the *achaete-cute* complex. *Trends Genet.* **8**, 202–8 (1992).

5. Jarman, A. P., Grell, E. H., Ackerman, L., Jan, L. Y. and Jan, Y. N. *atonal* is the proneural gene for *Drosophila* photoreceptors. *Nature* **369**, 398–400 (1994).

6. Jarman, A. P., Grau, Y., Jan, L. Y. and Jan, Y. N. *atonal* is a proneural gene that directs chordotonal organ formation in the *Drosophila* peripheral nervous system. *Cell* **73**, 1307–21 (1993).

7. Huang, M.-L., Hsu, C.-H. and Chien, C.-T. The proneural gene *amos* promotes multiple dendritic neuron formation in the *Drosophila* peripheral nervous system. *Neuron* **25**, 57–67 (2000).

8. Goulding, S. E., zur Lage, P. and Jarman, A. P. *amos*, a proneural gene for *Drosophila* olfactory sense organs that is regulated by lozenge. *Neuron* **25**, 69–78 (2000).

9. Murre, C. *et al.* Interactions between heterologous helix-loop-helix proteins generate complexes that bind specifically to a common DNA sequence. *Cell* **58**, 537–44 (1989).

10. Vaessin, H., Brand, A., Jan, L. Y. and Jan, Y. N. *daughterless* is essential for neuronal precursor differentiation but not for initiation of neuronal precursor formation in the *Drosophila* embryo. *Development* **120**, 935–45 (1994).

11. Cabrera, C. V. and Alonso, M. C. Transcriptional activation by heterodimers of the *achaete-scute* and *daughterless* gene products of *Drosophila. EMBO J.* **10**, 2965–73 (1991).

12. Van Doren, M., Bailey, A. M., Esnayra, J., Ede, K. and Posakony, J. W. Negative regulation of proneural gene activity: hairy is a direct transcriptional repressor of *achaete. Genes Dev.* **8**, 2729–42 (1994).

13. Skeath, J. B., Panganiban, G., Selegue, J. and Carroll, S. B. Gene regulation in two dimensions: the proneural *achaete* and *scute* genes are controlled by combinations of axis-patterning genes through a common intergenic control region. *Genes Dev.* **6**, 2606–19 (1992).

14. Phillips, R. G. and Whittle, J. R. S. *wingless* expression mediates determination of peripheral nervous system elements in late stages of *Drosophila* wing disc development. *Development* **118**, 427–38 (1993).

15. Leyns, L., Gomez-Skarmeta, J.-L. and Dambly-Chaudiere, C. *iroquois*: a prepattern gene that controls the formation of bristles on the thorax of *Drosophila. Mech. Dev.* **59**, 63–72 (1996).

16. Gomez-Skarmeta, J.-L., Diez del Corral, R., Calle-Mustienes, D. L., Ferres-Marco, D. and Modolell, J. *araucan* and *caupolican*, two members of the novel iroquois complex, encode homeoproteins that control proneural and vein-forming genes. *Cell* **85**, 95–107 (1996).

17. Simpson, P. Lateral inhibition and the development of the sensory bristles of the adult sensory nervous system of *Drosophila. Development* **109**, 509–19 (1990).

18. Ghysen, A., Dambly-Chaudiere, C., Jan, L. Y. and Jan, Y. N. Cell interactions and gene interactions in peripheral neurogenesis. *Genes Dev.* **7**, 723–33 (1993).

19. Campos-Ortega, J. Early neurogenesis in *Drosophila melanogaster*. In The development of *Drosophila melanogaster* (ed. M. Bate and A. Martinez-Arias), pp. 1091–129 (Cold Spring Harbor Laboratory Press, New York, 1993).

20. Artavanis-Tsakonas, S., R and, M. D. and Lake, R. J. Notch signaling: cell fate control and signal integration in development. *Science* **284**, 770–6 (1999).

21. Technau, G. and Campos-Ortega, J. Cell autonomy of expression of neurogenic genes of *Drosophila melanogaster*. *Proc. Natl. Acad. Sci. USA* **84**, 4500–4 (1987).

22. Artavanis-Tsakonas, S., Matsuno, K. and Fortini, M. E. Notch signalling. *Science* **268**, 225–32 (1995).

23. Kopan, R. and Turner, D. L. The Notch pathway: democracy and aristocracy in the selection of cell fate. *Curr. Opin. Neurobiol.* **6**, 594–601 (1996).

24. Schroeter, E. H., Kisslinger, J. A. and Kopan, R. Notch-1 signalling requires ligand-induced proteolytic release of intracellular domain. *Nature* **393**, 382–6 (1998).

25. Lecourtois, M. and Schweisguth, F. Indirect evidence for Delta dependent intracellular processing of notch in *Drosophila* embryos. *Curr. Biol.* **8**, 771–4 (1998).

26. Kidd, S., Lieber, T. and Young, M. W. Ligand-induced cleavage and regulation of nuclear entry of Notch in *Drosophila melanogaster* embryos. *Genes Dev.* **12**, 3728–40 (1998).

27. Lecourtois, M. and Schweisguth, F. The neurogenic Suppressor of Hairless DNA-binding protein mediates the transcriptional activation of the *Enhancer of split* complex genes triggered by Notch signalling. *Genes Dev.* **9**, 2598–608 (1995).

28. Qi, H. *et al.* Processing of the Notch ligand Delta by the metalloprotease Kuzbanian. *Science* **283**, 91–4 (1999).

29. Fleming, R. J., Gu, Y. and Hukriede, N. A. Serrate-mediated activation of Notch is specifically blocked by the product of the gene fringe in the dorsal compartment of the *Drosophila* wing imaginal disc. *Development* **124**, 2973–81 (1997).

30. Ghysen, A. and Dambly-Chaudiere, C. The specification of sensory neuron identity in *Drosophila*. *BioEssays* **15**, 293–8 (1993).

31. Hartenstein, V. and Posakony, J. W. A dual function of the *Notch* gene in *Drosophila* sensillum development. *Dev. Biol.* **142**, 13–30 (1990).

32. Parks, A. L. and Muskavitch, M. A. T. *Delta* function is required for bristle organ determination and morphogenesis in *Drosophila*. *Dev. Biol.* **157**, 484–96 (1993).

33. Rhyu, M., Jan, L. Y. and Jan, Y. N. Asymmetric distribution of numb protein during division of the sensory organ precursor cell confers distinct fates to daughter cells. *Cell* **76**, 477–91 (1994).

34. Knoblich, J. A., Jan, L. Y. and Jan, Y. N. Asymmetric segregation of Numb and Prospero during cell division. *Nature* **377**, 624–7 (1995).

35. Friese, E., Knoblich, J. A., Younger-Shepherd, S., Jan, L. Y. and Jan, Y. N. The *Drosophila* Numb protein inhibits signaling of the Notch receptor during cell–cell interaction in sensory organ lineage. *Proc. Natl. Acad. Sci. USA* **93**, 1–8 (1996).

36. Guo, M., Jan, L. Y. and Jan, Y. N. Control of daughter cell fate during asymmetric division: interaction of Numb and Notch. *Neuron* **17**, 27–41 (1996).

37. Spana, E. P. and Doe, C. Q. Numb antagonizes Notch signalling to specify sibling neuron cell fates. *Neuron* **17**, 21–6 (1996).

38. Guo, M., Bier, E., Jan, L. Y. and Jan, Y. N. *tramtrack* acts downstream of numb to specify distinct daughter cell fates during asymmetric cell divisions in the *Drosophila* PNS. *Neuron* **14**, 913–25 (1995).

39. Hartenstein, V. and Posakony, J. W. Sensillum development in the absence of cell division: the sensillum phenotype of the *Drosophila* mutant string. *Dev. Biol.* **138**, 147–58 (1990).

40. Doe, C. Q., Chu-La Graff, Q., Wright, D. M. and Scott, M. P. The *prospero* gene specifies cell fates in the *Drosophila* central nervous system. *Cell* **65**, 451–65 (1991).

41. Ikeshima-Kataoka, H., Skeath, J. B., Nabeshima, Y., Doe, C. Q. and Matsuzaki, F. Miranda directs Prospero to a daughter cell during *Drosophila* asymmetric divisions. *Nature* **390**, 625–29 (1997).

42. Shen, C.-P., Jan, L. Y. and Jan, Y. N. Miranda is required for the asymmetric localization of Prospero during mitosis in *Drosophila*. *Cell* **90**, 449–58 (1997).

43. Lu, B., Rothenberg, M., Jan, L. Y. and Jan, Y. N. Partner of Numb colocalizes with Numb during mitosis and directs Numb asymmetric localization in *Drosophila* neural and muscle progenitors. *Cell* **95**, 225–35 (1998).

44. Kraut, R., Chia, W., Jan, L. Y., Jan, Y. N. and Knoblich, J. A. Role of *inscuteable* in orienting asymmetric cell divisions in *Drosophila*. *Nature* **383**, 50–5 (1996).

45. Tio, M., Zavortink, M., Yang, X. and Chia, W. A functional analysis of *inscuteable* and its roles during *Drosophila* asymmetric cell divisions. *J. Cell Sci.* **112**, 1541–51 (1999).

46. Wodarz, A., Ramrath, A., Kuchinke, U. and Knust, E. Bazooka provides an apical cue for Inscuteable localization in *Drosophila* neuroblasts. *Nature* **402**, 544–7 (1999).

47. Schober, M., Schaefer, M. and Knoblich, J. Bazooka recruits Inscuteable to orient asymmetric cell divisions in *Drosophila* neuroblasts. *Nature* **402**, 548–51 (1999).

48. Bier, E., Vaessin, H., Younger-Shepherd, S., Jan, L. Y. and Jan, Y. N. *deadpan*, an essential pan-neural gene in *Drosophila*, encodes a helix–loop–helix protein similar to the *hairy* gene product. *Genes Dev.* **6**, 2137–51 (1992).

49. Brand, A., Jarman, A. P., Jan, L. Y. and Jan, Y. N. *asense* is a *Drosophila* neural precursor gene and is capable of initiating sense organ formation. *Development* **119**, 1–17 (1993).

50. Lee, J. E. Basic helix–loop–helix genes in neural development. *Curr. Opin. Neurobiol.* **7**, 13–20 (1997).

51. Guillemot, F. *et al.* Mammalian achaete–scute homolog 1 is required for the early development of olfactory and autonomic neurons. *Cell* **75**, 463–76 (1993).

52. Casarosa, S., Fode, C. and Guillemot, F. *Mash1* regulates neurogenesis in the ventral telencephalon. *Development* **126**, 525–34 (1999).

53. Ferreiro, B., Kintner, C., Zimmerman, K., Anderson, D. J. and Harris, W. A. *XASH1* genes promote neurogenesis in *Xenopus* embryos. *Development* **120**, 3649–55 (1994).

54. Ben-Aire, N. *et al.* Math1 is essential for genesis of cerebellar granule neurons. *Nature* **390**, 169–72 (1997).

55. Ma, Q., Kintner, C. and Anderson, D. J. *Neurogenin*, a vertebrate neuronal determination gene, acts upstream of *NeuroD* in a cascade. *Cell* **87**, 43–52 (1996).

56. Lee, J. E. *et al.* Conversion of *Xenopus* ectoderm into neurons by NeuroD, a basic helix–loop–helix protein. *Science* **268**, 836–44 (1995).

57. Marcus, E. A., Kintner, C. and Harris, W. A. The role of GSK3beta in regulating neuronla differentiation in *Xenopus laevis*. *Mol. Cell. Neurosci.* **12**, 269–80 (1998).

58. Ishibashi, M. *et al.* Targeted disruption of mammalian *hairy* and *Enhancer of split* homolog-1 (*HES-1*) leads to up-regulation of neural helix–loop–helix factors, premature neurogenesis, and sever neural tube defects. *Genes Dev.* **9**, 3136–48 (1995).

59. Ishibashi, M. *et al.* Persistent expression of helix–loop–helix factor HES-1 prevents mammalian neural differentiation in the central nervous system. *EMBO J.* **13**, 1799–805 (1994).

60. Chitnis, A., Henrique, D., Lewis, J., Ish-Horowicz, D. and Kintner, C. Primary neurogenesis in *Xenopus* embryos regulated by a homologue of the *Drosophila* neurogenic gene *Delta*. *Nature* **375**, 761–6 (1995).

61. Austin, C. P., Feldman, D. E., Ida, J. A. and Cepko, C. L. Vertebrate retinal ganglion cells are selected from competent progenitors by the action of Notch. *Development* **121**, 3637–50 (1995).

62. Dorsky, R. I., Rapaport, D. H. and Harris, W. A. *Xotch* inhibits cell differentiation in the *Xenopus* retina. *Neuron* **14**, 487–96 (1995).

63. Ma, Q., Chen, Z., del Barco Barrantes, I., de la Pompa, J. L. and Anderson, D. J. *neurogenin1* is essential for the determination of neuronal precursors for proximal cranial sensory ganglia. *Neuron* **20**, 469–82 (1998).

64. Fode, C. *et al.* The bHLH protein Neurogenin 2 is a determination factor for epibranchial placode-derived sensory neurons. *Neuron* **20**, 483–94 (1998).

65. Fode, C. *et al.* A role for neural determination genes in specifying the dorso-ventral identity of telencephalic neurons. *Genes Dev.* **14**, 67–80, 2000.

66. Szucsik, J. C. *et al.* Altered forebrain and hindbrain development in mice mutant for the *Gsh*-2 homeobox gene. *Dev. Biol.* **191**, 230–42 (1997).

67. Mizuseki, K., Kishi, M., Shiota, K., Nakanishi, S. and Sasai, Y. SoxD: an essential mediator of induction of anterior neural tissues in *Xenopus* embryos. *Neuron* **21**, 77–85 (1998).

68. Xuan, S. *et al.* Winged helix factor BF-1 is essential for the development of the cerebral hemispheres. *Neuron* **14**, 1141–52 (1995).

69. Bourguignon, C., Li, J. and Papalopulu, N. XBF-1, a winged helix transcription factor with dual activity, has a role in positioning neurogenesis in *Xenopus* competent ectoderm. *Development* **125**, 4889–900 (1998).

70. Bellefroid, E. J. *et al.* Xiro3 encodes a *Xenopus* homolog of the *Drosophila iroquois* genes and functions in neural specification. *EMBO J.* **17**, 191–203 (1998).

71. Morgan, R. and Sargent, M. G. The role in neural patterning of translation initiation factor eIF4AII; induction of neural fold genes. *Development* **124**, 2751–60 (1997).

72. Nagata, K., Nagai, T., Aruga, J. and Mikoshiba, K. *Xenopus* Zic3, a primary regulator both in neural and neural crest development. *Proc. Natl. Acad. Sci. USA* **94**, 11980–5 (1997).

73. Brewster, R., Lee, J. and Ruiz i Altaba, A. Gli/Zic factors pattern the neural plate by defining

domains of cell differentiation. *Nature* **393**, 579–83 (1998).

74. McDonald, J. A. *et al.* Dorsoventral patterning in the *Drosophila* central nervous system: the *vnd* homeobox gene specifies ventral column identity. *Genes Dev.* **12**, 3603–12 (1998).

75. Weiss, J. B. *et al.* Dorsoventral patterning in the *Drosophila* central nervous system: the intermediate neuroblasts defective homeobox gene specifies intermediate column identity. *Genes Dev.* **12**, 3591–602 (1998).

76. Chitnis, A. B. Control of neurogenesis— lessons from frogs, fish and flies. *Curr. Opin. Neurobiol.* **9**, 18–25 (1999).

77. Briscoe, J. *et al.* Homeobox gene *Nkx2.2* and specification of neuronal identity by graded Sonic hedgehog signalling. *Nature* **398**, 622–7 (1999).

78. Kimmel, C. B., Warga, R. M. and Kane, D. A. Cell cycles and clonal strings during formation of the zebrafish central nervous system. *Development* **120**, 265–76 (1994).

79. Dehay, C., Giroud, P., Berland, M., Smart, I. and Kennedy, H. Modulation of the cell cycle contributes to the parcellation of the primate visual cortex. *Nature* **366**, 464–6 (1993).

80. Lee, E. *et al.* Mice deficient for Rb are nonviable and show defects in neurogenesis and haematopoiesis. *Nature* **359**, 288–94 (1992).

81. Ross, M. E. and Risken, M. MN20, a D2 cyclin found in brain, is implicated in neural differentiation. *J. Neurosci.* **14**, 6384–91 (1994).

82. Lumsden, A., Clarke, J. D. W., Keynes, R. and Fraser, S. E. Early phenotypic choices by neuronal precursors, revealed by clonal analysis of the chick embryo hindbrain. *Development* **120**, 1581–9 (1994).

83. Edlund, T. and Jessell, T. M. Progression from extrinsic to intrinsic signaling in cell fate specification: a view from the nervous system. *Cell* **96**, 211–24 (1999).

84. Morrison, S. J., Shah, N. M. and Anderson, D. J. Regulatory mechanisms in stem cell biology. *Cell* **88**, 287–98 (1997).

85. Gao, W.-Q., Heintz, N. and Hatten, M. E. Cerebellar granule cell neurogenesis is regulated by cell–cell interactions *in vitro*. *Neuron* **6**, 705–15 (1991).

86. Ebens, A. J., Garren, H., Cheyette, B. N. and Zipursky, S. L. The *Drosophila* anachronism locus: a glycoprotein secreted by glia inhibits neuroblast proliferation. *Cell* **74**, 15–27 (1993).

87. LoTurco, J. J., Owens, D. F., Heath, M., Dvais, M. and Kriegstein, A. R. GABA and glutamate depolarize cortical progenitor cells and inhibit DNA synthesis. *Neuron* **15**, 1287–98 (1995).

88. Johe, K. K., Hazel, T. G., Muller, T., Dugich-Djordjevic, M. M. and McKay, R. D. Single factors direct the differentiation of stem cells from the fetal and adult central nervous system. *Genes Dev.* **10** (1996).

89. de Pablo, F. and de la Rosa, E. J. The developing CNS: a scenario for the action of proinsulin, insulin and insulin-like growth factors. *Trends Neurosci.* **18**, 143–50 (1995).

90. Dickinson, M. E., Krumlauf, R. and McMahon, A. P. Evidence for a mitogenic effect of Wnt-1 in the developing mammalian central nervous system. *Development* **120**, 1453–71 (1994).

91. Rowitch, D. H. *et al.* Sonic hedgehog regulates proliferation and inhibits differentiation of CNS precursor cells. *J. Neurosci.* **19**, 8954–65 (1999).

92. Qian, X., Goderie, S. K., Shen, Q., Stern, J. H. and Temple, S. Intrinsic programs of patterned cell lineages in isolated vertebrate CNS ventricular zone cells. *Development* **125**, 3143–52 (1998).

93. Huttner, W. B. and Brand, M. Asymmetric division and polarity of neuroepithelial cells. *Curr. Opin. Neurobiol.* **7**, 29–39 (1997).

94. Zhong, W., Feder, J. N., Jiang, M. M., Jan, L. Y. and Jan, Y. N. Asymmetric localization of a mammalian Numb homolog during mouse cortical neurogenesis. *Neuron* **17**, 43–53 (1996).

95. Zhong, W., Jiang, M.-M., Weinmaster, G., Jan, L. Y. and Jan, Y. N. Differential expression of mammalian Numb, Numblike and Notch1 suggests distinct roles during mouse cortical neurogenesis. *Development* **124**, 1887–97 (1997).

96. Chenn, A. and McConnell, S. K. Cleavage orientation and the asymmetric inheritance of Notch1 immunoreactivity in mammalian neurogenesis. *Cell* **82**, 631–41 (1995).

97. Roelink, H. *et al.* Floor plate and motor neuron induction by different concentrations of the amino-terminal cleavage product of sonic hedgehog autoproteolysis. *Cell* **81**, 445–55 (1995).

98. Ericson, J., Morton, S., Kawakami, A., Roelink, H. and Jessell, T. M. Two critical periods of Sonic hedgehog signaling required for the specification of zmotor neuron identity. *Cell* **87**, 661–73 (1996).

99. Tremblay, P., Pituello, F. and Gruss, P. Inhibition of floor plate differentiation by *Pax3*: evidence from ectopic expression in transgenic mice. *Development* **122**, 2555–67 (1996).

100. Ericson, J. *et al.* Pax6 controls progenitor cell identity and neuronal fate in response to graded SHH signaling. *Cell* **90**, 169–80 (1997).

101. Tanabe, Y., William, C. and Jessell, T. M. Specification of motor neuron identity by the MNR2 homeodomain protein. *Cell* **95**, 67–80 (1998).

102. Pfaff, S. L., Mendelsohn, M., Stewart, C. L., Edlund, T. and Jessell, T. M. Requirement for LIM homeobox gene Is11 in motor neuron generation

reveals a motor neuron-dependent step in inter-neuron differentiation. *Cell* **84**, 1–20 (1996).

103. Tsuchida, T. *et al.* Topographic organization of embryonic motor neurons defined by expression of LIM homeobox genes. *Cell* **79**, 957–70 (1994).

104. Sharma, K. *et al.* LIM homeodomain factors Lhx3 and Lhx4 assign subtype identities for motor neurons. *Cell* **95**, 817–28 (1998).

105. Lin, J. H. *et al.* Functionally related motor neuron pool and muscle sensory afferent subtypes defined by coordinate ETS gene expression. *Cell* **95**, 393–407 (1998).

106. Goulding, M. Specifying motor neurons and their connections. *Neuron* **21**, 943–6 (1998).

107. Eisen, J. S. Determination of primary motoneuron identity in developing zebrafish embryos. *Science* 569–72 (1991).

108. Eisen, J. S. Development of motoneuronal phenotype. *Annu. Rev. Neurosci.* **17**, 1–30 (1994).

109. Appel, B. *et al.* Motoneuron fate specification revealed by patterned LIM homeobox gene expression in embryonic zebrafish. *Development* **121**, 4117–25 (1995).

110. Tiret, L., Le Mouellic, H., Maury, M. and Brulet, P. Increased apoptosis of motoneurons and altered somatotopic maps in the brachial spinal cord of *Hoxc-8*-deficient mice. *Development* **125**, 279–91 (1998).

111. Ensini, M., Tsuchida, T., Belting, H.-G. and Jessell, T. M. The control of rostrocaudal pattern in the developing spinal cord: specification of motor neuron subtype identity is initiated by signals from paraxial mesoderm. *Development* **125**, 969–82 (1998).

112. Eiden, L. E. The cholinergic gene locus. *J. Neurochem.* **70**, 2227–40 (1998).

113. Zetterstrom, R. H. *et al.* Dopamine neuron agenesis in *Nurr-1*-deficient mice. *Science* **276**, 248–50 (1997).

114. Saucedo-Cardenas, O. *et al.* Nurr1 is essential for the induction of the dopaminergic phenotype and the survival of ventral mesencephalic late dopaminergic precursor neurons. *Proc. Natl. Acad. Sci. USA* **95**, 4013–18 (1998).

115. Hirsch, M.-R., Tiveron, M.-C., Guillemot, F., Brunet, J.-F. and Goridis, C. Control of noradrenergic differentiation and Phox2a expression by MASH1 in the central and peripheral nervous system. *Development* **125**, 599–608 (1998).

116. Lo, L., Tiveron, M. C. and Anderson, D. J. MASH1 activates expression of the paired homeodomain transcription factor Phox2a, and couples pan-neuronal and subtype specific components of autonomic neuronal identity. *Development* **125**, 609–20 (1998).

117. Morin, X. *et al.* Defects in sensory and autonomic ganglia and absence of locus coeruleus in mice deficient for the homeobox gene *Phox2a*. *Neuron* **18**, 411–23 (1997).

118. Harris, W. A. and Hartenstein, V. Cellular determination. In *Fundamental neuroscience* (ed. M. J. Zigmond, F. Bloom, S. C. Landis, J. L. Roberts and L. R. Squire), pp. 481–517 (Academic Press, San Diego, 1999).

119. Matsuzaki, F. Asymmetric division of *Drosophila* neural stem cells: a basis for neural diversity. *Curr. Opin. Neurobiol.* **10**, 38–44 (2000).

120. Chan, Y.-M. and Jan, Y. N. Conservation of neurogenic genes and mechanisms. *Curr. Opin. Neurobiol.* **9**, 582–8 (1999).

5
The Neural Crest

The majority of cells contributing to the peripheral nervous system (PNS) in vertebrates arise at the lateral margins of the neural plate, from a narrow zone of cells
called the neural crest that appears between the future neural tube and the epidermis. The neural crest is a uniquely vertebrate character, not found even in other
chordates. The remainder of the PNS arises from placodes, isolated patches of ectoderm in the head region that delaminate neurons directly into the cranial sensory
ganglia forming beneath them, in a process that more closely reflects PNS development in *Drosophila*.

The neural crest provides one of the most striking examples of cell migration and
diversification during early development. It has a well-defined, focal origin at the
edge of the neural plate where cells undergo an epithelial-to-mesenchymal transition
in form and behaviour, becoming highly migratory and invading many regions of the
early embryo where they finally adopt a wide variety of fates. These include neurons
and glial cells of the peripheral nervous system (sensory, sympathetic and parasympathetic ganglia, sheath (Schwann) cells of nerves), pigment cells (melanocytes),
neuroendocrine cells of the adrenal medulla, and connective tissue forming cells of
the craniofacial region. In addition, there is a small population of neural crest cells
that remains within the dorsal neural tube, which produces the proprioceptive sensory neurons of the mesencephalic trigeminal nucleus.[1] Some authors believe that the
primary sensory neurons of fish and tadpoles (Rohon–Beard cells), which reside
within the dorsal neural tube rather than in dorsal root ganglia, may also originate
from non-migratory neural crest cells.

The crest is specified during neural induction but the timing of its emigration
varies with species and with axial level within a species. Although classically regarded
as being cells derived from the neural folds, as is the case for amphibian and higher
vertebrate embryos, this definition would exclude the neural crest of teleost fishes
such as the zebrafish. A peculiarity of neurulation in teleosts is that the tube forms by
cavitation of an initially solid mass of neurectoderm, the neural keel, while the
neural crest cells originate by direct delamination from the surface ectoderm flanking
the neural keel. In chick, however, where the crest forms stereotypically within
neural folds, emigration begins at or soon after neural tube closure as the surface
ectoderm on either side of the embryo establishes continuity across the dorsal
midline (Fig. 5.1). Between the dorsal pole of the neural tube and surface ectoderm is a

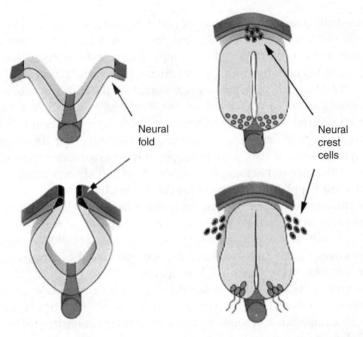

Figure 5.1 Neural crest cells form within the lips of the neural folds (black) as these begin to close on each other during neurulation. As the two sides of the neural plate fuse dorsally and the epidermal ectoderm establishes continuity across the dorsal midline, the neural crest cells detach and migrate away.

small gap that rapidly becomes filled by neural crest cells as they detach from the mid-dorsal neural tube. To leave the neuroepithelium, neural crest cells must lose their epithelial characteristics and take on the properties of migratory mesenchymal cells. The mechanisms that regulate this dramatic change in cell behaviour are poorly understood, but are thought to require a major restructuring of cell–cell contacts, and in particular the downregulation of molecules and organelles that serve an adhesive or cohesive function for epithelial cells. The basal lamina bounding the external surface of the neural tube is also digested in preparation for the escape of neural crest cells into the periphery.

Early determination and individuation of the neural crest

The generation of neural crest cells appears to result from inductive interactions shared with the early epidermis and the neural plate, involving members of the TGFβ superfamily, especially BMP2, BMP4 and BMP7. Analysis of zebrafish mutants for BMPs or their antagonists has suggested that a gradient of BMP activity, high laterally and low medially, specifies epidermal, neural crest and neural plate development at successively lower thresholds (Fig. 5.2, see also Chapter 2).[2,3] Consistent with these observations, it has been shown also for higher vertebrate embryos that BMPs can induce crest differentiation from competent neurectoderm.[4] Local WNT signalling within the dorsal neuroectoderm is also important for the early stages of neural crest development, since mice double-mutant for *Wnt1* and *Wnt3a* show a marked deficiency in neural crest derivatives.[5] Injection of BMP4-expressing cells into the neural tube upregulates *Wnt1* and *Wnt3a* expression, suggesting that the WNT pathway operates downstream of BMP signalling, possibly to expand or maintain the crest population. Other genes that may act downstream of BMPs in regulating the extent of the neural crest population have been considered in Chapter 4.

Against this concept of an early role for BMPs is an earlier view that argued for the importance of local interactions between neural and epidermal regions. For example, crest cells, as well as molecular markers such as *Wnt1* and *Wnt3a*, appear at the interface between these tissues when they are juxtaposed experimentally.[6–8] Furthermore, experiments in which Sonic hedgehog (SHH)-secreting or BMP antagonist (noggin)-secreting cells are grafted to neurulating chick embryos have shown that the early steps of neural crest specification are blocked by SHH but not by noggin.[9] This challenges the importance of a BMP gradient in defining the territory of the ectoderm that will adopt the neural crest cell fate.

The epithelial–mesenchymal switch in emerging crest cells is accompanied by the onset of expression of the zinc finger transcription factor Slug, whose expression is maintained during the phase of crest cell migration.[10] Individuation of crest cells from the neural tube also depends on the modulation of cell–cell adhesion. Two cell

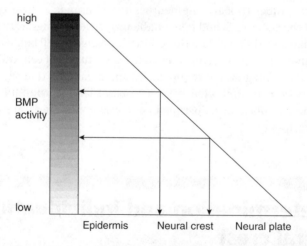

Figure 5.2 A gradient of BMP activity which is high laterally and low medially may be responsible for locating the neural crest between the epidermis and the neural plate and for determining the mediolateral width of the crest-producing region. Neural differentiation is inhibited by high levels of BMP signalling but permitted by low levels. This model is based primarily on analysis of a zebrafish mutant (*somitabun*) whose expanded crest domain could be explained in terms of a shallower BMP gradient. After Chitnis.[76]

adhesion molecules, N-CAM and N-cadherin (see Chapter 9), are expressed by cells of the neural tube, and E-cadherin is expressed by the epidermal ectoderm right up to the neural plate boundary. Expression of these adhesion molecules is lost from presumptive neural crest cells as they appear in the neural folds. At this stage, the neural fold cells express another cadherin (cad-6B), but this is also downregulated at the onset of cell migration.[11] Crest cells then re-express N-CAM and N-cadherin once they stop migrating, coalesce and differentiate, for example in dorsal root ganglia, while a subpopulation of cells, mainly restricted to the dorsal and ventral roots, express cadherin-7.[11-13] This modulation of adhesion molecule expression appears to be required for neural crest cell detachment and migration, which is prevented by the overexpression of N-cadherin or cadherin-7.[14] The *Snail* gene of mice has an expression pattern and dynamics that are similar to chick *Slug* and has been shown to mediate the epithelial to mesenchymal transition of cell lines by repressing E-cadherin expression.[15] Another player in the process of delamination is the intracellular signalling molecule rhoB, a GTP-binding protein, which is expressed in the premigratory and early migrating neural crest. Inhibition of rhoB prevents crest emigration but not differentiation.[16]

Trunk neural crest

Migration pathways

The migratory pathways of the crest are stereotyped and have been defined by labelling experiments using, for example, grafts of Japanese quail crest into chick embryos,[17] immunostaining for cell surface markers such as the HNK-1 carbohydrate epitope, or marking the crest with fluorescent vital dyes such as DiI. In the trunk region of birds and mammals, crest cells arise from the dorsal neural tube underneath the ectoderm and adjacent to the mesodermal somites. From this position they take one of two principal routes. The first is ventral, initially between the somites while they remain epithelial, and then into the anterior (rostral) part of the somite-derived sclerotome.[18] Crest cells that remain in the anterior half-sclerotome aggregate to form the dorsal root ganglia, becoming primary sensory neurons and associated glia, while cells that penetrate further ventrally adopt autonomic (sympathetic postganglionic and adrenal medullary phenotypes. The second route is dorsal, between the surface ectoderm (epidermis) and the dermatome derivative of the somite (future dermis); cells that take this path differentiate into melanocytes (Figs 5.3 and 5.4A). How the decision is made to enter one or other pathway and whether this also involves early specification of neurogenic or melanogenic fate is poorly understood. However, there is evidence from zebrafish that cells are specified for one or other fate

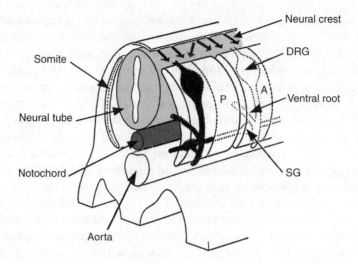

Figure 5.3 Major components of the embryonic axis at spinal cord levels. The peripheral nerves associated with the cord are segmentally reiterated in register with the somites: both the sensory dorsal root ganglia (DRG) and the motor ventral roots are aligned with the anterior (A) half of the somite, as are the ganglia of the sympathetic chain (SG). The posterior halves of somites (P) are inhibitory to the entry of neuronal growth cones and the neural crest cells that make the peripheral ganglia.

before they leave the neural crest primordium; high WNT signalling is thought to induce melanogenic precursors with a dorsal migration preference whereas lower WNT levels are associated with the development of neurogenic precursors.[19]

Guidance molecules

A variety of molecular systems have been identified in the local environment of the crest that may direct crest migration. Foremost among these are the constituents of the extracellular matrix, comprising motility-promoting permissive molecules as well as repulsive or motility-inhibiting molecules. Laminin (see also Chapter 9) is a good example of the former class, one of its isoforms ($\alpha1\beta1\gamma1$) being widespread along crest migratory paths, correlating with its ability to promote crest migration *in vitro*. Other permissive matrix molecules found on migration pathways are fibronectin and collagen types I, IV and VI, while candidate non-permissive molecular systems include a number of chondroitin sulphate proteoglycans, for example collagen type IX and versican, and the tenascins.[20] Molecules known to be repulsive for growing axons (for example, members of the collapsin/semaphorin and ephrin families, see Chapter 9) have also been implicated in crest guidance, by defining no-go areas from which the migrating cells would be repelled. Consistent with this, *in vivo* time-lapse studies of zebrafish trunk neural crest cells have shown that their filopodia can collapse following contact with neighbouring somite cells in their pathway,

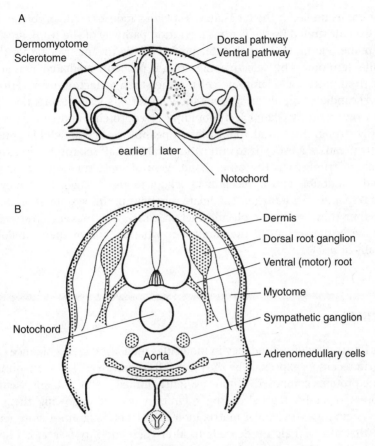

Figure 5.4 Transverse sections through the trunk of young (A) and older (B) chick embryos showing the emergence, pathways and final locations of neural crest cells. As they leave the dorsal neural tube, crest cells enter either the dorsal pathway, above the somites, or the ventral pathway, between the somites and the neural tube (A, left). As the inner, sclerotomal region of the somite de-epithelializes, liberating cells that will accumulate around the notochord to form vertebrae, ventrally migrating crest cells accumulate to form a dorsal root ganglion (A, right). In B, the stippled structures either contain crest derivatives (the dermis, and later the epidermis, fills with melanocytes that reach the skin via the dorsal pathway; the ventral root motor axons are ensheathed by Schwann cells) or are made entirely by crest cells.

suggesting that crest cells undergo a repulsive response similar to that shown by axon growth cones.[21]

Segmental crest migration through the somites

The large number of candidate molecules, and the attendant potential for functional complexity and redundancy, has made it difficult to pinpoint any one as being critical in directing crest migration in a particular region of the embryo; the crest migrates normally, for example, in the tenascin-C knockout mouse.[22] The problem of redundancy is well-illustrated by the ventral migration pathway of the trunk crest cells in the somite mesoderm, when they enter preferentially the anterior rather than posterior half-sclerotome. This selective migration is probably mediated by repulsion of the crest from posterior sclerotome cells, rather than attraction by anterior cells[23] and several candidate repulsion systems show posterior-specific expression. The case for the involvement of peanut lectin-binding glycoproteins and certain ephrins is particularly strong, since local application of peanut lectin[24] or soluble ephrinB1 or its receptor[25] causes crest cells to enter the posterior half-sclerotome in explants of chick embryo trunks. On the other hand, ventral crest migration is apparently unaffected in a double ephrin receptor knockout mouse.[26] The extracellular matrix molecule F-Spondin[27] is a further candidate repellent in this system. It remains to be seen whether these various molecules act in concert to prevent crest cells from entering the posterior half of the somite, or whether one of them predominates functionally *in vivo*.

Integrins

A further illustration of redundancy in molecules mediating crest guidance concerns the integrin receptors expressed by the crest cells themselves. These are dimeric cell membrane proteins composed of non-covalently linked α and β chains. Neural crest cells express several integrins during migration *in vivo*, endowing them with a receptor system for extracellular matrix molecules (such as laminin, fibronectin and tenascin) that also signals inside cells to alter their motility (see also Chapter 9). Consistent with an important role for integrins in crest motility, function-blocking antibodies to the β_1-class integrins inhibit avian crest cell motility *in vitro*, and prevent cranial crest migration *in vivo* when injected locally into the hindbrain region of the embryo.[28] Moreover, at least three distinct β_1-class integrins have been implicated in the interaction of crest cells with laminin and fibronectin.[29] However, mice harbouring genetic deletions of a variety of individual integrin subunits show normal migration and development of the crest derivatives, perhaps due to functional compensation by the remaining integrins, so it is difficult to be certain that any individual subtype is truly indispensable.

Neural crest cell differentiation

Once neural crest cells have left the neural tube, they encounter cues in their migration pathway and at their final destination which influence their proliferation and survival, as well directing their choice of differentiation fate (Fig. 5.4). In addition, there is some evidence to suggest that the neural crest is initially heterogeneous with respect to its differentiation potential, with a range of more or less committed precursors already delineated within the neural crest primordium. Thus, cell type differentiation appropriate to position in the embryo may involve not only the instructive induction of uncommitted cells but also the selective survival of precursors that are committed to particular lineages and reach the right destination, together with the selective elimination of those that end up in the wrong place. For further discussion on the issue of multipotency versus commitment in neural crest cells, the reader is referred to Le Douarin and Kalcheim.[17]

Dorsal root gangliogenesis

Neural crest cells that accumulate in the ventral sclerotome form dorsal root ganglia (DRG), consisting of various subtypes of sensory neuron together with satellite (glial) cells. Although fate-restricted precursor cells have been detected within the crest that migrates to the DRG, it is generally held that cell fate is progressively acquired by interaction with the local environment.[17] The differentiation of sympathetic neurons under the influence of BMPs secreted by the aorta has provided an example of this process, as discussed below. However, for the sensory ganglia, it is unclear how the environment contributes to fate restriction within the neurogenic crest, and whether interaction between the neural crest cells themselves might also be involved. The latter possibility has been examined by studies of chick embryo DRG, which have shown that Notch signalling is involved in the neuron/glial cell decision.[30] In forming DRG, Notch-1 is expressed preferentially by cells in the outer shell of the ganglion whereas the expression of Delta-1, and early neuronal markers, is localized to the core region (Fig. 5.5). In cultures of quail DRG cells, Notch activation prevents neuronal differentiation and keeps cells in an undifferentiated, actively proliferating state, although they can ultimately form glia. During cell divisions *in situ*, the Notch antagonist Numb is localized to a cytoplasmic crescent, suggesting that divisions are asymmetrical and fate-determining; as for sense organ precursors in the *Drosophila* PNS (Chapter 4), Numb is segregated to the neuronal daughters of these divisions. The outer region appears to be a proliferative zone in which young neurons are produced that then migrate to the core, while glia accumulate in the shell. These later migrate among and sheathe the neurons, possibly in response to Neuregulin signalling. Thus, cell fate diversification within forming DRG involves mechanisms that are autonomous to the crest population, including Notch-mediated lateral specification and asymmetric division.

Development of sympathetic neurons

The best worked example of neuronal differentiation from neural crest precursors concerns the neurons of sympathetic chain ganglia. These arise from cells that migrate beyond the DRG to reach the surface of the dorsal aorta, where they begin to

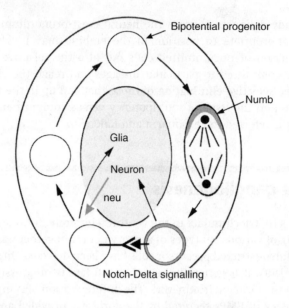

Figure 5.5 A model for intrinsic control of neurogenesis and gliogenesis within the dorsal root ganglion. The shell region of the forming ganglion contains proliferating bipotential precursors. The core region contains differentiating neurons and, later, differentiating glia. Asymmetric distribution of Numb in dividing progenitors suppresses Notch activation in one daughter, which expresses Delta and becomes a sensory neuron, whereas Notch activation in the other daughter prevents neuronal differentiation. These cells can then either divide again or, under the influence of neuregulin (neu) signalling from neurons, differentiate into glial (satellite) cells. Data from Wakamatsu et al.[30]

express the transcriptional regulator Mash1 and enzymes that are involved in synthesis of the neurotransmitter noradrenaline (NA). As we have seen in Chapter 4, Mash1 is a bHLH transcription factor which acts as a determinant of the neuronal state, and in the sympathetic nervous system it is an important regulator of the noradrenergic phenotype of these cells. Downstream targets regulated by Mash1 include the homeobox gene *Phox2a*,[31] whose protein products bind directly to the regulatory elements in the promoter of the NA-synthesizing enzyme dopamine β-hydroxylase (DBH). Most peripheral noradrenergic (NA) neurons of the *Mash1*$^{-/-}$ mouse fail to express *DBH*. When *Phox2a* is overexpressed, either in tissue culture cells or in embryos, tyrosine hydroxylase (TH) expression is dramatically upregulated, representing the imposition of an early step in the NA synthesis pathway.[32] *Phox2a* overexpression can also induce the generation of neurons that express pan-neuronal, noradrenergic and cholinergic genes characteristic of sympathetic neurons.[33]

A number of lines of evidence suggest that the positional signal regulating NA differentiation in presumptive sympathetic neurons is a BMP (4 or 7) produced by the aorta itself.[34,35] In particular, neural crest cells are induced to express *Mash1*, followed by *Phox2a* and components of the NA pathway when they are cultured in the presence of BMPs, and ectopic TH[+] cells form around fibroblasts expressing BMPs implanted near the sympathetic ganglia in chick embryos.[35] Our knowledge of the hierarchy of genetic control leading to NA differentiation is extensive, but it has yet to be shown that BMP expression is necessary to induce *Mash1* and *Phox2a* in sympathetic neurons. The cascade of actions following Mash1 induction in sympathetic neurons is certainly among the best evidence so far that vertebrate proneural genes control both pan-neuronal and neuron subtype-specific differentiation.[31]

The neurons generated by BMP signalling *in vitro* express an autonomic lineage-specific marker, but not the catecholamine biosynthetic enzymes associated with the sympathetic neurotransmission, and it is likely that further environmental signals are needed for expression of the full neurotransmitter repertoire of an individual neuronal phenotype. It has been shown that the transmitter phenotype of sympathetic neurons can be switched from noradrenergic to cholinergic by culture medium conditioned by heart cells[36] and this effect can be replicated by application of ciliary neurotrophic factor (CNTF) or the cytokine leukaemia inhibitory factor (LIF).[37]

An attractive possibility is that the targets of sympathetic cholinergic innervation, such as the sweat glands, induce cholinergic differentiation in their innervating neurons by the secretion of such factors. The innervation of sweat glands in the developing rat footpad is initially noradrenergic, but becomes cholinergic during maturation, and this switch depends on the presence of the target sweat glands.[38,39] A soluble 'sweat gland factor', distinct from LIF and CNTF, has been identified that reproduces this switch in cultured sympathetic neurons, and its production by gland cells has been shown to depend in turn on the presence of sympathetic neuro-transmitters.[40,41] A similar example is provided by the neural crest-derived chro-maffin cell, whose differentiation *in vitro* depends on the presence of glucocorticoid hormones, mimicking the presumed influence of the adrenal cortex *in vivo*.[42] It seems likely that axon targets and glial cells express instructive factors for neurotransmitter phenotype more generally throughout the nervous system[43] and other molecular candidates for this activity include the various neurotrophins (see Chapter 12). Nerve growth factor (NGF), for example, has been shown to induce selectively the expres-sion of particular neuropeptides in sensory neurons,[44] and Brain-derived neuro-trophic factor (BDNF) can induce somatostatin and neuropeptide Y expression in rat cortical neurons.[43]

Ligand–receptor systems involved in migration, proliferation and survival

Several ligand–receptor systems have been identified that are critical for the development of subpopulations of the neural crest. In each case the receptor system is a member of the receptor tyrosine kinase superfamily, and is expressed by the crest cells, while the ligand is present in the local crest environment. The evidence that these molecules are critical for crest development comes principally from showing that particular crest derivatives fail to appear in the relevant mouse mutants, and this could result from a failure of crest migration, proliferation and/or survival.

The *c-ret* proto-oncogene product is expressed by particular subpopulations of the cranial crest, and its targeted ablation in the mouse results in the absence of the superior cervical (sympathetic) ganglia and of enteric ganglia at mid- and hindgut levels.[45] Heterozygous *c-ret* mutations in humans cause Hirschsprung's disease, a condition due to absence of enteric ganglia in the distal colon resulting in large bowel obstruction.[46] *In situ* hybridization for mouse *c-ret*, combined with lineage analysis of vagal and trunk crest using DiI labelling, shows that the *ret*-dependent cells of the enteric and sympathetic lineages together originate from the vagal crest, deriving in turn from the post-otic hindbrain; the majority of the foregut enteric nervous system (ENS) and remainder of the sympathetic ganglia derive from a separate crest lineage migrating from the trunk level. Is *c-ret* required for migration of progenitor crest cells into the sites of terminal differentiation, or solely for subsequent proliferation and/or survival at the differentiation site? Mutant enteric crest cells can be detected in the foregut but fail to migrate further along the embryonic gastrointestinal tract, suggesting a need for *c-ret* function in this particular migration. On the other hand, crest cells do colonize the site of differentiation of the superior cervical ganglion, so here the requirement for *c-ret* is presumably to promote proliferation and/or survival rather than migration.[47]

The ligand for c-ret has turned out to be a complex of GDNF (glial cell line derived neurotrophic factor, originally identified as trophic for midbrain dopaminergic neurons; see Chapter 12) with a further protein, GDNFRa.[48,49] This complex can be secreted or GPI-anchored (via GDNFRa) to the cell surface, and while GDNF is expressed in the developing gut cells close to the nascent enteric ganglia, it is uncertain whether GDNFRa is coexpressed with c-ret by the enteric crest or derives instead from surrounding gut cells. GDNF knockout mice completely lack an ENS, further emphasizing the importance of GDNF–GDNFRa–c-ret signalling in its development.[50] Null mutation of the homeobox gene *Phox2b*, which is essential for the expression of c-ret, also results in the absence of autonomic ganglia, suggesting that *Phox2b* induces *c-ret* in autonomic precursors, thereby enabling transduction of the GDNF signal. Upstream control may be exerted by BMP2, which has been shown to induce *Mash1*, *Phox2* and *c-ret* in neural crest cells.

Another well-known ligand–receptor tyrosine kinase system has been implicated in the proliferation and survival of crest-derived neuronal lineages, namely the neurotrophins and their trk receptors. Their trophic functions are discussed in Chapter 12 but, although plausible, there is no definitive evidence that the system is also involved in directing the migration of the crest. The same argument applies to the neuregulin–ErbB receptor system; as described in Chapter 6, neuregulin signalling is essential for the normal development of Schwann cells in association with peripheral axons, and of the crest-derived components of the cranial ganglia, but whether it mediates long-distance attraction of crest cells towards these sites is less clear.

Lastly, the migration of the melanocyte progenitors along the dorsolateral pathway, between the surface ectoderm and the dermomyotome, is regulated by a further ligand–receptor system, stem cell factor (SCF, also known as Steel factor) and the receptor tyrosine kinase c-kit. Melanocyte progenitors express c-kit as they leave the neural tube, while SCF is expressed by cells of the dermatome and ectoderm before the onset of crest migration between these tissues. In *Steel* mutant mice, lacking functional SCF, the progenitors appear alongside the neural tube but fail to migrate; a secreted form of SCF is needed to promote their migration along the dorsolateral pathway, while a membrane-bound form is required for their survival.[51] This result suggests a chemoattractive role for secreted SCF in directing the migration of *c-kit*-expressing cells, as can be demonstrated *in vitro*, and detailed mutant analysis is consistent in showing that migration patterns vary according to the local availability of SCF.[52] A factor that appears to be important for melanocyte differentiation and/or survival is the transcription factor Mitf, which marks what may be melanocyte precursors in the dorsal neural tube.

Cranial neural crest

In the head region, crest cells leaving the caudal diencephalon, midbrain and hindbrain neural folds invade a variety of peripheral territories, including most of the presumptive facial and branchial region where they have a wide range of mesenchymal fates in addition to the neurogenic and melanogenic fates of the trunk crest. The mesenchyme that derives from the neural crest is referred to as ectomesenchyme to distinguish it from the otherwise similar tissue of mesodermal origin. Caudal diencephalic and midbrain-derived ectomesenchyme contributes to the cartilages of anterior cranial base (trabeculae cranii/mesethmoid) middle ear elements (malleus and incus), and Meckel's cartilage (first branchial arch), together with the dermal bones of the calvaria and ensheathing bones of the face (e.g. maxilla and mandible). Neural derivatives of forebrain and midbrain crest include parasympathetic ganglia (otic, sphenopalatine), neurons of the dorsomedial (DM) half of the trigeminal (sensory) ganglion and the Schwann cells of the rostral cranial nerves. Hindbrain crest also contributes to parasympathetic ganglia and to the DM regions of the remaining cranial sensory ganglia, and the Schwann cell population. Its ectomesenchyme joins midbrain crest in making the jaws and other first-arch structures (e.g. the ear ossicles, including the stapes) but contributes exclusively to their more caudal segmental homologues (second- and third-arch skeletal and connective tissues). Crest cells from the vagal region (the post-otic hindbrain, opposite the most rostral somites) migrate in several directions: some go towards the cardiac outflow tract, contributing smooth muscle cells to the arterial walls, some invade the developing pharynx and gut to contribute to the ENS, some migrate dorsolaterally to generate melanocytes, while others migrate locally to produce neurons and glia of the IXth and Xth cranial nerve ganglia and the superior cervical (sympathetic) ganglion.

How the cranial neural crest came to acquire its mesenchymal range of fates (connective tissue, cartilage, bone, dentine, etc.), and thereby usurp the expected role of the mesodermal germ layer, is a matter for conjecture. Presumably it happened in early vertebrates, close to their origin from chordates. The rostral expansion of the neural plate to provide sufficient precursor material for the enlarged brain may have left little room for the development of mesoderm (whose principal contribution is to head muscles) and a secondary source of mesenchymal cells was recruited. Indeed, there is more than a superficial resemblance between mesoderm formation in the primitive streak and neural crest formation. In mammals, the cranial neural crest begins its migration long before the neural tube closes, possibly as a consequence of the relatively large size of the mammalian brain, already obvious at the neural plate stage, and its correspondingly retarded neurulation.

However, it is not yet clear that the difference in fate between trunk and head actually reflects a difference in the potential of their respective neural crest populations. It remains possible that the neural crest of the two regions has identical or closely similar potentials but that in the head there is an additional source of emigrating cells, distinct from the neural crest itself. Fate mapping studies in chick have revealed that single cells in the surface ectoderm lateral to the cranial neural folds generate cell clones that populate exclusively the mesenchymal tissues, whereas single cells that lie in the cranial neural folds themselves generate exclusively ganglion cells and melanocytes.[53] Although these results suggest a distinction between the neural fold and the epidermal ectoderm as separate sources of migratory cells, tissue culture studies are needed to examine the range of potential of these different regions. However, what is suggested is that the evolutionary origin of head ectomesenchyme may have been distinct from that of the neural crest proper. Consistent with ectomesenchyme and neural crest lineages being distinct, the zebrafish *colourless* mutation results in severe defects to derivatives of the neural crest proper (neurons, glia and melanocytes) but leaves the ectomesenchyme untouched.[54] This phenotype suggests that there would be a precursor that is restricted to neural and melanogenic fates, consistent with the notion that ectomesenchyme and neural crest may indeed be distinct cell lineages.

Prepatterning of the cranial crest

Heterotopic grafting experiments using chick–quail chimeras have suggested that the neural crest at hindbrain levels is specified morphogenetically prior to its migration from the neural primordium.[55] When presumptive first (mandibular) arch crest is grafted in place of second (hyoid) arch crest, the embryo develops a tandem set of first-arch cartilages in place of hyoid structures, together with a reduplicated arrangement of first-arch musculature and connective tissues. This suggests not only that the axial identity of the crest must be determined at a premigratory stage but also that the neural crest cells dictate pattern to the surrounding mesoderm from which the muscle cells are derived. That the mesoderm is indeed a passive player in branchial patterning is also shown by the phenotype of the zebrafish *chinless* mutant[56] and by avian chimeras in which trunk somites are grafted alongside the hindbrain in place of the unsegmented paraxial mesoderm.[57] Here, presumably under the patterning influence of the resident cranial neural crest, the transplanted cells make morphologically normal extrinsic ocular muscles which receive normal oculomotor, trochlear and abducens innervation.

Candidates for encoding the prepattern exhibited by cranial neural crest populations are the *Hox* genes, which display appropriate expression in the parent rhombencephalon and which, through gain- or loss-of-function experiments, have been shown to be essential regulators of head development. For example, loss of *Hoxa2* function in mice produces a craniofacial phenotype that is similar to that of the reduplicated first-arch experiment referred to above—in the absence of *Hoxa2*, the second arch develops a complete set of proximal first-arch structures, including malleus, incus and tympanic bone, in tandem position (but mirror image orientation) with the normal first-arch structures.[58]

Migration of the cranial neural crest into the branchial arches

The finding that the cranial neural crest is prepatterned, and that it imposes patterning information on tissues in its migration environment, predicts that its migration would be orchestrated sufficiently for this patterning information to be faithfully retained during the process. In order to produce the segmental series of cranial ganglia that flank the hindbrain (Fig. 3.9A), together with their associated branchial arch tissues, there would be expected to exist some mechanism for maintaining the AP position of origin of the crest as it flows ventrally, and for preventing the mixing between adjacent streams of cells. Because there are no somites anterior to the otocyst, the segmental patterning of neural crest derivatives cannot be based on a mechanism involving somite polarity, as is the case for the dorsal root ganglia. Instead, it appears that the crest outflow from the hindbrain neural folds is itself segmented, in direct correspondence with the pronounced segmentation of its parent neuroepithelium into an iterated series of rhombomeres (see Chapter 3). In chick and mouse embryos, crest cells are formed by rhombomeres 1 and 2 (contributing to the trigeminal ganglion and the first branchial arch ectomesenchyme), rhombomere 4 (facial and vestibuloacoustic ganglia and second branchial arch ectomesenchyme) and rhombomeres 6 and 7 (superior and jugular ganglia and third branchial arch ectomesenchyme).[59–61] Between these crest-producing rhombomeres are two rhombomeres, 3 and 5, that produce little migratory neural crest.[59] Thus, in the rhombencephalon the neural crest originates from three discontinuous levels and migrates ventrally in three distinct streams (Fig. 5.6).

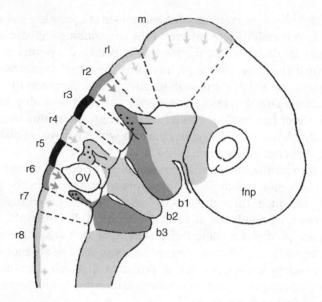

Figure 5.6 The branchial neural crest originates from midbrain and hindbrain levels of the neuraxis, with each rhombomere (r) of origin contributing crest cells to a specific branchial arch territory (b), and to the cranial ganglia associated with the arches. Although the branchial crest is produced in a continuous column from rhombomere 8 up to the midbrain, the majority of crest cells produced by r3 and r5 are removed by apoptosis before migration. Remnant cells from these rhombomeres (black dots) can be found in the ganglia. Crest from the posterior diencephalon (not shown) migrates above the eye to the frontonasal process (fnp).

   The dorsal median aspect of r3 and r5 is associated with elevated levels of cell death, suggesting that neural crest cell production is continuous along the neuraxis but that many crest cells are eliminated from r3 and r5 before emigration, consistent with the small number of r3- or r5-derived cells that contribute to the pharyngeal region.[61,62] *In vitro* studies have shown that odd-numbered rhombomeres will produce neural crest if they are freed from the influence of even-numbered rhombomeres.[63] Thus, even-numbered rhombomeres appear to exert a repressive effect upon the production of neural crest by odd-numbered rhombomeres, most likely through the induction of cell death. The apoptotic elimination of neural crest cells in r3 and r5 involves the induction of high-level BMP4 expression in the neural crest primordium, which stimulates expression of the homeobox gene *Msx2*.[64] Thus, the sculpting of the neural crest into discrete streams which populate and pattern the branchial arches involves a mechanism that is intrinsic to the neuroepithelium with a contribution by local signalling between rhombomeres (Fig. 5.7). The use of BMP4 as a death signal for cranial crest cells would seem a curious reversal of its earlier role as an inducer of the neural crest and as an agent involved in sympathetic crest cell differentiation. However, the competence state of the cell and its available intracellular signalling pathways change during development; cell death is an alternative fate for rhombencephalic crest cells at this stage. It is pertinent to consider that probably thousands of proteins are involved in *intracellular* signalling,

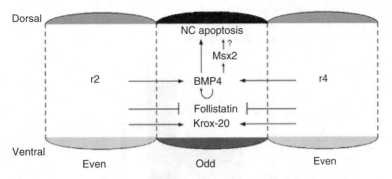

Figure 5.7 An interactive mechanism controls the expression of BMP4 and Msx2 in rhombomeres 3 and 5 and subsequent apoptosis of their neural crest cells. Expression of the transcription factor Krox-20 in r3 is controlled by a separate interaction with the even-numbered rhombomeres, as is repression of the BMP antagonist follistatin.[77]

whereas those available for *intercellular* signalling number only in the tens; the same signal molecules must be used repeatedly for different functions.

The significance of the sculpting process whereby cell death leaves the emergent crest divided into discrete segmental streams that would simply migrate ventrally into appropriate arches is that it suggests a way the embryo might retain the fidelity of patterning information during its transfer from the hindbrain. In chick, the adjacent streams are initially separated by gaps due to cell death, so there may be little opportunity for mixing between the streams.[65] In other species, such as *Xenopus*, where the loss of crest cells in r3 and r5 is less prominent, there is another mechanism that acts to prevent such mixing. This involves the ephrin–Eph receptor system that has also been implicated in the migration of neural crest cells through the somite sclerotome.

In *Xenopus*, the receptors EphA4 and EphB1 are expressed in the neural crest and mesoderm of the third arch, while the cognate ligand ephrin-B2 is expressed in the crest and mesoderm of the neighbouring second arch. Blocking receptor function (by injecting RNA encoding truncated receptor lacking the intracellular kinase domain into the two-cell embryo) results in third-arch crest cells migrating aberrantly in the second and fourth arches.[66] In accordance with the repulsion model of ephrin–Eph receptor interaction (see Chapter 9), this suggests that adjacent streams of the cranial crest may be prevented from intermingling as they migrate into branchial arch territory by mutual repulsion between cells at the borders of the streams (Fig. 5.8).

The anteroposterior identity of premigratory cranial neural crest cells appears to be preprogrammed in the context of the cellular community—that is, pre-specification is manifested by a group of cells in the dorsal hindbrain in contact with neighbours of like specification. When single or dispersed neural crest cells are transplanted heterotopically, they are isolated from any community effect with their normal neighbours and become labile, adopting the molecular expression and fitting into the pattern dictated by their new neighbours.[67] However, it is

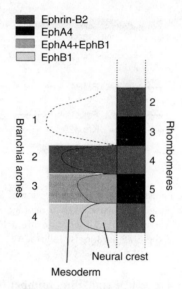

Figure 5.8 A model for restricted migration of neural crest cells to the branchial arches of *Xenopus*. EphA4 receptors are expressed in rhombomeres 3 and 5; their ephrin-B2 ligands are expressed in r2, r4 and r6. Ephrin-B2 is also expressed in second-arch neural crest and mesoderm whereas these cells express both EphB1 and EphA4 in the third arch. Repulsive interaction at the interface between ligand- and receptor-bearing cells serves to segregate second- and third-arch cells. After Smith *et al.*[66]

uncertain what significance can be attached to such findings, other than that determination in respect of branchial pattern is a property of the segmental crest subpopulation as a whole. As we have described for forebrain neurons (Chapter 3), a community effect, whereby similar cells enjoy mutual reinforcement of their specification state, seems to be required to maintain nascent regional identity.

Influence of the local environment on cell type differentiation

The above discussion has focused on the early determination of the cranial neural crest with respect to pattern, that is the spatial arrangement of cells, and has avoided the question of how diverse cell types are ultimately produced by the immigrant neural crest population. Here, it is clear that premigratory cells are not determined but remain multipotent for a range of possible ectomesenchymal fates. Local signals in the environment are necessary to elicit cell type differentiation in the branchial arches. For example, mutation of either the ligand Endothelin-1 (Et-1, secreted by the mesodermal central core of the arches, surface ectoderm and pharyngeal endoderm) or its type A receptor (EndrA, expressed on postmigratory neural crest cells) results in loss or hypoplasia of the arch cartilages.[68,69] Prior to the manifestation of defective chondogenesis, the branchial neural crest cells of both mutants fail to express the bHLH transcription factor dHAND.[70] Thus, neural crest cells must normally receive Et-1 signals from their local surroundings in order to translate nascent pattern into differentiated structure.

Neurogenic placodes

Neurogenic placodes are the major source of primary sensory neurons in the heads of vertebrate embryos.[71,72] All of the neurogenic placodes are focal thickenings of the surface ectoderm, forming bilaterally, but three distinct types can be recognized on the basis of position and developmental origin—olfactory, dorsolateral and epibranchial. The olfactory placodes are the most anterior, lying on either side of the rostral tip of the forebrain vesicle, and give rise to the olfactory epithelium and its sensory neurons. The dorsolateral placodes form directly alongside the hindbrain and include the trigeminal placode, which contributes neurons to the ventrolateral (VL) portion of the trigeminal ganglion, and the otic placode, which produces the inner ear and its associated sensory cells, together with the vestibular and auditory ganglia. In aquatic lower vertebrates, the dorsolateral series is augmented by placodes of the lateral line system which develop both rostral and caudal to the otic placode and form the mechanosensory neuromast organs. The epibranchial placodes form further ventrolaterally, each at the dorsal corner of a branchial cleft, and their neurons are distinct from those of the dorsolateral placodes in that they express the homeobox gene *Phox2a*.[73] In amniotes, the epibranchial series includes the geniculate, the petrosal and the nodose placodes, which form, respectively, the inferior ganglia of the VIIth, IXth and Xth cranial nerves (Fig. 5.9). The main function of epibranchial placode-derived sensory neurons is to relay branchial and pharyngeal sensation, including gustation, to hindbrain nuclei. In fishes, which have a more extensive series of branchial arches, the epibranchial series extends further caudally. For the cranial nerve sensory ganglia as a whole, placode-derived neurons appear before those of the neural crest, and contribute a much greater number of neurons.[74]

Although neurogenic placodes share a superficially similar origin, as transient ectodermal thickenings arising in isolation from the neural plate, they have different developmental and evolutionary origins. The olfactory placodes form through a series of inductive interactions between ectoderm and the forebrain, with some involvement of adjacent ectomesenchyme. Similarly, otic placode induction requires contact or proximity to the hindbrain (see Chapter 8) together with signalling (FGF19) from the underlying mesenchyme.[75], while trigeminal placode induction remains poorly understood.

The epibranchial placodes develop in proximity to neural crest ectomesenchyme and pharyngeal endoderm, both of which have been proposed as inducing tissues[74] despite an earlier observation, recently confirmed using molecular markers,[73] that

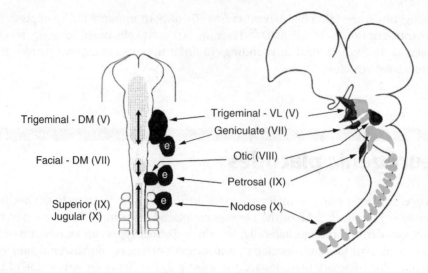

Figure 5.9 The majority of neurons of the cranial sensory ganglia develop from neurogenic ectodermal placodes (black). The rest of the neurons and all of the glia develop from neural crest cells (stippled/grey). The trigeminal placode forms the ventrolateral neurons of the Vth nerve ganglion, whereas the dorsomedial half contains neurons of rhombomere 1 and 2 neural crest origin. The Otic placode forms the otocyst, its sensory epithelium and the neurons of the VIIIth nerve ganglia. The remaining three placodes are epibranchial (e) and contribute neurons to the ventral ganglia of the VIIth, IXth and Xth nerves. The dorsal ganglia of these nerves contain neurons of crest origin. After D'Amico-Martel and Noden[72] and Le Douarin.[78]

epibranchial placodes and their neurons form normally after crest ablation. Furthermore, this study[73] has shown that pharyngeal endoderm can induce placodal neurons to form in cranial ectoderm but that trunk ectoderm is refractory to the inducer. A feature common to all neurogenic placodes is that each forms at a specific location within an ectodermal sheet which is broadly competent. Because most of the cranial ectoderm is competent to make neurogenic placodes of one form or other, it would seem likely that the inducing tissues both provide the focus of the induction and decide the choice of fate. Meeting these expectations is the signalling molecule BMP7, which is expressed at the specific site where cranial ectoderm meets pharyngeal endoderm at the tops of the branchial clefts, and can induce $Phox2a^+$ placodal sensory neurons in isolated cranial ectoderm, an effect which can be blocked by the BMP antagonist follistatin.

Key points

1 Neural crest cells contribute the major part of the peripheral nervous system (neurons and glia) as well as differentiating into a wide variety of non-neural cell types, including melanocytes and (in the head region only) connective tissue, cartilage and bone-forming cells.

2 Emergence of crest cells from the neural folds involves an epithelial to mesenchymal transition marked by a change in the expression of adhesion molecules.

3 A gradient of BMP activity across the mediolateral axis of the ectoderm is thought to be responsible for inducing the neural crest (within a particular range of concentration) and for positioning the crest domain between epidermal ectoderm and the neural plate. Local signals are probably also involved.

4 In the trunk region, the neural crest migrates along two distinct pathways. The first of these is ventral, between the neural tube and somites, where derivatives include dorsal root and sympathetic ganglia. The second is dorsal, beneath the epidermal ectoderm, where the crest cells differentiate into melanocytes.

5 Cell fate decisions depend on local interactions in the migration site, as for the action of BMPs produced by the aorta in inducing sympathetic neurons.

6 Several ligand–receptor systems exist that are crucial for the migration, proliferation and survival of crest cell lineages. A well-worked example is the action of environmental GDNF on c-ret receptor-bearing crest cells in the developing enteric nervous system.

7 The choice of neuron versus glia in the dorsal root ganglia may depend on Notch–Delta signalling and lateral specification interactions taking place within the crest cell population itself.

8 Sympathetic neurons differentiate from neural crest cells that have been exposed to BMPs emanating from the dorsal aorta.

9 Hindbrain level neural crest contributes to the cranial sensory ganglia and its ectomesenchyme fills the branchial arches. Both neurogenic and ectomesen-chymal crest populations have a segmental origin from specific rhombomeres and are morphogenetically prespecified before leaving the neural tube.

10 Two mechanisms are known that segregate the streams of branchial crest cells and prevent their mixing—patterned apoptosis depletes crest cells in rhombomeres 3 and 5; Eph–ephrin interaction causes repulsion between adjoining streams.

11 The majority of neurons of cranial sensory ganglia (but not the glia) arise from ectodermal placodes. Those placodes that form in the branchial clefts, the epibranchial placodes, are induced in competent ectoderm by endodermal BMP7 signalling.

General reading

■ Le Douarin, N. M. and Kalcheim, C. *The neural crest*, 445pp (Cambridge University Press, 1999).

References

1. Narayanan, C. H. and Narayanan, Y. Determination of the embryonic origin of the mesencephalic nucleus of the trigeminal nerve in birds. *J. Embryol. Exp. Morphol.* **43**, 85–105 (1978).

2. Marchant, L., Linker, C., Ruiz, P., Guerrero, N. and Mayor, R. The inductive properties of mesoderm suggest that the neural crest cells are specified by a BMP gradient. *Dev. Biol.* **198**, 319–29 (1998).

3. Nguyen, V. H. *et al.* Ventral and lateral regions of the zebrafish gastrula, including the neural crest progenitors, are established by a bmp2b/swirl pathway of genes. *Dev. Biol.* **199**, 93–110 (1998).

4. Liem, K. F., Tremml, G., Roelink, H. and Jessell, T. M. Dorsal differentiation of neural plate cells induced by BMP-mediated signals from epidermal ectoderm. *Cell* **82**, 969–79 (1995).

5. Ikeya, M., Lee, S. M., Johnson, J. E., McMahon, A. P. and Takada, S. Wnt signalling is required for expansion of neural crest and CNS progenitors. *Nature* **389**, 966–70 (1997).

6. Moury, J. D. and Jacobson, A. G. The origins of neural crest cells in the axolotl. *Dev. Biol.* **141**, 243–53 (1990).

7. Dickinson, M. E., Sellecek, M., McMahon, A. P. and Bronner-Fraser, M. Dorsalization of the neural tube by the non-neural ectoderm. *Development* **121**, 2099–106 (1995).

8. Selleck, M. and Bronner-Fraser, M. Origins of the avian neural crest: the role of neural plate–epidermal interactions. *Development* **121**, 525–38 (1995).

9. Selleck, M., Garcia-Castro, M. I., Artinger, K. B. and Bronner-Fraser, M. Effects of Shh and Noggin on neural crest formation demonstrate that BMP is required in the neural tube but not ectoderm. *Development* **125**, 4919–30 (1998).

10. Nieto, M. A., Sargent, M. G., Wilkinson, D. G. and Cooke, J. Control of cell behavior during vertebrate development by *Slug*, a zinc finger gene. *Science* **264**, 835–9 (1994).

11. Nakagawa, S. and Takeichi, M. Neural crest cell–cell adhesion controlled by sequential and subpopulation-specific expression of novel cadherins. *Development* **121**, 1321–32 (1995).

12. Edelman, G. M. Cell adhesion molecules. *Science* **219**, 450–7 (1983).

13. Hatta, K., Takagi, S., Fujisawa, H. and Takeichi, M. Spatial and temporal expression pattern of N-cadherin cell adhesion molecules

correlated with morphogenetic processes of chicken embryos. *Dev. Biol.* **120**, 215–27 (1987).

14. Nakagawa, S. and Takeichi, M. Neural crest emigration from the neural tube depends on regulated cadherin expression. *Development* **125**, 2963–71 (1998).

15. Cano, A. *et al.* The transcription factor Snail controls epithelial–mesenchymal transitions by repressing E-cadherin expression. *Nat. Cell Biol.* **2**, 76–83 (2000).

16. Liu, J.-P. and Jessell, T. M. A role for rhoB in the delamination of neural crest cells from the dorsal neural tube. *Development* **125**, 5055–67 (1998).

17. Le Douarin, N. M. and Kalcheim, C. *The neural crest* (Cambridge University Press, 1999).

18. Rickmann, M., Fawcett, J. W. and Keynes, R. J. The migration of neural crest cells and the growth of motor axons through the rostral half of the chick somite. *J. Embryol. Exp. Morphol.* **90**, 437–55 (1985).

19. Dorsky, R. I., Moon, R. T. and Raible, D. W. Control of neural crest cell fate by the Wnt signalling pathway. *Nature* **396**, 370–2 (1998).

20. Perris, R. The extracellular matrix in neural crest cell migration. *Trends Neurosci.* **20**, 23–31 (1997).

21. Jesuthasan, S. Contact inhibition/collapse and pathfinding of neural crest cells in the zebrafish trunk. *Development* **122**, 381–9 (1996).

22. Saga, Y., Yagi, T., Ikawa, Y., Sakakura, T. and Aizawa, S. Mice develop normally without tenascin. *Genes Dev.* **6**, 1821–31 (1992).

23. Keynes, R. J., Johnson, A. R., Pini, A., Tannahill, D. and Cook, G. Spinal nerve segmentation in higher vertebrates: axon guidance by repulsion and attraction. *Semin. Neurosci.* **8**, 339–45 (1996).

24. Krull, C. E., Collazo, A., Fraser, S. E. and Bronner-Fraser, M. Segmental migration of trunk neural crest: time-lapse analysis reveals a role for PNA-binding molecules. *Development* **121**, 3733–43 (1995).

25. Krull, C. E. *et al.* Interactions of Eph-related receptors and ligands confer rostrocaudal pattern to trunk neural crest migration. *Curr. Biol.* **7**, 571–80 (1997).

26. Wang, H. U. and Anderson, D. J. Eph family transmembrane ligands can mediate repulsive guidance of trunk neural crest migration and motor axon outgrowth. *Neuron* **18**, 383–96 (1997).

27. Debby-Brafman, A., Burstyn-Cohen, T., Klar, A. and Kalcheim, C. F-Spondin, expressed in somite regions avoided by neural crest cells, mediates inhibition of distinct somite domains to neural crest migration. *Neuron* **22**, 475–88 (1999).

28. Bronner-Fraser, M. Alterations in neural crest migration by a monoclonal antibody that affects cell adhesion. *J. Cell Biol.* **101**, 610–17 (1985).

29. Kil, S. H., Lallier, T. and Bronner-Fraser, M. Inhibition of cranial neural crest adhesion *in vitro* and migration *in vivo* using integrin antisense oligonucleotides. *Dev. Biol.* **179**, 91–101 (1996).

30. Wakamatsu, Y., Maynard, T. M. and Weston, J. A. Fate determination of neural crest cells by NOTCH-mediated lateral inhibition and asymmetrical cell division during gangliogenesis. *Development* **127**, 2811–21 (2000).

31. Lo, L., Tiveron, M. C. and Anderson, D. J. MASH1 activates expression of the paired homeodomain transcription factor Phox2a, and couples pan-neuronal and subtype specific components of autonomic neuronal identity. *Development* **125**, 609–20 (1998).

32. Goridis, C. and Brunet, J.-F. Transcriptional control of neurotransmitter phenotype. *Curr. Opin. Neurobiol.* **9**, 47–53 (1999).

33. Stanke, M. *et al.* The Phox2 homeodomain proteins are sufficient to promote the development of sympathetic neurons. *Development* **126**, 4087–94 (1999).

34. Shah, N. M., Groves, A. K. and Anderson, D. J. Alternative neural crest cell fates are instructively promoted by TGFbeta superfamily members. *Cell* **85**, 332–43 (1996).

35. Reissman, E. *et al.* Involvement of bone morphogenetic protein-4 and BMP-7 in the differentiation of the adrenergic phenotype in developing sensory neurons. *Development* **122**, 2079–88 (1996).

36. Patterson, P. H. and Chun, L. L. Y. The induction of acetylcholine synthesis in primary cultures of dissociated rat sympathetic neurons. *Dev. Biol.* **56**, 263–80 (1977).

37. Yamamori, T. *et al.* The cholinergic neuronal differentiation factor from heart cells is identical to leukaemia inhibitory factor. *Science* **246**, 1412–16 (1989).

38. Schotzinger, R. J. and Landis, S. C. Cholinergic phenotype developed by noradrenergic sympathetic neurons after innervation of a novel cholinergic target *in vivo*. *Nature* **335**, 637–9 (1988).

39. Guidry, G. and Landis, S. C. Target-dependent development of the vesicular acetylcholine transporter in rodent sweat glands. *Dev. Biol.* **199**, 175–84 (1998).

40. Habecker, B. A. and Landis, S. C. Noradrenergic regulation of cholinergic differentiation. *Science* **264**, 1602–4 (1994).

41. Francis, N. J. and Landis, S. C. Cellular and molecular determinants of sympathetic neuron development. *Annu Rev Neurosci*, **22**, 541–66 (1999).

42. Doupe, A., Patterson, P. H. and Landis, S. C. Environmental influences in the development of neural derivatives: glucocorticoids, growth factors and chromaffin cell plasticity. *J. Neurosci.* **5**, 2119–42 (1985).

43. Patterson, P. H. and Nawa, H. Neuronal differentiation factors/cytokines and synaptic plasticity. *Cell/Neuron Suppl.* **72/10**, 123–37 (1993).

44. Lindsay, R. M. and Harmar, A. J. Nerve growth factor regulates expression of neuropeptide genes in adult sensory neurons. *Nature* **337**, 362–4 (1989).

45. Schuchardt, A., D'Agati, V., Larsson-Blomberg, L., Constantini, F. and Pachnis, V. Defects in the kidney and enteric nervous system of mice lacking the tyrosine kinase receptor Ret. *Nature* **367**, 380–3 (1994).

46. Edery, P. *et al.* Mutations of the RET proto-oncogene in Hirschsprung's disease. *Nature* **367**, 378–80 (1994).

47. Durbec, P. L., Larsson-Blomberg, L. B., Schuchardt, A., Constantini, F. and Pachnis, V. Common origin and developmental dependence on c-ret of subsets of enteric and sympathetic neuroblasts. *Development* **122**, 349–69 (1996).

48. Treanor, J. *et al.* Characterization of a multicomponent receptor for GDNF. *Nature* **382**, 80–3 (1996).

49. Jing, S. *et al.* GDNF-induced activation of the Ret protein tyrosine kinase is mediated by GDNFR-alpha, a novel receptor for GNDF. *Cell* **85**, 1113–24 (1996).

50. Moore, M. W. *et al.* Renal and neuronal abnormalities in mice lacking GDNF. *Nature* **382**, 76–9 (1996).

51. Wehrle-Haller, B. and Weston, J. A. Soluble and cell-bound forms of steel factor activity play distinct roles in melanocyte precursor dispersal and survival on the lateral neural crest migration pathway. *Development* **121**, 731–42 (1995).

52. Wehrle-Haller, B. and Weston, J. A. Receptor tyrosine kinase-dependent neural crest migration in response to differentially localized growth factors. *BioEssays* **19**, 337–45 (1997).

53. Adams, N., Lumsden, A. and Weston, J. A. Origin of cranial ectomesenchyme distinct from the neural crest. In preparation.

54. Kelsh, R. N. and Eisen, J. S. The zebrafish colourless gene regulates development of

non-ectomesenchymal neural crest derivatives. *Development* **127**, 515–25 (2000).

55. Noden, D. The role of the neural crest in patterning of avian cranial skeletal, connective and muscle tissue. *Dev. Biol.* **96**, 144–65 (1983).

56. Schilling, T. F., Walker, C. and Kimmel, C. B. The chinless mutation and neural crest interactions in zebrafish jaw development. *Development* **122**, 1417–26 (1996).

57. Noden, D. Patterning of avian craniofacial muscles. *Dev. Biol.* **116**, 347–56 (1996).

58. Rijli, F. M. A homeotic transformation is generated in the rostral branchial region of the head by disruption of Hoxa-2, which acts as a selector gene. *Cell* **75**, 1333–49 (1993).

59. Lumsden, A., Sprawson, N. and Graham, A. Segmental origin and migration of neural crest cells in the hindbrain region of the chick embryo. *Development* **113**, 1281–91 (1991).

60. Serbedzija, G., Fraser, S. E. and Bronner-Fraser, M. Vital dye analysis of cranial neural crest migration in the mouse embryo. *Development* **118**, 691–703 (1992).

61. Koentges, G. and Lumsden, A. Rhombencephalic neural crest segmentation is preserved throughout craniofacial ontogeny. *Development* **122**, 3229–42 (1996).

62. Sechrist, J., Serbedzija, G., Scherson, T., Fraser, S. E. and Bronner-Fraser, M. Segmental migration of the hindbrain neural crest does not arise from its segmental generation. *Development* **118**, 691–703 (1993).

63. Graham, A., Heyman, I. and Lumsden, A. Even-numbered rhombomeres control the apoptotic elimination of neural crest cells from odd-numbered rhombomeres in the chick hindbrain. *Development* **119**, 233–45 (1993).

64. Graham, A., Francis-West, P., Brickell, P. and Lumsden, A. The signalling molecule BMP4 mediates apoptosis in the rhombencephalic neural crest. *Nature* **372**, 684–6 (1994).

65. Kulesa, P. M. and Fraser, S. E. In ovo time-lapse analysis of chick hindbrain neural crest cell migration shows cell interactions during migration to the branchial arches. *Development* **127**, 1161–72 (2000).

66. Smith, A., Robinson, V., Patel, K. and Wilkinson, D. G. The EphA4 and EphB1 receptor tyrosine kinases and ephrin-B2 ligand regulate targeted migration of branchial neural crest cells. *Curr. Biol.* **7**, 561–70 (1997).

67. Trainor, P. and Krumlauf, R. Plasticity in mouse neural crest cells reveals a new patterning role for cranial mesoderm. *Nat. Cell Biol.* **2**, 96–102 (2000).

68. Kurihara, Y. *et al.* Elevated blood pressure and craniofacial abnormalities in mice deficient in endothelin-1. *Nature* **368**, 703–10 (1994).

69. Clouthier, D. E. *et al.* Cranial and cardiac neural crest defects in endothelin-A receptor-deficient mice. *Development* **125**, 813–24 (1998).

70. Thomas, T. *et al.* A signalling cascade involving endothelin-1, dHAND, and Msx1 regulates development of neural crest-derived branchial arch mesenchyme. *Development* **125**, 3005–14 (1998).

71. Ayer-Le Lievre, C. and Le Douarin, N. M. The early development of cranial sensory ganglia and the potentialities of their component cells in quail–chick chimeras. *Dev. Biol.* **94**, 291–310 (1982).

72. D'Amico-Martel, A. and Noden, D. M. Contributions of placodal and neural crest cells to avian cranial peripheral ganglia. *Am. J. Anat.* **166**, 445–68 (1983).

73. Begbie, J., Brunet, J.-F., Rubenstein, J. and Graham, A. Induction of the epibranchial placodes. *Development* **126**, 895–902 (1999).

74. Webb, J. F. and Noden, D. M. Ectodermal placodes: contributions to the development of the vertebrate head. *Am. Zool.* **33**, 434–47 (1993).

75. Ladher, R. K., *et al.*, Identification of synergistic signals initiating inner ear development. *Science* **290**, 1965–8 (2000).

76. Chitnis, A. B. Control of neurogenesis—lessons from frogs, fish and flies. *Curr. Opin. Neurobiol.* **9**, 18–25 (1999).

77. Graham, A. and Lumsden, A. Interactions between rhombomeres modulate Krox-20 and follistatin expression in the chick embryo hindbrain. *Development* **122**, 473–80 (1996).

78. Le Douarin, N. Cephalic placodes and neurogenesis. *Trends Neurosci.* **9**, 175–80 (1986).

6

Glia and Myelination

As well as making contacts with other neurons at synapses, nerve cells interact intimately with glial cells. Most axons have a close association with glial cells and usually each axon has a near-complete covering of glial cells throughout its length. Exceptionally in vertebrates, the smallest unmyelinated CNS axons are not ensheathed by glial processes and these axons lie directly next to one another.[1] The axon-associated glia of the vertebrate peripheral nervous system are the Schwann cells. These are derived from the neural crest, with a small additional contribution from the ventral neural tube, and their precursors migrate into the periphery (see Chapter 4) to differentiate into adult Schwann cells under the control of axons (see below). Also derived from the neural crest are the satellite cells associated with the peripheral ganglia, and the enteric glia. The equivalent central glia are the oligo-dendrocytes and the astrocytes, which originate from progenitor cells in the ventri-cular zone of the neural tube (see Chapter 1). The CNS also contains the microglia, the resident macrophages of the nervous system, and these derive from a population of mesoderm cells of the monocyte lineage which enter the developing CNS during early development.[2] Axons and glia develop together in maturing peripheral nerves and central pathways, and influence each other's phenotype (and probably survival) throughout life. Glia also associate with the cell bodies of neurons and the synaptic regions of the CNS.

Glia are essential for the working of the nervous system. By separating axons from each other they prevent electrical excitation of axons by nerve impulses in their neighbours, and myelination speeds impulse propagation by altering axon cable properties. Astrocytes possess ligand-gated ion channels, are electrically coupled by gap junctions, and can propagate long-range changes in intracellular calcium ion concentration, so they may contribute to information processing in the CNS. By participating in the formation of the blood–brain and blood–nerve barriers, glia also help to keep the environment of the nervous system relatively well protected from chemical fluctuations in the blood, and they act as a sink for excess potassium ions and transmitters (especially glutamate) liberated during nervous activity. Glia prob-ably control the entry of inflammatory cells into the CNS, thus minimizing the likelihood of potentially damaging inflammation. Recent evidence suggests that they have important trophic effects on neurons, and during development specialized glial cells are involved in guiding migrating neurons (see Chapter 7). Following injury in the adult they have profound effects on the success (Schwann cells) or failure (oligodendrocytes and astrocytes) of reinnervation by regrowth of cut axons (see Chapter 17).

Determination of glial fate in the CNS

The study of glial differentiation in the rat optic nerve provides a good example of the analytical power of the *in vitro* approach in studying the control of neural cell fate in the vertebrate nervous system. Progenitor cells can be harvested from the neonatal nerve as homogeneous populations of almost 100 per cent purity, and their environment can be manipulated more precisely than *in vivo*.[3] A variety of markers can be used to distinguish three different glial phenotypes: oligodendrocytes (which myelinate the optic axons), and type 1 and type 2 astrocytes (Fig. 6.1). Oligodendrocytes and type 2 astrocytes derive postnatally from a bipotential precursor cell, the O-2A progenitor, while type 1 astrocytes arise before birth from a different precursor. O-2A proliferation can be driven *in vitro* by conditioned medium derived from type 1 astrocytes, and by the growth factors PDGF, NT-3 and IGF-1, which are synthesized by astrocytes, but after a maximum of about eight rounds of division the cells exit the cell cycle and differentiate. The culture conditions also influence cell fate, low serum

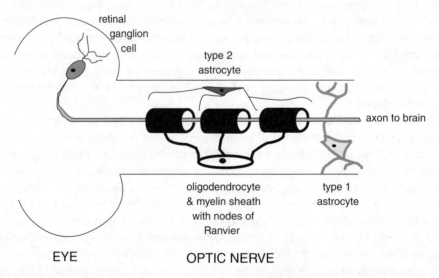

Figure 6.1 Glial cells in the developing rat optic nerve. Oligodendrocytes myelinate the retinal ganglion cell axons, while processes from type 2 astrocytes associate with the nodes of Ranvier.

concentrations favouring oligodendrocyte differentiation and certain growth factors, such as CNTF, favouring astrocyte differentiation. The decision to become postmitotic is further dependent on the presence of small hydrophobic molecules such as thyroid hormone and retinoic acid, for O-2A proliferation continues unchecked without them.[4] Such behaviour suggests the existence in O-2A cells of a mitogen-dependent clock that determines the readiness of cells to exit the cycle; a cell can differentiate provided its time has come, and provided the hydrophobic effector signals are also present. However, just what form the clock takes is unknown. It does not work through counting the number of cell divisions, for O-2A cells stop dividing and differentiate after fewer divisions when cultured at 33°C rather than 37°C.[5] Instead, it may involve the decay of a cell cycle stimulator such as a cyclin or cyclin-dependent kinase, and/or accumulation to a critical threshold level of an inhibitor, such as the cyclin-dependent kinase inhibitor, p27, whose concentration builds up in O2-A cells as they proliferate.[6]

Whether the intrinsic timer of O2-A cells operates *in vivo* is less certain at present, but the importance of an adequate supply of PDGF for oligodendrocyte development has been confirmed by the phenotype of PDGF knockout mice (specifically, the isoform PDGF-AA). These animals die shortly after birth, with accompanying CNS dysmyelination, and their spinal cords contain less than 10 per cent of the normal population of O2-A progenitors.[7] The CNS is hypomyelinated, moreover, in *Igf1* null mutant mice.[8] *In vivo* it is likely that axons also provide mitogenic signals for the oligodendrocyte lineage, and both neuronally-derived PDGF[9] and neuregulin signalling by axons[10] (see below) have been implicated here. Another critical factor may be the level of electrical activity in axons; intraocular injection of tetrodotoxin (which blocks activity in optic axons) reduces proliferation of oligodendrocyte progenitors by some 80 per cent, and one mechanism could be that electrical activity augments mitogen production by astrocytes.[11]

Different CNS tracts in an individual species are myelinated reliably on schedule during development, so the precise timing of oligodendrocyte differentiation and myelination is presumably subject to rigorous control. It is perhaps not surprising, then, that axons also appear to exert negative regulation on oligodendrocyte differentiation through the Notch signalling pathway (see Chapter 4). In the developing rat optic nerve, oligodendrocytes and their precursors express Notch1 receptors, while retinal axons simultaneously express Jagged1, a Notch1 ligand. As myelination proceeds, expression of Jagged1 decreases on a parallel time course, a correlation consistent with the possibility that axons inhibit oligodendrocyte differentiation by Notch activation until a critical stage is reached when myelination can proceed. Such a mechanism could serve to ensure that the stock of available oligodendrocyte precursor cells is not exhausted prematurely, and could also help to maintain small numbers of precursor cells in the adult brain (see Chapter 17).[12]

Glial origins and migration in the neural tube

The question of the precise anatomical origins of glial lineages has been studied in the spinal cord. When the early developing rat spinal cord is divided into dorsal and ventral regions and cultured *in vitro*, only the ventral region furnishes oligodendrocytes.[13] The availability of markers for the O-2A progenitors, such as the PDGF alpha-receptor (PDGFRα), has revealed that the earliest progenitors may originate as a distinct subset of cells close to the floor plate of the neural tube, extending into the hindbrain, midbrain and ventral diencephalon.[14-16] Moreover, like motor neurons and some interneurons (see Chapter 3), their specification depends on signals derived from the floor plate, and these can be mimicked by Sonic hedgehog (SHH) protein.[17] This raises in turn the possibility that motor neurons and oligodendrocytes share a common precursor in the ventral neural tube,[18] as suggested also by lineage analysis of the chick spinal cord using retroviral labelling (Fig. 6.2).[19] The anatomy of oligodendrocyte origins in the spinal cord has proved somewhat controversial, however. Fate-mapping studies using quail–chick grafting have favoured a wider origin,

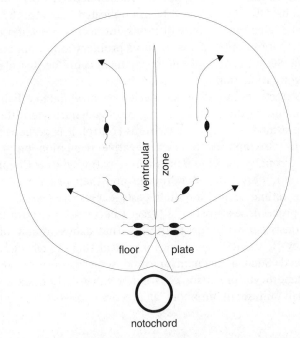

Figure 6.2 Origin of oligodendrocytes from the ventral part of the developing spinal cord, in the ventricular zone just dorsal to the floor plate. Cells subsequently migrate (*arrows*) to colonize the rest of the spinal cord.

including dorsal regions of the neural tube,[20] and the same conclusion comes from experiments using transplants into the neonatal mouse CNS of fragments of embryonic mouse neural tube genetically engineered to express *lacZ* exclusively in oligodendrocytes.[21] A more recent study using chick–quail grafting has confirmed, nevertheless, that only ventral grafts generate oligodendrocytes, while astrocytes arise from both dorsal and ventral regions of the neural tube.[22] Whether different astrocyte subtypes derive from regionally restricted domains of the neuroepithelium remains to be determined.

A localized origin for the oligodendrocyte lineage would imply that these cells must migrate long distances to reach their target axons in the developing white matter. Migration in the radial direction could be guided by radial glial cells, while migration in the dorsoventral and longitudinal axes could be guided by earlier-developing axon tracts. A good example is provided by the oligodendrocyte precursors of the optic nerve, which originate at the ventral midline of the third ventricle and migrate in the developing nerve in close association with axons.[23] Precursor cells, but not mature oligodendrocytes, are motile in culture, and it is likely that migrating cells *in vivo* are also proliferative, in contrast to migrating neuroblasts which are postmitotic. Oligodendrocyte progenitors express a sub-population of integrin receptors that may mediate interactions with the extra-cellular matrix of the developing CNS,[24] and their migration *in vitro* is inhibited by removal of polysialic acid from NCAM and by Tenascin-C.[25] Much, however, remains to be learned about this process.

Control of glial numbers in the CNS

The same growth factors that are mitogens for oligodendrocyte progenitors also promote their survival, and the study of this system has emphasized the parallel role of cell death (see Chapter 13) in determining final numbers of differentiated oligo-dendrocytes. Excess numbers of oligodendrocytes are generated during normal development and undergo elimination by apoptosis.[26] Overall population size may be controlled by mitogen availability from neighbouring astrocytes and neurons, in combination with competition among newly-differentiated oligodendrocytes for axon- and astrocyte-derived survival signals (Fig. 6.3).[3] Consistent with this, over-expression of PDGF-A in transgenic mice markedly increases the size of the O2-A population, but the excess cells continue to undergo apoptosis to yield normal numbers of mature oligodendrocytes.[7] This latter finding implies that cell-survival controls dominate cell-proliferation controls in determining final cell numbers. The importance of axons is underscored by the finding that transection of the optic nerve during development severely reduces oligodendrocyte numbers,[27] presumably reflecting the requirement of the lineage for axon-derived signals such as PDGF and neuregulins (see below) for both proliferation and survival.

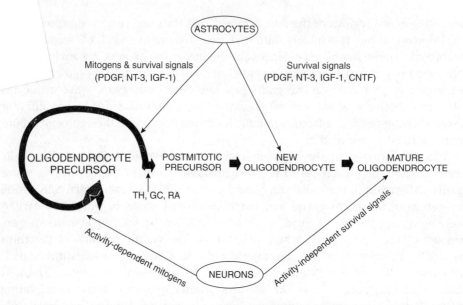

Figure 6.3 Scheme for control of the size of the oligodendrocyte population. Astrocytes and neurons provide mitogens, and newly-differentiated oligodendrocytes also compete for axon- and astrocyte-derived survival signals. After Barres and Raff.[3]

Astrocyte proliferation in the rat optic nerve is also regulated by local cell inter-actions, particularly with retinal ganglion cell axons. Section of the neonatal optic nerve blocks astrocyte division, as does the intraocular injection of colchicine, which disrupts fast axonal transport. The molecular basis for this is uncertain, but may involve the provision by axons of a member of the FGF family; only bFGF, of all signalling molecules known to be synthesized by ganglion cells, is mitogenic for cultured optic nerve astrocytes. Retinal astrocytes, on the other hand, express PDGFRα, and their numbers can be modulated by experimental perturbation of PDGF signalling by retinal neurons.[28]

Unlike oligodendrocytes, electrical activity in optic axons does not influence astrocyte proliferation, for proliferation is unaffected by intraocular injection of tetrodotoxin.[29] The further finding that neurons inhibit astrocyte proliferation in hippocampal cultures also raises the possibility that regulation, if not stimulation, of astrocyte division by axons may be general throughout the CNS.[30]

Schwann cells and the neuregulins

Schwann cells and their neural crest-derived progenitors need to interact with axons for proliferation, survival and terminal differentiation, as can be shown *in vitro*.[31,32]

The migration of progenitor cells is also arrested when they encounter axons.[33] Control of Schwann cells by the axon presumably ensures an appropriate number of glial cells for the amount of axonal membrane that needs to be encased, and it is mediated by both peptide/protein growth factors and electrical signals. In particular, members of the neuregulin family and their receptors have been implicated in these critical stages of development.

One of the first neuregulins to be identified, glial growth factor (GGF), was originally purified from bovine brain and pituitary as a Schwann cell mitogen.[34] The neuregulins are EGF-related proteins derived from alternative splicing of mRNA transcribed from a single gene, and constitute an important molecular signalling pathway active during neural and cardiac development, and in mammary carcinogenesis (the role of the neuregulin ARIA in neuromuscular synapse formation is discussed in Chapter 11). Some of the neuregulin isoforms are expressed as a transmembrane precursor, while others are secreted, and a second family of neuregulin-like ligands (termed NRG2 and transcribed from a separate gene) has also been described.[35,36] The neuregulins are transduced by the ErbB family receptors, a set of EGF receptor-related protein tyrosine kinases which operate through coexpression of ErbB2 (the product of the c-neu proto-oncogene) with ErbB3 and/or ErbB4. Ligand-induced receptor dimerization results in some 10 possible homo- and heterodimeric receptor combinations, and causes receptor autophosphorylation and intracellular signalling primarily through the Ras–Raf–MAP-kinase pathway.[36,37]

Neuregulins are expressed in motor neurons and the neurons of differentiating peripheral ganglia *in vivo*,[38] and are therefore well placed to instruct adjacent uncommitted neural crest cells to become glia rather than neurons, as discussed in Chapter 5. A critical role for neuregulin signalling in sensory ganglion development is further indicated by the profound loss of crest-derived components of cranial sensory ganglia seen in both neuregulin and ErbB2 knockout mice.[39,40] Neuregulin signalling also stimulates Schwann cell proliferation at later stages of development, for antibodies directed against membrane-bound neuregulin and ErbB2 block Schwann cell division induced by axonal contact.[41] It is less clear what brakes operate to prevent Schwann cells from multiplying continually when in contact with mitogen-bearing axons. One mechanism may be an autocrine system in which Schwann cells secrete a metalloprotease (stromelysin) that generates anti-mitotic peptide fragments from fibronectin.[42]

A survival-promoting effect of neuregulins on Schwann cells has also been described in several studies. Neuregulin administration can prevent Schwann cell death in culture,[43] and rescue those that would normally die in developing postnatal rodent peripheral nerves.[44,45] Death can be also induced at the neuromuscular junction by neonatal axotomy, and again this is preventable by neuregulin.[46] Consistent with the actions of neuregulins in promoting Schwann cell fate, mitosis and survival, neuregulin knockout mice show reduced numbers of Schwann cells in their peripheral nerves.[39]

ciation of axons with Schwann cells

Precisely how axons become so closely associated with Schwann cells remains unclear. When axons are growing to their targets they associate closely (fasciculate) with one another by means of homophilic adhesion molecules (see Chapter 9).[47,48] Presumably later the adhesion between axons and glial cells is stronger, to allow the separation and electrical insulation of axons from one another by their enclosure within invaginations of the glial membrane. In the absence of glia there is a tendency for active nerve fibres to excite their neighbours,[49] although in the CNS the fact that the smallest unmyelinated axons are not usually enclosed in glial processes does not apparently cause problems.

Axons cause changes in gene expression in the Schwann cells with which they are associated. For example, the ErbB2 receptor for neuregulin, the low-affinity NGF receptor and NGF itself are all downregulated. If, in addition, Schwann cells start to myelinate axons, there are further changes in gene expression which are described below.

Myelination

In mammals all axons greater than about 1 μm in diameter are myelinated. This is of great functional significance for it improves the electrical cable properties of the axon so that impulses can be propagated passively between the nodes of Ranvier with considerable gain in speed and saving in ionic transfer.

The process of myelin formation is an extraordinary feat of cell biology. Observations made *in vitro* have shown that the wrapping process that encases the axon in myelin cannot be accounted for by rotation of the Schwann cell body around the axon, and it would not be possible for the axon to rotate within the Schwann cell. Rather, the innermost membrane of the Schwann cell nearest to the axon moves over its surface, extending beneath the previous layers which are gradually displaced outwards (Fig. 6.4),[50] and continues to do so as long as new membrane material is supplied. During this process, the Schwann cell elaborates a basal lamina which encloses the entire Schwann cell–axon complex. This acellular coat is needed if the Schwann cells are to myelinate their axons successfully,[51] and it provides a persistent scaffold after nerve degeneration to confine dividing Schwann cells and guide regrowing axons (see Chapter 17).

Cross-suture experiments between nerves in which most axons are myelinated and nerves whose axons are largely unmyelinated show that the axons, rather than the glial cells, control the onset of myelination.[52] There is also a good correlation between

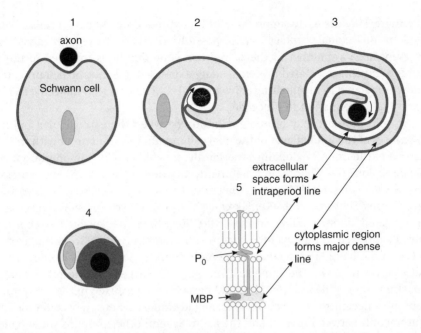

Figure 6.4 The formation of myelin in the peripheral nervous system (steps 1–4). In step 5, the distribution of two of its associated proteins, P_0 and MBP (myelin basic protein), occurs in the myelin of the peripheral nervous system.

myelin thickness (the number of layers of Schwann cell membrane) and axon diameter.[53] This is vividly demonstrated by the development of ectopic myelin around the normally unmyelinated axons of postganglionic sympathetic neurons if their diameters are increased experimentally using NGF.[54] Raising the levels of cAMP in Schwann cells can trigger some expression of myelin specific proteins (e.g. P_0, see below), but the only way found so far to induce Schwann cells to synthesize myelin is to associate them with large axons.

A simple lipid bilayer cannot make compact myelin. Both peripheral and central myelin contain specific proteins associated with the bilayer, two of which, P_0 and MBP, are illustrated in Fig. 6.4, and their presence in the right amounts and proportions is essential if compact myelin is to form. Once oligodendrocytes have differentiated, these proteins are expressed regardless of the presence or absence of axons,[55] but their expression by Schwann cells is controlled by axons and is normally absent until myelination begins.[56] Indeed, it seems likely that axon-derived signals, possibly neuregulins, actively repress P_0 expression by Schwann cells before the onset of myelination.[57]

The gene *Krox-20*, which encodes a zinc-finger transcription factor, may also participate in the overall control of the myelination programme in Schwann cells, for *Krox-20* knockout mice lack myelinated axons and do not express myelin-associated proteins (see below).[58] During development, *Krox-20* is first expressed in the glial cells associated with the dorsal and ventral roots ('boundary cap cells'), and is then activated along the entire length of peripheral nerves as the Schwann cell progenitors differentiate. Like the early suppression of P_0, expression in Schwann cells *in vitro* is dependent on axonal contact, again possibly through neuregulin signalling.[59] Conversely *Pax3*, a member of the paired box gene family, is involved in the suppression of myelin-associated proteins, being expressed in Schwann cell progenitors and downregulated in myelinating Schwann cells.[60] The adhesion molecule L1 is also necessary for myelination to proceed.[61]

The myelin proteins may promote adhesion between the extracellular and intracellular faces of the lipid bilayer of the glial cell membrane. Consistent with this, P_0 is a member of the immunoglobulin superfamily, to which many homophilic adhesion molecules belong (see Chapter 9).[56] Before myelination, all Schwann cells express the adhesion molecules N-CAM and L1 but afterwards they are absent except in the unmyelinating Schwann cells (Remak cells).[62] As these two adhesion molecules are downregulated, another adhesion molecule, MAG (myelin-associated glycoprotein), becomes expressed in regions of Schwann cell membrane away from the axon and adjacent to the basal lamina (abaxonal) where there is no compact myelin, and the protein periaxin shows the same distribution.[63,64] Earlier, on the other hand, as compact myelin begins to form, MAG and periaxin are localized in the Schwann cell membrane adjacent to the axon membrane (adaxonal), where they could modulate the interaction between myelin and the axon. Several other proteins show regional expression in the Schwann cell membrane on myelination, for example certain integrins (abaxonal) and the cytoskeletal proteins F-actin and spectrin (adaxonal), making the point that Schwann cells are highly specialized, polarized epithelial cells. Yet more specifically, the carbohydrate epitope HNK1 is present on the P_0 glycoprotein only of motor axons and is absent from the myelin around sensory axons.[65] Both myelinated and unmyelinated Schwann cells express N-cadherin.[66]

Although much is known about the structure and localization of proteins expressed during myelination, less is known about their functions and interactions during myelination. There exist several naturally occurring and artificially generated mutations in the genes coding for myelin-associated proteins, and several of these are associated with severe defects in myelination which are summarized at the end of this chapter. Such phenotypes certainly tell us that roles exist for these proteins in myelination, and the challenge now is to define those roles more precisely.

Ion channels

Following myelination the voltage-gated ion channels become restricted to the nodal and paranodal region of axons, a change with clear functional benefits. This process is probably dictated by the Schwann cells because continuous conduction (which requires restoration of ion channels to the internodal region) is re-established in some mature axons if they are demyelinated with diphtheria toxin.[67] Moreover, when dorsal root ganglion cells are cultured alone, sodium channels remain uniformly distributed along their axons, while in the presence of Schwann cells they become clustered;[68] oligodendrocytes, but not astrocytes, likewise induce clustering of sodium channels in retinal axons.[69] The molecules mediating such local influences of glia on axons have not been characterized, although Tenascin-R is a candidate channel clustering factor.[70,71]

Myelination by oligodendrocytes

Although these cells perform the same important function as Schwann cells by myelinating axons in the CNS, they differ from them in several respects. Astonishingly, each oligodendrocyte is able to myelinate several axons,[1] a feat which Schwann cells are unable to perform. Nor is CNS/oligodendrocyte myelin identical in composition to that made by Schwann cells, for example containing relatively more proteolipid protein (PLP, see below), but the importance of this is not known. Although the synthesis of MBP is upregulated during brain development,[72] mature oligodendrocytes appear to control their gene expression more independently of axons than Schwann cells. There is evidence, nevertheless, that mature oligodendrocytes can dedifferentiate and proliferate when axons degenerate.[73] Remyelination in disease states such as multiple sclerosis may be carried out by these cells, or via a population of oligodendrocyte precursor cells resident in the white matter.[74] Which of these sources of remyelination predominates in the adult mammalian CNS is unresolved, and is a question of potential clinical importance.

Trophic interactions between Schwann cells and neurons

One of the reasons for the widespread association of axons and glial cells is probably to facilitate trophic interactions between them, and glia produce a range of proteins with known trophic action on neurons.[71] Following axonal degeneration Schwann cells are known to synthesize NGF and BDNF (members of the neurotrophin family of trophic factors—see Chapter 12),[75] as well as insulin-like growth factor (IGF1). These are probably important in stimulating axon regeneration (Chapter 17). Myelinated Schwann cells also synthesize LIF and CNTF (members of the neurokine family of trophic factors) but, unlike the others, CNTF is downregulated when Schwann cells become dissociated from axons.[76]

Recent studies have revealed the importance of these factors in neuronal survival during the postnatal period. For example, both exogenous CNTF and BDNF are able to prevent the axotomy-induced death of motor neurons in neonatal mice.[77,78] Even more significantly, in CNTF null-mutant mice there is a gradual loss of motor neurons with increasing age.[79] Not surprisingly in view of this dependence on CNTF, motor neurons express the α-component of the CNTF receptor which is essential for its action.[80] The Schwann cell-derived factors that promote the survival of axons before the stage of target innervation remain uncertain, and both GDNF and NT3 have been implicated as candidates.[71]

It seems likely that, reciprocally, neurons are necessary for the long-term survival of Schwann cells: if axons are cut and prevented from regenerating, the Schwann cells gradually atrophy and eventually degenerate.[81] The action of neuregulins in promoting the survival of Schwann cells and their progenitors is discussed above. In the shorter term, however, the survival of Schwann cells in the absence of their axons is critical for the success of peripheral nerve regeneration, and there is evidence that Schwann cells are able to do this by their establishment of an autocrine survival loop.[82]

Perineurium

Another cell type found in peripheral nerves is the perineurial cell. These form the impermeable perineurium, a layer around the outside of each major nerve and nerve bundle which, together with the impermeable nature of the capillaries, provides the axons with a protected environment. Perineurial cells arise from fibroblasts as a result of an interaction with both axons and Schwann cells.[83] A member of the hedgehog family of signalling molecules, Desert Hedgehog, has been implicated here as a secreted product of Schwann cells which triggers surrounding fibroblasts to organize the perineurium.[71] Apart from its protective function the perineurium is also of practical importance in nerve repair for it provides surgeons with a layer of tissue that can be used to stitch together the two stumps of a cut nerve (Chapter 17). There are no perineurial sheaths within the CNS.

The blood–brain barrier

The capillaries in the brain, unlike those in other tissues, do not have clefts or gaps between individual endothelial cells. There are both tight and adherens junctions between the cells and these create a continuous permeability barrier between blood and the extracellular fluid around the cells of the brain. This is the 'blood–brain barrier',[84] and it is of considerable importance in providing the environment needed for the normal working of the brain; it isolates neurons and glia from ionic fluctuations in the extracellular fluid of the body as a whole, and reduces the access of bacteria and macrophages, polymorphs and lymphocytes. The water-soluble nutrients needed for the brain, which would, if the brain capillaries were like those in other tissues, diffuse through the intercellular clefts, instead gain access to the brain extracellular fluid by means of specific transporter mechanisms in the endothelial cell membranes.

The blood–brain barrier is not an intrinsic property of the capillaries that invade the brain during development. The tight junctions that form between the cells of the capillary endothelium are gradually induced by astrocytes, whose foot processes cover the surface of the capillaries.[85] Since the foot processes are separated from the outer surface of the endothelial cells by the basal lamina, the inducing agent is probably a secreted molecule. In keeping with this view, it has been found possible to generate high-resistance junctions between endothelial cells in culture by exposing them to astrocyte-conditioned medium if, at the same time, the level of cAMP within the cells is raised.[86]

Glial mutations in mouse and man

The study of myelin mutants has the potential for illuminating the biology of myelination and certain human diseases. Several mouse mutations affect genes encoding proteins expressed in Schwann cells or oligodendrocytes which are necessary for the formation of compact myelin.[87] The outcome is impaired myelin formation with consequent defects in nerve conduction and motor performance. Very similar conditions are found in humans and other mammals. The murine mutants are *jimpy* (*jp*), *shiverer* (*shi*) and *Trembler* (*Tm*). Table 6.1 lists five of the major proteins associated with myelin, either in the PNS or in the CNS, and the phenotypes of the related mutants.

The *jimpy* mutation is in the gene coding for PLP, a major component of compact CNS myelin, and the human equivalent is Pelizaeus–Merzbacher disease. Patients have impaired central myelin formation and suffer a variety of defects including psychomotor retardation, spasticity, ataxia and optic atrophy, dying before middle age. It is still uncertain, however, just how these mutations cause disease. The finding that targeted PLP knockout mice make virtually normal compact CNS myelin suggests that the dysmyelination seen in Pelizaeus–Merzbacher disease arises from a long-term requirement for PLP in stabilizing rather than forming myelin.[88] PLP is also likely to play a role in peripheral myelin formation, since human PLP null mutations can also cause a demyelinating peripheral neuropathy.[89]

shiverer mutant mice fail to produce normal myelin basic protein,[90] and *trembler* mice have a deficiency in peripheral myelin protein 22 (PMP-22).[91] It is probable that a disease of the human peripheral nervous system, Charcot–Marie–Tooth (CMT) disease (type 1), in which there is progressive onset of weakness starting in the distal parts of the limbs, is also due to mutations affecting PMP-22.[91] The majority of cases result from a duplication of the gene, leading by unknown mechanisms (possibly involving an early *increase* in myelin thickness) to axonal atrophy and demyelination.[92] In

Table 6.1 Mutations in myelin associated-proteins

Protein	CNS	PNS	Mutational effect
P_0	−	+ + + +	*Null mutant* → myelin and axon degeneration in PNS Mutations found in some cases of *Charcot–Marie–Tooth Type I* neuropathy
PLP	+ + + +	+ / −	*jimpy* → segment deletion → no CNS myelin *jp*^{msd} → amino acid substitution → no CNS myelin *rump shaker* → gene defect unknown *Pelizaeus–Merzbacher disease in humans* → amino acid substitution *shaking pup* → amino acid substitution
MBP	+ + +	+ +	*shiverer mouse* → gene deletion → little CNS myelin
PMP-22	+ / −	+ +	*trembler mouse* → point mutation → little PNS myelin + continuous Schwann cell proliferation *Charcot–Marie–Tooth Type 1 in humans*
MAG	+	+	*Null mutant* → nearly normal myelin formation but myelin and axon degeneration in old age

another group of patients with CMT, mutations affect a gap junction protein (connexin-32),[93] although it is unclear why only the PNS is involved for the same connexin is present in oligodendroglia. In yet other patients with CMT disease there may instead be a mutation in the gene coding for the major peripheral myelin-associated protein, P_0.[94] When the P_0 gene is eliminated in null mutant mice, myelin formation is severely impaired and axons, and their neurons, die in the peripheral nervous system.[95] In MAG knockout mice the initial formation of myelin is only slightly abnormal in the CNS, but by the time the animals reach 8 months (quite middle-aged for a mouse), myelin starts to degenerate and axons are lost.[96] This result shows that gene defects may take some time to manifest themselves even if a normal constituent is absent from conception as a result of a null mutation.

Other mutant mice in which glial–axon relationships are impaired are known, but the reasons for the failure are not so clear as in the mutants just described. In *quaking* (*qk*) there is also failure of myelin formation, possibly due to defective lipid production;[97] the *qk* product is predicted to have both signal-transducing and RNA-binding properties.[98] In *dystrophia muscularis* (*dy*) myelination of spinal nerve roots is especially poor compared with other regions, apparently because of the absence here of Schwann cells.[99] Where myelin is formed in *dy* mice it appears to be normal, so the essential problem may be inadequate generation, migration or survival of Schwann cells specifically in the region of the spinal roots.

Neurofibromatosis (Von Recklinghausen's disease) is a human disease inherited as an autosomal dominant. In type I neurofibromatosis, individuals develop benign tumours comprised of Schwann cells and fibroblasts along the length of their peripheral nerves around adolescence. The gene encodes a large protein, neurofibromin, which has a wide tissue expression but is especially abundant in Schwann cells, oligodendrocytes and neurons.[100] The protein may act as a tumour suppressor by regulating the cellular proto-oncogene *ras*. Interestingly, mice lacking functional neurofibromin die at embryonic day 13.5, but neural crest cells taken from them can survive well without neurotrophic factors, possibly because the ras signalling pathway is constitutively active, having escaped from negative regulation by neurofibromin.[101] In type II neurofibromatosis, tumours appear especially in the VIIIth cranial nerve (acoustic neuroma). The gene has been found to encode a large protein, schwannomin, which is associated with the cell membrane and attached to integrin and the cytoskeleton.[102]

Key points

1 The glial cells of the CNS are the oligodendrocytes, astrocytes and microglia; the glia of the PNS are the Schwann cells. Oligodendrocytes and Schwann cells ensheath axons and, for axons above 1 μm diameter, provide the thick myelin sheath which is critical for saltatory propagation of the nerve impulse. Amongst other things, astrocytes help to control the internal environment of the brain by controlling capillary permeability (their action on endothelial cells enables the blood–brain barrier to form) and providing a sink for ion accumulation. Microglia are transformed macrophages. All glial cells probably provide trophic support for neurons.

2 The common progenitor cells of oligodendrocytes and type 2 astrocytes (O-2A cells) mostly originate from a restricted group of cells close to the floor plate of the neural tube. These precursors are motile and migrate to other parts of the brain. Type 1 astrocytes arise from a separate group of precursors cells.

3 *In vitro* studies of O-2A cells isolated from neonatal rat optic nerve have revealed that proliferation and final differentiation depend on various growth factors (e.g. PDGF, NT-3 and IGF-1) and small hydrophobic molecules (e.g. retinoic acid and thyroid hormone), acting in combination with an internal cell clock. The importance of PDGF signalling has been confirmed *in vivo*: PDGF-knockout mice die shortly after birth, with little CNS myelin and few O-2A progenitors in the spinal cord.

4 Oligodendrocytes are generated in excess, and their numbers are controlled by death of those cells unable to acquire survival signals from axons or astrocytes.

5 The proliferation, survival and final differentiation of the neural crest-derived Schwann cell precursors is determined by interaction with axons of peripheral neurons. Among other factors, these supply EGF-related proteins, neuregulins, whose actions are transduced by a receptor protein tyrosine kinase (ErbB).

6 Myelin is formed by Schwann cells or oligodendrocytes inserting successive layers of their cell membranes around axons, adding each new layer from the inside. The layers becomes compacted, excluding cytoplasm, with the aid of proteins specific to myelin whose expression is controlled by signals from the axon. Overall

control is also exerted by a transcription factor encoded by the *Krox-20* gene. The protein composition of CNS myelin is not identical to peripheral myelin, and oligodendrocytes also differ from Schwann cells in being able to myelinate more than one axon and in controlling their gene expression more independently of axons. Table 6.1 summarizes the clinical consequences of mutations in genes coding for myelin-specific proteins.

7 The important trophic actions of Schwann cells, their role in neuronal survival and axon regeneration following peripheral nerve injury, and the negative effects of oligodendrocytes and astrocytes on CNS regeneration are all discussed in Chapter 17.

General reading

- Burden, S. and Yarden, Y. Neuregulins and their receptors: a versatile signaling module in organogenesis and oncogenesis. *Neuron* **18**, 847–55 (1997).

- Durand, B. and Raff, M. A cell-intrinsic timer that operates during oligodendrocyte development [in process citation]. *BioEssays* **22**, 64–71 (2000).

- Jessen, K. R. and Mirsky, R. Schwann cells and their precursors emerge as major regulators of nerve development. *Trends Neurosci.* **22**, 402–10 (1999).

- Jessen, K. R. and Richardson, W. D. (eds) *Glial cell development.* (Oxford University Press, Oxford, 2001).

References

1. Bunge, R. P. Glial cells and the central myelin sheath. *Physiol. Rev.* **48**, 197–251 (1968).

2. Perry, V. *Macrophages and the nervous system* (CRC Press, 1994).

3. Barres, B. A. and Raff, M. C. Control of oligodendrocyte number in the developing rat optic nerve. *Neuron* **12**, 935–42 (1994).

4. Barres, B. A., Lazar, M. A. and Raff, M. C. A novel role for thyroid hormone, glucocorticoids and retinoic acid in timing oligodendrocyte development. *Development* **120**, 1097–108 (1994).

5. Gao, F. B., Durand, B. and Raff, M. Oligodendrocyte precursor cells count time but not cell divisions before differentiation. *Curr. Biol.* **7**, 152–5 (1997).

6. Durand, B. and Raff, M. A cell-intrinsic timer that operates during oligodendrocyte development [in process citation]. *BioEssays* **22**, 64–71 (2000).

7. Calver, A. R. *et al.* Oligodendrocyte population dynamics and the role of PDGF *in vivo. Neuron* **20**, 869–82 (1998).

8. Beck, K. D., Powell-Braxton, L., Widmer, H. R., Valverde, J. and Hefti, F. Igf1 gene disruption results in reduced brain size, CNS hypomyelination, and loss of hippocampal granule and striatal parvalbumin-containing neurons. *Neuron* **14**, 717–30 (1995).

9. Yeh, H. J. *et al.* PDGF A-chain gene is expressed by mammalian neurons during development and in maturity. *Cell* **64**, 209–16 (1991).

10. Canoll, P. D. *et al.* GGF/neuregulin is a neuronal signal that promotes the proliferation and survival and inhibits the differentiation of oligodendrocyte progenitors. *Neuron* **17**, 229–43 (1996).

11. Barres, B. A. and Raff, M. C. Proliferation of oligodendrocyte precursor cells depends on electrical activity in axons. *Nature* **361**, 258–60 (1993).

12. Wang, S. *et al.* Notch receptor activation inhibits oligodendrocyte differentiation. *Neuron* **21**, 63–75 (1998).

13. Warf, B. C., Fok-Seang, J. and Miller, R. H. Evidence for the ventral origin of oligodendrocyte

precursors in the rat spinal cord. *J. Neurosci.* **11**, 2477–88 (1991).

14. Pringle, N. P. and Richardson, W. D. A singularity of PDGF alpha-receptor expression in the dorsoventral axis of the neural tube may define the origin of the oligodendrocyte lineage. *Development* **117**, 525–33 (1993).

15. Noll, E. and Miller, R. H. Oligodendrocyte precursors originate at the ventral ventricular zone dorsal to the ventral midline region in the embryonic rat spinal cord. *Development* **118**, 563–73 (1993).

16. Miller, R. H. Oligodendrocyte origins. *Trends Neurosci.* **19**, 92–6 (1996).

17. Pringle, N. P. *et al.* Determination of neuroepithelial cell fate: induction of the oligodendrocyte lineage by ventral midline cells and sonic hedgehog. *Dev. Biol.* **177**, 30–42 (1996).

18. Richardson, W. D., Pringle, N. P., Yu, W. P. and Hall, A. C. Origins of spinal cord oligodendrocytes: possible developmental and evolutionary relationships with motor neurons. *Dev. Neurosci.* **19**, 58–68 (1997).

19. Leber, S. M., Breedlove, S. M. and Sanes, J. R. Lineage, arrangement, and death of clonally related motoneurons in chick spinal cord. *J. Neurosci.* **10**, 2451–62 (1990).

20. Cameron-Curry, P. and Le Douarin, N. M. Oligodendrocyte precursors originate from both the dorsal and the ventral parts of the spinal cord. *Neuron* **15**, 1299–310 (1995).

21. Hardy, R. J. and Friedrich, V. L., Jr. Oligodendrocyte progenitors are generated throughout the embryonic mouse brain, but differentiate in restricted foci. *Development* **122**, 2059–69 (1996).

22. Pringle, N. P., Guthrie, S., Lumsden, A. and Richardson, W. D. Dorsal spinal cord neuroepithelium generates astrocytes but not oligodendrocytes. *Neuron* **20**, 883–93 (1998).

23. Ono, K., Yasui, Y., Rutishauser, U. and Miller, R. H. Focal ventricular origin and migration of oligodendrocyte precursors into the chick optic nerve. *Neuron* **19**, 283–92 (1997).

24. Milner, R. and ffrench-Constant, C. A developmental analysis of oligodendroglial integrins in primary cells: changes in alpha v-associated beta subunits during differentiation. *Development* **120**, 3497–506 (1994).

25. Wang, C., Rougon, G. and Kiss, J. Z. Requirement of polysialic acid for the migration of the O-2A glial progenitor cell from neurohypophyseal explants. *J. Neurosci.* **14**, 4446–57 (1994).

26. Barres, B. A. *et al.* Cell death and control of cell survival in the oligodendrocyte lineage. *Cell* **70**, 31–46 (1992).

27. David, S., Miller, R. H., Patel, R. and Raff, M. C. Effects of neonatal transection on glial cell development in the rat optic nerve: evidence that the oligodendrocyte-type 2 astrocyte cell lineage depends on axons for its survival. *J. Neurocytol.* **13**, 961–74 (1984).

28. Fruttiger, M. *et al.* PDGF mediates a neuron-astrocyte interaction in the developing retina. *Neuron* **17**, 1117–31 (1996).

29. Burne, J. F. and Raff, M. C. Retinal ganglion cell axons drive the proliferation of astrocytes in the developing rodent optic nerve. *Neuron* **18**, 223–30 (1997).

30. Gasser, U. E. and Hatten, M. E. Neuron–glia interactions of rat hippocampal cells *in vitro*: glial-guided neuronal migration and neuronal regulation of glial differentiation. *J. Neurosci.* **10**, 1276–85 (1990).

31. Wood, P. M. and Bunge, R. P. Evidence that sensory axons are mitogenic for Schwann cells. *Nature* **256**, 662–4 (1975).

32. Ratner, N., Hong, D. M., Lieberman, M. A., Bunge, R. P. and Glaser, L. The neuronal cell-surface molecule mitogenic for Schwann cells is a heparin-binding protein. *Proc. Natl. Acad. Sci. USA* **85**, 6992–6 (1988).

33. Bhattacharyya, A., Brackenbury, R. and Ratner, N. Axons arrest the migration of Schwann cell precursors. *Development* **120**, 1411–20 (1994).

34. Brockes, J. P., Lemke, G. E. and Balzer, D. R. Purification and preliminary characterization of a glial growth factor from the bovine pituitary. *J. Biol. Chem.* **255**, 8374–7 (1980).

35. Lemke, G. Neuregulins in development. *Mol. Cell. Neurosci.* **7**, 247–62 (1996).

36. Burden, S. and Yarden, Y. Neuregulins and their receptors: a versatile signaling module in organogenesis and oncogenesis. *Neuron* **18**, 847–55 (1997).

37. Carraway, K. L. and Cantley, L. C. A neu acquaintance for erbB3 and erbB4: a role for receptor heterodimerization in growth signaling. *Cell* **78**, 5–8 (1994).

38. Ho, W. H., Armanini, M. P., Nuijens, A., Phillips, H. S. and Osheroff, P. L. Sensory and motor neuron-derived factor. A novel heregulin variant highly expressed in sensory and motor neurons. *J. Biol. Chem.* **270**, 26722 (1995).

39. Meyer, D. and Birchmeier, C. Multiple essential functions of neuregulin in development. *Nature* **378**, 386–90 (1995).

40. Lee, K. F. *et al.* Requirement for neuregulin receptor erbB2 in neural and cardiac development. *Nature* **378**, 394–8 (1995).

41. Morrissey, T. K., Levi, A. D., Nuijens, A., Sliwkowski, M. X. and Bunge, R. P. Axon-induced mitogenesis of human Schwann cells involves heregulin and p185erbB2. *Proc. Natl. Acad. Sci. USA* **92**, 1431–5 (1995).

42. Muir, D. and Manthorpe, M. Stromelysin generates a fibronectin fragment that inhibits Schwann cell proliferation. *J. Cell Biol.* **116**, 177–85 (1992).

43. Dong, Z. *et al.* Neu differentiation factor is a neuron–glia signal and regulates survival, proliferation, and maturation of rat Schwann cell precursors. *Neuron* **15**, 585–96 (1995).

44. Syroid, D. E. *et al.* Cell death in the Schwann cell lineage and its regulation by neuregulin. *Proc. Natl. Acad. Sci. USA* **93**, 9229–34 (1996).

45. Grinspan, J. B., Marchionni, M. A., Reeves, M., Coulaloglou, M. and Scherer, S. S. Axonal interactions regulate Schwann cell apoptosis in developing peripheral nerve: neuregulin receptors and the role of neuregulins. *J. Neurosci.* **16**, 6107–18 (1996).

46. Trachtenberg, J. T. and Thompson, W. J. Schwann cell apoptosis at developing neuromuscular junctions is regulated by glial growth factor. *Nature* **379**, 174–7 (1996).

47. Thanos, S., Bonhoeffer, F. and Rutishauser, U. Fiber–fiber interaction and tectal cues influence the development of the chicken retinotectal projection. *Proc. Natl. Acad. Sci. USA* **81**, 1906–10 (1984).

48. Rutishauser, U. and Landmesser, L. Polysialic acid in the vertebrate nervous system: a promoter of plasticity in cell–cell interactions. *Trends Neurosci.* **19**, 422–7 (1996).

49. Huizar, P., Kuno, M. and Miyata, Y. Electrophysiological properties of spinal motoneurones of normal and dystrophic mice. *J. Physiol. (London)* **248**, 231–46 (1975).

50. Bunge, R. P., Bunge, M. B. and Bates, M. Movements of the Schwann cell nucleus implicate progression of the inner (axon-related) Schwann cell process during myelination. *J. Cell Biol.* **109**, 273–84 (1989).

51. Sanes, J. R. Extracellular matrix molecules that influence neural development. *Annu. Rev. Neurosci.* **12**, 491–516 (1989).

52. Bray, D. and Gilbert, D. Cytoskeletal elements in neurons. *Annu. Rev. Neurosci.* **4**, 505–23 (1981).

53. Friede, R. L. Control of myelin formation by axon caliber (with a model of the control mechanism). *J. Comp. Neurol.* **144**, 233–52 (1972).

54. Voyvodic, J. T. Target size regulates calibre and myelination of sympathetic axons. *Nature* **342**, 430–3 (1989).

55. Zeller, N. K., Behar, T. N., Dubois-Dalcq, M. E. and Lazzarini, R. A. The timely expression of myelin basic protein gene in cultured rat brain oligodendrocytes is independent of continuous neuronal influences. *J. Neurosci.* **5**, 2955–62 (1985).

56. Lemke, G. Unwrapping the genes of myelin. *Neuron* **1**, 535–43 (1988).

57. Cheng, L. and Mudge, A. W. Cultured Schwann cells constitutively express the myelin protein P0. *Neuron* **16**, 309–19 (1996).

58. Topilko, P. *et al.* Krox-20 controls myelination in the peripheral nervous system. *Nature* **371**, 796–9 (1994).

59. Murphy, P. *et al.* The regulation of Krox-20 expression reveals important steps in the control of peripheral glial cell development. *Development* **122**, 2847–57 (1996).

60. Kioussi, C., Gross, M. K. and Gruss, P. Pax3: a paired domain gene as a regulator in PNS myelination. *Neuron* **15**, 553–62 (1995).

61. Wood, P. M., Schachner, M. and Bunge, R. P. Inhibition of Schwann cell myelination *in vitro* by antibody to the L1 adhesion molecule. *J. Neurosci.* **10**, 3635–45 (1990).

62. Jessen, K. R., Mirsky, R. and Morgan, L. Myelinated, but not unmyelinated axons, reversibly down-regulate N-CAM in Schwann cells. *J. Neurocytol.* **16**, 681–8 (1987).

63. Gillespie, C. S., Sherman, D. L., Blair, G. E. and Brophy, P. J. Periaxin, a novel protein of myelinating Schwann cells with a possible role in axonal ensheathment. *Neuron* **12**, 497–508 (1994).

64. Scherer, S. S., Xu, Y. T., Bannerman, P. G., Sherman, D. L. and Brophy, P. J. Periaxin expression in myelinating Schwann cells: modulation by axon–glial interactions and polarized localization during development. *Development* **121**, 4265–73 (1995).

65. Martini, R. and Schachner, M. Immunoelectron microscopic localization of neural cell adhesion molecules (L1, N-CAM, and myelin-associated glycoprotein) in regenerating adult mouse sciatic nerve. *J. Cell Biol.* **106**, 1735–46 (1988).

66. Shibuya, Y., Mizoguchi, A., Takeichi, M., Shimada, K. and Ide, C. Localization of N-cadherin in the normal and regenerating nerve fibers of the chicken peripheral nervous system. *Neuroscience* **67**, 253–61 (1995).

67. Bostock, H. and Sears, T. A. The internodal axon membrane: electrical excitability and continuous conduction in segmental demyelination. *J. Physiol. (London)* **280**, 273–301 (1978).

68. Joe, E. H. and Angelides, K. Clustering of voltage-dependent sodium channels on axons depends on Schwann cell contact. *Nature* **356**, 333–5 (1992).

69. Kaplan, M. R. *et al.* Induction of sodium channel clustering by oligodendrocytes. *Nature* **386**, 724–8 (1997).

70. Salzer, J. L. Clustering sodium channels at the node of Ranvier: close encounters of the axon-glia kind. *Neuron* **18**, 843–6 (1997).

71. Jessen, K. R. and Mirsky, R. Schwann cells and their precursors emerge as major regulators of nerve development. *Trends Neurosci.* **22**, 402–10 (1999).

72. Haas, S. *et al.* A 39-kD DNA-binding protein from mouse brain stimulates transcription of myelin basic protein gene in oligodendrocytic cells. *J. Cell Biol.* **130**, 1171–9 (1995).

73. Ludwin, S. K. Proliferation of mature oligodendrocytes after trauma to the central nervous system. *Nature* **308**, 274–5 (1984).

74. Gensert, J. M. and Goldman, J. E. Endogenous progenitors remyelinate demyelinated axons in the adult CNS. *Neuron* **19**, 197–203 (1997).

75. Meyer, M., Matsuoka, I., Wetmore, C., Olson, L. and Thoenen, H. Enhanced synthesis of brain-derived neurotrophic factor in the lesioned peripheral nerve: different mechanisms are responsible for the regulation of BDNF and NGF mRNA. *J. Cell Biol.* **119**, 45–54 (1992).

76. Friedman, B. *et al.* Regulation of ciliary neurotrophic factor expression in myelin-related Schwann cells *in vivo*. *Neuron* **9**, 295–305 (1992).

77. Sendtner, M., Kreutzberg, G. W. and Thoenen, H. Ciliary neurotrophic factor prevents the degeneration of motor neurons after axotomy. *Nature* **345**, 440–1 (1990).

78. Sendtner, M., Holtmann, B., Kolbeck, R., Thoenen, H. and Barde, Y. A. Brain-derived neurotrophic factor prevents the death of motoneurons in newborn rats after nerve section. *Nature* **360**, 757–9 (1992).

79. Masu, Y. *et al.* Disruption of the CNTF gene results in motor neuron degeneration. *Nature* **365**, 27–32 (1993).

80. Ip, N. Y. *et al.* The alpha component of the CNTF receptor is required for signaling and defines potential CNTF targets in the adult and during development. *Neuron* **10**, 89–102 (1993).

81. Weinberg, H. J. and Spencer, P. S. The fate of Schwann cells isolated from axonal contact. *J. Neurocytol.* **7**, 555–69 (1978).

82. Meier, C., Parmantier, E., Brennan, A., Mirsky, R. and Jessen, K. R. Developing Schwann cells acquire the ability to survive without axons by establishing an autocrine circuit involving insulin-like growth factor, neurotrophin-3, and platelet-derived growth factor-BB. *J. Neurosci.* **19**, 3847–59 (1999).

83. Bunge, M. B., Wood, P. M., Tynan, L. B., Bates, M. L. and Sanes, J. R. Perineurium originates from fibroblasts: demonstration *in vitro* with a retroviral marker. *Science* **243**, 229–31 (1989).

84. Rubin, L. L. and Staddon, J. M. The cell biology of the blood–brain barrier. *Annu. Rev. Neurosci.* **22**, 11–28 (1999).

85. Janzer, R. C. and Raff, M. C. Astrocytes induce blood–brain barrier properties in endothelial cells. *Nature* **325**, 253–7 (1987).

86. Rubin, L. L. *et al.* A cell culture model of the blood–brain barrier. *J. Cell Biol.* **115**, 1725–35 (1991).

87. Griffiths, I. R. Myelin mutants: model systems for the study of normal and abnormal myelination. *BioEssays* **18**, 789–97 (1996).

88. Klugmann, M. *et al.* Assembly of CNS myelin in the absence of proteolipid protein. *Neuron* **18**, 59–70 (1997).

89. Garbern, J. Y. *et al.* Proteolipid protein is necessary in peripheral as well as central myelin. *Neuron* **19**, 205–18 (1997).

90. Readhead, C. *et al.* Expression of a myelin basic protein gene in transgenic shiverer mice: correction of the dysmyelinating phenotype. *Cell* **48**, 703–12 (1987).

91. Suter, U., Welcher, A. A. and Snipes, G. J. Progress in the molecular understanding of hereditary peripheral neuropathies reveals new insights into the biology of the peripheral nervous system. *Trends Neurosci.* **16**, 50–6 (1993).

92. Hanemann, C. O. and Muller, H. W. Pathogenesis of Charcot–Marie–Tooth 1A (CMT1A) neuropathy. *Trends Neurosci.* **21**, 282–6 (1998).

93. Bergoffen, J. *et al.* Connexin mutations in X-linked Charcot–Marie–Tooth disease. *Science* **262**, 2039–42 (1993).

94. Hayasaka, K. *et al.* Charcot–Marie–Tooth neuropathy type 1B is associated with mutations of the myelin P0 gene. *Nat. Genet.* **5**, 31–4 (1993).

95. Martini, R., Zielasek, J., Toyka, K. V., Giese, K. P. and Schachner, M. Protein zero (P0)-deficient mice show myelin degeneration in peripheral nerves characteristic of inherited human neuropathies. *Nat. Genet.* **11**, 281–6 (1995).

96. Fruttiger, M., Montag, D., Schachner, M. and Martini, R. Crucial role for the myelin-associated glycoprotein in the maintenance of axon–myelin integrity. *Eur. J. Neurosci.* **7**, 511–15 (1995).

97. Lyon, M. F. and Searle, A. G. *Genetic variants and strains of the laboratory mouse* (Oxford University Press, 1989).

98. Ebersole, T. A., Chen, Q., Justice, M. J. and Artzt, K. The quaking gene product necessary in embryogenesis and myelination combines features of RNA binding and signal transduction proteins. *Nat. Genet.* **12**, 260–5 (1996).

99. Stirling, C. A. Abnormalities of Schwann cell sheaths on spinal nerve roots of dystrophic mice. *J. Anat.* **119**, 169–80 (1975).

100. Gutmann, D. H. and Collins, F. S. The neurofibromatosis type 1 gene and its protein product, neurofibromin. *Neuron* **10**, 335–43 (1993).

101. Vogel, K. S., Brannan, C. I., Jenkins, N. A., Copeland, N. G. and Parada, L. F. Loss of neurofibromin results in neurotrophin-independent survival of embryonic sensory and sympathetic neurons. *Cell* **82**, 733–42 (1995).

102. Kinzler, K. W. and Vogelstein, B. Cancer: A gene for neurofibromatosis 2. *Nature* **363**, 495–6 (1993).

7
Development of Cerebral Cortex and Cerebellar Cortex

Because of the importance and complexity of their function, the mammalian cerebral cortex and cerebellar cortex have received special attention from developmental neurobiologists seeking to identify how individual areas of the CNS develop. In the cerebral neocortex, for example, outstanding questions concern how the proliferating neuroepithelium generates an ordered stacking of cells into six layers, each with appropriate local and long-distance connections, and how different regions of the cortical sheet become structurally and functionally diversified. The early patterning of the developing brain has been discussed in Chapter 3, including the roles of the mammalian homologues of the *Drosophila* homeobox genes *orthodenticle* (*Otx1* and *Otx2*) and *empty spiracles* (*Emx1* and *Emx2*), which are expressed in nested domains in the rostral neural tube, and the importance of the isthmus signalling system in creating the merging structures comprising midbrain, hindbrain and cerebellum. In this chapter we will consider in more detail related events in the development of the cerebral and cerebellar cortex, particularly the factors regulating cortical neurogenesis and neuronal migration, as well as those that underlie cortical regionalization and morphogenesis.

Development of cerebral cortex

The cerebral cortex arises from paired evaginations of the early forebrain vesicle, the telencephalic vesicles. These also give rise to the basal ganglia/striatum, olfactory bulbs and amygdala, and the mechanisms involved in their early regionalization are discussed in Chapter 3. The six-layered neocortex develops from the major, dorsolateral part of each vesicle, while the more ancient paleocortex and three-layered archicortex (presumptive hippocampus) arise, respectively, from the lateral and medial portions of the vesicle. The mechanisms involved in the individuation of these broad phylogenetic subdivisions are uncertain, but one interesting possibility is that cells located at the extreme medial edge of the vesicle constitute a signalling region that patterns the hippocampal cortex and distinguishes it from the neighbouring epithelium of the choroid plexus. This region of the telencephalic epithelium, the 'cortical hem', expresses several members of the *Wnt* gene family, suggesting parallels with the isthmus signalling centre.[1]

Proliferation and production of cortical neurons

At the height of its development the human brain has been estimated to generate several hundred thousand new nerve cells per minute, much of which can be attributed to the cerebral cortex. The germinal layer of the cerebral cortex is the ventricular zone (VZ), the neuroepithelium that lines the lateral ventricular cavities of the developing telencephalon (Fig. 7.1). Cells in this zone undergo massive proliferation, generating postmitotic cells which then migrate through the intermediate zone to their definitive sites of terminal differentiation. The earliest-born cells colonize the preplate, the first layer of neurons, and this becomes divided into

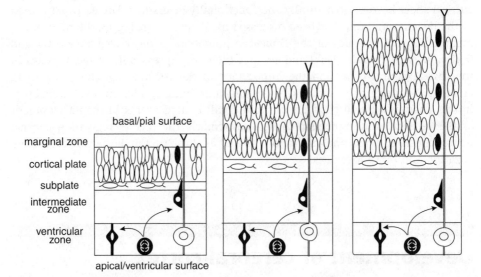

Figure 7.1 Development of the cerebral cortex. Neurons become layered in the cortical plate, the first layer to form being the deepest, the last to form being the outer layer next to the pial surface. Postmitotic neurons migrate along radial glial cells from the ventricular zone, where they are generated, to their final destination, while sibling cells in the ventricular zone remain to divide again. Lineage tracing shows that clonally-related neurons can be found in any cortical layer. After Chenn *et al.*[117]

the subplate and marginal zone by the developing neurons of the cortical plate. In regions of the CNS such as the cerebral and cerebellar cortex, where cells are stacked in superimposed layers, these layers are usually generated by migration of post-mitotic cells in a ventricular-to-pial ('inside-out') direction. The earliest migrating neurons of the cortical plate become the deepest layer of the definitive cerebral cortex, and ensuing waves of migrating neurons pass their predecessors, stopping when they reach the marginal zone to form successively more superficial layers. The granular layers of the hippocampal dentate gyrus and cerebellar cortex are exceptions to this rule, developing on an 'outside-in' basis. Cortical neurogenesis is a largely prenatal process, the hippocampus being an exception, and it is supplanted in the postnatal period by the generation of glial cells. Most glia are derived from the subventricular zone, a second germinal layer of cells that persists into the adult.

Studies using tritiated thymidine labelling of proliferating cortical cells originally suggested that the extensive proliferation of VZ cells required to expand the initial pool of precursor cells is likely to involve symmetrical cell divisions, each daughter cell having the same fate. On the other hand, radiolabelling studies also suggested that postmitotic cortical neurons arise from asymmetrical divisions, in which the sibling cells remain in the proliferating state (Fig. 7.2).[2] Consistent with this, lineage-tracing studies using replication-defective retrovirus vectors have shown that the progeny of single labelled progenitor cells occupy multiple layers of the cortex, a result that is hard to interpret exclusively in terms of symmetrical divisions.[3,4] *In vitro* studies of the progeny of isolated cortical progenitor cells have also shown that neural progenitors can generate reproducible asymmetrical division patterns, while glial progenitors undergo prolonged symmetrical divisions.[5]

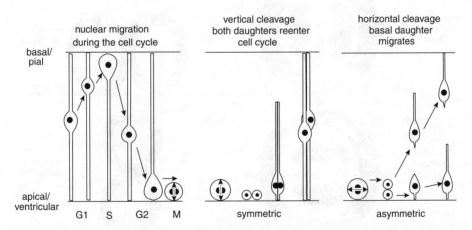

Figure 7.2 Nuclear migrations accompanying cell division in the ventricular zone (*left*). The different results of symmetric, vertically-orientated mitosis (*middle*) and asymmetric, horizontally-oriented mitosis (*right*) are shown. Asymmetric division delivers different cytoplasmic contents to the two daughters, so one cell becomes postmitotic and migrates, while the other remains in the proliferative state in the ventricular zone.

Direct evidence for asymmetrical divisions of progenitor cells has been provided by time-lapse studies of DiI-labelled progenitor cells in slice cultures of ferret cortex. During the initial phase of expansion of the progenitor cell population, divisions are seen to be mainly symmetrical and 'vertical', with a plane of cleavage orthogonal to the ventricular surface. Later in development, however, asymmetrical horizontal divisions are seen with increasing frequency: one daughter cell remains attached to the ventricular surface of the neural epithelium and continues to proliferate, while the other (presumably postmitotic) daughter migrates away (Fig. 7.2).[6] Towards the end of development it is possible that the terminal divisions of the VZ progenitor cells are again symmetrical, generating two postmitotic daughters, but this remains to be established.

As discussed in Chapter 4, several proteins have been identified in *Drosophila* that are distributed asymmetrically in dividing neuronal precursor cells, including the products of *numb* and *prospero*, and these are important in establishing different fates for the daughter cells following asymmetrical cell division. Similar mechanisms may operate in the developing mammalian cerebral cortex. In the ferret, for example, Notch1 protein is concentrated in the basal part of VZ cells as they enter mitosis, and is partitioned equally to the daughters following symmetrical division but preferentially to the basal daughter after asymmetrical division.[6] Numb protein, by contrast, is localized in the apical part of the cell, and therefore segregates to the apical daughter following asymmetrical division (Fig. 7.3).[7] Numb has been shown to antagonize Notch signalling in *Drosophila* (see Chapter 4), raising the possibility that Notch signalling is disinhibited in the basal daughters of asymmetrically dividing VZ

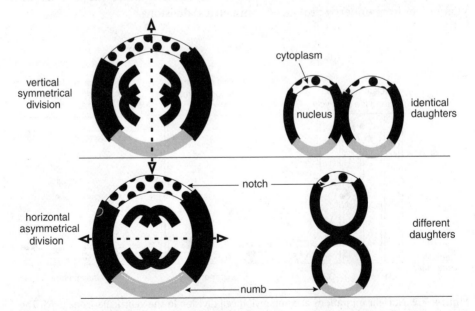

Figure 7.3 Notch and numb protein are asymmetrically distributed in progenitor cells in such a way that vertical cell division gives roughly equal amounts to each daughter cell, but horizontal cleavage gives all notch to the basal/pial daughter and all numb to the apical/ventricular daughter. After Chenn *et al.*[117]

cells by the loss of numb. This appears somewhat paradoxical, since *Notch* expression generally correlates with the *suppression* of neurogenesis, whereas the basal daughter cells are undergoing neuronal differentiation. Perhaps Notch signalling allows the basal cell to ignore other local signals directing it to re-enter the cell cycle. It has also been shown that the basal cells do express *numb*, as well as its homologue *numblike*, but only after migration through the intermediate zone to the cortical plate, and this may suppress residual Notch activity to permit terminal neuronal differentiation.[8] At all events, while the similarities between neuronal specification mechanisms in *Drosophila* and the mammalian neocortex are certainly impressive, the higher degree of diversity of neuronal types in the vertebrate CNS suggests that drawing direct parallels may prove to be oversimplistic.

As for other systems such as the neural crest (Chapter 5) and retina (Chapter 8), numerous exogenous factors have been identified that appear to control the proliferation of progenitor cells in the developing cerebral cortex. It has been shown, for example, that addition of FGF2 (bFGF) to cultures of dissociated rat progenitor cells promotes their proliferation.[9] Moreover, cortical progenitor cells differentiate prematurely when cultured in isolation, but are stimulated to proliferate when cultured in contact with other cortical cells or astrocytes, or when cultured in the presence of astrocyte membrane homogenates. Again, FGF2 is a strong candidate mitogen, being expressed in the cerebral cortex throughout neurogenesis and associated with the cell surface. Consistent with this, a single microinjection of FGF2 into the cerebral ventricles of rat embryos at the onset of cortical neurogenesis nearly doubles the number of neurons in the adult cerebral cortex; and cortical cell numbers (neurons and glia) are reduced in FGF2 knockout mice.[10] Additional factors are likely to be involved, however, since serum is also required to stimulate cortical cell division *in vitro*.[11] Moreover, the neurotransmitters GABA and glutamate have been implicated as antimitogens, suggesting a possible feedback mechanism whereby the maturing neuropil could influence progenitor cells to differentiate.[12]

Exogenous factors are also likely to promote the differentiation of cortical cells, and a good such candidate is the neurotrophin NT-3, which accelerates neuronal differentiation in FGF2-expanded cortical cultures.[9,13] The neurotrophin does not affect the final number of neurons produced in these cultures, so it probably promotes the differentiation of already-committed progenitor cells rather than stimulating the production of extra neuronal progenitor cells from a multipotential precursor. Cortical neurogenesis appears to be unaffected, on the other hand, in mice with targeted disruptions of NT-3 and its receptor TrkC (or other neurotrophins, see Chapter 12), and considerable redundancy seems likely in the environmental triggers for cortical neuronal differentiation. One important endogenous regulator of the proliferation/differentiation process is the winged helix transcription factor BF-1, whose expression is restricted to the developing telencephalon. Cortical progenitor cells differentiate precociously in BF-1 mutant mice, depleting the overall population so that the telencephalon is much reduced in size. Whether BF-1 facilitates the action of mitogens such as FGF2 or acts directly on the cell cycle is unclear, but it provides a good example of a regionally-restricted influence on cell proliferation and morphogenesis in the CNS.[14]

Migration of cortical neurons

As noted above, a key feature of the development of both cerebral and cerebellar cortex is the migration of newly postmitotic neurons from the ventricular zone to their final, often distant sites of terminal differentiation in the cortical plate (see reference 15 for review). Abnormalities of migration have been suggested to underlie a number of developmental anomalies of the human brain, and these are discussed below. Radial (inside-out) migration was originally seen in thymidine birthdating studies of cortical development,[16] and shown to be directed by *radial glial cells* whose processes span the full thickness of the cortex. These cells form close contacts with the migrating cells that can be seen electron microscopically.[17]

The predominantly radial migration of postmitotic cells suggested that region-specific differences in the cerebral cortex (e.g. sensory versus motor cortex) might be specified early in development, in the form of a 'protomap' in the ventricular zone that is maintained as cells maintain their relative positions during subsequent migration (see below).[18] It is now recognized, however, that a significant proportion of postmitotic cortical cells also undertake extensive non-radial ('tangential') migrations. In studies using retroviral markers to follow the lineage of cortical precursor cells, it has become clear that the clonal progeny of single cells can be widely dispersed throughout the cerebral cortex.[19] The same conclusion has been reached by another study adopting a transgenic approach, using X-inactivation to label approximately half the population of cortical progenitors randomly with β-galactosidase.[20] Lastly, long distance, tangential migration of postmitotic cells within the ventricular and subventricular zones has been detected by fluorescent (DiI) labelling in the early postnatal ferret, a species in which cortical neurogenesis continues for some 2 weeks after birth.[21] In the latter study migration was seen to be confined to postmitotic cells, as assessed by the absence of bromodeoxyuridine (BrdU) incorporation and the presence of a neuron-specific marker, and involved up to one-third of migrating cells. Other studies, however, have suggested that progenitor cells can also move tangentially within the ventricular zone.[22,23]

The relative significance of the two migration routes within developing cortex, radial and tangential, remains uncertain. As discussed below, it appears that the patterns of cortical connectivity are largely determined after the migration stage, possibly by incoming thalamic axons, so the regional origin of the migrating cells seems unlikely to be critical. It may turn out, nevertheless, that different types of cortical neuron, such as pyramidal/projection neurons and interneurons, take different migratory routes to their final cortical destinations. A study of chimeric mice has suggested that some radial migrations are linked to the pyramidal neuronal lineage, while tangential migrations are linked predominantly to GABAergic interneurons.[24] Moreover, GABAergic neurons have been shown to undergo an extensive tangential invasion of the neocortex from the lateral ganglionic eminence (LGE) and developing striatum, across the corticostriatal boundary into the neocortical

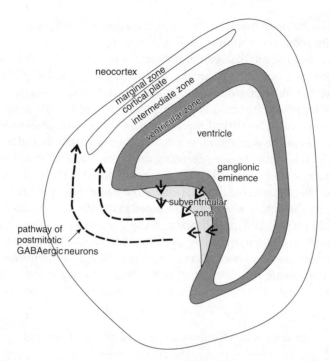

Figure 7.4 Coronal section through the early rodent telencephalic vesicle, showing tangential migration of GABAergic neurons into the neocortex from the ventricular and subventricular zones of the lateral ganglionic eminence (future striatum). After Pearlman *et al.*[39]

marginal and intermediate zones (Fig. 7.4; see also Chapter 3). Separation of the neocortex from the adjacent LGE/striatum in slice cultures substantially reduces the number of GABAergic neurons that appear throughout the neocortex.[25] The LGE may therefore be an important source of neocortical interneurons, and the same appears to apply to the MGE.[26] It has also been shown to give rise to cells that colonize the primary olfactory cortex.[27] A further example is the subpial granule cell layer of the human neocortex, whose neurons appear to originate from a proliferative region in the anterior frontal lobe and migrate tangentially throughout the marginal zone.[28] Finally, there is evidence that neurotrophins (see Chapter 12) can regulate tangential migration, since the number of GABAergic interneurons seen in the rat cortical marginal zone increases dramatically after exogenous application of NT-4 in the absence of changes in cell death or proliferation.[29]

Cortical lamination and differentiation

Lamination appears to have arisen during brain evolution as a means of enhancing neuronal communication within a given area of neuropil receiving a large afferent input. In at least one case, the laminated vagal lobe of the goldfish hindbrain, its evolution seems to have involved the reorganization of existing neuronal populations, rather than the generation of new connectivity.[30]

In the case of the mammalian cerebral cortex, how are the distinct layers of cells, each containing neurons with particular morphology, connectivity and functional properties, generated during development? Retroviral lineage studies have shown that early cortical progenitor cells are multipotent, giving rise to clones of daughter cells that occupy multiple cortical layers. On the other hand, heterochronic transplantation studies in the postnatal ferret have shown that laminar identity is sealed during the cell cycle immediately preceding the terminal division of the progenitor cell. If progenitors of deep cortical layers are transplanted early in the cycle (S phase) into the ventricular zone of older hosts, where the upper layers are being generated, they migrate to the upper layers and change their fate appropriately. But if the terminal division has already taken place in the donor, cells migrate to the deeper layers and maintain their normal fate as deep layer neurons (Fig. 7.5).[31] The implication is that final cortical neuronal fates are determined by environmental signals in the ventricular zone operating during the terminal cell cycle of the progenitors. Plasticity of cortical progenitor fates is not absolute, however. In the reverse

presumptive layer 6 neurons transplanted into older host brains

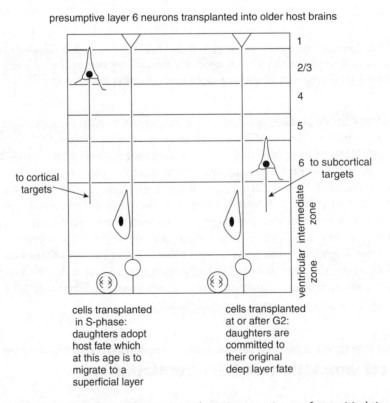

cells transplanted
in S-phase:
daughters adopt
host fate which
at this age is to
migrate to a
superficial layer

cells transplanted
at or after G2:
daughters are
committed to
their original
deep layer fate

Figure 7.5 Evidence from heterochronic transplantation experiments for a critical time window during the S phase of the cell cycle when cortical progenitor cells can receive instructional signals that determine their fate. After Chenn et al.[117]

paradigm, where late progenitor cells, destined for upper layers, are grafted into younger cortex generating deeper layers, they still migrate to the upper layers and maintain their original fates. This suggests that the differentiation potential of cortical neurons becomes progressively restricted as development proceeds.[32] Such restriction is presumably underlain by lamina-specific gene expression, and such patterns have been detected. Expression of the homeobox gene *Otx1*, for example, is confined to neurons of layers 5 and 6, and their progenitors.[33]

Alongside laminar position, cortical neurons also acquire their characteristic morphology, neurotransmitter phenotype and connectivity. Pyramidal neurons, for example, release excitatory amino acids such as glutamate, and project to distant or local targets, while non-pyramidal neurons are primarily GABA-releasing interneurons. As discussed above, there is evidence that these two main classes of cortical neuron may have distinct progenitors, taking different migration routes and differentiating as individual clones with uniform phenotype. A further study, using a library of genetically tagged retroviruses to identify clonal siblings, has argued that such clones may be the terminal branches of a more widespread lineage, since about half the clones were seen to be widely distributed in the cortex, comprising multiple neuronal or glial types.[22] Much remains to be discovered regarding the factors, both intrinsic and external, that determine cortical cell phenotypes. *In vitro* experiments have suggested that their neurotransmitter phenotype is specified by local environmental factors,[34] as for the peripheral nervous system (Chapter 5). The assembly of cortical circuits, involving the development of appropriate horizontal and vertical projections from neurons lying in any particular layer, is discussed further in Chapters 10 and 14.

Reeler mice, reelin and human abnormalities of migration/lamination

Important insights into cortical development have come from the analysis of a mutant mouse, *reeler*, first described nearly 50 years ago. These animals, so-called because they lack motor control and fall over, have disordered lamination of the cerebral neocortex, hippocampus and cerebellar cortex, as well as abnormal neuronal arrangements in the retina and in several brainstem nuclei. In the neocortex the early phases of cell proliferation and migration are normal but the cortical plate does not form within the preplate, and so fails to divide it into the marginal zone and subplate. Instead, cortical plate neurons pile up in a disorganized manner underneath the undivided preplate ('superplate');[35] later-formed neurons fail to migrate past their predecessors and come to occupy successively deeper levels of the neuropil.

The *reeler* gene has turned out to encode a large extracellular matrix-like protein, reelin, which is not secreted in the mutant.[36] Reelin contains EGF-like repeats similar to those found in other extracellular matrix molecules, and its amino-terminus is homologous to F-spondin, a protein secreted from the floor plate which regulates growth of commissural axons.[37] During normal cortical development it is expressed preferentially by cells in the outer part of the preplate which later become a subset of cells in the marginal zone, also known as Cajal–Retzius neurons,[38] but its exact function is unclear at present. One possibility is that it provides (or binds and stabilizes) a cue for migrating neurons directing them to stop migration and differentiate,[39,40] and a similar role has been suggested in the cerebellar cortex (see below). It has been shown, for example, that reelin binds $\beta 1$ integrin, thereby modulating integrin-mediated cell–cell adhesion.[41] The neurotrophin BDNF (Chapter 12) has also been shown to be a negative regulator of reelin expression by Cajal–Retzius neurons,[42] providing one possible mechanism for control of cortical development by neurotrophins. Expression is further regulated by thyroid hormone, and this may partly explain the well-known dependence of postnatal cortical development on adequate levels of the hormone.[43,44] Reelin is expressed later in cortical development by cortical plate cells, and its role in the development of hippocampal connections is discussed in Chapter 7.

Mutations in the murine gene *mdab1*, homologous to the gene *disabled* in *Drosophila*, also have a *reeler*-like phenotype. *mdab1* is expressed by migrating cortical neurons, and encodes a cytoplasmic adapter protein that may bind and facilitate the function of cytoplasmic tyrosine kinases, possibly as a component of an intracellular signalling cascade triggered in migrating neurons by their interaction with extracellular reelin.[45] Candidate receptors for reelin have also been identified, namely the ApoE receptor 2 and the very low-density lipoprotein receptor, which may be functionally redundant, and a family of cadherin-like proteins.[46] Overall, of course, a variety of molecular mechanisms are likely to act in concert to regulate cortical neuronal migration, as strongly suggested by the number (over 25) of distinct human syndromes that appear to involve abnormal cortical migration/lamination.[39,46,47] Examples include the congenital malformation *lissencephaly*, where the cerebral cortex is smooth, and *microgyria*, where it shows an increased number of small folds. A gene *LIS-1*, which is mutated in some lissencephalic patients, encodes the non-catalytic subunit of platelet-activating factor acetylhydrolase,[48] a protein with homologies to the β-subunit of G proteins.[49] A further gene associated with human lissencephaly is *doublecortin*, which encodes a novel microtubule-associated protein expressed in migrating brain neurons,[46,50,51] but precisely how these mutations result in lissencephaly remains uncertain. It has also been speculated that major neuropsychiatric disorders such as schizophrenia may result from abnormal cortical cell migration. Abnormal cortical layering has been described in the brains of schizophrenics,[52] but the evidence that this condition has its origins in such early developmental processes is not yet strong.[53]

Migration of olfactory bulb precursors

A unique population of tangentially migrating neurons has been identified that originates in the subventricular zone of the cerebral cortex adjacent to the anterior tip of the lateral ventricle. Retroviral labelling experiments have shown that these cells

migrate further forwards, in 'chains' parallel to the pial surface, for several millimetres into the developing olfactory bulb. Here they migrate radially and differentiate into interneurons (Fig. 7.6). Many divide during migration, so they are
progenitor cells rather than postmitotic, presumptive neurons. In the rat most of the
migration takes place during the early postnatal stage, but some cells continue to
migrate throughout the life of the animal,[54] providing an exception to the general
rule that there is no stem cell renewal of neurons in the adult mammalian brain (see
also Chapter 17).

This migration, known as the 'rostral migratory stream', is dependent on the presence in the pathway of the highly polysialated form of the cell adhesion molecule
NCAM (see Chapter 9). Targeted deletion of this NCAM isoform in mice results in a
small olfactory bulb, and cells accumulate in the migratory pathway.[55] The defect is
also phenocopied by specific cleavage of polysialic acid (PSA) from NCAM after intracranial injection of the enzyme endoneuraminidase N into neonatal mice,[56] and PSA
removal is thought to block migration by increasing cell–cell adhesion. In transplantation experiments, cells from the anterior subventricular zone (aSVZ) of mutant mice
migrate normally when placed in the aSVZ of normal mice, but not vice versa, con-
firming the importance of the cell environment in facilitating migration.[57] *In vivo* the
migrating cell chains are ensheathed by glial cells, but these may not be critical since
migrating cell chains can be seen in explant cultures of aSVZ cells in the absence of

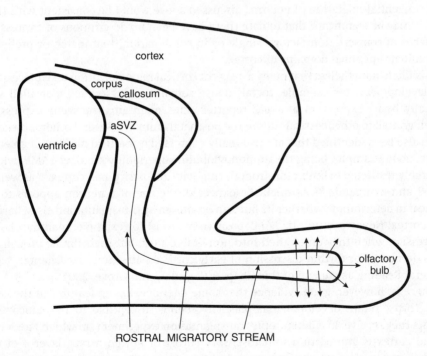

Figure 7.6 Lengthy 'horizontal' migration of olfactory bulb interneuron precursors from the
anterior subventricular zone (aSVZ). Once in the olfactory bulb, cells migrate radially. After
O'Rourke.[118]

glia.[58] Presumably the production by migrating cells themselves of PSA–NCAM is important for their movement, while the extensive contacts they make with each other during migration also suggest that mutually cooperative interactions are critical.

The factors that guide the migration are less clear, although there is evidence that diffusible repellent molecules may be released by the midline septum.[59] One such repellent has been identified as the diffusible protein Slit,[60] also involved in axon guidance at the body midline in flies and vertebrates (see Chapter 9), and the same molecule has been implicated in another tangential migration, from the lateral ganglionic eminence to the developing neocortex (see above).[61]

Regionalization of cerebral cortex

A key feature of the mammalian cerebral cortex is its regionalization into distinct areas with individual functions, cytoarchitecture and patterns of connectivity. Since the function of any area is critically dependent on the modality (e.g. visual, somatosensory) of its thalamic input, one possibility would be that this input also imprints regional character on the cortex during development. In the extreme, the early cortical plate might represent a 'tabula rasa' waiting for further instruction from thalamic axons, rather than a protomap (see above) of already-determined subregions. The tangential migration of neurons discussed above would be consistent with this, and it may be significant that to date there have been no descriptions of expression patterns of transcription factors, single or in combination, that match or prefigure individual functional domains of cortex.

It is likely nonetheless that many aspects of cortical regionalization take place early in development: for example, foetal mouse somatosensory cortex, identified specifically by its expression of a *lacZ* reporter gene, maintains transgene expression when grafted to other cortical sites in the postnatal animal.[62] Several other molecules have also been identified that are regionally expressed by cortical neurons at an early stage, good examples being the immunoglobulin superfamily member LAMP, which is largely restricted to limbic (prefrontal, cingulate and perirhinal) cortex,[63] as well as FGF-7 and neuregulin.[64] As might be expected, the age of a neuron appears to be critical in determining whether its fate can be altered by transplantation elsewhere in the cortex. Newly postmitotic LAMP-positive neurons, for example, maintain LAMP expression when they are grafted into non-limbic sites, but their limbic progenitor cells do not.[64] For further discussion of early cortical patterning, see Chapter 3 and General Reading at the end of this Chapter (Ragsdale and Grove, 2001).

There is, however, good evidence that some later-developing features of the cerebral cortex retain developmental plasticity, being susceptible to the subcortical inputs they receive. In a heterotopic transplantation experiment, in which late foetal visual cortex is grafted into somatosensory cortex of newborn rats, layer 4 of the grafted cortex changes character and develops typical 'barrels' of cells processing input from individual whiskers (see Chapter 14), presumably under the influence of the ingrowing whisker-related thalamic afferents.[65] Long-distance cortical efferent connections are also determined late, since frontoparietal cortex grafted to an occipital position makes subcortical connections typical of its new position.[66] Finally, if retinal axons are made to innervate auditory or somatosensory cortex in neonatal rodents, these regions of cortex can process the visual input in a behaviourally appropriate way.[67] Such results may be consistent with the phylogenetic importance of cerebral cortex as a mediator of CNS plasticity, and the activity-dependence of cortical connectivity seen at later postnatal stages (Chapter 14) is a further reflection of this remarkable property.

Cortical morphogenesis

Gyri, sulci and folia are characteristic anatomical features of the human cerebral and cerebellar cortex, allowing a large surface area of grey matter to fit within the restricted cranial volume, and it is interesting to ask how they arise. Sulci are classified into primary, secondary and tertiary, and while the primary sulci are invariant in all members of a species, the others (particularly tertiary sulci) show greater variability, even in identical twins. The generation of cortical neurons ends before birth in monkeys, and presumably in humans, and gyri are not prominent until between 26 and 28 weeks of human gestation. Tertiary sulci appear during the last 2 months of human gestation, probably after the phase of neuronal production, and become fully developed in the first year after birth. Even though the human brain continues to undergo extensive growth to reach maturity, multiplying its neonatal weight some fourfold as glia proliferate, neurons enlarge their arbors and axons are myelinated, the final morphology is established early.

One explanation for cortical folding is that it arises from unequal rates of cell proliferation and/or migration in the different layers and regions of the cortex, and this has been advanced to account for lissencephaly and microgyria, as discussed above. It has also been suggested that mechanical tension along axons in the cerebral cortical white matter, counterbalanced by hydrostatic pressure, might pull strongly interconnected regions together while allowing more weakly interconnected regions to drift apart. Consistent with this possibility, neurites can generate mechanical tension on an adhesive substrate, and show viscoelastic properties under sustained stretching. Such tension-based morphogenesis could also contribute to the marked folding of the mammalian cerebellar cortex, which takes place primarily along the axis of the parallel fibres, perhaps because they too are under tension.[68]

Development of cerebellar cortex

The regularity and comparative simplicity of the cerebellar cortex, which contains only five main neuronal types, makes it an attractive system for analysing the

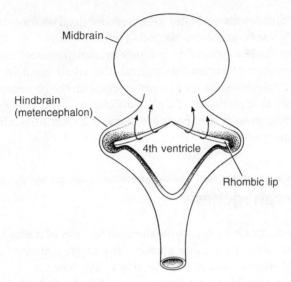

Figure 7.7 Dorsal view of the early mammalian cerebellum, showing the developing rhombic lips. Arrows show the anterior migratory path of cells from the rhombic lips forming the external granular layer. After Hatten and Heintz.[85]

specification and assembly of cortical circuitry (reviewed in reference 69). The cerebellum develops in the alar plate of rhombomere 1 and the isthmus, under the influence of the isthmic signalling centre (see Chapter 3), and quail–chick embryonic grafting experiments have shown that while the bulk of the cerebellum is derived from the anterior (rostral) hindbrain, some mediodorsal cells also originate from the midbrain epithelium.[70,71] Its primordium becomes visible after a thinning of the dorsal neural tube combines with the ventral curvature created by the pontine flexure (see Fig. 1.8) to form a rhomboid-shaped roof plate. As this structure buckles ventrally, its two anterior margins, now known as the *rhombic lips*, extend in the mediolateral axis so that cells originally lying posterior in the dorsal midline come to lie laterally, and the structure develops in a lateral-to-medial (posterior-to-anterior) sequence (Fig. 7.7).

Granule cell differentiation

The majority of cells in the three-layered cerebellar cortex develop in an inside-out sequence from the ventricular zone of the early epithelium, above the precursors of the earlier-arising deep cerebellar nuclei. The cerebellar granule cells are anomalous, however, as Cajal first recognized. They originate from cells of the rhombic lip which migrate anteriorly over the surface of the cerebellar primordium to establish the external germinal layer (EGL), effectively forming a displaced germinal zone on the pial side of the epithelium (Fig. 7.7). In mammals, the EGL cells proliferate during the early postnatal period (the layer persists for almost 2 years in humans),[72] and the population undergoes a massive clonal expansion. This proliferation has been shown to be regulated by the protein sonic hedgehog (SHH), which is produced by cerebellar Purkinje cells,[73,74] and enhanced SHH signalling has been implicated in the development of human cerebellar medulloblastoma, a malignant tumour that is thought to arise in granule cell precursors.[75]

EGL cells give rise exclusively to granule neurons,[76] even when implanted into postnatal cerebellum,[77] and are characterized by the expression of the zinc finger transcription factor, *RU49*.[78] Interestingly, *RU49* is also expressed in the granule cell lineages of the dentate gyrus and olfactory bulb, and EGL cells grafted into the developing hippocampus can adopt a hippocampal granule cell fate,[79] suggesting that the morphological identification of granule cells in different brain regions is matched by a common developmental origin. A further transcription factor, *Math1*, has been identified as essential for granule cell differentiation and is also expressed in the rhombic lip. *Math1* is the mouse homologue of the *Drosophila* gene *atonal*, a basic helix–loop–helix transcription factor essential for generating chordotonal organs, proprioceptors and R8 photoreceptor precursor cells, and *Math1* mutant mice are born without cerebellar granule cells.[80]

Granule cell migration and radial glia

Newly postmitotic granule neurons undergo a characteristic differentiation pattern to reach their mature phenotype. After descending into the deeper part of the EGL, each cell extends two axons from opposite poles of the cell body (the future parallel fibres), and the cell body then migrates 'outside-in' through the molecular layer along the radially-aligned Bergmann glial fibres, with which it makes close apposition.[81,82] It finally settles in the internal granular layer beneath the Purkinje cells, having trailed a further axon process behind it (Fig. 7.8).

In vitro assays of granule cell migration on Bergmann glia have allowed the characterization of several molecules that may mediate this interaction. Migration is inhibited by antibodies against the neuronal cell surface glycoprotein astrotactin,[83] a member of a novel family of adhesion molecules containing EGF repeats and fibronectin type III domains,[84] and expression studies of astrotactin mRNA and protein have confirmed that astrotactin is expressed maximally by granule cells during the migration phase.[85] Astrotactin is also expressed by migrating cells in the cerebral cortex and olfactory bulb, and so may be important for the generation of laminated cortex more generally. Other adhesion molecules implicated in granule cell migration include the 'adhesion molecule on glia' (AMOG)[86] and cytotactin/tenascin,[87] while mutation in a mammalian homologue of UNC-5, a protein that mediates repulsive migration responses to UNC-6/netrin (see Chapter 9), has been shown to underlie the migration defects seen in the mouse cerebellar mutant *rostral cerebellar malformation*.[88] In the latter case, netrin expression in regions surrounding the cerebellum may serve to constrain migrating neurons to cerebellar territory. Lastly, the neuregulin–erbB receptor system (see Chapter 6) has been shown to play a critical

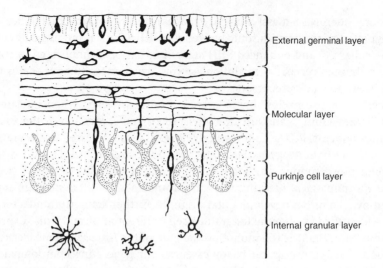

External germinal layer

Molecular layer

Purkinje cell layer

Internal granular layer

Figure 7.8 Granule cell differentiation and migration. Precursor cells proliferate in the superficial part of the external granular layer (EGL). Each postmitotic neuron descends into the deeper part of the EGL and extends two axons from opposite poles of the cell body (the future parallel fibres). The cell body continues to migrate deeper, through the molecular layer, and settles in the internal granular layer beneath the Purkinje cells, having trailed a further axon process behind it. After Jacobson.[44]

role in migration in cerebellar cortex[89] as well as cerebral cortex.[90] Granule cells express neuregulin during the migration phase, and Bergmann glia correspondingly express the neuregulin receptor erbB4; when radial glial erbB receptors are blocked *in vitro* by transfection with a dominant negative erbB4 receptor, migration on them of cocultured granule neurons is slowed significantly.[89] Based on the timing of expression, neuregulin signalling appears to operate earlier than astrotactin, but precisely how these systems interact in mediating and controlling neuronal migration is unknown.

Neuregulin signalling is also involved in generating the radial glial phenotype: granule cells are known to induce a radial glial morphology in cultured cerebellar astroglial cells,[91] and this effect can be mimicked by soluble neuregulin and blocked by glial expression of the dominant negative erbB4 receptor.[89] Neuregulin may trigger the expression of glial molecules such as BLBP, which is necessary for maintaining radial glial differentiation; BLBP is a member of a lipid-binding protein family whose other members (such as cellular retinoic acid-binding protein) convey small hydrophobic signalling molecules (such as retinoids) between cellular compartments.[92]

Purkinje cell migration and differentiation

The analysis of *reeler* mice has indicated a role for reelin in the migration of Purkinje cells, which form clusters deep in the cortical neuropil in the mutant instead of the normal, more superficial layer of cells occupying the middle stratum of the three-layered cortex. The *reeler* phenotype can be replicated in explant cultures of normal cerebellar cortex by the addition of a neutralizing antibody to reelin, and rescued when normal granule cells are added.[93] Reelin is secreted by granule cells during their premigratory phase in the EGL, and one possibility is that (as for cerebral cortex) it conveys a stop-signal (e.g. repulsive or excessively adhesive) for migrating Purkinje cells, causing them to position themselves just deep to the EGL before the phase of granule cell migration. This, however, remains to be confirmed.

The cerebellum has also been a useful system for examining the dependence of neuronal differentiation on interaction with other innervating cells. It might be anticipated, for example, that Purkinje cell differentiation is influenced by the connection of Purkinje cell dendrites with granule cell-derived parallel fibres. The early stages of Purkinje cell differentiation in fact take place in the absence of granule cells, whether in *weaver* mutant mice (see below) or X-irradiated cerebellum,[94,95] or *in vitro*.[96] On the other hand, the development of the Purkinje cell dendritic spines is dependent on interaction between the parallel fibres and the Purkinje cell dendritic arbor.[85] The autonomy of Purkinje cell development is also well demonstrated in *reeler* mice where, despite abnormal placement of the cell bodies within the cortex, the Purkinje cell phenotype persists and the cells receive normal synaptic input.[97]

Cerebellar compartments

The study of a variety of protein and glycolipid markers in the adult cerebellum has shown a striking expression pattern of seven pairs of sagittally-oriented bands, with adjacent non-expressing interbands, on either side of the midline.[98] This is exemplified by the expression of the Purkinje cell-specific antigens recognized by the antibodies Zebrin I and Zebrin II,[99] and corresponds closely to the patterns of afferent segregation in the cerebellar cortex.[100] Similar banded patterns have been seen in the developing cerebellum using *in situ* hybridization for members of several gene families implicated in early pattern formation, for example *En*, *Wnt* and *Pax*,[101] which disappear by the time the adult pattern is established. It has been suggested that some of these patterns of cortical subdivision, together with further banded patterns in the anterior–posterior axis of the cerebellum, could reflect the deployment of lineage restriction compartments of the kind defined in *Drosophila* and seen in the rhombomeres of the developing hindbrain (see Chapter 3).[102] It is interesting to speculate on the relation, for example, between compartition mechanisms and the development of functional subdivisions of the cerebellum, such as the flocculonodular lobe (vestibulocerebellum), and individual cortical lobules, but at present there is no definitive evidence for or against this possibility.

Mutations affecting cerebellar development

The motor disturbances caused by developmental abnormalities of the cerebellum are readily detected, as a result of which more than 30 separate mutations affecting cerebellar development have been described in the mouse. Examples include *reeler*, *weaver*, *staggerer*, *lurcher*, *swaying*, *Purkinje cell degeneration*, *agitans*, *hyperspiny Purkinje cell*, *meander tail*, *nervous* and *stumbler* (see reference 103 for review). In some cases the mutation affects other brain regions besides the cerebellum, a good example being *reeler* (see above). There are also several genetically-determined cerebellar ataxias in humans, some of which may be equivalent to the mouse mutations.

The detailed analysis of these mutants holds the promise of further insights into cerebellar development, and several have been now characterized at the molecular level. In *weaver*, the EGL undergoes normal proliferation but granule cell differentiation and migration subsequently fail.[104] The *weaver* mutation has been identified as a point mutation in a G-protein-gated inwardly rectifying potassium channel, GIRK2,[105] which results in constitutive sodium entry through the channel and chronic depolarization of the cell.[106,107] Differentiation and migration of *weaver* cells proceed normally if they are reaggregated with wild-type cells,[108] or implanted into wild-type EGL *in vivo*,[109] so the mutation is non-autonomous, raising the question of how wild-type cells suppress the function of the *weaver* channel. GIRK2 is also expressed more widely in the developing nervous system than predicted by the regional specificity of the *weaver* phenotype, again suggesting the additional involvement of environmental factors in modulating the function of the channel when mutant.[110]

In the case of *staggerer* (*sg*), homozygotes show marked cerebellar ataxia due to a cell-autonomous defect in Purkinje cell development, with dendritic atrophy, and decreased granule cell proliferation. These mice have a deletion within the RORα gene, which encodes a member of the nuclear hormone-receptor superfamily. The mutation prevents translation of the ligand-binding homology domain, and may retard Purkinje cell maturation by blocking the thyroid hormone signalling pathway, which is well known to be important for normal cerebellar maturation.[111] In heterozygotes of *lurcher*, a cell-autonomous mutation, Purkinje cells undergo apoptosis following their maturation in postnatal cerebellum.[112] Homozygotes die shortly after birth, and show extensive degeneration of mid- and hindbrain neurons during late embryonic development.[113] The mutation has been identified as a point mutation in the δ2 glutamate receptor which induces a large constitutive inward current, resulting in a form of cell death closely related to the excitotoxic death caused by excess glutamate.[114]

Some of the cerebellar mutations discussed above may have their counterparts in congenital human cerebellar ataxias. A further example in humans is Friedreich's ataxia, which has a prevalence of 1 in 50,000. It has an onset in childhood and is due to a recessive mutation on chromosome 9. Besides the cerebellum, degeneration in this condition affects many other parts of the brain and the peripheral nervous system. The mutation consists of an expansion of a trinucleotide repeat sequence

(GAA) which is located, surprisingly, in an intron site.[115] The normal gene codes for a phosphatidyl inositol-4-phosphate 5-kinase, and its alteration may cause a defect in vesicular trafficking or synaptic transmission.[116]

In summary, the analysis of cerebellar mutants has turned out to be somewhat fickle in terms of yielding insights into developmental mechanisms. On the other hand, examples such as *reeler* provide notable exceptions and show the power of the approach.

Key points

1 Key features of the development of cerebral and cerebellar cortex include the control of cell numbers, the layered organization, the variety of cell types and the regional differences between areas. The development of cortical connectivity is discussed in Chapters 8 and 10.

2 Mitosis occurs in cells closest to the ventricles (the ventricular zone). During the initial phase of expansion, cell divisions of the progenitor population are symmetrical and the plane of cleavage is 'vertical', so that both daughter cells remain close to the ventricle and continue dividing. Later divisions are more frequently 'horizontal' and asymmetric, causing unequal allocation to the two daughter cells of cytoplasmic proteins involved in establishing different fates. For example, more Notch-1 protein is delivered to basal cells and more Numb protein to the apical daughter.

3 Proliferation is dependent on mitogens such as FGF2, and on factors that regulate the timing of differentiation such as BF-1, a winged helix transcription factor whose expression is restricted to the developing telencephalon. The neurotransmitters GABA and glutamate have also been shown to inhibit mitosis, so reducing proliferation as cells differentiate.

4 The layers of cerebral cortex are formed by cells migrating radially along processes of radial glial cells from the ventricular zone. The earliest-born layer of neurons becomes separated into the subplate and marginal zone by the cells of the cortical plate, the definitive cerebral cortex. Cells become committed to migrate to particular layers according to the timing of their generation in the ventricular zone, their fate probably being determined by environmental signals. Lamina-specific expression of homeobox genes has been detected. Within layers there is evidence that pyramidal and non-pyramidal cells may originate from distinct precursor clones.

5 Some cells also migrate horizontally ('tangentially') in the developing cortex. For example, GABAergic neurons enter the cortex from the developing striatum, and olfactory bulb neurons migrate several millimetres from the anterior tip of the lateral ventricle, parallel to the pial surface, into the olfactory bulb; the latter process is dependent upon the polysialated form of the cell adhesion molecule NCAM.

6 Migration and layering is disrupted in many brain areas in *reeler* mice. Cortical neurons pile up in a disorganized manner as cells fail to migrate past earlier-formed ones. The gene codes for a large extracellular matrix protein, reelin, whose function is not yet clear. Other genes affecting migration have been identified, and are implicated in disorders of the developing human brain.

7 Distinct cerebral cortical areas are not known to be presaged by patterned expression of genes encoding position, and an important role is likely to played by incoming thalamic afferents at later stages of cortical formation. Certain areas, however, can be identified before thalamic inputs arrive by expressing particular proteins.

8 It has been suggested that the morphogenesis of cortical gyri and sulci may depend on different rates of cell division in particular loci, or possibly on relative degrees of tethering of different areas generated by the extent of their neuronal interconnections. Although the human brain continues growth long after birth by glial proliferation, neuronal arbor enlargement and myelination of axons, cortical gyri appear at about 28 weeks of gestation and are fully developed by the first year, so the final morphology is established relatively early.

9 The cerebellum develops from the first rhombomere of the hindbrain with a smaller contribution from the posterior midbrain.

10 All cell types except the granule cells arise conventionally in the ventricular zone and migrate outwards. The Purkinje cells require reelin in order to migrate properly, but their typical shape is largely normal in *reeler* mutant mice in spite of their misplacement deep in the cerebellum. Spines, however, fail to form on the dendrites.

11 Granule cells form from precursors which migrate over the developing structure to form a secondary, intensely active proliferative zone beneath the pia which, unusually, continues to produce granule cell neurons for some time postnatally. Granule cells migrate inwards, develop the two precursor axons of the parallel fibres, and then continue migrating outside-in by travelling along the surface of Bergman glial cells until they have passed deep to the Purkinje cell layer, spinning out their axon behind them.

12 Several factors are known to be important for granule cell migration: astrotactin (a cell surface glycoprotein), AMOG, cytotactin/tenascin, the protein homologue of the nematode *unc5* gene, neuregulin (present in granule cells) and erbB-4 (present on the Bergman glial cells).

13 Cerebellar granule cells share markers with granule cells in other parts of the brain, in particular two transcription factors: RU-49, and the product of the *Math 1* gene, a homologue of the *Drosophila* gene *atonal* which is essential for development of various sensory receptors in that species.

14 During development, a banded expression of several gene families implicated in early pattern formation can be seen to presage the intriguing series of seven sagittally-oriented stripes or bands on each side of the cerebellum. These can be visualized in the adult cerebellum by antibody staining against the Purkinje cell markers Zebrin I and II.

15 As motor disturbances arising from abnormalities of cerebellar development are readily conspicuous, more than 30 separate mouse mutations affecting cerebellar development have been documented. Several have now been characterized at the molecular level, and some such as *reeler* have illuminated the mechanisms of cerebellar development.

General reading

- Cowan, W. M., Jessell, T. M. and Zipursky, S. L. (ed.) *Molecular and cellular approaches to neural development*, 563pp. (Oxford University Press, New York, 1997).

- Hatten, M. E. and Heintz, N. Mechanisms of neural patterning and specification in the developing cerebellum. *Annu. Rev. Neurosci.* **18**, 385–408 (1995).

- Hatten, M. E. Central nervous system neuronal migration. *Annu. Rev. Neurosci.* **22**, 511–39 (1999).

- Ragsdale, C. W. and Grove, E. A. Patterning the mammalian cerebral cortex. *Curr. Opin. Neurobiol.* **11**, 50–8 (2001).

- Wingate, R. J. T. The rhombic lip and early cerebellar development. *Curr. Opin. Neurobiol.* **11**, 82–8 (2001).

References

1. Grove, E. A., Tole, S., Limon, J., Yip, L. and Ragsdale, C. W. The hem of the embryonic cerebral cortex is defined by the expression of multiple Wnt genes and is compromised in Gli3-deficient mice. *Development* **125**, 2315–25 (1998).

2. Rakic, P. Neurons in rhesus monkey visual cortex: systematic relation between time origin and eventual disposition. *Science* **183**, 425–7 (1974).

3. Price, J. and Thurlow, L. Cell lineage in the rat cerebral cortex: a study using retroviral-mediated gene transfer. *Development* **104**, 473–82 (1988).

4. Luskin, M. B., Pearlman, A. L. and Sanes, J. R. Cell lineage in the cerebral cortex of the mouse studied *in vivo* and *in vitro* with a recombinant retrovirus. *Neuron* **1**, 635–47 (1988).

5. Qian, X., Goderie, S. K., Shen, Q., Stern, J. H. and Temple, S. Intrinsic programs of patterned cell lineages in isolated vertebrate CNS ventricular zone cells. *Development* **125**, 3143–52 (1998).

6. Chenn, A. and McConnell, S. K. Cleavage orientation and the asymmetric inheritance of Notch1 immunoreactivity in mammalian neurogenesis. *Cell* **82**, 631–41 (1995).

7. Zhong, W., Feder, J. N., Jiang, M. M., Jan, L. Y. and Jan, Y. N. Asymmetric localization of a mammalian numb homolog during mouse cortical neurogenesis. *Neuron* **17**, 43–53 (1996).

8. Zhong, W., Jiang, M. M., Weinmaster, G., Jan, L. Y. and Jan, Y. N. Differential expression of mammalian Numb, Numblike and Notch1 suggests distinct roles during mouse cortical neurogenesis. *Development* **124**, 1887–97 (1997).

9. Ghosh, A. and Greenberg, M. E. Distinct roles for bFGF and NT-3 in the regulation of cortical neurogenesis. *Neuron* **15**, 89–103 (1995).

10. Vaccarino, F. M. *et al.* Changes in cerebral cortex size are governed by fibroblast growth factor during embryogenesis. *Nat. Neurosci.* **2**, 246–53 (1999).

11. Kilpatrick, T. J. and Bartlett, P. F. Clones multipotential precursors from the mouse cerebrum require FGF-2, whereas glial restricted precursors are stimulated with either FGF-2 or EGF. *J. Neurosci.* **15**, 3653–61 (1995).

12. LoTurco, J. J., Owens, D. F., Heath, M. J., Davis, M. B. and Kriegstein, A. R. GABA and glutamate

depolarize cortical progenitor cells and inhibit DNA synthesis. *Neuron* **15**, 1287–98 (1995).

13. Vicario-Abejon, C., Johe, K. K., Hazel, T. G., Collazo, D. and McKay, R. D. Functions of basic fibroblast growth factor and neurotrophins in the differentiation of hippocampal neurons. *Neuron* **15**, 105–14 (1995).

14. Xuan, S. *et al*. Winged helix transcription factor BF-1 is essential for the development of the cerebral hemispheres. *Neuron* **14**, 1141–52 (1995).

15. Hatten, M. E. Central nervous system neuronal migration. *Annu. Rev. Neurosci.* **22**, 511–39 (1999).

16. Angevine, J. and Sidman, R. Autoradiographic study of cell migration during histogenesis of cerebral cortex in the mouse. *Nature* **192**, 766–8 (1961).

17. Rakic, P. Mode of cell migration to the superficial layers of fetal monkey neocortex. *J. Comp. Neurol.* **145**, 61–83 (1972).

18. Rakic, P. Specification of cerebral cortical areas. *Science* **241**, 170–6 (1988).

19. Walsh, C. and Cepko, C. L. Widespread dispersion of neuronal clones across functional regions of the cerebral cortex. *Science* **255**, 434–40 (1992).

20. Tan, S. S. *et al*. Cell dispersion patterns in different cortical regions studied with an inactivated transgenic marker. *Development* **121**, 1029–39 (1995).

21. O'Rourke, N. A., Chenn, A. and McConnell, S. K. Postmitotic neurons migrate tangentially in the cortical ventricular zone. *Development* **124**, 997–1005 (1997).

22. Reid, C. B., Liang, I. and Walsh, C. Systematic widespread clonal organization in cerebral cortex. *Neuron* **15**, 299–310 (1995).

23. Fishell, G., Mason, C. A. and Hatten, M. E. Dispersion of neural progenitors within the germinal zones of the forebrain. *Nature* **362**, 636–8 (1993) [published erratum appears in *Nature* **363**, 286 (1993)].

24. Tan, S. S. *et al*. Separate progenitors for radial and tangential cell dispersion during development of the cerebral neocortex. *Neuron* **21**, 295–304 (1998).

25. Anderson, S. A., Eisenstat, D. D., Shi, L. and Rubenstein, J. L. Interneuron migration from basal forebrain to neocortex: dependence on *Dlx* genes. *Science* **278**, 474–6 (1997).

26. Lavdas, A. A., Gregoriou, M., Pachnis, V. and Parnavelas, J. G. Medial ganglionic eminence gives rise to a population of early neurons in the developing cerebral cortex. *J. Neurosci.* **99**, 7881–8 (1999).

27. de Carlos, J. A., Lopez-Mascaraque, L. and Valverde, F. Dynamics of cell migration from the lateral ganglionic eminence in the rat. *J. Neurosci.* **16**, 6146–56 (1996).

28. Meyer, G. and Gonzalez-Hernandez, T. Developmental changes in layer I of the human neocortex during prenatal life: a DiI-tracing and AChE and NADPH-d histochemistry study. *J. Comp. Neurol.* **338**, 317–36 (1993).

29. Brunstrom, J. E., Gray-Swain, M. R., Osborne, P. A. and Pearlman, A. L. Neuronal heterotopias in the developing cerebral cortex produced by neurotrophin-4. *Neuron* **18**, 505–17 (1997).

30. Finger, T. Feeding patterns and brain evolution in ostariophysean fishes. *Acta Physiol. Scand. Suppl.* **638**, 59–66 (1997).

31. McConnell, S. K. and Kaznowski, C. E. Cell cycle dependence of laminar determination in developing neocortex. *Science* **254**, 282–5 (1991).

32. Frantz, G. D. and McConnell, S. K. Restriction of late cerebral cortical progenitors to an upper-layer fate. *Neuron* **17**, 55–61 (1996).

33. Frantz, G. D., Weimann, J. M., Levin, M. E. and McConnell, S. K. Otx1 and Otx2 define layers and regions in developing cerebral cortex and cerebellum. *J. Neurosci.* **14**, 5725–40 (1994).

34. Götz, M. and Bolz, J. Differentiation of transmitter phenotype in rat cerebral cortex. *Eur. J. Neurosci.* **6**, 18–32 (1994).

35. Caviness, V. S. and Rakic, P. Mechanisms of cortical development: a view from mutations in mice. *Annu. Rev. Neurosci.* **1**, 297–326 (1978).

36. D'Arcangelo, G. and Curran, T. Reeler: new tales on an old mutant mouse. *BioEssays* **20**, 235–44 (1998).

37. D'Arcangelo, G. *et al*. A protein related to extracellular matrix proteins deleted in the mouse mutant reeler. *Nature* **374**, 719–23 (1995).

38. Marin-Padilla, M. Cajal-Retzius cells and the development of the neocortex. *Trends Neurosci.* **21**, 64–71 (1998).

39. Pearlman, A. L., Faust, P. L., Hatten, M. E. and Brunstrom, J. E. New directions for neuronal migration. *Curr. Opin. Neurobiol.* **8**, 45–54 (1998).

40. Sheppard, A. M. and Pearlman, A. L. Abnormal reorganization of preplate neurons and their associated extracellular matrix: an early manifestation of altered neocortical development in the reeler mutant mouse. *J. Comp. Neurol.* **378**, 173–9 (1997).

41. Dulabon, L. *et al*. Reelin binds beta 1 integrin and inhibits neuronal migration. *Neuron* **27**, 33–44 (2000).

42. Ringstedt, T. *et al*. BDNF regulates reelin expression and Cajal-Retzius cell development in the cerebral cortex. *Neuron* **21**, 305–15 (1998).

43. Alvarez-Dolado, M. *et al*. Thyroid hormone regulates reelin and dab1 expression during and brain development. *J. Neurosci.* **19**, 6979–93 (1999).

44. Jacobson, M. *Developmental neurobiology* (Plenum Press, London, 1991).

45. Howell, B. W., Hawkes, R., Soriano, P. and Cooper, J. A. Neuronal position in the developing brain is regulated by mouse disabled-1. *Nature* **389**, 733–7 (1997).

46. Gleeson, J. G. and Walsh, C. A. Neuronal migration disorders: from genetic diseases to developmental mechanisms. *Trends Neurosci.* **23**, 352–9 (2000).

47. Walsh, C. A. Genetic malformations of the human cerebral cortex. *Neuron* **23**, 19–29 (1999).

48. Hattori, M., Adachi, H., Tsujimoto, M., Arai, H. and Inoue, K. Miller–Dieker lissencephaly gene encodes a subunit of brain platelet-activating factor acetylhydrolase [corrected]. *Nature* **370**, 216–8 (1994) [published erratum appears in *Nature* **370**, 391 (1994)].

49. Reiner, O. *et al.* Isolation of a Miller–Dieker lissencephaly gene containing G protein beta-subunit-like repeats. *Nature* **364**, 717–21 (1993).

50. Gleeson, J. G. *et al.* Doublecortin, a brain-specific gene mutated in human X-linked lissencephaly and double cortex syndrome, encodes a putative signaling protein. *Cell* **92**, 63–72 (1998).

51. Gleeson, J. G., Lin, P. T., Flanagan, L. A. and Walsh, C. A. Doublecortin is a microtubule-associated protein and is expressed widely by migrating neurons. *Neuron* **23**, 257–71 (1999).

52. Akbarian, S. *et al.* Maldistribution of interstitial neurons in prefrontal white matter of the brains of schizophrenic patients. *Arch. Gen. Psychiatry* **53**, 425–36 (1996).

53. Raedler, T. J., Knable, M. B. and Weinberger, D. R. Schizophrenia as a developmental disorder of the cerebral cortex. *Curr. Opin Neurobiol.* **8**, 157–61 (1998).

54. Lois, C. and Alvarez-Buylla, A. Long-distance neuronal migration in the adult mammalian brain. *Science* **264**, 1145–8 (1994).

55. Tomasiewicz, H. *et al.* Genetic deletion of a neural cell adhesion molecule variant (N-CAM-180) produces distinct defects in the central nervous system. *Neuron* **11**, 1163–74 (1993).

56. Ono, K., Tomasiewicz, H., Magnuson, T. and Rutishauser, U. N-CAM mutation inhibits tangential neuronal migration and is phenocopied by enzymatic removal of polysialic acid. *Neuron* **13**, 595–609 (1994).

57. Hu, H., Tomasiewicz, H., Magnuson, T. and Rutishauser, U. The role of polysialic acid in migration of olfactory bulb interneuron precursors in the subventricular zone. *Neuron* **16**, 735–43 (1996).

58. Wichterle, H., Garcia-Verdugo, J. M. and Alvarez-Buylla, A. Direct evidence for homotypic, glia-independent neuronal migration. *Neuron* **18**, 779–91 (1997).

59. Hu, H. and Rutishauser, U. A septum-derived chemorepulsive factor for migrating olfactory interneuron precursors. *Neuron* **16**, 933–40 (1996).

60. Wu, W. *et al.* Directional guidance of neuronal migration in the olfactory system by the protein Slit. *Nature* **400**, 331–6 (1999).

61. Zhu, Y., Li, H., Zhou, L., Wu, J. Y. and Rao, Y. Cellular and molecular guidance GABAergic neuronal migration from an extracortical origin to the neocortex. *Neuron* **23**, 473–85 (1999).

62. Cohen-Tannoudji, M., Babinet, C. and Wassef, M. Early determination of a mouse somatosensory cortex marker. *Nature* **368**, 460–3 (1994).

63. Levitt, P. A monoclonal antibody to limbic system neurons. *Science* **223**, 299–301 (1984).

64. Levitt, P., Barbe, M. F. and Eagleson, K. L. Patterning and specification of the cerebral cortex. *Annu. Rev. Neurosci.* **20**, 1–24 (1997).

65. Schlaggar, B. L. and O'Leary, D. D. Potential of visual cortex to develop an array of functional units unique to somatosensory cortex. *Science* **252**, 1556–60 (1991).

66. O'Leary, D. D. and Stanfield, B. B. Selective elimination of axons extended by developing cortical neurons is dependent on regional locale: experiments utilizing fetal cortical transplants. *J. Neurosci.* **9**, 2230–46 (1989).

67. Frost, D. O. and Metin, C. Induction of functional retinal projections to the somatosensory system. *Nature* **317**, 162–4 (1985).

68. Van Essen, D. C. A tension-based theory of morphogenesis and compact wiring in the central nervous system. *Nature* **385**, 313–8 (1997).

69. Goldowitz, D. and Hamre, K. The cells and molecules that make a cerebellum. *Trends Neurosci.* **21**, 375–82 (1998).

70. Le Douarin, N. M. Embryonic neural chimaeras in the study of brain development. *Trends Neurosci.* **16**, 64–72 (1993).

71. Wingate, R. J. T. and Hatten, M. E. Cerebellar rhombic lip derivatives. *Development* **126**, 4395–404 (1999).

72. Raaf, J. and Kernohan, J. A study of the external granular layer in the cerebellum. *Am. J. Anat.* **75**, 151–72 (1944).

73. Wechsler-Reya, R. J. and Scott, M. P. Control of neuronal precursor proliferation in the cerebellum by Sonic Hedgehog. *Neuron* **22**, 103–14 (1999).

74. Dahmane, N. and Ruiz-i-Altaba, A. Sonic hedgehog regulates the growth and patterning of the cerebellum. *Development* **126**, 3089–100 (1999).

75. Goodrich, L. V., Milenkovic, L., Higgins, K. M. and Scott, M. P. Altered neural cell fates and medulloblastoma in mouse patched mutants. *Science* **277**, 1109–13 (1997).

76. Hallonet, M. E., Teillet, M. A. and Le Douarin, N. M. A new approach to the development of the cerebellum provided by the quail–chick marker system. *Development* **108**, 19–31 (1990).

77. Alder, J., Cho, N. K. and Hatten, M. E. Embryonic precursor cells from the rhombic lip are specified to a cerebellar granule neuron identity. *Neuron* **17**, 389–99 (1996).

78. Yang, X. W., Zhong, R. and Heintz, N. Granule cell specification in the developing mouse brain as defined by expression of the zinc finger transcription factor RU49. *Development* **122**, 555–66 (1996).

79. Vicario-Abejon, C., Cunningham, M. G. and McKay, R. D. Cerebellar precursors transplanted to the neonatal dentate gyrus express features characteristic of hippocampal neurons. *J. Neurosci.* **15**, 6351–63 (1995).

80. Ben-Arie, N. *et al.* Math1 is essential for genesis of cerebellar granule neurons. *Nature* **390**, 169–72 (1997).

81. Sidman, R. L. and Rakic, P. Neuronal migration, with special reference to developing human brain: a review. *Brain Res.* **62**, 1–35 (1973).

82. Rakic, P. Neuron–glia relationship during granule cell migration in developing cerebellar cortex. A Golgi and electronmicroscopic study in Macacus Rhesus. *J. Comp. Neurol.* **141**, 283–312 (1971).

83. Edmondson, J. C., Liem, R. K., Kuster, J. E. and Hatten, M. E. Astrotactin: a novel neuronal and cell surface antigen that mediates neuron–astroglial interactions in cerebellar microcultures. *J. Cell Biol.* **106**, 505–17 (1988).

84. Zheng, C., Heintz, N. and Hatten, M. E. CNS gene encoding astrotactin, which supports neuronal migration along glial fibers. *Science* **272**, 417–19 (1996).

85. Hatten, M. E. and Heintz, N. Mechanisms of neural patterning and specification in the developing cerebellum. *Annu. Rev. Neurosci.* **18**, 385–408 (1995).

86. Antonicek, H., Persohn, E. and Schachner, M. Biochemical and functional characterization of a novel neuron–glia adhesion molecule that is involved in neuronal migration. *J. Cell Biol.* **104**, 1587–95 (1987).

87. Chuong, C. M., Crossin, K. L. and Edelman, G. M. Sequential expression and differential function of multiple adhesion molecules during the formation of cerebellar cortical layers. *J. Cell Biol.* **104**, 331–42 (1987).

88. Ackerman, S. L. *et al.* The mouse rostral cerebellar malformation gene encodes an UNC-5-like protein. *Nature* **386**, 838–42 (1997).

89. Rio, C., Rieff, H. I., Qi, P., Khurana, T. S. and Corfas, G. Neuregulin and erbB receptors play a critical role in neuronal migration. *Neuron* **19**, 39–50 (1997).

90. Anton, E. S., Marchionni, M. A., Lee, K. F. and Rakic, P. Role of GGF/neuregulin signaling in interactions between migrating neurons and radial glia in the developing cerebral cortex. *Development* **124**, 3501–10 (1997).

91. Hatten, M. E. Neuronal regulation of astroglial morphology and proliferation *in vitro*. *J. Cell Biol.* **100**, 384–96 (1985).

92. Feng, L., Hatten, M. E. and Heintz, N. Brain lipid-binding protein (BLBP): a novel signaling system in the developing mammalian CNS. *Neuron* **12**, 895–908 (1994).

93. Miyata, T., Nakajima, K., Mikoshiba, K. and Ogawa, M. Regulation of Purkinje cell alignment by reelin as revealed with CR-50 antibody. *J. Neurosci.* **17**, 3599–609 (1997).

94. Llinas, R., Hillman, D. E. and Precht, W. Neuronal circuit reorganization in mammalian agranular cerebellar cortex. *J. Neurobiol.* **4**, 69–94 (1973).

95. Sotelo, C. Formation of presynaptic dendrites in the rat cerebellum following neonatal X-irradiation. *Neuroscience* **2**, 275–83 (1977).

96. Baptista, C. A., Hatten, M. E., Blazeski, R. and Mason, C. A. Cell–cell interactions influence survival and differentiation of purified Purkinje cells *in vitro*. *Neuron* **12**, 243–60 (1994).

97. Rakic, P. and Sidman, R. Synaptic organisation of displaced and disoriented cerebellar cortical neurons in reeler mice. *J. Neuropathol. Exp. Neurol.* **31**, 192 (1972).

98. Oberdick, J., Baader, S. L. and Schilling, K. From zebra stripes to postal zones: deciphering patterns of gene expression in the cerebellum. *Trends Neurosci.* **21**, 383–90 (1998).

99. Hawkes, R., Brochu, G., Dore, L., Gravel, C. and Leclerc, N. Zebrins: molecular markers of compartmentation in the cerebellum. In *The cerebellum revisited* (ed. R. Llinas and C. Sotelo), pp. 22–55 (Springer-Verlag, New York, 1992).

100. Gravel, C. and Hawkes, R. Parasagittal organization of the rat cerebellar cortex: direct comparison of Purkinje cell compartments and the organization of the spinocerebellar projection. *J. Comp. Neurol.* **291**, 79–102 (1990).

101. Millen, K. J., Hui, C. C. and Joyner, A. L. A role for En-2 and other murine homologues of *Drosophila* segment polarity genes in regulating positional information in the developing cerebellum. *Development* **121**, 3935–45 (1995).

102. Herrup, K. and Kuemerle, B. The compartmentalization of the cerebellum. *Annu. Rev. Neurosci.* **20**, 61–90 (1997).

103. Goldowitz, D. and Eisenman, L. M. Genetic mutations affecting murine cerebellar structure and function. In *Genetically defined models of neurobehavioural dysfunctions* (ed. P. Driscoll), pp. 66–88 (Birkhauser, Boston, 1992).

104. Sotelo, C. and Changeux, J. P. Bergmann fibers and granular cell migration in the cerebellum of homozygous weaver mutant mouse. *Brain Res.* **77**, 484–91 (1974).

105. Patil, N. *et al.* A potassium channel mutation in weaver mice implicates membrane, excitability in granule cell differentiation. *Nat. Genet.* **11**, 126–9 (1995).

106. Kofuji, P. *et al.* Functional analysis of the weaver mutant GIRK2 K^+ channel and rescue of weaver granule cells. *Neuron* **16**, 941–52 (1996).

107. Slesinger, P. A. *et al.* Functional effects of the mouse weaver mutation on G protein-gated inwardly rectifying K^+ channels. *Neuron* **16**, 321–31 (1996).

108. Gao, W. Q., Liu, X. L. and Hatten, M. E. The weaver gene encodes a nonautonomous signal for CNS neuronal differentiation. *Cell* **68**, 841–54 (1992).

109. Gao, W. Q. and Hatten, M. E. Neuronal differentiation rescued by implantation of Weaver granule cell precursors into wild-type cerebellar cortex. *Science* **260**, 367–9 (1993).

110. Hess, E. J. Identification of the weaver mouse mutation: the end of the beginning. *Neuron* 16, 1073–6 (1996).

111. Hamilton, B. A. *et al.* Disruption of the nuclear hormone receptor RORalpha in staggerer mice. *Nature* **379**, 736–9 (1996) [published erratum appears in *Nature* **381**, 346 (1996)].

112. Norman, D. J. *et al.* The lurcher gene induces apoptotic death in cerebellar Purkinje cells. *Development* **121**, 1183–93 (1995).

113. Cheng, S. S. W. and Heintz, N. Massive loss of mid- and hindbrain neurons during embryonic development of homozygous lurcher mice. *J. Neurosci.* **17**, 2400–7 (1997).

114. Zuo, J. *et al.* Neurodegeneration in Lurcher mice caused by mutation in delta2 glutamate receptor gene. *Nature* **388**, 769–73 (1997).

115. Campuzano, V. *et al.* Friedreich's ataxia: autosomal recessive disease caused by an intronic GAA triplet repeat expansion. *Science* **271**, 1423–7 (1996).

116. Carvajal, J. J. *et al.* The Friedreich's ataxia gene encodes a novel phosphatidylinositol-4-phosphate 5-kinase. *Nat. Genet.* **14**, 157–62 (1996).

117. Chenn *et al.* Development of the cerebral cortex: mechanisms controlling cell fate, laminar and areal patterning, and axonal connectivity. In *Molecular and cellular approaches to neural development* (ed. W. M. Cowan, T. M. Jessell and S. L. Zipursky), pp. 440–73 (Oxford University Press, New York, 1997).

118. O'Rourke, N. A. Neuronal chain gangs: homotypic contacts support migration into the olfactory bulb. *Neuron* **16**, 1061–4 (1996).

8

Development of Sense Organs

The eye

The compound eye of the fly and some evolutionary considerations

The compound eye of the fly has provided a powerful model system for analysing the mechanisms of inductive signalling and cell interactions in determining cell fate in the nervous system. In developing tissues such as the neurogenic region of the fly, where the signalling and receiving cells start out as equivalent, cell fates are established through lateral specification, as discussed in Chapter 4. In the compound eye, by contrast, the participating cells start out with non-equivalent properties. Genetic mosaic studies in the 1970s showed that despite the well-ordered development of the different classes of neuron and support cell in the eye, there are no strict lineage relationships between them, suggesting an important role for cell interactions.[1,2] The development of one particular neuron, the R7 photoreceptor, then became the subject of intense interest. Mutant screens identified genes involved in determining the R7 fate, and mosaic analysis was used to assess whether their products are involved in the transmission or reception of the relevant signals between interacting cells.[3] More generally, the validity of this system as a model for other neuronal determination pathways has been vindicated by the finding that the molecules involved in R7 determination are highly conserved between insects and vertebrates. With the advantage of hindsight this is perhaps not surprising, for despite strikingly different patterns of eye morphogenesis between the compound eyes of insects and the camera eyes of vertebrates, and the long-standing belief that the two systems evolved independently, studies of the earlier stages of eye development have also revealed remarkable homologies in a number of critical regulatory components, suggesting descent from a common ancestral eye. This is exemplified by the *Drosophila* gene *eyeless*, which encodes a nuclear protein expressed in the eye imaginal disc, containing both a homeodomain and a paired domain. Loss of *eyeless* function results in deleted eye structures, while its misexpression in other imaginal discs causes ectopic eyes to develop on the antennae, wings and legs;[4] strikingly, its mouse homologue, *Pax6*, is also essential for normal eye development (see below),[5] and *Pax6* can also induce ectopic compound eyes when misexpressed in *Drosophila*.

At least five *Drosophila* genes whose mutations result in eye loss have now been characterized. Further examples are provided by *eyes absent* (*eya*), a gene that is essential for eye formation by *eyeless*, and which can be functionally replaced by a vertebrate *Eya* homologue;[6] and the homeobox gene *sine oculis*, in mutants of which the optic lobes and ommatidia fail to develop,[7] and whose mammalian homologue, *Six3*, is involved in lens development (see below). In *Drosophila* these genes can induce ectopic eyes, alone or in combination, and function at several stages of eye development, from initial determination of the eye primordium to photoreceptor differentiation. Their products appear to operate through an interactive network involving reciprocal feedback, or through a linear hierarchy, depending on the developmental stage.[8] Whether their vertebrate homologues act similarly in a conserved genetic pathway remains to be determined.

Another argument favouring common ancestry is that light absorption by opsins and phototransduction via a G-protein-linked signalling cascade are common to insects, cephalopods and vertebrates, presumably having evolved from a simple ancestral photosensitive cell. One possibility would be that the common ancestral eye consisted only of such photoreceptors; since *eyeless* is re-expressed during terminal photoreceptor differentiation in *Drosophila*, and its homologues control expression of rhodopsin genes through a highly conserved binding site found in the rhodopsin promoters of most species,[9] it has been suggested that this was its ancestral role. Perhaps it was subsequently co-opted for each upstream developmental stage as the eye diverged in evolution. *Pax6* is not expressed, however, in vertebrate or cephalopod photoreceptors.[10] Alternatively, if different metazoan eyes did evolve independently, it would have to be argued that they recruited similar signalling pathways for the purpose, with genes such as *Pax6* and *Six3* playing an earlier role in patterning other anterior head structures.[10,11]

Photoreceptor differentiation

The compound eye is a lattice of some 800 hexagonally-arranged reiterated units known as ommatidia, each ommatidium containing an invariant number of cells comprising eight photoreceptor neurons and 12 additional non-neuronal cells (cone cells, which secrete the lens, and pigment cells). In the eye imaginal disc of the late larval stage, ommatidial differentiation is initiated in a structure known as the morphogenetic furrow, a groove which progresses in a posterior-to-anterior direction within the disc as increasing numbers of ommatidia are assembled (Fig. 8.1). The

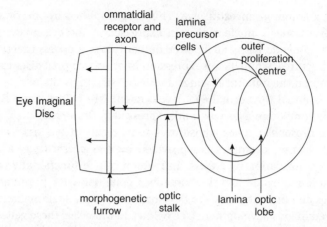

Figure 8.1 Lateral view of the developing *Drosophila* eye and optic lobe. Photoreceptor cells in the eye imaginal disc differentiate in the morphogenetic furrow and trigger further receptor differentiation by secreting Hedgehog protein, so the furrow moves forward (arrows). Receptor cell axons traverse the optic stalk and trigger lamina precursor cells to differentiate while new precursor cells are recruited from the outer proliferative zone. Receptor axons 1 to 6 terminate retinotopically in the lamina, but axons from receptors 7 and 8 advance further into the medulla (not shown). After Cutforth and Gaul.[122]

photoreceptors differentiate in a fixed sequence (R8, then sequential pairings of R2 and R5, R3 and R4, R1 and R6, and finally R7). As they do so, they secrete Hedgehog protein (Hh), which is thought to perpetuate movement of the furrow by triggering differentiation of neighbouring, anteriorly-placed cells,[12-14] a process that also involves the Dpp signalling pathway.[15,16]

A variety of mutations affecting R7 development have been identified, prominent among them being the *sevenless* (*sev*)[17,18] and *bride of sevenless* (*boss*)[19] genes. In null *sev* and *boss* mutants, R7 is transformed into a non-neuronal cone cell, and mosaic analysis shows that the *sev* product is required in R7, and the *boss* product in R8, for R7 to develop successfully. The implication is that the *boss* product is a signal generated by R8 that interacts with an appropriate receptor on R7, the *sev* product, to induce normal R7 development. Consistent with this, the *sevenless* gene encodes a receptor tyrosine kinase (RTK),[20] and the protein is localized immunohistochemically in R7 (as well as R3 and R4) precisely where it abuts R8 but not other cells.[21] Expression appears in R7 several hours before overt differentiation, and its expression needs to continue for several hours for R7 induction to be effective.[22] Also consistent with the model, the *boss* sequence encodes a transmembrane protein which localizes on the R8 cell membrane, and is expressed for the duration of the period required for *sev* activity.[19] Finally, expression of a truncated, constitutively active version of Sev protein rescues the sevenless (and boss) phenotype, and transforms cone cell precursors into supernumerary R7 cells.[23]

Direct evidence for boss–sevenless interaction has come from *in vitro* transfection experiments using a *Drosophila* cell line: *sev*-expressing cells aggregate with *boss*-expressing cells when the two cell types are mixed together, accompanied by a rapid increase in tyrosine phosphorylation on Sev protein, but both cell types form single-cell suspensions when cultured alone.[24,25] Boss–Sev interaction *in vivo* appears to be followed by transfer of Boss protein from R8 to R7 and its internalization via receptor-mediated endocytosis (although the latter process is not essential for R7 development to proceed normally).

What events are triggered by activated Sev tyrosine kinase that direct the cell towards the R7 fate? To answer this, the advantages of the genetic approach have been elegantly exploited in *Drosophila*, with a systematic screen for dominant enhancers of Sev function.[26] Flies carrying a temperature-sensitive *sev* allele were incubated at a temperature just sufficient to keep Sev activity above the threshold for R7 formation (that is, with some 80 per cent of ommatidia generating an R7 cell). With Sev signalling critically poised in this way, it was anticipated that small reductions in the activity of other signals in the pathway might further reduce R7 formation substantially. A screen could therefore be carried out for genes where inactivation of both alleles might be embryo-lethal, but where inactivation of only one copy (reducing the level of gene product by half) might have detectable effects on R7 development. One of the loci so-revealed was the *Ras1* gene, encoding a p21*ras* protein, the *Drosophila* homologue of vertebrate ras. As for other developmental signalling pathways (e.g. vulval development in *Caenorhabditis elegans*), Ras1 activation turns out to be a key component of the Sev signalling pathway; like activated Sev, for example, constitutively activated (but not wild-type) Ras1 protein under Sev gene control rescues the *sevenless* phenotype.[27]

Ras activity is regulated by bound guanine nucleotides, being active in the GTP-bound state and inactive in the GDP-bound state. The relative levels of active versus inactive Ras are further determined by the intrinsic GTPase activity of Ras [which inactivates GTP:Ras, a process stimulated by RasGTPase activating (RasGAP) protein] and, in reverse, by the exchange of bound GDP for GTP on Ras protein (stimulated by guanine nucleotide exchange factors, or GNEFs). Consistent with this model of Ras function in the determination of R7, a further gene identified in the Sev/dominant enhancer screen, *Son of sevenless* (*Sos*), shows significant GNEF sequence homology. Other modulators have also been identified, for example Drk, which may link Sev and Sos in a signalling complex,[28,29] and Gap1, a RasGAP protein that acts as a negative regulator of Ras1.[30] Rather less is known about events downstream of Ras, but there is good evidence that, as in vertebrates, the product of the c-raf proto-oncogene is involved,[31] and the product of *seven in absentia* (*sina*), a nuclear protein, may act still further downstream, or alternatively in parallel with the Sev pathway.[32] Figure 8.2 shows a summary scheme for R7 determination based on these genetic studies.[33]

Sev is simultaneously expressed in several ommatidial cells alongside the R7 precursor, so why does only one cell assume the R7 fate? If Boss is expressed in all presumptive ommatidial cells under the hsp 70 promoter, the cone cell precursors acquire an R7 fate, suggesting that the spatial localization of Boss is an important determinant of R7 patterning.[34] It is not the only factor, however, for the other photoreceptor precursor cells fail to adopt an R7 fate under these conditions, suggesting that they are already committed to non-R7 fates. Mutations of genes such as *seven-up* (encoding a member of the steroid receptor superfamily)[35] and *rough*

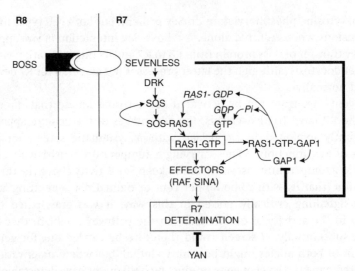

Figure 8.2 Signal transduction pathways downstream of Sevenless that determine the ommatidial R7 receptor. Activating pathways are shown by arrows and inhibitory pathways by thick black lines. See text for details. After Zipursky and Rubin.[33]

(encoding a homeodomain protein)[36] cause some of the R1–R6 precursors to transform into R7, implicating them in determining these alternative fates, and the R7 signalling pathway is suppressed in uncommitted cells by intrinsic negative regulators such as Gap1 (see above) and the transcription factor *yan*.[36] Finally, the Notch signalling pathway is also important in determining cell fates in the compound eye.[37] Misexpression of activated Notch under the control of the *sev* promoter transforms R3 and R4 precursors into R7, while R7 itself becomes a cone cell. These transformations are identical to those produced by *seven-up* and *rough* for R3 and R4, and *sev* and *boss* for R7, so they may represent the default differentiation pathways for these cells when their normal determination is perturbed. In turn, Notch signalling may help to maintain cells in an undetermined state and prevent them from responding to environmental cues until the appropriate time (see also below).[38]

It is striking that all the genes so far identified as critical for the formation of *non*-R7 photoreceptors encode nuclear products, representing transcription factors, rather than signalling molecules like Sev and Boss that might provide unique codes for individual photoreceptors. The Ras pathway, moreover, is needed in all photoreceptors,[26] so how is it triggered in these cells? The *Drosophila* EGF receptor, DER, may play a crucial role, being essential for the formation of all photoreceptors.[39] The use of a dominant-negative, truncated form of the receptor has shown that DER is required for the initial determination not only of photoreceptors but also of cone and pigment cells, suggesting that all ommatidial cells are determined by a similar mechanism.[40] The products of two further genes, *spitz* and *argos*, are also involved. The *spitz* product, which is similar to mammalian TGF-α, is a transmembrane protein bearing an extracellular EGF motif, the latter being released by proteolytic cleavage to generate the main activating ligand for DER.[41–43] The *argos* product, by contrast, is a secreted protein with an EGF-like motif that acts as an *inhibitor* of DER, and whose expression is itself triggered by DER activation.[44] A model for the operation of this system, based on the short-range concentric diffusion of the activator, Spitz, and longer-range diffusion of the inhibitor, Argos, is shown in Fig. 8.3. It helps to explain how the sequential determination of the various ommatidial cell fates may be achieved by the reiterative use of the same signalling molecules.[45] The parallel between inhibition of DER signalling by Argos (which interacts directly with the receptor) and inhibition of BMP signalling during neural induction in *Xenopus* (where the antagonists interact with the ligand rather than the receptor, see Chapter 2) is also worth noting.

Like Sev, DER is a receptor tyrosine kinase and activates the Ras pathway, so while R7 determination may need two bursts of Ras activation, perhaps to take it above some critical threshold, DER activation alone may suffice to trigger determination in the remaining cells. In either case, however, how can such apparently non-specific signalling between ommatidial cells generate the *differences* between them? The critical factor here may be one of timing, with the read-out of cell fate in response to Ras activation changing progressively as development (and the subset of transcription factors expressed within cells) also changes.[45] Such shifts in cell ground-state could be regulated internally by cells and/or by external signals derived from neighbouring cells (cf. Notch signalling discussed above), and would imply that DER–sev–Ras signalling is not so much instructive as selective or permissive of cell fates. At all events, this serves as a reminder that, alongside the importance of cell interactions in prescribing phenotypes in this system, cell-intrinsic factors remain critical, and highlights the continual interplay between cell-intrinsic and cell-extrinsic signals in generating the final pattern.

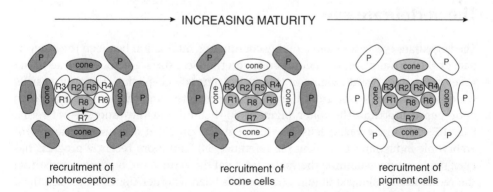

Figure 8.3 A model for ommatidial development in which secretion of Spitz protein (short range of action, light grey cells) triggers differentiation of neighbouring cells (white) but not more distant ones (dark grey). The latter are inhibited by argos protein, manufactured by each cell as it is determined and acting over a long range. R1–R8, receptor cells; P, pigment cells. In the left-hand diagram R7 formation also requires Boss–sevenless interaction as depicted by the arrow. After Freeman.[45]

Influence of axons on neurogenesis in retinal target tissues

Studies in the visual system of *Drosophila* have also revealed an important influence of axons on target cell proliferation patterns. The eight photoreceptor axons of each ommatidium fasciculate together and grow into the ipsilateral optic lobes of the CNS; R1–R6 terminate in the lamina while R7 and R8 project to deeper targets in the medulla (Fig. 8.1). Axons that have newly arrived in the lamina are necessary both for the completion of the final cell division of lamina precursor cells[46] and for their subsequent differentiation.[47] In the absence of innervation, cell division can be driven by ectopic expression of Hedgehog protein in lamina cells, Hh being normally transported anterogradely along the photoreceptor axons to serve as an inductive signal in the developing brain.[48,49] The subsequent stages of lamina neuron differentiation have been shown to be dependent on the expression of *Spitz* (see above), itself induced by hedgehog signalling.[50]

Such modulation of target cell differentiation by axons may have its counterpart in the vertebrate CNS. For example, cell survival and laminar segregation in the chick optic tectum depend on retinal innervation,[51,52] and cell cycle kinetics in the developing olfactory bulb is influenced by ingrowing primary olfactory axons.[53] The process can also be contrasted with the regulation of neuronal survival in populations of vertebrate neurons by the *retrograde* axonal transport of neurotrophic signals from their targets (see Chapter 12).

The vertebrate eye

The vertebrate eye arises from a highly coordinated interaction between the anterior part of the neural plate, the neural crest and the local surface ectoderm. The retina develops as an outward bulging of the ventrolateral diencephalon, the optic vesicle, which induces lens tissue from the overlying ectoderm, and then involutes into an optic cup comprising the outer pigment epithelium and the inner neural retina (Fig. 1.5). For many years, lens development has provided a classical example of embryonic induction (for review see reference 54), and more recently progress has been made in understanding the specification of the various cell types that constitute the retina itself. A long-standing question has been whether the two eyes originate from a single primordial field of cells which then splits in two, or from two bilaterally symmetrical primordial fields.[55,56] A recent study in *Xenopus* has helped to resolve this question: a member of the T-domain protein family of transcription factors, ET, is expressed initially as a continuous band in the anterior neural plate, and subsequently resolves into two retinal primordia. The same pattern is seen in the expression of *Pax6* (see below). The critical factor in splitting the primordial field

Dorsal view of anterior neural plate

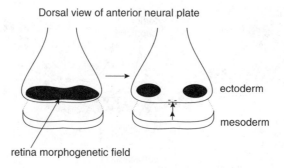

ectoderm

mesoderm

retina morphogenetic field

Figure 8.4 Formation of two eyes by the inhibitory action of the prechordal plate mesoderm acting on the original single retina morphogenetic field in the anterior neural plate. After Li *et al.*[57]

arises from the mesoderm underlying the midline of the anterior neural plate, the prechordal plate, because transplantation of prechordal plate mesoderm in chick embryos can suppress *Pax6* expression, while ablation of the mesoderm leads to the development of a single retina (Fig. 8.4).[57] It seems likely, therefore, that the prechordal mesoderm normally prevents retinal development in the midline, at least in birds and amphibia; studies of the *cyclops* mutant in zebrafish embryos have suggested that in this species the midline cells of the neural plate may also be involved in mediating midline suppression of retinal development.[58]

The signalling molecule initiating suppression is probably Sonic hedgehog (SHH), which is expressed not only in the notochord and floor plate, but also in the prechordal plate mesoderm.[59] Most strikingly, SHH knockout mice have a cyclops phenotype, with a single midline optic vesicle that remains poorly developed.[60] This phenotype is included in a rare human syndrome of congenital malformations known as holoprosencephaly, and mutations in the human *Shh* gene are known to cause this.[61] The role of SHH signalling in forebrain patterning is considered further in Chapter 3.

Besides suppressing eye development in the midline, SHH signalling probably exerts a proximo-distal patterning influence directly on the early eye primordia. Studies of *Pax* gene expression in the zebrafish have shown that ventral midline-derived SHH upregulates *Pax2* expression in the adjacent precursor cells of the developing optic stalk, while simultaneously suppressing *Pax6* to restrict its expression to the more distal parts of the optic vesicle.[62] In *cyclops* mutant embryos, for example, the presumptive retinae are expanded, along with expanded *Pax6* expression and restricted *Pax2* expression, while the reverse is seen in *Shh*-injected embryos (Fig. 8.5). Like its *Drosophila* homologue *eyeless* (see above), *Pax6* is known to be critical for normal eye development in vertebrates: it is expressed in the developing lens, neural retina and pigment epithelium,[63] and *Pax6* mutations cause the severe eye defects found in *Small eye* mutant mice[5] as well as the aniridia syndrome in humans.[64] Precisely how *Pax6* functions in normal eye development remains to be established, and one possibility is that it is involved in specifying an essential signal in the lens placode area that is critical for subsequent development of the optic vesicle.[11] Its widespread expression

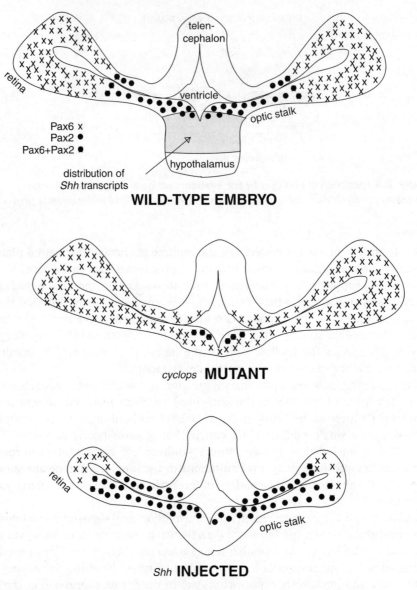

Figure 8.5 Distribution of Pax6 and Pax2 protein in wild-type, *cyclops* and *shh*-injected zebrafish embryos. See text for details. After Macdonald *et al.*[62]

not only in eye development but also in the developing brain and spinal cord suggests that it carries out multiple functions in early pattern formation and the determination of a variety of cell phenotypes, as discussed in Chapter 3.

Not surprisingly, other genes have also been implicated in the early regional specification of the eye, for example the homeobox genes *Msx*, *Rx* and *Otx2*,[65–67] but precisely how their products function is unclear at present. In the case of the mammalian homologue of *Drosophila sine oculis*, *Six3*, which is expressed in the anterior neural plate and prospective eye field, ectopic expression in fish embryos promotes ectopic lens formation in the otic placode. This suggests a role for *Six3* in the pathway that determines the lens placodal ectoderm, and also supports the view that placodal ectoderm in different regions of the head is equipotential early in its development.[11]

Subsequent stages of eye development involve the determination of its axes and the patterning of its cell types. A variety of molecular markers show graded expression patterns in the dorsoventral and nasotemporal axes, reflecting such determination, a good example being the nasotemporal gradient of the Eph receptor tyrosine kinase, EphA3 (see also Chapter 10).[68] How these gradients are established, and how they are linked to the more general process of early axis formation in the embryo, is discussed in Chapter 3.

Like the compound eye of the fly, the specification of individual cell fates in the vertebrate retina appears to mediated by sequential cell–cell interactions rather than the early appearance of cell-autonomous lineages. Since the original studies using tritiated thymidine to work out the sequence of cell fates in the developing retina,[69] it has been clear that the generation of retinal cell layers follows a rather precise, stereotyped programme. Ganglion cells, horizontal cells and cones arise first, followed by amacrine cells, bipolar cells, rods and finally glia. Cell birthdays overlap nonetheless, and at any given time multiple cell types are being generated. Studies using retroviral markers in rodents[70] and injected lineage tracers in *Xenopus*[71,72] have shown that individual labelled retinal precursor cells can generate most retinal cell phenotypes, and that cell fates are not determined irreversibly until around the stage of the final mitosis. Normal phenotypes arise in *Xenopus* eyes even when cell division and DNA synthesis are inhibited at early gastrulation,[73] so there is no obligatory requirement for precursor cells to proliferate through a set number of cycles before differentiation, again consistent with a lineage-independent mechanism.

The most extreme interpretation of these findings is that dividing retinal progenitor cells remain totipotent throughout development, and their postmitotic progeny are instructed to adopt the various retinal fates by changing environmental signals. Another possibility would be that the progenitors do undergo changes in differentiation potential with time, as seen in the fly eye, and studies of the fates of subpopulations of progenitor cells identified by specific antibodies are consistent with this.[74]

The vertebrate homologues of the *Drosophila* Notch–Delta signalling pathway, discussed in Chapter 4, are also involved in retinal development. In the developing rat retina, for example, the Notch pathway genes *Notch1*, *Notch2*, *Delta* and *Jagged* are expressed in the areas undergoing cell fate determination and differentiation.[75] The *Xenopus Notch* homologue *Xotch* is expressed by the progenitor cells and newly-postmitotic cells of the neural retina, but not by early stem cells fated to become both neural retina and pigment epithelium, or by differentiated neurons and glia. The last cells to express *Xotch* become Müller glial cells, the final phenotype to appear in the developing retina, and retinoblasts transfected with an activated form of *Xotch* retain a neuroepithelial morphology, failing to express molecular markers of differentiated neurons. These observations imply that *Xotch* may function normally to delay or inhibit cell differentiation, maintaining cells in an undifferentiated state.[76] The

Xenopus Delta homologue, *X-Delta-1*, is expressed in the same retinal cell populations as *Xotch*, and a detailed analysis of the fates of Delta-misexpressing cells at different stages of retinal development suggests a model in which Delta expression by a cell controls its competence to respond to the local environmental signals that determine its fate.[77] Following the *Drosophila* model for Notch–Delta signalling discussed in Chapter 4, Delta expression by a cell might simultaneously activate Notch expression in neighbouring cells, preventing their differentiation and keeping them in the pool of progenitor cells (Fig. 8.6).

The importance of environmental signals in determining retinal cell fates has been confirmed by retinal culture experiments. For example, the proportion of rods that differentiate in cultures of early retina can be increased by co-culture with retinal cells from older developmental stages,[78-80] while *Xenopus* rod determination *in vitro* requires at least two cell interaction steps.[81] Such experiments have also shown that retinal progenitor cells are intrinsically different at different developmental stages, and that they respond to external cues with a limited range of options. The neonatal rat retina, for example, harbours both an autoinhibitory signal produced by amacrine cells that suppresses amacrine production and a signal that generates the cone

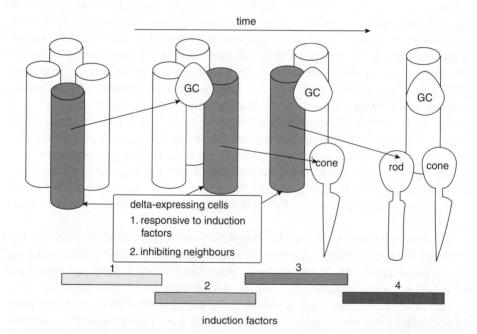

Figure 8.6 Model for vertebrate retinal cell differentiation. Those progenitor cells expressing delta protein (dark shading) are (1) able to respond to the current induction factor and (2) prevent other neighbouring cells from doing so. Once these cells have matured, other cells express delta protein in turn, and can respond to any new induction factor then present; the factors in states 1, 2 and 3 induce delta-expressing cells to form, respectively, ganglion cells (GCs), cones and then rods (*arrows*). After Dorsky *et al.*[77]

fate.[82] Several environmental factors have been implicated in vertebrate retinal development. These include SHH, which promotes the proliferation of mouse retinal precursor cells,[83] FGF signalling, which can redirect the developing retinal pigment epithelium to adopt a neural retinal fate[84] and influence cell fates in the neural retina,[85] and EGF or TGF signalling, which can also modulate retinal cell fates.[86] Receptor tyrosine kinase activation therefore appears to be critical in establishing cell fates in the vertebrate retina, as for the compound eye of the fly. A further signal may be the cytokine CNTF, which causes a marked reduction in rod differentiation in favour of a bipolar cell phenotype when added to postnatal rat retinal explants, and is able to respecify even postmitotic, presumptive rods.[87] The commitment of progenitor cells to individual retinal cell fates is also regulated by members of the basic helix–loop–helix family of transcription factor genes (see Chapter 4),[88] and by genes such as the *Otx*-like homeobox gene, *Crx*, whose product binds to conserved DNA sequences found upstream of several photoreceptor-specific sequences. *Crx* mutations also cause an inherited cone–rod dystrophy in humans.[89]

Normal retinal development also involves cell death, and this has been detected in two distinct periods that together regulate the final number of retinal cells. The first coincides with the onset of neuronal birth and migration, and has been shown, surprisingly, to be triggered by microglia-derived NGF acting through the p75 receptor.[90,91] It is also counteracted by BDNF,[92] and both neurotrophins are expressed in the early retinal epithelium. The second period corresponds to target (tectal) innervation, as discussed in Chapter 13. Lastly, the presence of melanin in the retinal pigment epithelium, which lies adjacent to the mitotic layer of the neural retina, is necessary in some way for normal retinal development. The pattern of retinal maturation is delayed in albino rats, with a deficit of rods, and there are associated abnormalities of retinal axon guidance at the optic chiasm.[93]

The inner ear

The labyrinth of chambers comprising the vertebrate inner ear is derived, like several other special sense organs, from a thickening of the head surface ectoderm, or placode. The otic placode appears adjacent to the hindbrain rhombomeres 5 and 6, and invaginates and pinches off to form the epithelial otic vesicle (otocyst). This undergoes a complex series of morphogenetic movements to acquire the three-dimensional arrangement of chambers of the adult inner ear (Fig. 8.7). Simultaneously, the epithelial cells acquire a variety of different fates, including the mechanosensory hair cells and their supporting cells, the sensory neurons of the VIIIth cranial nerve ganglia, and the specialized cells of the mammalian stria vascularis that secrete the endolymphatic fluid.

These different stages in the development of the inner ear are not well understood. Classical embryological experiments have shown that the otic placode is induced by

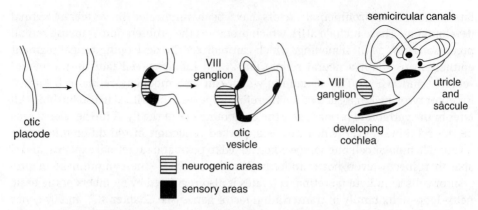

Figure 8.7 Inner ear development. The otic placode invaginates to form first a vesicle and then the complex endolymph-filled labyrinth. The neurons of the VIIIth cranial nerve and the areas giving rise to hair cells for both the cochlea and vestibular apparatus arise from localized areas of the otic vesicle. After Fekete.[101]

neighbouring tissues,[94] and transplantation studies in *Xenopus* suggest that determination of the otic vesicle occurs early, even before the appearance of the neural plate. Mesoderm underlying the presumptive otic area at the midgastrula stage is able to induce otic vesicles in unbiased ectoderm.[95] The hindbrain is thought to act as a later inducer, influencing the polarity of the inner ear, and a candidate inducing signal here is FGF3, which is expressed adjacent to the otic vesicle in rhombomeres 5 and 6, and within the vesicle itself. Although an *in vitro* study has suggested that hindbrain-derived FGF3 acts as a vesicle inducer,[96] the detailed analysis of two mouse mutants that show perturbed inner ear development argues that FGF3 is actually required later, for correct patterning within the vesicle. In FGF3 knockout mice,[97] and in *kreisler* mutants in which r5 and r6 are defective and lack localized FGF3 expression,[98] otic vesicles still form but generate a deficient endolymphatic sac and duct. The inducing signals for otic placode development have recently been identified as FGF19 and WNT8c.

The mechanisms that enable individual regions of the otic vesicle to acquire their region-specific fates are also unclear, although some generalizations can be made. Experiments involving early rotations of the chick otic vesicle *in ovo* have shown that patterning of sensory organs in the inner ear is first specified along the anteroposterior axis of the vesicle, followed by the dorsoventral axis.[99] This suggests that, as might be expected, different types of sensory organ are specified by multiple steps rather than a single inductive event. Gene expression studies have revealed that a number of transcriptional regulators (e.g. homeobox genes, POU-domain transcription factors) and developmental signalling molecules (e.g. FGF3, WNT, BMP4/5, Eph receptors, RET, Notch, Delta) are regionally expressed within the early otic vesicle. Such patterns suggest that the various cell fates of the inner ear may be specified at an early stage, and raise the possibility of mechanisms such as lateral specification of hair cells through Notch–Delta signalling.[100,101] Detailed information correlating these expression patterns with cell lineage is not available at present, and it will be interesting to see how cell diversification in the placodal ectoderm-derived inner ear turns out to compare with that of the neural ectoderm-derived retina. Studies of zebrafish mutations of the inner ear identified in a systematic screen,[102] and of mouse mutants,[103] should also be revealing.

Lastly, cell death is an important further influence affecting inner ear development. It is involved extensively in the morphogenesis of inner ear structures, for example in the formation of the semicircular canals, and its reduction in chick embryos by retrovirus-mediated overexpression of human *bcl-2* (see Chapter 13) leads to abnormal ear morphogenesis.[104] The survival of the sensory neurons of the vestibuloacoustic ganglion is influenced by both BDNF and NT-3. Nearly all of these neurons die prenatally in mice with targeted deletions of the genes for both neurotrophins, and for their receptors TrkB and TrkC. In mice lacking BDNF or TrkB, vestibular innervation to the semicircular canals is depleted by more than 80 per cent, while a similar degree of depletion is seen in cochlear innervation in NT-3- or TrkC-deficient animals (see also Chapter 12).[105]

Development of the lateral line

The lateral line is a sensory system found in fishes and amphibia for the detection of water motion close to the animal, and mediates a variety of behaviours such as prey and predator detection, shoaling, and the avoidance of obstacles. The lateral line organs comprise the *neuromasts*, which resemble the sensory patches of the inner ear; they contain both hair cells and supporting cells, together with afferent connections (projecting to the ipsilateral Mauthner cell) and efferent connections (from the hindbrain).[106] Like the inner ear, neuromasts and their afferent neurons develop from placodal ectoderm, and it was suggested last century that the inner ear derives phylogenetically from the lateral line, although this remains to be firmly established. It is interesting, for example, that most mutations affecting ear morphogenesis in a zebrafish screen do not affect the development of the lateral line.[102] In the zebrafish, the primordial cells of the lateral line are first detectable using Nomarski optics immediately adjacent to the developing acoustic ganglion. The primordium migrates caudally and rapidly (some 100 µm per hour) as a visible bump within the epidermis, at the level of the horizontal myoseptum in the midbody line, reaching a final position near the base of the caudal fin. As it migrates, it deposits clusters of cells at precise, constant positions that develop into mature neuromasts. The growth cones of the afferent sensory neurons also migrate with the primordium, but are never seen to lead it, suggesting that the primordial cells are the pathfinders and that the sensory axons follow.[107] The molecular basis for primordium migration is not well understood, but cues provided by the horizontal myoseptum may be important: in zebrafish mutants that lack a myoseptum, posterior lateral line organs are displaced ventrally.[108]

Development of taste buds

The development of the vertebrate taste system has been relatively understudied compared with other sensory systems. It was originally suggested that taste buds derive from placodal ectoderm, specifically from epibranchial placodes that lie in a ventrolateral position alongside the developing pharyngeal pouches. These placodes are very well developed, for example, in embryonic catfishes, correlating with a remarkable extension of the taste bud field to cover the entire body in this species. Transplantation experiments in axolotls have shown, however, that the epibranchial placodes give rise to gustatory afferent neurons but not the taste buds themselves.[109] Similar experiments have also ruled out an alternative origin, the neural crest, so it is likely that taste buds arise directly from the developing lingual epithelium derived from the pharyngeal endoderm. This has been confirmed in axolotls by fluorescent labelling of the early endoderm, and also by a mosaic analysis of transgenic mice expressing a *lacZ* reporter gene.[110]

The special sensory afferent axons from the VIIth (facial), IXth (glossopharyngeal) and Xth (vagus) cranial nerves invade the lingual epithelium before taste bud differentiation, so it is possible that they play an inductive role in taste bud development. Taste buds do not mature if the IXth nerve is cut bilaterally in early postnatal rats, by which time incipient taste buds have appeared,[111] and they are well known to atrophy following lingual denervation in the adult. It has also been shown that reinnervation of a denervated tongue in the adult by non-gustatory afferents can also restore the normal morphology of taste buds,[112] so at this stage the necessary signals are not specific to gustatory axons. While such observations suggest that innervation plays an essential role in maintaining the differentiated state, they do not address the question whether axons might directly instruct the differentiation of taste buds from a uniform population of precursor cells.

There is in fact good evidence that taste bud cells can develop independently of gustatory axons. Grafts of presumptive axolotl lower jaw/lingual tissue, taken before the stage of axon invasion, develop well-differentiated taste buds both *in vivo* (when placed in the trunk region) and *in vitro*, in both cases in the absence of close contacts with axons. Moreover, in mice with targeted deletions of the neurotrophin BDNF, or its receptor trkB, the number of gustatory afferents is substantially reduced, yet taste buds continue to differentiate in these animals. The capacity of the pharyngeal endoderm to generate taste buds is probably determined as early as the end of gastrulation, but the underlying molecular mechanisms have yet to be elucidated.[113] It also remains unclear how the central projections of taste afferents are mapped onto the cerebral cortex.

Development of olfactory receptors

The receptors and neurons of the olfactory system develop from invagination of the most rostrally placed placodes, the olfactory placodes, but little is known about the mechanisms leading to their individuation and differentiation. The mapping of their axon projections to the olfactory bulb represents a remarkable example of topographic specificity, and is discussed in Chapter 10. It has also been shown that the hypothalamic neurons that secrete gonadotrophin-releasing hormone (GnRH) originate from olfactory epithelial cells (the vomeronasal organ), migrating into the brain to reach their final sites for terminal differentiation.[114] This migration, and that of the primary olfactory axons, fails in patients with *Kallmann syndrome*, a rare X- linked disorder characterized by anosmia and sterility with atrophy of the olfactory bulbs and gonads. The related gene encodes a member of the immunoglobulin superfamily which is presumably involved in mediating the migration.[115] A further migration critical for the development of the olfactory system concerns the olfactory bulb interneurons, whose pathway from the forebrain ventricular zone is discussed in Chapter 7.

Development of peripheral sense organs

The sensory receptors in the skin, muscle, joints and connective tissue are formed from an association between the peripheral terminals of sensory axons, whose cell bodies lie in the sensory ganglia adjacent to the brainstem and spinal cord, and specialized receptor cells. These receptor cells transduce the sensory stimulus into electrical impulses and determine the sensitivity and pattern of impulse discharge in the sensory axon. Like synapse formation, the development of the nerve terminal and the associated cells involves mutual interactions between the growth cone of the sensory axon and the innervated cells; the sensory axon must be induced to stop growing and the receptor cells induced to differentiate. However, apart from supplying the relevant neurotrophin for survival and maintenance of the innervating sensory nerve cell (see Chapter 12), little is known about the action of the receptor cells on the sensory axons, and this account is therefore restricted to the effects of sensory axons on receptor cell differentiation.

At one end of the spectrum, the sensory axon seems to be able to alter the normal differentiation pathway of the cells it innervates and irreversibly change their phenotype. For example, muscle spindles, with their specialized intrafusal muscle fibres, cannot be detected in the adult rat if the afferents are removed at birth.[116] The sensory axons reach developing muscles before any motor axons,[117] and myotubes that are contacted by these afferents develop into the specialized, thin, weakly contractile intrafusal muscle fibres (Fig. 8.8). If the entry of afferents into developing muscle is delayed but not prevented, hybrid muscle fibres develop: the centre of the fibre in contact with the sensory axon has the typical appearance of an intrafusal fibre but the poles are large, like normal extrafusal fibres.[118] So in the case of intrafusal muscle fibres, the large-diameter primary afferent fibre can convert a myotube that would normally develop into a large extrafusal fibre into an altogether different sort of fibre.

A different scenario is evident in the case of Merkel's discs (specialized slowly adapting touch receptors in the skin), for the specific receptor cells are already present before the arrival of the nerve,[119] and the Merkel cell afferent seeks them out, although it is unclear whether this is done by chemotropism or by random searching followed by contact-based recognition.[120] While the sensory axon is not needed to induce the Merkel cells from undifferentiated epidermal cells, it is necessary for their complete maturation. It has also been shown that the mechanical sensitivity of this system is reduced some tenfold in mice with targeted deletion of the neurotrophin BDNF (see Chapter 12), in the absence of any obvious morphological abnormalities of the Merkel cells or their afferent terminals.[121] The mechanism of dependence of the sensory transduction apparatus on BDNF is uncertain, but this observation serves as a further reminder that the interactions between receptor cell and innervating axon are likely to be reciprocal.

The overall conclusion from these experiments is that sensory nerves are essential both for the development of sensory end organs and for their maintenance in the adult. The signals that mediate these actions are not yet known.

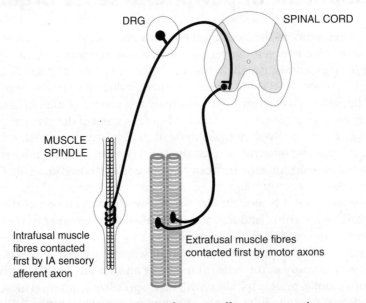

Figure 8.8 The different inductive actions of sensory afferent axons and motor axons on the fates of developing myotubes.

Key points

1 The development of the invertebrate compound eye, the vertebrate eye and ear, lateral line organs of amphibia and fish, taste buds and peripheral sensory receptors such as Merkel's discs in the skin and muscle spindles have all been intensively investigated.

2 Despite major structural differences between the compound eyes of insects and the camera-lens eyes of vertebrates, remarkable homologies exist in a number of critical components of mechanisms controlling their development. For example, the product of the *Pax6* gene, which is necessary for eye development in the mouse, can induce ectopic formation of compound eyes in *Drosophila* in the same way as the fly gene *eyeless*, and there are several other insect genes needed for eye formation with vertebrate homologues.

3 The mechanisms involved in the specification of the different cell types in each ommatidium of the *Drosophila* compound eye have been intensively analysed by the study of mutants. This has revealed a complex interplay of intrinsic and extrinsic factors.

4 All ommatidial cells need a functioning Ras signalling pathway for normal development, and this is activated by a fly homologue of vertebrate TGFα (encoded by the *spitz* gene). The EGF-like sequence of this protein activates a receptor tyrosine kinase DER, a fly homologue of the vertebrate EGF receptor. Cell secrete Hedgehog (Hh) protein as they differentiate, and this is thought to trigger the differentiation of nearby anterior cells.

5 Within the ommatidium the eight photoreceptor cells develop in strict sequence with R7, which has been the most investigated, last. The earlier-developing photoreceptors become committed to their fates by the action of genes such as *seven-up* (encoding a steroid receptor superfamily member) and *rough* (encoding a homeodomain protein). Misexpression of activated Notch protein delays this commitment. R7 development, however, is triggered by activation of a receptor tyrosine kinase on its surface encoded by the gene *sevenless*. The signal comes from a transmembrane protein present on its already-formed neighbour, R8, and this protein is encoded by the gene *bride of sevenless*. The result is activation again of the ras pathway, and several mutants disrupting R7 development are known in which the affected gene encodes a protein required downstream on this signalling pathway (e.g. *son of sevenless*).

6 The axons of the photoreceptor cells are important for the development of the cells in the optic lobe, and this is mediated by axonal transport of Hedgehog protein.

7 The vertebrate retina develops as an outward bulging of the ventrolateral diencephalon, the optic vesicle, which induces lens formation from the overlying ectoderm and then involutes into an optic cup comprising the outer pigment epithelium and the inner neural retina. The *Pax6* gene is critical for normal eye evelopment in vertebrates, with mutations causing severe eye defects in mice and humans. It is expressed in developing lens, neural retina and pigment epithelium.

Several homeobox genes are also implicated in the early regional specification of the eye.

8 The presence of two eyes results from the early inhibitory action of midline mesoderm which suppresses *Pax6* in the midline, thus converting the continuous band of *Pax6* expressing, and hence eye-destined, anterior neural plate into two separate halves. The inhibitory signal is the protein product of the *Sonic hedgehog* gene, which is also important in setting up proximo-distal gradients in the developing eye. A variety of molecular markers show graded expression patterns in the dorsoventral and nasotemporal axes but how they are established is not yet clear.

9 *In vivo* labelling studies with retroviral markers and *in vitro* studies have shown that, as in the fly, different cell types in the retina arise by sequential cell–cell interactions, with progenitors undergoing progressive changes in differentiation potential with time. Also similar is the role of Notch in holding cells in an undifferentiated state, while Delta controls competence to respond to environmental signals. Amongst agents known to affect fate are: SHH protein, which controls proliferation of precursors; FGF, which can redirect retinal epithelium to a neural fate; CNTF, which favours bipolar cell formation over that of rods; the pigment melanin; and EGF or TGF signalling, which also modulate fate. Final commitment to a particular fate may be regulated by a homeobox gene *Crx*.

10 Cell population size in the retina is partly controlled by cell death, occurring in two phases: first, while cells are being born and migrating, triggered surprisingly by the neurotrophin NGF acting on its p75 receptor; second, at the time of synapse formation (see Chapter 13).

11 The vertebrate inner ear is derived from a thickening of the head surface ectoderm, the otic placode, adjacent to rhombomeres 5 and 6, which invaginates and pinches off to form the epithelial otic vesicle (otocyst). This undergoes a complex series of morphogenetic movements to acquire the three-dimensional arrangement of chambers of the adult inner ear. Simultaneously, the epithelial cells acquire a variety of different fates, including the mechanosensory hair cells and their supporting cells, the sensory neurons of the VIIIth cranial nerve ganglion, and the specialized cells of the mammalian stria vascularis that secrete the endolymphatic fluid.

12 The signals inducing otic vesicle formation emanate first from the mesoderm and later from the hindbrain. They are not yet known, nor is it certain how the different regions differentiate, although a number of transcriptional regulators and signalling molecules are regionally expressed in the early otic vesicle. Cell death is involved extensively in the morphogenesis of inner ear structures, and the population size of vestibuloacoustic neurons is regulated by neurotrophin-regulated cell death (BDNF and NT-3).

13 In the case of peripheral sensory receptors, the afferent sensory axon is critical in either inducing differentiation of the specialized cells which it innervates and/or stimulating the further development and survival of an already-differentiated precursor.

General reading

- Cepko, C. L. The roles of intrinsic and extrinsic cues and bHLH genes in the determination of retinal cell fates. *Curr. Opin. Neurobiol.* **9**, 37–46 (1999).

- Freeman, M. Cell determination strategies in the *Drosophila* eye. *Development* **124**, 261–70 (1997).

- Whitfield, T., Haddon, C. and Lewis, J. Intercellular signals and cell fate choices in the developing inner ear: origins of global and of fine-grained pattern. *Semin. Cell Dev. Biol.* **8**, 239–47 (1997).

- Zipursky, S. L. and Rubin, G. M. Determination of neuronal cell fate: lessons from the R7 neuron of *Drosophila*. *Annu. Rev. Neurosci.* **17**, 373–97 (1994).

References

1. Lawrence, P. A. and Greene, S. M. Cell lineage in the developing retina of *Drosophila*. *Dev. Biol.* **71**, 142–52 (1979).

2. Ready, D. F., Hanson, T. E. and Benzer, S. Development of the *Drosophila* retina, a neurocrystalline lattice. *Dev. Biol.* **53**, 217–40 (1976).

3. Lawrence, P. *The making of a fly* (Blackwell Scientific Publications, Oxford, 1992).

4. Halder, G., Callaerts, P. and Gehring, W. J. Induction of ectopic eyes by targeted expression of the eyeless gene in *Drosophila*. *Science* **267**, 1788–92 (1995).

5. Hill, R. E. *et al.* Mouse small eye results from mutations in a paired-like homeobox-containing gene. *Nature* **354**, 522–5 (1991) [published erratum appears in *Nature* **355**, 750 (1992)].

6. Bonini, N. M., Bui, Q. T., Gray-Board, G. L. and Warrick, J. M. The *Drosophila* eyes absent gene directs ectopic eye formation in a pathway conserved between flies and vertebrates. *Development* **124**, 4819–26 (1997).

7. Cheyette, B. N. *et al.* The *Drosophila* sine oculis locus encodes a homeodomain-containing protein required for the development of the entire visual system. *Neuron* **12**, 977–96 (1994).

8. Desplan, C. Eye development: governed by a dictator or a junta? *Cell* **91**, 861–4 (1997).

9. Sheng, G., Thouvenot, E., Schmucker, D., Wilson, D. S. and Desplan, C. Direct regulation of rhodopsin 1 by Pax-6/eyeless in *Drosophila*: evidence for a conserved function in photoreceptors. *Genes Dev.* **11**, 1122–31 (1997).

10. Harris, W. A. Pax-6: where to be conserved is not conservative. *Proc. Natl. Acad. Sci. USA* **94**, 2098–100 (1997).

11. Oliver, G. and Gruss, P. Current views on eye development. *Trends Neurosci.* **20**, 415–21 (1997).

12. Heberlein, U., Wolff, T. and Rubin, G. M. The TGF beta homolog dpp and the segment polarity gene *hedgehog* are required for propagation of a morphogenetic wave in the *Drosophila* retina. *Cell* **75**, 913–26 (1993).

13. Ma, C., Zhou, Y., Beachy, P. A. and Moses, K. The segment polarity gene *hedgehog* is required for progression of the morphogenetic furrow in the developing *Drosophila* eye. *Cell* **75**, 927–38 (1993).

14. Burke, R. and Basler, K. Hedgehog signaling in *Drosophila* eye and limb development—conserved machinery, divergent roles? *Curr. Opin. Neurobiol.* **7**, 55–61 (1997).

15. Heberlein, U. and Moses, K. Mechanisms of *Drosophila* retinal morphogenesis: the virtues of being progressive. *Cell* **81**, 987–90 (1995).

16. Pignoni, F. and Zipursky, S. L. Induction of *Drosophila* eye development by decapentaplegic. *Development* **124**, 271–8 (1997).

17. Tomlinson, A. and Ready, D. *Sevenless*: a cell specific homeotic mutation of the *Drosophila* eye. *Science* **231**, 400–2 (1986).

18. Tomlinson, A. and Ready, D. Cell fate in the *Drosophila* ommatidium. *Dev. Biol.* **123**, 264–75 (1987).

19. Reinke, R. and Zipursky, S. L. Cell–cell interaction in the *Drosophila* retina: the *bride of sevenless* gene is required in photoreceptor cell R8 for R7 cell development. *Cell* **55**, 321–30 (1988).

20. Hafen, E., Basler, K., Edstroem, J. E. and Rubin, G. M. *Sevenless*, a cell-specific homeotic gene of *Drosophila*, encodes a putative transmembrane receptor with a tyrosine kinase domain. *Science* **236**, 55–63 (1987).

21. Tomlinson, A., Bowtell, D. D., Hafen, E. and Rubin, G. M. Localization of the sevenless protein, a putative receptor for positional information, in the eye imaginal disc of *Drosophila*. *Cell* **51**, 143–50 (1987).

22. Mullins, M. C. and Rubin, G. M. Isolation of temperature-sensitive mutations of the tyrosine kinase receptor sevenless (sev) in *Drosophila* and their use in determining its time of action. *Proc. Natl. Acad. Sci. USA* **88**, 9387–91 (1991).

23. Basler, K., Christen, B. and Hafen, E. Ligand-independent activation of the sevenless receptor tyrosine kinase changes the fate of cells in the developing *Drosophila* eye. *Cell* **64**, 1069–81 (1991).

24. Kramer, H., Cagan, R. L. and Zipursky, S. L. Interaction of bride of sevenless membrane-bound ligand and the sevenless tyrosine-kinase receptor. *Nature* **352**, 207–12 (1991).

25. Hart, A. C., Kramer, H. and Zipursky, S. L. Extracellular domain of the boss transmembrane ligand acts as an antagonist of the sev receptor. *Nature* **361**, 732–6 (1993).

26. Simon, M. A., Bowtell, D. D., Dodson, G. S., Laverty, T. R. and Rubin, G. M. Ras1 and a putative guanine nucleotide exchange factor perform crucial steps in signaling by the sevenless protein tyrosine kinase. *Cell* **67**, 701–16 (1991).

27. Fortini, M. E., Simon, M. A. and Rubin, G. M. Signalling by the sevenless protein tyrosine kinase is mimicked by Ras1 activation. *Nature* **355**, 559–61 (1992).

28. Olivier, J. P. *et al.* A *Drosophila* SH2–SH3 adaptor protein implicated in coupling the sevenless tyrosine kinase to an activator of Ras guanine nucleotide exchange, Sos. *Cell* **73**, 179–91 (1993).

29. Simon, M. A., Dodson, G. S. and Rubin, G. M. An SH3–SH2–SH3 protein is required for p21Ras1 activation and binds to sevenless and Sos proteins *in vitro*. *Cell* **73**, 169–77 (1993).

30. Gaul, U., Mardon, G. and Rubin, G. M. A putative Ras GTPase activating protein acts as a negative regulator of signaling by the Sevenless receptor tyrosine kinase. *Cell* **68**, 1007–19 (1992).

31. Dickson, B., Sprenger, F., Morrison, D. and Hafen, E. Raf functions downstream of Ras1 in the Sevenless signal transduction pathway. *Nature* **360**, 600–3 (1992).

32. Carthew, R. W. and Rubin, G. M. *seven in absentia*, a gene required for specification of R7 cell fate in the *Drosophila* eye. *Cell* **63**, 561–77 (1990).

33. Zipursky, S. L. and Rubin, G. M. Determination of neuronal cell fate: lessons from the R7 neuron of *Drosophila*. *Annu. Rev. Neurosci.* **17**, 373–97 (1994).

34. Van Vactor, D. L., Jr., Cagan, R. L., Kramer, H. and Zipursky, S. L. Induction in the developing compound eye of *Drosophila*: multiple mechanisms restrict R7 induction to a single retinal precursor cell. *Cell* **67**, 1145–55 (1991).

35. Mlodzik, M., Hiromi, Y., Weber, U., Goodman, C. S. and Rubin, G. M. The *Drosophila seven-up* gene, a member of the steroid receptor gene superfamily, controls photoreceptor cell fates. *Cell* **60**, 211–24 (1990).

36. Lai, Z. C. and Rubin, G. M. Negative control of photoreceptor development in *Drosophila* by the product of the *yan* gene, an ETS domain protein. *Cell* **70**, 609–20 (1992).

37. Cagan, R. L. and Ready, D. F. Notch is required for successive cell decisions in the developing *Drosophila* retina. *Genes Dev.* **3**, 1099–112 (1989).

38. Fortini, M. E., Rebay, I., Caron, L. A. and Artavanis-Tsakonas, S. An activated Notch receptor blocks cell-fate commitment in the developing *Drosophila* eye. *Nature* **365**, 555–7 (1993).

39. Xu, T. and Rubin, G. M. Analysis of genetic mosaics in developing and adult *Drosophila* tissues. *Development* **117**, 1223–37 (1993).

40. Freeman, M. Reiterative use of the EGF receptor triggers differentiation of all cell types in the *Drosophila* eye. *Cell* **87**, 651–60 (1996).

41. Rutledge, B. J., Zhang, K., Bier, E., Jan, Y. N. and Perrimon, N. The *Drosophila spitz* gene encodes a putative EGF-like growth factor involved in dorsal–ventral axis formation and neurogenesis. *Genes Dev.* **6**, 1503–17 (1992).

42. Schweitzer, R., Shaharabany, M., Seger, R. and Shilo, B. Z. Secreted Spitz triggers the DER signaling pathway and is a limiting component in embryonic ventral ectoderm determination. *Genes Dev.* **9**, 1518–29 (1995).

43. Tio, M. and Moses, K. The *Drosophila* TGF alpha homolog Spitz acts in photoreceptor recruitment in the developing retina. *Development* **124**, 343–51 (1997).

44. Schweitzer, R., Howes, R., Smith, R., Shilo, B. Z. and Freeman, M. Inhibition of *Drosophila* EGF receptor activation by the secreted protein Argos. *Nature* **376**, 699–702 (1995).

45. Freeman, M. Cell determination strategies in the *Drosophila* eye. *Development* **124**, 261–70 (1997).

46. Selleck, S. B., Gonzalez, C., Glover, D. M. and White, K. Regulation of the G1-S transition in postembryonic neuronal precursors by axon ingrowth. *Nature* **355**, 253–5 (1992).

47. Selleck, S. B. and Steller, H. The influence of retinal innervation on neurogenesis in the first optic ganglion of *Drosophila*. *Neuron* **6**, 83–99 (1991).

48. Huang, Z. and Kunes, S. Hedgehog, transmitted along retinal axons, triggers neurogenesis in the developing visual centers of the *Drosophila* brain. *Cell* **86**, 411–22 (1996).

49. Kunes, S. Axonal signals in the assembly of neural circuitry. *Curr. Opin. Neurobiol.* **10**, 58–62 (2000).

50. Huang, Z., Shilo, B. Z. and Kunes, S. A retinal axon fascicle uses spitz, an EGF receptor ligand, to construct a synaptic cartridge in the brain of *Drosophila*. *Cell* **95**, 693–703 (1998).

51. Kelly, J. P. and Cowan, W. M. Studies on the development of the chick optic tectum. III. Effects of early eye removal. *Brain Res.* **42**, 263–88 (1972).

52. Yamagata, M., Herman, J.-P. and Sanes, J. R. Lamina-specific expression of adhesion molecules in developing chick optic tectum. *J. Neurosci.* **15**, 4556–71 (1995).

53. Gong, Q. and Shipley, M. T. Evidence that pioneer olfactory axons regulate telencephalon cell cycle kinetics to induce the formation of the olfactory bulb. *Neuron* **14**, 91–101 (1995).

54. Saha, M. S., Servetnick, M. and Grainger, R. M. Vertebrate eye development. *Curr. Opin. Genet. Dev.* **2**, 582–8 (1992).

55. Adelmann, H. B. The problem of cyclopia. Pt. I. *Q. Rev. Biol.* **11**, 161–82 (1936).

56. Adelmann, H. B. The problem of cyclopia. Pt. II. *Q. Rev. Biol.* **11**, 284–304 (1936).

57. Li, H., Tierney, C., Wen, L., Wu, J. Y. and Rao, Y. A single morphogenetic field gives rise to two retina primordia under the influence of the prechordal plate. *Development* **124**, 603–15 (1997).

58. Hatta, K., Puschel, A. W. and Kimmel, C. B. Midline signaling in the primordium of the zebrafish anterior central nervous system. *Proc. Natl. Acad. Sci. USA* **91**, 2061–5 (1994).

59. Marti, E., Takada, R., Bumcrot, D. A., Sasaki, H. and McMahon, A. P. Distribution of Sonic hedgehog peptides in the developing chick and mouse embryo. *Development* **121**, 2537–47 (1995).

60. Chiang, C. *et al.* Cyclopia and defective axial patterning in mice lacking Sonic hedgehog gene function. *Nature* **383**, 407–13 (1996).

61. Roessler, E. *et al.* Mutations in the human Sonic hedgehog gene cause holoprosencephaly. *Nat. Genet.* **14**, 357–60 (1996).

62. Macdonald, R. *et al.* Midline signalling is required for *Pax* gene regulation and patterning of the eyes. *Development* **121**, 3267–78 (1995).

63. Walther, C. and Gruss, P. *Pax-6*, a murine paired box gene, is expressed in the developing CNS. *Development* **113**, 1435–49 (1991).

64. Jordan, T. *et al.* The human PAX6 gene is mutated in two patients with aniridia. *Nat. Genet.* **1**, 328–32 (1992).

65. Monaghan, A. P. *et al.* The *Msh*-like homeobox genes define domains in the developing vertebrate eye. *Development* **112**, 1053–61 (1991).

66. Mathers, P. H., Grinberg, A., Mahon, K. A. and Jamrich, M. The *Rx* homeobox gene is essential for vertebrate eye development. *Nature* **387**, 603–7 (1997).

67. Matsuo, I., Kuratani, S., Kimura, C., Takeda, N. and Aizawa, S. Mouse Otx2 functions in the formation and patterning of rostral head. *Genes Dev.* **9**, 2646–58 (1995).

68. Cheng, H. J., Nakamoto, M., Bergemann, A. D. and Flanagan, J. G. Complementary gradients in expression and binding of ELF-1 and Mek4 in development of the topographic retinotectal projection map. *Cell* **82**, 371–81 (1995).

69. Sidman, R. Histogenesis of the mouse retina studied with tritiated thymidine. In *The structure of the eye* (ed. G. Smelser), pp. 487–505 (Academic Press, New York, 1961).

70. Turner, D. L., Snyder, E. Y. and Cepko, C. L. Lineage-independent determination of cell type in the embryonic mouse retina. *Neuron* **4**, 833–45 (1990).

71. Holt, C. E., Bertsch, T. W., Ellis, H. M. and Harris, W. A. Cellular determination in the *Xenopus* retina is independent of lineage and birth date. *Neuron* **1**, 15–26 (1988).

72. Wetts, R. and Fraser, S. E. Multipotent precursors can give rise to all major cell types of the frog retina. *Science* **239**, 1142–5 (1988).

73. Harris, W. A. and Hartenstein, V. Neuronal determination without cell division in *Xenopus* embryos. *Neuron* **6**, 499–515 (1991).

74. Alexiades, M. R. and Cepko, C. L. Subsets of retinal progenitors display temporally regulated and distinct biases in the fates of their progeny. *Development* **124**, 1119–31 (1997).

75. Bao, Z. Z. and Cepko, C. L. The expression and function of *Notch* pathway genes in the developing rat eye. *J. Neurosci.* **17**, 1425–34 (1997).

76. Dorsky, R. I., Rapaport, D. H. and Harris, W. A. *Xotch* inhibits cell differentiation in the *Xenopus* retina. *Neuron* **14**, 487–96 (1995).

77. Dorsky, R. I., Chang, W. S., Rapaport, D. H. and Harris, W. A. Regulation of neuronal diversity

in the *Xenopus* retina by Delta signalling. *Nature* **385**, 67–70 (1997).

78. Reh, T. A. Cellular interactions determine neuronal phenotypes in rodent retinal cultures. *J. Neurobiol.* **23**, 1067–83 (1992).

79. Watanabe, T. and Raff, M. C. Diffusible rod-promoting signals in the developing rat retina. *Development* **114**, 899–906 (1992).

80. Altshuler, D. and Cepko, C. A temporally regulated, diffusible activity is required for rod photoreceptor development *in vitro. Development* **114**, 947–57 (1992).

81. Harris, W. A. and Messersmith, S. L. Two cellular inductions involved in photoreceptor determination in the *Xenopus* retina. *Neuron* **9**, 357–72 (1992).

82. Belliveau, M. J. and Cepko, C. L. Extrinsic and intrinsic factors control the genesis of amacrine and cone cells in the rat retina. *Development* **126**, 555–66 (1999).

83. Jensen, A. M. and Wallace, V. A. Expression of Sonic hedgehog and its putative role as a precursor cell mitogen in the developing mouse retina. *Development* **124**, 363–71 (1997).

84. Pittack, C., Jones, M. and Reh, T. A. Basic fibroblast growth factor induces retinal pigment epithelium to generate neural retina *in vitro. Development* **113**, 577–88 (1991).

85. McFarlane, S., Zuber, M. E. and Holt, C. E. A role for the fibroblast growth factor receptor in cell fate decisions in the developing vertebrate retina. *Development* **125**, 3967–75 (1998).

86. Anchan, R. M., Reh, T. A., Angello, J., Balliet, A. and Walker, M. EGF and TGF-alpha stimulate retinal neuroepithelial cell proliferation *in vitro. Neuron* **6**, 923–36 (1991).

87. Ezzeddine, Z. D., Yang, X., DeChiara, T., Yancopoulos, G. and Cepko, C. L. Postmitotic cells fated to become rod photoreceptors can be respecified by CNTF treatment of the retina. *Development* **124**, 1055–67 (1997).

88. Cepko, C. L. The roles of intrinsic and extrinsic cues and bHLH genes in the determination of retinal cell fates. *Curr. Opin. Neurobiol.* **9**, 37–46 (1999).

89. Furukawa, T., Morrow, E. M. and Cepko, C. L. *Crx*, a novel otx-like homeobox gene, shows photoreceptor-specific expression and regulates photoreceptor differentiation. *Cell* **91**, 531–41 (1997).

90. Frade, J. M., Rodriguez-Tebar, A. and Barde, Y. A. Induction of cell death by endogenous nerve growth factor through its p75 receptor. *Nature* **383**, 166–8 (1996).

91. Frade, J. M. and Barde, Y. A. Microglia-derived nerve growth factor causes cell death in the developing retina. *Neuron* **20**, 35–41 (1998).

92. Frade, J. M. *et al.* Control of early cell death by BDNF in the chick retina. *Development* **124**, 3313–20 (1997).

93. Jeffery, G. The albino retina: an abnormality that provides insight into normal retinal development. *Trends Neurosci.* **20**, 165–9 (1997).

94. Harrison, R. Experiments on the development of the internal ear. *Science* **59**, 448 (1924).

95. Gallagher, B. C., Henry, J. J. and Grainger, R. M. Inductive processes leading to inner ear formation during *Xenopus* development. *Dev. Biol.* **175**, 95–107 (1996).

96. Represa, J., Leon, Y., Miner, C. and Giraldez, F. The int-2 proto-oncogene is responsible for induction of the inner ear. *Nature* **353**, 561–3 (1991).

97. Mansour, S. L., Goddard, J. M. and Capecchi, M. R. Mice homozygous for a targeted disruption of the proto-oncogene int-2 have developmental defects in the tail and inner ear. *Development* **117**, 13–28 (1993).

98. McKay, I. J., Lewis, J. and Lumsden, A. The role of FGF-3 in early inner ear development: an analysis in normal and *kreisler* mutant mice. *Dev. Biol.* **174**, 370–8 (1996).

99. Wu, D. K., Nunes, F. D. and Choo, D. Axial specification for sensory organs versus non-sensory structures of the chicken inner ear. *Development* **125**, 11–20 (1998).

100. Whitfield, T., Haddon, C. and Lewis, J. Intercellular signals and cell fate choices in the developing inner ear: origins of global and of fine-grained pattern. *Semin. Cell Dev. Biol.* **8**, 239–247 (1997).

101. Fekete, D. M. Cell fate specification in the inner ear. *Curr. Opin. Neurobiol.* **6**, 533–41 (1996).

102. Whitfield, T. *et al.* Mutations affecting development of the zebrafish inner ear and lateral line. *Development* **123**, 241–54 (1996).

103. Steel, K. P. Inherited hearing defects in mice. *Annu. Rev. Genet.* **29**, 675–701 (1995).

104. Fekete, D. M., Homburger, S. A., Waring, M. T., Riedl, A. E. and Garcia, L. F. Involvement of programmed cell death in morphogenesis of the vertebrate inner ear. *Development* **124**, 2451–61 (1997).

105. Fritzsch, B., Silos-Santiago, I., Bianchi, L. M. and Farinas, I. The role of neurotrophic factors in regulating the development of inner ear innervation. *Trends Neurosci.* **20**, 159–64 (1997).

106. Metcalfe, W. K., Kimmel, C. B. and Schabtach, E. Anatomy of the posterior lateral line system in young larvae of the zebrafish. *J. Comp. Neurol.* **233**, 377–89 (1985).

107. Metcalfe, W. K. Sensory neuron growth cones comigrate with posterior lateral line

primordial cells in zebrafish. *J. Comp. Neurol.* **238**, 218–24 (1985).

108. van Eeden, F. J. *et al.* Mutations affecting somite formation and patterning in the zebrafish, *Danio rerio. Development* **123**, 153–64 (1996).

109. Barlow, L. A. and Northcutt, R. G. Embryonic origin of amphibian taste buds. *Dev. Biol.* **169**, 273–85 (1995).

110. Stone, L. M., Finger, T. E., Tam, P. P. and Tan, S. S. Taste receptor cells arise from local epithelium, not neurogenic ectoderm. *Proc. Natl. Acad. Sci. USA* **92**, 1916–20 (1995).

111. Hosley, M. A., Hughes, S. E. and Oakley, B. Neural induction of taste buds. *J. Comp. Neurol.* **260**, 224–32 (1987).

112. Zalewski, A. A. Regeneration of taste buds after reinnervation of a denervated tongue papilla by a normally nongustatory nerve. *J. Comp. Neurol.* **200**, 309–14 (1981).

113. Northcutt, R. G. and Barlow, L. A. Amphibians provide new insights into taste-bud development. *Trends Neurosci.* **21**, 38–43 (1998).

114. Schwanzel-Fukuda, M. and Pfaff, D. W. Origin of luteinizing hormone-releasing hormone neurons. *Nature* **338**, 161–4 (1989).

115. Franco, B. *et al.* A gene deleted in Kallmann's syndrome shares homology with neural cell adhesion and axonal path-finding molecules. *Nature* **353**, 529–36 (1991).

116. Zelena, J. Development, degeneration and regeneration of receptor organs. *Prog. Brain Res.* **13**, 175–213 (1964).

117. Milburn, A. The early development of muscle spindles in the rat. *J. Cell Sci.* **12**, 175–95 (1973).

118. Werner, J. K. Mixed intra- and extrafusal muscle fibers produced by temporary denervation in newborn rats. *J. Comp. Neurol.* **150**, 279–302 (1973).

119. Scott, S., Cooper, E. and Diamond, J. Merkel cells as targets of the mechanosensory nerves in salamander skin. *Proc. R. Soc. Ser. B* **211**, 455–70 (1981).

120. English, K. B., Burgess, P. R. and Kavka-Van Norman, D. Development of rat Merkel cells. *J. Comp. Neurol.* **194**, 475–96 (1980).

121. Carroll, P., Lewin, G. R., Koltzenburg, M., Toyka, K. V. and Thoenen, H. A role for BDNF in mechanosensation. *Nat. Neurosci.* **1**, 42–6 (1998).

122. Cutforth, T. and Gaul, U. The genetics of visual system development in *Drosophila*: specification, connectivity and asymmetry. *Curr. Opin. Neurobiol.* **7**, 48–54 (1997).

9

Growth and Guidance of Axons and Dendrites

The typical tree-like form of a mature neuron arises as the axon and dendrites grow out from the cell body and the biochemical, physiological and functional differences between the axon and dendrites emerge. These developments allow synaptic connections to form and establish the differences in shape and size between nerve cells of different sorts. This chapter considers three main topics:

1. The mechanism of axonal and dendritic lengthening. The key element here is the growth cone, the specialized terminal region of growing axons and dendrites where material transported from the cell body becomes incorporated into the lengthening neurites.

2. The factors that permit growth cones to find their proper targets. Experiments have shown that the ordered patterns of neural connections so characteristic of mature nervous systems are made possible because neurons have identities which are expressed as molecular labels; these allow the growth cones to respond specifically to guidance cues of various kinds along their pathways.

3. The development of the differences between axons and dendrites.

4. The following chapter considers the mechanisms that allow axons to make the correct connections within their target areas, generating ordered topographic maps in the vertebrate CNS, while Chapters 13 and 14 complete the description of connection formation in the brain by showing that the initial, quite well-ordered connections laid down by a detailed in-built development programme are further refined by competition. This occurs at the level both of whole neurons, some of which die, and of individual nerve terminal branches, some of which are removed while new branches are added elsewhere. It is at this stage that interactions of the developing animal with the environment can help to adapt the nervous system in detail to optimize its performance.

The axon growth cone

At the end of the last century Ramon y Cajal recognized that the terminal enlargement of growing axons is a special region where elongation might occur, and he named this structure the growth cone.[1] This conclusion was drawn from examination of fixed silver-stained preparations of embryonic tissue, but advancing living growth cones were soon observed in the first tissue culture experiments[2] and then later in the tails of live tadpoles.[3] In culture and *in vivo* axons can lengthen at a rate of many tens of micrometres an hour or a few millimetres a day. Growth cones navigating through living tissue may grow rapidly and straight in parts of their course, but they tend to grow slowly at places where changes in direction are made. At such places the growth cone is more swollen.[4,5] As advance continues, the region behind the growth cone differentiates rapidly into a typical axon. Growth ultimately stops when an appropriate location for synapse formation is found and the highly specialized presynaptic terminal differentiates (see Chapter 11). The terminal region of the axon, unlike that of the dendrite, maintains a separate identity from the rest of the axon.

Axons rarely branch as they grow between their source and target, but when they reach their destination they do so and this ensures some innervation of all target cells. The pattern of branching is modified subsequently by the addition of extra branches. This occurs both within particular parts of the target and, in some parts of the developing brain, outside the original target. Growth of extra branches within the target area always occurs and is accompanied by loss of some branches; such modifications are described in Chapter 14. Outside the target, new growth cones can arise from the axon and innervate additional targets. These new branches are probably attracted by chemotropic factors (see later),[6] and the phenomenon ('interstitial branching') is discussed further in Chapter 10.

The growth cone is thus able not only to lengthen axons but also to respond to local cues; these are used either to dictate the direction of growth and branching pattern or to bring growth to a halt. The growth cone also transduces, or itself generates, signals that are used to control gene expression in the cell body (see Chapters 11 and 16); it secretes proteolytic enzymes[7] and other transported proteins,[8] and probably releases transmitter even before synapses form. In short, the growth cone contains the machinery for both elongation and control of the pace and direction of growth.

Composition of the growth cone

Electron microscopy shows that the body of a growth cone does not have the ordered cytoskeleton of a mature axon. It contains mitochondria, numerous vesicles, microfilaments and a central bundle of microtubules but no neurofilaments (Fig. 9.1). Projecting from its margins are both broad extensions (lamellipodia) and fine

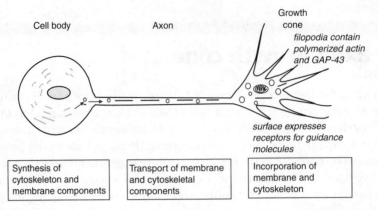

Figure 9.1 Simplified diagram of the roles of the cell body, the axon and the growth cone in axon extension. New material is synthesized in the cell body, transported down the axon and incorporated in the growth cone. The latter has the ability to respond to guidance and target recognition molecules. The diagram exaggerates the sizes of the axon and growth cone relative to the body of the nerve cell.

processes called filopodia (or microspikes). In tissue culture these can be seen to extend rapidly for distances of up to 50 μm. They either adhere to the surface or are quickly withdrawn, and the dynamic nature of the growth cone gives the impression of continuous sampling and decision making. The filopodia contain bundles of microfilaments which can be stained with antibodies to actin and myosin,[9] and filopodial protrusion may be powered by the rapid polymerization of actin into rods. Cytochalasin, a drug that inhibits actin polymerization, and colchicine, which interferes with microtubule polymerization, both slow or stop axonal advance on most growth surfaces.[10-12] Cytochalasin, applied at doses that block filopodia formation, also disrupts axon pathfinding in the grasshopper limb bud[13] and the amphibian retinotectal projection,[14] suggesting a critical role for regulation of the actin cytoskeleton in axon guidance. Certainly filopodia are more than structures thrown out at random and used to advance and stick down the growth cone; individual filopodia cut off from the very large growth cones of neurons from the pond snail can respond to neurotransmitters with elevated levels of calcium ions,[15] so they are likely to contribute to the ability of the growth cone to react to external stimuli.

The growth cone has molecules (see below) on its surface membrane to enable it to recognize molecules on other axons and cells and in the extracellular matrix. Concentrated in the growth cone and associated with the cytoplasmic face of the membrane are both the heterotrimeric G protein, G_o,[16] which links membrane receptors to effector systems within cells, and also a phosphoprotein called GAP-43.[17,18] GAP-43 (synonyms include B50, F1, pp46, P57 and neuromodulin) is a substrate for phosphorylation by protein kinase C, binds calmodulin and can stimulate GTP binding to G_o, an event usually triggered by activation of receptors on the cell surface. Molecularly engineered expression of GAP-43 can induce the formation of filopodia in non-neural cells.[19] GAP-43 expression generally correlates with axon regenerative ability and nerve terminal plasticity, but while it appears to be involved in the regulation of the growth cone cytoskeleton in some way, its precise function remains unclear (one suggestion is that it regulates the sensitivity of axon growth cones to repulsive ligands).[20] Its importance is also shown by the fact that null mutant mice die in the early postnatal period. The brain, however, is grossly normal in appearance and growth cones of neurons taken from these mice advance at a normal rate *in vitro*, although *in vivo* they may be sluggish at places where turning decisions have to be made, such as the optic chiasm.[21] Transgenic mice over-expressing chicken GAP-43 develop spontaneous sprouts from motor endplates, and following nerve section axons regenerate more vigorously and collateral sprouts occur sooner and more abundantly.[22]

Material is added to growing axons mainly at the growth cone

New axon membrane is added near the growing axon tip, since marks placed on the membrane proximal to the growth cone do not generally move forward.[23-25] Indeed, membrane may move backwards from the growth cone as excess is added at the tip and becomes accommodated by moving towards the cell body.[26,27] It has also been shown that membrane inside growth cones isolated from developing brain can be added to the surface membrane if the internal calcium ion concentration is raised,[28] so the machinery for membrane incorporation clearly exists in growth cones. Newly synthesized proteins also first appear in the membrane of the growth cone.[29] It is likely that neurite elongation is dependent on the continuous transport of membrane components from the cell body: for example, blocking vesicle transport along the axon by laser optical tweezers inhibits axon outgrowth within minutes.[30] One model of neurite elongation proposes a large-scale endocytotic cycle in growing axons, in which membrane components are transported from the cell body and exocytosed at the growth cone, followed by diffusion back in the plasma membrane towards the cell body.[26]

Similar observations have been made for the cytoskeleton. A fluorescently marked segment of the microtubule cytoskeleton in the axon proximal to the growth cone remains stationary, in the mouse at least[31] (but see reference 32), showing that microtubules at the nerve terminal cannot be derived by transport of whole tubules assembled more proximally. This argues that they must, therefore, be assembled locally in or near the terminal. There is also more direct evidence that new microtubules are assembled in the terminal[33] and that very low doses of vinblastine, which prevents microtubule dynamics, also prevents net forward movement while not stopping all growth cone motility.[34] Finally, direct proof that the growth cone contains all the machinery needed for axon lengthening is that growth cones continue to elaborate axons for some time after being isolated from the cell body of the neuron both *in vitro*[35] and *in vivo*.[36] Although it is clear that new material is transported down the axon and is added in the region of the growth cone, the precise site of addition and the mechanisms that trigger it are not certain.[37] Administration of antisense oligonucleotides to SNAP-25, a receptor for the intracellular vesicle fusion proteins NSF (N-ethylmaleimide-sensitive fusion protein) and SNAP (soluble NSF attachment protein),[38] inhibits neurite elongation by rat cortical neurons,[39] so the mechanism of membrane addition during growth may be similar, at least initially, to the temporary addition that occurs during transmitter liberation from synaptic vesicles. In relation to this, it is interesting that the concentration of calcium ions within the growth cone needs to be neither too high nor too low if growth cones are to advance normally (see below),[40,41] as rises in calcium are the trigger for transmitter vesicle fusion with nerve terminals.

The role of adhesion in growth cone advance

Attachment of growth cone filopodia to substrates accompanies axonal growth[42] and can generate tension in the axon behind.[43] This may stimulate the insertion of new membrane and trigger the assembly of cytoskeleton; certainly adult axons can be elongated and incorporate new membrane if they are stretched (see below). Growth cones grow well on surfaces to which they can adhere strongly, and they can show a graded preference among a range of different surfaces in culture.[44] Strong adhesion has often been held to be an important factor controlling the direction of axon growth and determining the pattern of branching, but tension generation does not always accompany elongation on very adhesive surfaces so it may not be essential for lengthening. Moreover, direct measurements of the force of adhesion of filopodia on a range of substrates have not shown greater adhesion to those which encouraged the best growth.[45] It therefore seems likely that factors other than, or additional to, the strength of adhesion may determine whether a surface is a good one for supporting growth cone advance, and it appears in particular that effects on growth cone dynamics are mediated by activation of intracellular second messengers (see below).

Intercalated axonal growth

Axons form synapses with their targets long before an animal has reached full size. As an animal grows, its axons must, therefore, lengthen so that contact can be maintained between neurons and synapses. Such lengthening depends on the addition of new material throughout the length of the already-formed axon. There is evidence from *in vitro* experiments that the stimulus for incorporation of such new material is tension.[46] Furthermore, if a nerve in an adult rabbit is stretched slowly enough, it can be lengthened considerably over the course of some weeks without loss of function.[47] Axons also grow in diameter, a process that needs insertion of new membrane into the mature axon, and the number of neurofilaments further increases while the number of microtubules does not change. How tension-induced lengthening brings about the insertion of new membrane, or the addition of extra neurofilaments, is unknown.

Factors affecting the rate and direction of axon growth

Numerous observations and experiments have shown that axons do not grow in random directions during development. Rather, the characteristic anatomical patterns of nerves and axon pathways in the mature animal result from the operation of a range of guidance mechanisms that enable the growth cones to steer themselves along well-defined routes—see Fig. 9.2.

- Rapid and sustained axon growth depends on the synthetic machinery of the neuron cell body, which is responsible for supplying the building materials that are needed.

- Axon trajectories are often subdivided into shorter segments, interrupted by intermediate targets (choice points) where axons make critical guidance decisions.

- Late-developing axons often grow along bundles of axons that developed at an earlier stage (fasciculation), sometimes switching between fascicles at specific choice points (selective fasciculation).

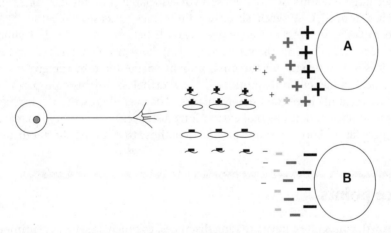

Figure 9.2 Simplified scheme to summarize how a growth cone can be guided to its correct target by a combination of attractants (+), both attached to cells and extracellular matrix lying between the neuron and its target (A) and also released from the target to provide a graded diffusible chemotropic lure (chemoattraction), and repellents (−), generated by locally attached molecules and also diffusing from inappropriate targets (B; chemorepulsion). Molecules that are attractive to the growth cone may be repulsive to the growth cones of other neurons, and those that are repulsive may be attractive to others.

- Growth can be promoted and guided by factors bound to extracellular matrix or present on the surfaces of other cells and their processes (contact attraction).

- Growth cones can also be attracted by diffusible molecules released by other cells (chemotropism or chemoattraction) and by electrical fields of the appropriate sign (galvanotropism).

- Guidance is also provided by molecules that prevent axon advance in particular directions. These may be surface bound (contact repulsion) or diffusible (chemorepulsion). Such molecules can be 'bifunctional', mediating attraction or repulsion depending on the receptor-mediated response of the growth cone.

- Many of the growth-promoting and growth-inhibitory molecules found in vertebrates are structurally related to those carrying out similar functions in various invertebrate phyla.

- Growing axons are probably programmed to use a succession of different guidance cues as they advance towards their specific targets.

An account of these factors and how they might interact with the growth cone is given in the following sections.

The role of the nerve cell body in axonal growth

The nerve cell body supplies the growth cone with essential building materials for the membrane and cytoskeleton, and while axons and dendrites are lengthening it expresses large amounts of so-called growth-associated proteins (GAPs). After axon growth has stopped, GAP synthesis either diminishes or ceases altogether.[48] Among the known GAPs are GAP-43 (see above), class II beta tubulin, the $T\alpha1$ subunit of tubulin[49] and actin.[50] While the production of all these proteins is necessary for rapid growth it is not sufficient, for the environment encountered by the growth cone is also a critical influence on its motility.[51,52] Nevertheless, intrinsic properties of the neuron are certainly important determinants of its overall growth rate: for example, chick cranial sensory neurons that extend long distances in the embryo to reach their targets grow faster, both *in vivo* and *in vitro*, than those that extend shorter distances.[53]

Choice points

Axon growth cones often navigate long distances, as much as several centimetres, to reach their targets in the embryo. This seemingly formidable task is simplified by the fragmentation of their journey into shorter steps interrupted by intermediate targets, known as choice points, where other cells provide critical guidance cues that direct growth cones on the next stage of their trajectory. A good example is provided by the specialized cells comprising the CNS midline in both insects and vertebrates. In the latter case, the ventral midline floor plate of the spinal cord and brainstem provides an intermediate target for commissural axons, whose task is to cross from one side of the CNS to the other. The floor plate secretes a chemoattractant, netrin, that directs commissural axons towards it in a dorsoventral trajectory, as discussed below. A further example in the vertebrate CNS is the subplate of the developing cerebral cortex, which provides an intermediate target for axons navigating between the thalamus and the cerebral cortex (see Chapter 7).

Choice points are also provided by smaller, isolated groupings of 'guidepost' cells, which may be neurons themselves. These have been well characterized in the developing insect nervous system and in their absence, for example following laser ablation, the earliest pioneer growth cones often make pathfinding errors.[54-56]

Fasciculation

Axons that navigate their pathways after the pioneer axons ('followers') may be guided to and from choice points by selective fasciculation on the pioneers. A clear example is seen in the developing grasshopper CNS, whose longitudinal tracts are pioneered by the axons of two 'A' and three 'P' neurons per hemisegment. The follower 'G' axon fasciculates selectively on the P axons rather than the A axons, and stalls when all three P neurons are laser-ablated.[57] Studies in both zebrafish and insect embryos have shown, however, that in some cases the follower axons are still capable of reaching their targets in the absence of the pioneers, suggesting that the requirement for pioneer neurons in axon guidance need not be absolute. The developing longitudinal axon tracts in the CNS of *Drosophila* are pioneered, for example, by four axons per hemisegment, and tracts are thinned and disrupted if all four (but not individual) axons are ablated genetically, but some follower axons can still navigate longitudinal pathways.[58] Such results also serve to emphasize that, *in vivo*, guidance cues are likely to be multiple and redundant.

An important component of axon guidance involves selective fasciculation and defasciculation of growth cones at critical stages in their trajectories. These processes appear to driven by the balance of attractive/adhesive and repulsive interactions between axons themselves and between axons and surrounding cells. The underlying molecular mechanisms will be discussed below, in the context of the major classes of molecules that mediate guidance.

The precision of axon guidance, brought about by the differing decisions of growth cones navigating at choice points, is well illustrated in the vertebrate CNS by the pattern of axon bundles that develop in the early zebrafish brain. By the end of the first day of embryonic development a precise, stereotyped scaffold of axon bundles has appeared, and projection errors are not seen. A collection of axon fascicles runs longitudinally in the ventral diencephalon, merging with the medial longitudinal fasciculus caudally in the midbrain, and joined rostrally by other fascicles originating from neuronal clusters sited at discrete positions in the forebrain (Fig. 9.3). Such 'twig-to-trunk' development of axon branching patterns in the CNS has been aptly contrasted with the trunk-to-twig growth of a tree.[59]

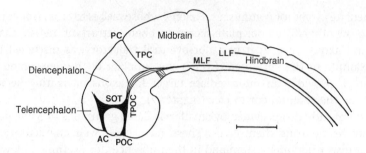

Figure 9.3 The pattern of axon bundles arising during the first embryonic day in the zebrafish brain (left side view). AC, anterior commissure; POC, post-optic commissure; SOT, supraoptic tract; TPOC, tract of the post-optic commissure; TPC, tract of the posterior commissure; PC, posterior commissure; MLF, medial longitudinal fasciculus; LLF, lateral longitudinal fasciculus. Scale bar 100 μm. After Kimmel.[59]

Axon guidance by attraction

Adhesion molecules and axon growth—CAMs, extracellular matrix molecules and integrins

Growth cones can advance either on the surfaces of other cells or on the substratum provided by the extracellular matrix. The molecules on the surfaces of other cells which make this possible are the cell adhesion molecules (CAMs), and the molecules in the extracellular matrix are surface or substrate adhesion molecules (SAMs). Adhesion molecules are so-called because some of the cell surface molecules known to promote axonal growth were first discovered in the search for the molecular basis of cell–cell adhesion. It has turned out, however, that promoting cell adhesion is only part of their role. A better term would be *recognition* molecule, because this is their prime function;[60] the *consequences* of the recognition (cell migration, cell adhesion, axon growth, growth cone adhesion/attraction or repulsion) depend on the state of the responding cell.

Table 9.1 lists some CAMs and SAMs of importance, and Fig. 9.4 illustrates their interactions with the growth cone in a diagrammatic way. Critical amino acid sequences in proteins with important functional roles tend to be conserved during evolution, so that several vertebrate adhesion molecules have been found to be homologues of those found in invertebrates.

Many of the CAMs involved in axon growth (exceptions include N-cadherin and fasciclin I) are members of a larger group, the immunoglobulin superfamily,[61] because they have variable numbers of extracellular domains whose sequences are related to those present in immunoglobulins (Fig. 9.5). These CAMs frequently adopt multiple forms generated by alternative mRNA splicing. The CAM on the growth cone

Table 9.1 Some adhesion molecules involved in axon growth

Name	Similar/identical molecules	Comments
Cell adhesion molecules (CAMs)		
N-cadherin (mouse)	N-CalCAM (chick) A-CAM (chick)	Calcium-dependent
NCAM	BSP-2	Immunoglobulin superfamily
L1 (mouse)	NILE* (rat) G4, Ng-CAM, 8D9 (chick) Nr-CAM, neurofascin Neuroglian (insects)	Immunoglobulin superfamily
TAG-1 (rat)	Axonin-1, F11	Immunoglobulin superfamily
Fasciclins		Insects. Fasciclin II is the orthologue of NCAM
Substrate adhesion molecules (SAMs)		
Laminin		Binds to Integrin
Fibronectin		Binds to Integrin
Tenascin	Cytotactin, J1, myotendinous antigen	
Collagen		

*Nerve growth factor-inducible large external glycoprotein.

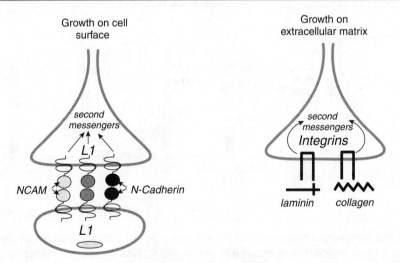

Figure 9.4 A few well-known adhesion/recognition molecules which help axons to grow and navigate on the surfaces of other cells and on the extracellular matrix. These and other molecules are described in the text. Many of the molecules mediating intercellular communication are 'homophilic', that is they recognize identical molecules on the surface of other cells. They bring about their effects not simply by providing temporary attachment sites for the filopodia of growth cones but by acting as ligand and receptor in the first stage of a signalling pathway. The same is true for integrins, the binding of which to material in the extracellular matrix can activate intracellular signalling pathways.

IMMUNOGLOBULIN SUPERFAMILY MEMBERS MODULATING AXON GROWTH BY ACTING AS LIGANDS OR RECEPTORS IN AXON GUIDANCE

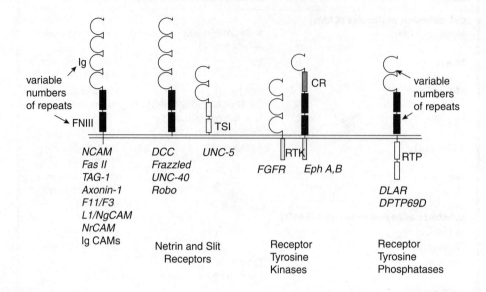

LAMININ, NETRIN, SEMAPHORIN AND NEUROPILIN GUIDANCE MOLECULES

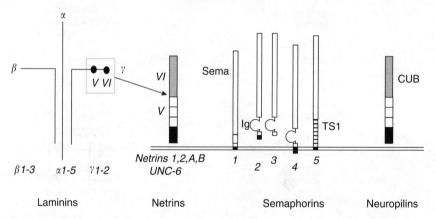

Figure 9.5 Summary of molecules that control axon growth by acting as attractants or repellents, either attached or unattached to cells or extracellular matrix. The horizontal double line represents the plasma membrane. See text for more information on individual molecules. Many (top row) belong to the immunoglobulin superfamily. Numbers of immunoglobulin (Ig) repeats differ, as do the number of fibronectin type III (FNIII) repeats. TSI, thrombospondin type I domain; CR, cysteine-rich region; RTK, receptor tyrosine kinase domain; RTP, receptor tyrosine phosphatase domain. In the bottom row are illustrated laminin, the distantly-related netrins, the semaphorins and their co-receptors, the neuropilins. Sema, semaphorin domain; CUB, complement-binding domains. These molecules are conserved in structure and function in invertebrates (nematodes and insects) and vertebrates. After Tessier-Lavigne and Goodman.[142]

and the binding partner on the other cell are often identical, so-called homophilic adhesion, and the homophilic binding site for NCAM has been localized to its third immunoglobulin domain.[62] As already discussed, however, it seems likely that growth stimulation is mediated not simply by providing attachment for the growth cone and its filopodia, allowing them to exert tension; several soluble fragments of different domains of both NCAM and L1 have been shown to support axon growth *in vitro*,[63] so a more important effect of CAMs is probably to trigger a cascade of molecular changes via second messengers acting within the growth cone (see below).

The evidence that any individual adhesion molecule is involved in growth cone advance and guidance comes from several sources: first, it is expressed in the embryo at the right place at the right time; second, antibodies directed against it can interfere with growth *in vitro* and *in vivo*; third, its loss-of-function, arising genetically or following chemical treatment, interferes with growth; and fourth, ectopic expression in cells which do not normally express it can greatly accelerate axon growth across the cell surface *in vitro*, and alter axon growth patterns *in vivo*. Examples are given below.

In mammals, most of the adhesion molecules are widely distributed, and there appears to be some redundancy of function among them because antibodies to several CAMs (N-CAM, N-cadherin) and SAMs (integrin) may need to be applied simultaneously to block axon growth completely.[64] Although this argues for a generally permissive growth-promoting role, selective guidance of particular groups of axons could be achieved theoretically by quite weak preferential affinities.[65] In invertebrates the distribution of CAMs is often sharply restricted to subsets of axon fascicles, and so each CAM could, and some do, have a unique part to play in pathfinding of specific axons (Fig. 9.6).[66]

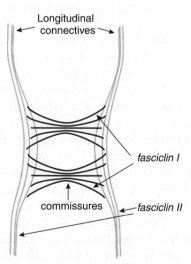

Figure 9.6 The differential distribution of two members of the fasciclin family of recognition molecules on the longitudinal connectives and transverse commissures of the developing nervous system of the grasshopper. Such specific labelling allows axons to make choices about where to grow during development. After Bastiani *et al.*[256]

Examples of individual adhesion molecules

NCAM (neural cell adhesion molecule)[67] was the first cell–cell adhesion molecule to be characterized. It is present on most neurons, in embryonic and denervated adult skeletal muscle and at the normal adult neuromuscular junction. There are several neural isoforms with differing molecular weights and membrane linkages, generated by alternative RNA splicing and by post-translational modifications. There are also differences between neural and muscle NCAM. NCAM is likely to be important as a general facilitator of axon growth and fasciculation. Ingrowth of motor axons to muscle coincides with the appearance of NCAM on the muscle fibres.[68] Antibodies to NCAM prevent motor axons growing on myotubes in culture[69] and reduce sprouting of motor axons in paralysed muscles,[70] and they also disrupt the fasciculation of retinal axons growing into the tectum.[71] NCAM is expressed by Schwann cells providing they are not programmed by axon contact to make myelin[72] and may therefore assist axon regrowth following Wallerian degeneration (see Chapter 17). An element of specificity may also result, because Schwann cells previously associated with motor axons have the HNK1 (human natural killer) carbohydrate epitope associated with their NCAM and L1, and this may enable motor axons to regenerate preferentially back along their old pathways.[73]

NCAM is unique among adhesion molecules because it is associated covalently with polysialic acid (PSA), a polymer of N-acetyl neuraminic acid otherwise found as part of the coating of some bacterial cell walls.[74] The amount of PSA linked to NCAM can be high (H or embryonic form) or low (L or adult form). Selective removal of PSA by treatment of chick embryos with endosialidase interferes with the sorting of motor axons near the spinal cord at the site of the future limb plexus, with the result that some axons innervate the wrong limb muscles.[75] A possible explanation is that PSA, being a bulky molecule, creates a charge cloud that keeps neighbouring axon membranes further apart than usual, so reducing interaction between neighbouring CAMs.[74] Its removal from motor axons at the plexus may encourage such strong fasciculation that interaction with other guidance molecules, normally leading to defasciculation, is less effective. This suggestion is borne out by the finding that reducing the axon fasciculation with antibodies to L1 (see below) overcomes the enzyme-induced misrouting.[76] In normal avian muscles there is more nerve branching in those parts of the muscles in which motor axon NCAM is highly sialylated, probably because in these regions motor axons defasciculate more readily and send branches to the muscle fibres.[77]

Perhaps surprisingly, only one conspicuous abnormality of axon pathfinding has been detected in NCAM knockout mice (e.g. NCAM-180),[78] namely defasciculation and targeting errors in the hippocampal mossy fibre pathway.[79] These mice also have impaired migration of precursor olfactory bulb cells from their birthplace at the lateral ventricle to the bulb, a defect that can be phenocopied in wild-type mice by local injection of endosialidase (see also Chapter 7),[80] and they show impaired long-term potentiation in the hippocampus (see Chapter 15).[81]

Fasciclin II, the *Drosophila* homologue of NCAM, is normally restricted to certain longitudinally running fascicles in the developing CNS, as well as motor axons and their growth cones (Fig. 9.6). Its overexpression on motor axons shows that it is necessary for selective fasciculation decisions but not necessarily for controlling the overall direction of outgrowth.[82] Some axons, for example, fail to defasciculate from their parent intersegmental nerve at a choice point region, so bypassing their normal muscle target, yet they do reach their targets at later times of development. Similarly, Fas II loss-of-function prevents CNS fascicles from forming normally, yet growth cones again can reach their targets under these conditions.[82] Fas II also controls synaptic stabilization and growth (see Chapter 11).

Several genes have been identified in *Drosophila* whose products appear to regulate Fas II function by inhibitory mechanisms, so their loss-of-function results in a fasciculation phenotype similar to that of Fas II gain-of-function. These include certain receptor tyrosine phosphatases (see below), and a small secreted protein (Beat) expressed by motor axons.[83] Precisely how they regulate fasciculation is unknown at present, although Beat appears to work by decreasing interaxonal adhesion mediated by Fas II.

L1-type molecules (L1, Nr-CAM, Ng-CAM and neurofascin in vertebrates, neuroglian in insects) are dynamically expressed on various neurons and glial cells during development, and expression may even be localized to parts of axons. They may interact homophilically, and also heterophilically with several other Ig superfamily molecules (e.g. DM-GRASP, TAG-1/axonin-1) and with extracellular matrix molecules. Antibodies to L1 can prevent axon fasciculation and slow axonal growth.[84] Several domains of the L1 molecule facilitate axon growth, but the intact molecule is more effective than individual parts.[85] Levels of L1 expression in cultured sensory neurons can also be varied simply by altering the pattern of applied electrical stimulation, high frequencies favouring high expression.[86] L1 mutations in humans have been linked to a set of overlapping hereditary syndromes associated with brain malformations (stenosis of the aqueduct of Sylvius with hydrocephalus, hypoplasia of the pyramidal tract, dysgenesis of the corpus callosum, spastic paraplegia and mental retardation),[87] although it is unclear at present precisely how L1 dysfunction brings these about.[88] In L1 knockout mice, reduced numbers of corticospinal axons cross the midline in the caudal medulla (the so-called 'pyramidal' or motor decussation), so L1 dysfunction may also affect this decussation in humans.[89]

TAG-1 is less widespread and is more fleetingly expressed than L1. It is found, for example, on commissural axons which project from the dorsal to ventral spinal cord and then cross the midline floor plate. At the time of crossing, neurons downregulate TAG-1 and instead express L1 as they run longitudinally alongside the floor plate on the contralateral side.[90]

This change in neuronal expression of adhesion molecules as axons elongate is intriguing. It may be triggered by interaction of axons with the floor plate cells, and may contribute to the turning decision of axons in this region of the spinal cord. In the chick embryo, for example, spinal commissural axons and growth cones express the TAG-1 homologue axonin-1, while the floor plate cells express the L1 homologue Nr-CAM; these bind to each other heterophilically, and their perturbation by neutralizing antibodies prevents many axons from crossing the midline, running instead alongside the floor plate on the ipsilateral side.[91]

N-cadherin is an integral membrane glycoprotein, so-called because it uses calcium ions to promote intercellular adhesion. It is a member of a family of cadherins that play major roles in intercellular adhesion, especially during morphogenesis (see Chapter 1).[92] N-cadherin is also widely distributed on axons, where it may promote fasciculation, and on astrocytes.[93] It provides an excellent substrate for axonal growth when expressed by cells grown in monolayers, and the rate of growth is linearly related to the density of N-cadherin. This is unlike the growth promotion produced by monolayers transfected to express NCAM, when the growth rate is independent of NCAM density once a threshold value is reached.[94] N-cadherin is needed for retinal axonal outgrowth *in vivo*; when a dominant-negative N-cadherin construct is transfected into the embryonic *Xenopus* eye, initiation and outgrowth of retinal axons are impaired.[95]

Extracellular matrix molecules (SAMs) and integrins

Molecules in the extracellular matrix can affect axonal extension. Material released from cells in culture is also an excellent growth substrate for axons when it becomes bound to the surface of the culture dish,[96] and such release may partly explain why axons growing out from explants turn towards similar explants growing in the same dish.[97] Molecules present in the extracellular matrix and known to affect axon growth (see Table 9.1) include laminin, J1/tenascin,[98] collagens, proteoglycans and oligosaccharides.[99] Association with proteoglycans may be important for optimal functioning of both laminin[100] and NCAM.[101]

Laminin is a dagger-shaped molecule comprising three polypeptide chains[102] and is a component of basal laminae (Fig. 9.5). Laminin is in general an excellent substrate for axonal growth,[103] and its application to growth cones already advancing slowly on another substrate leads to acceleration of movement within a few minutes.[104] There are in fact several laminin isoforms, and these are preferentially recognized by the axons of different populations of nerve cells.[105] Laminin also has a domain which has growth factor activity.[106] It is expressed in appropriate places *in vivo*, both in the peripheral nervous system (e.g. the basal lamina of Schwann cells)[107] and in the CNS (e.g. at the site of the developing corpus callosum).[108] In vertebrates it remains unclear whether laminin imparts specific guidance cues preferentially to some groups of axons over others, although the diverse expression patterns of different laminin isoforms suggest that this could be the case for subsets of peripheral axons in vertebrate embryos.[109] Molecules with subunits homologous to the three laminin subunit chains are also present in invertebrates, both in insects (the A, B1 and B2 chains)[110] and in nematode worms (the B2 chain).[111] A critical requirement for laminin A during axon pathfinding in *Drosophila* has been revealed in *LamA* hypomorphic mutants, in which photoreceptor (ocellar) axons extending from the eye–antenna imaginal disc stall short of the brain.[112] Mutations in the nematode gene coding for the B1 homologue (*unc6*, where *unc* denotes uncoordinated movements) prevent axons navigating correctly around the body wall (see also netrins, below).[113]

Adhesion to molecules such as laminin in the extracellular matrix is carried out by integrins, integral cell membrane proteins composed of non-covalently linked α and β chains. The integrins in nerve cells usually have a β_1 chain,[114] but the α chain can vary making it possible for different neural integrins to recognize different molecules in the extracellular matrix. In general, integrins recognize ECM molecules that possess the tripeptide Arg-Gly-Asp (the RGD sequence), but neuronal integrins may recognize laminin differently, at a site near the end of its long arm.[115,116] Antibodies against integrins inhibit extension of axons on laminin.[93]

Work in other systems has shown that integrins do not act simply as mechanical attachment sites for cells and their processes but also as signalling receptors. There is evidence, for example, that integrins can modulate a tyrosine kinase (focal adhesion kinase, FAK) and can induce changes in intracellular calcium ion concentration;[117,118] such signalling may be triggered by clustering of integrins. So integrins, like CAMs, are likely to affect growth cone behaviour by means other than simple adhesion.

Chemotropism

Guidance by concentration gradients of diffusible molecules that attract growth cones at a distance (chemotropism) was first proposed by Cajal as a result of his observations of the growth patterns of axons, but lacked strong experimental support until relatively recently. Evidence that a specific molecule could exert a tropic action was provided by the finding that local administration of nerve growth factor (NGF, see Chapter 12) in the brainstem of neonatal rats caused a massive ingrowth of axons from the sympathetic ganglia into the spinal cord and up to the site of injection.[119] NGF was also shown to attract growth cones of sensory nerve cells *in vitro*.[120]

These experiments showed that molecular gradients can influence growth cones, but NGF, an essential trophic factor for a wide range of neurons, is not itself a good candidate as a specific chemotropic molecule as it is not usually expressed by target cells until after they have become innervated.[121] Furthermore, the innervating neurons do not become sensitive to it and dependent upon it until then. There is evidence, however, that other molecules are released at times that are appropriate to attract axons. By culturing epithelial cells of the first branchial (maxillary) arch of mice next to trigeminal ganglion neurons suspended in a collagen gel, it has been shown that the epithelial cells secrete an activity (originally known as max factor) that attracts the sensory axons growing from the ganglion (Fig. 9.7).[122] The activity is released only at embryonic day 10, corresponding to the stage when maxillary nerve axons are susceptible to it, and a part of its activity has been identified as a combination of the neurotrophins BDNF and NT-3 (see Chapter 12).[123]

There is now good evidence that chemotropism also directs the outgrowth of axons in the developing vertebrate CNS. During development, a group of commissural

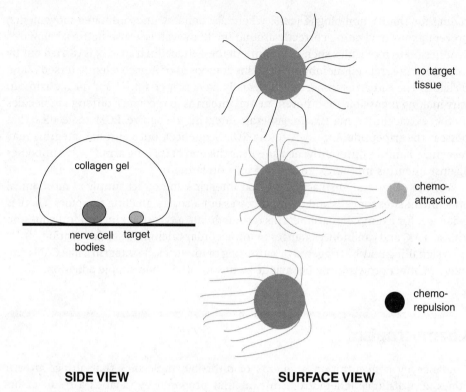

no target
tissue

collagen gel

chemo-
attraction

nerve cell   target
bodies

chemo-
repulsion

SIDE VIEW   SURFACE VIEW

Figure 9.7 Technique for the *in vitro* detection of chemoattractive and chemorepulsive molecules.[122] The cell bodies of the neurons under study are cultured together with potential sources of repulsive or attractive molecules in a collagen gel (left, side view). The small drop of gel (a few mm across) provides an environment which successfully stabilizes diffusion gradients and so mimics the real situation in the developing CNS. On the right are shown in surface view the patterns of axonal outgrowth in the absence of a target and when there is a source of diffusible attractant or repellent. The pattern of axon growth towards the target suggests true tropic directional attraction rather than general nutritive (trophic) support.

sensory axons navigates from the dorsal to ventral spinal cord, crosses the midline floor plate and then turns to form a longitudinal tract running alongside the floor plate on the opposite side of the cord. Floor plate cells have been found specifically to attract these axons when the two tissues (dorsal spinal cord and floor plate) are explanted near to each other in collagen gels.[124] Other examples of axon chemo-attraction have been described, a further one concerning the motor axons of the Vth, VIIth and IXth cranial nerves, which may be attracted to leave the brainstem by a chemoattractive source situated near to rhombomeres 2, 4 and 6.[125] Chemotropism probably also accounts for 'interstitial branching' of new growth cones from axon shafts, as discussed in Chapter 10.

Identity and mode of action of chemoattractant molecules

The search for the molecular basis of chemoattraction came to fruition in 1994, when the purification from chicken brain of the floor plate proteins that attract commissural axons was achieved (Fig. 9.8).[126,127] These proteins have been named netrins 1 and 2 (after a Sanskrit word meaning 'guiding'). Molecular cloning revealed that the sequence has 50 per cent homology to *unc6*, a nematode gene with homology to the B2 subunit of laminin which, like the netrins, is part of a system guiding axon growth

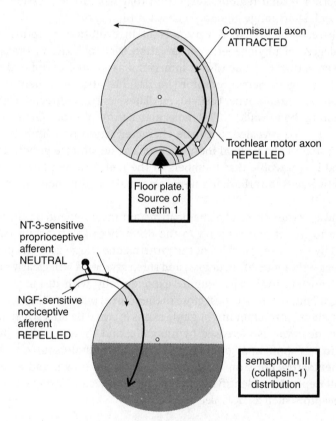

Figure 9.8 Chemoattraction and chemorepulsion in the developing spinal cord of vertebrates. *Top*: netrin-1 secreted from the floor plate attracts axons of commissural neurons from the dorsal spinal cord into the ventral spinal cord. Netrin-1 also acts *in vitro* as a chemorepellent for the axons of ventral-originating trochlear motor neurons in the developing brainstem, and these grow away from the floor plate. *Bottom*: semaphorin III (collapsin-1) is expressed in the ventral half of the developing spinal cord. This molecule repels NGF-sensitive nociceptive afferents which terminate in the dorsal horn. NT-3-sensitive afferents from muscle receptors are not repelled and can grow into the ventral spinal cord to connect with motor neurons and interneurons.

and cell migrations in the dorsoventral body axis (Fig. 9.5). Its importance for normal vertebrate development is shown by the death of netrin-knockout mice within 2 days after birth.[128] In these animals the ventral commissural axons frequently fail to reach the floor plate and, strikingly, the corpus callosum and other forebrain commissures are absent. A netrin receptor has been identified in mammals and is encoded by the DCC gene, originally characterized as a tumour suppressor gene lost in colorectal cancer. It is related to the immunoglobulin superfamily (Fig. 9.5) and is expressed in those neurons known to be sensitive to netrins;[129,130] again, the CNS phenotype in DCC-knockout mice is remarkably similar to that of the netrin knockout.[131] A further defect is seen in the developing eye of netrin- and DCC-deficient mice, where many axons fail to exit the retina into the optic nerve. They reach the optic disc but grow past it into other retinal regions, suggesting that netrin-1 expression by disc cells provides a local, short-range guidance cue for retinal axons.[132]

The netrin–receptor system is very ancient in evolutionary terms, showing an impressive degree of phylogenetic conservation. Netrins exist in *Drosophila*, where they have been shown to guide CNS commissural axons and peripheral axons,[133,134] and a DCC-homologous netrin receptor (*frazzled*) has also been identified.[135] Again, the nematode DCC homologue, UNC-40, mediates ventrally-directed cell migrations in the developing body wall.[136] The molecular nature of other chemoattractants is also beginning to be revealed, with the characterization of a limb-derived chemo-attractant for mammalian spinal motor neurons as hepatocyte growth factor/scatter factor,[137] and it is possible that members of the neurotrophin family provide local chemoattractive cues for arborizing nerve terminals within their target regions (see also Chapter 12).[138]

Growth towards the source of a chemoattractant must depend on the ability of the growth cone to detect and respond to the differences in attractant concentration encountered by the different sides of the growth cone. Large growth cones (a typical growth cone is only some 20 μm across) and steep gradients will clearly aid detection. Also, if the concentration falls roughly exponentially with distance from a point source, the gradient will be steepest close to the source, placing a limit on the distance over which a chemoattractant might guide axons *in vivo*. The effective diameter of the growth cone, however, is increased by filopodia, and these could be important for orientation in an exponential gradient generated by a distant source.[139] The mode of action of chemoattractants on the growth cone is unknown, and a deeper under-standing will depend on identifying the detailed molecular events activated down-stream of receptors such as DCC (see also below).

Interstitial axon branching

Chemotropism is able to guide the growth cones at the end of growing axons. It probably also triggers de novo sprouting of growth cones from the shaft of axons which later grow into side branches of some size, and which come to innervate nearby nuclei in the brain.[6] Such a process has been identified at several sites in the vertebrate CNS, and provides a means of targeting axons to innervate a series of different nuclei at staggered times so that branching decisions do not always have to be made at the terminal growth cone. It may also help to account for development of *topographic* targeting *within* a single nucleus, and is discussed further in Chapter 10.

Axon guidance by repulsion

Further guidance for axons seeking their targets comes from molecules that prevent rather than encourage growth in particular directions.[140-142] Repulsion of growth cones may result from direct contact between the surface of the growth cone and another cell, or from diffusible molecules secreted by the repellent source (chemorepulsion),[143] and several repulsion systems have been identified. In vertebrates, for example, contact *in vitro* between growth cones and axons of peripheral and central neurons induces, respectively, the collapse and withdrawal of central and peripheral growth cones (Fig. 9.9),[144] and such mutual repulsion could help to bundle growing axons of common origin or destination into groups and tracts. In higher vertebrates, spinal motor axons are channelled after leaving the spinal cord into the anterior (rostral) half of each somite by a contact-repulsive factor present in the posterior half.[145] Spinal sensory axons are flanked *in vivo* by tissues (such as the somite-derived

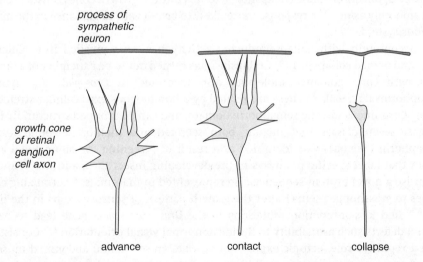

Figure 9.9 Axon growth cone collapse as seen *in vitro*. When the filopodia of the retinal ganglion cell growth cone contact the sympathetic axon, the growth cone shrinks rapidly and withdraws its filopodia so that only one filopodium remains attached to the sympathetic axon. The growth cone can remain quiescent for an hour or so before advancing again. After Kapfhammer and Raper.[144]

dermomyotome and notochord) that chemorepel them *in vitro*, and this 'surround-repulsion' may orient their dorsoventral trajectory *in vivo*.[146] Optic axons from ganglion cells in the temporal retina of the chick, which project to the anterior tectum, are repelled *in vitro* by a membrane glycoprotein expressed transiently in the posterior tectum (see also Chapter 10).[147] Finally, in the adult CNS it is known that axon regrowth following injury is inhibited by mature oligodendrocytes.[148] When antibodies to the inhibitory material are administered to *developing* rats, axon bundling patterns are somewhat disordered,[149] and if myelin formation is prevented by X-irradiation from destroying oligodendrocyte precursors in the optic nerve, ganglion cell axons sprout additional branches.[150] It seems possible, therefore, that inhibition of growth cones by oligodendrocytes and their myelin may be important as a means of suppressing unwanted axon sprouting in the mature brain.[151] Another factor that may be involved in suppressing unwanted growth in the adult is the smallest member of the immunoglobulin superfamily, Thy-1, which appears on terminal axons after connections have been made.[152]

Identity and mode of action of repulsion molecules

In the culture dish, growth cone repulsion appears to be an active process because the axon's advance is not simply halted. Instead, the growth cone shrinks, pulls in its filopodia and withdraws, resulting in a collapsed appearance (Fig. 9.9). Whether full collapse of growth cones takes place during normal development is unclear; small localized application of one collapsing factor to cultured growth cones causes them to turn smoothly aside,[153] a response more likely to be relevant to guidance in the intact nervous system.

A glycoprotein with collapse-inducing activity has been purified from chicken brain and named collapsin-1.[154] Collapsin-1 has turned out to be a member of a family of growth cone guidance molecules also identified in *Drosophila* and named semaphorins (Fig. 9.5).[155] These are related by a homologous extracellular stretch of some 500 amino acids, the semaphorin domain, and can be grouped structurally into at least seven classes that include both secreted and membrane-bound forms. Semaphorin I (sema1) was identified as a result of screening for monoclonal antibodies that label specific pathways in the developing insect CNS, and was found to comprise a novel protein sequence also represented in mammals. Neutralizing antibodies to grasshopper sema1 alter the growth pattern of sensory axons in the limb bud,[156] and loss-of-function mutations in the *Drosophila sema2* gene lead to behavioural defects such as inability to fly and abnormal visual orientation.[155] Consistent with a repulsive role, ectopic expression of *sema2* in segmental abdominal muscles causes some motor axons to stall short of their target muscles.[157] In vertebrates, collapsin-1/sema3 expressed by cells in the ventral spinal cord appears to repel the ingrowth of axons of NGF-dependent nociceptive afferents, so confining them to the dorsal layers of the spinal cord;[158,159] NT-3-dependent proprioceptive afferents from muscle spindles are not repelled by collapsin-1/sema3 *in vitro*, correlating with their ability to grow into the ventral horn and synapse directly with motor neurons (Fig. 9.8).

Many other members of the collapsin/semaphorin family have been identified in vertebrates (over 25 members have been identified thus far in mammals), and they show diverse expression patterns during neural development. *In vitro* they can act as both repellents and attractants, depending on the molecular subtype of semaphorin and anatomical subtype of axon; cortical axons, for example, are repelled or attracted by different class 3 semaphorins.[160] Their precise functions during axon guidance *in vivo* are less certain, however, and remain to be elucidated in detail.[161]

The neuropilins (Fig. 9.5) have been identified as class 3 semaphorin-binding proteins. Neuropilin-1, for example, is expressed on the neuronal surface and mediates collapsin-1/sema3A-induced growth cone collapse;[162,163] neuropilin-2 likewise mediates sema3F- and sema4-induced repulsion.[164-166] The neuropilins may be essential components of a receptor complex mediating the action of collapsin/semaphorins,[167] although they do not appear to mediate transmembrane signalling itself.[165,168] Members of the plexin family[169] have been identified as additional constituents of this receptor complex. Certain plexins may act alone as semaphorin receptors; in *Drosophila*, for example, *PlexA* and *Sema1a* loss-of-function mutants show strikingly similar axon guidance phenotypes, consistent with a model in which these proteins function as an interacting pair mediating axon defasciculation.[170] But there is also evidence that plexins and neuropilins can associate together to form a stable complex that acts as a receptor for class 3 semaphorins. It is possible that plexins are receptors for all semaphorin classes, either alone or in combination with neuropilins.[171]

Another example of a multigene family that mediates repulsive interactions during axon guidance is the Eph family of receptor tyrosine kinases (Fig. 9.5) and their ligands, the ephrins. This system is involved in the repulsive guidance of retinal axons during the formation of an ordered topographic map between the retina and the midbrain tectum (see Chapter 10), and also in the development of forebrain commissures and spinal nerve segmentation.[172] In the EphB2 knockout mouse, axons fail to navigate the anterior commissure, connecting the temporal cortex on either side of the forebrain, and instead grow aberrantly into the ventral forebrain, a phenotype which can be interpreted in terms of loss of repulsion of commissural axons by EphB2-expressing ventral forebrain cells.[173] During the outgrowth of spinal axons in the anterior half-somite, two transmembrane ephrins, ephrin-B2 in the rat and ephrin-B1 in the chick, are expressed by posterior but not anterior somite cells, and *in vitro* assays of motor axon outgrowth have shown that these ephrins can guide axons by repulsion.[174] The same system has been implicated in the restriction of migrating trunk neural crest cells to the anterior half-somite (see Chapter 5),[175] although a critical function for the Eph receptor–ephrin system in mediating spinal nerve segmentation has yet to be confirmed *in vivo*.

Bifunctional axon guidance molecules

As mentioned above, different members of a family of axon guidance molecules may be attractive or repulsive to growth cones (e.g. semaphorins above), and it has also become clear that individual guidance molecules may have a dual or 'bifunctional' role, repelling some growth cones while being simultaneously attractive to others. The *Drosophila* protein connectin, for example, is expressed on subsets of motor axons and muscles in the fly, and may mediate attractive–adhesive interactions between them, but it may be simultaneously repulsive for motor neurons destined for other muscles.[176] Sema3A has also been shown to be a repellent for the axons of cerebral cortical pyramidal neurons and an attractant for their dendrites, and its asymmetrical expression in the developing cortex may help to explain how the growth of the apical dendrites of these neurons is orientated towards the pial surface.[177] A further example of a bifunctional molecule is provided by netrin-1; while it attracts commissural axons (see above), *in vitro* it also repels the axons of trochlear motor neurons which grow away from the floor plate (Fig. 9.8).[178] Its nematode homologue, UNC-6, likewise attracts some cells migrating in the body wall and repels others, the response probably depending on the nature of the receptors expressed by the particular cell.[136] The ability of a guidance molecule to elicit both attractive and repulsive responses implies considerable subtlety on the part of the signal transduction mechanisms within growth cones, and the possible mechanisms underlying such flexibility are considered further below.

Axon guidance at the embryonic midline: analysis by genetic screens

In recent years large-scale mutant screens have been carried out in a variety of organisms to identify novel genes that regulate axon guidance and target innervation. Examples already mentioned include the *unc5*, *unc6* and *unc40* mutants in *C. elegans*, and *Drosophila* mutants showing guidance defects during neuromuscular innervation. The guidance of axons at the body midline of the fly provides a further system, where two mutants, *commissureless* (*comm*) and *roundabout* (*robo*), have been characterized in which axons behave abnormally in deciding whether or not to cross the CNS midline.[179] In *robo*, growth cones that would normally confine their trajectory to one side of the embryo cross the midline, sometimes back and forth, and the gene encodes a transmembrane protein (a member of the immunoglobulin superfamily) that participates in the reception of a midline repulsive signal (Fig. 9.5).[142,180]

This repellent has been identified as the product of the *slit* gene, first described as a gene affecting the larval cuticle pattern. Slit protein is secreted by the midline glial cells, and the phenotypes of *slit* and *robo* double mutants suggest that Slit and Robo act in the same pathway.[181] Biochemical experiments have also shown that Slit protein binds to Robo with high affinity.[182,183]

The opposite phenotype is seen in *comm* mutants, where axons fail to cross the midline. The *comm* gene encodes a transmembrane protein that is expressed by the CNS midline glia, and that is actually transferred to commissural axons as they contact and traverse the midline (the significance of this is unclear, and the phenomenon is similar to the transfer of the entire transmembrane BOSS protein to *sevenless*-expressing cells in the developing fly retina, see Chapter 8).[184] The precise function of *comm* is uncertain, but the finding that double mutants of *comm* and *robo* have a *robo* rather than a *comm* phenotype shows that in the absence of *robo* there is no absolute requirement for *comm* expression when axons cross the midline. This suggests that the normal function of Comm is to antagonize Robo signalling, for example by downregulation or degradation of Robo, although other interpretations are also possible.[185]

The operation of this short-range system at the midline complements the function of the longer-range netrin–frazzled system, which is involved in orienting growth cones towards the midline, much in the same way that axonin-1/Nr-CAM and netrin/DCC provide short- and long-range guidance cues at the vertebrate CNS midline. Moreover, like the netrin system, the Slit–Robo system shows phylogenetic conservation. Two *robo* homologues are expressed in the rat spinal cord, where they may control midline crossing,[180] and mutations in a *C. elegans* homologue, *sax3*, also cause repeated midline crossing of ventral cord axons.[180] At least three Slit isoforms have been identified in mammals, and have been shown to be chemorepulsive for Robo-expressing motor axons[182,183] and olfactory axons.[183,186] They are therefore candidates for mediating the chemorepulsion of motor axons by floor plate,[187] and of olfactory bulb axons by midline septum,[143,188] shown previously in collagen gel experiments. It is also interesting that mammalian Slit2 protein *promotes* the branching of primary sensory axons *in vitro*;[189] Slit proteins may be bifunctional, like several other molecular systems discussed above (see reference 190 for review).

The zebrafish provides an excellent model system for large-scale genetic screens in a vertebrate, and a variety of mutants have been identified with abnormalities of axon guidance and targeting in the retinotectal projection. The molecular cloning and functional analysis of mutants such as *bashful*, *grumpy* and *sleepy*, in which retinal axons projecting to the opposite tectum make errors after crossing the midline, should be revealing.[191,192]

The growth cone response

How do growth cones respond to external axon guidance molecules, whether by attraction or repulsion? The overall shape and hence the trajectory of the growth cone are critically dependent on the state of its internal cytoskeleton, so the response must involve the adjustment of cytoskeletal dynamics following the reception of an external signal by the growth cone. It seems likely that the attractive or repulsive nature of any particular guidance cue is determined by the cytoplasmic domain of the relevant growth cone receptor. It has been shown, for example, that netrins induce repulsive responses in flies when the intracellular domain of the Frazzled receptor (see above) is replaced by the intracellular domain of the Robo receptor; conversely, a chimeric receptor comprising the extracellular domain of Robo and the intracellular domain of Frazzled induces attractive responses to Slit.[193] The task, then, is to identify the molecular events triggered by interaction between guidance molecules and their receptors in the growth cone membrane. To date, calcium ions, cyclic nucleotides and small GTP-binding proteins of the Rho subfamily (Rho-like GTPases) have emerged as key mediators between signal reception and the cytoskeleton, although many details remain to be clarified.[194]

Focal increases in internal calcium ion concentration within cultured growth cones have been associated with local filopodial responses[195] and with growth cone turning,[196] and deviations from an optimal internal calcium level have been suggested to inhibit growth cone motility.[197] Consistent with this, growth cone collapse induced by myelin-based proteins (see above) is preceded by a release of calcium from internal stores and an acute rise in cytoplasmic calcium ion concentration.[198] On the other hand, homophilic interactions between CAMs are also followed by rises in internal calcium, and calcium channel blockers prevent CAM-induced growth stimulation.[63,199] Such apparently conflicting findings are not easy to reconcile; it is possible, for example, that small changes in internal calcium levels promote the formation of filopodial protrusions and growth, while larger changes inhibit the process, but this remains uncertain.[200] Whether growth cones show attractive or repulsive turning responses *in vitro* does appear to depend critically on the *pattern* of calcium elevation within growth cones. For example, local elevation of calcium levels within one side of a growth cone induces a turning response to that side, but this is converted into an opposite, repulsive response if the resting calcium level within the growth cone is lowered.[201] Conversion of attraction to repulsion in the presence of reduced calcium signals has also been seen in the *in vitro* turning response to netrin-1, and these experiments have further suggested an important role for calcium-induced calcium release from internal stores within the growth cone.[202]

The importance of growth cone calcium signalling has been confirmed in one *in vivo* system, the frog spinal cord, where the ambient level of ionized calcium in growing axons has been imaged. When axons grow rapidly, calcium levels show little change within the growth cone, but when growth stalls the cytoplasm shows wave-like pulses of calcium at some 5–15 waves per hour. Critically, photoinduced release of a 'caged' calcium chelator within the growth cone initiates growth, while release of caged calcium inhibits it.[203] Similar calcium waves have been seen in many other cell types, where they are generally thought to represent waves of calcium-induced calcium release from internal stores.[204] The same may be true for the growth cone, where influx through growth cone membrane calcium channels may also contribute, but their precise significance is unknown.[200]

When motility is increased by homophilic CAM binding at the growth cone membrane, a further route to calcium entry may involve activation of the fibroblast growth factor receptor (FGFR) tyrosine kinase.[199,205] NCAM, L1 and N-cadherin can stimulate neurite growth via FGFR activation, and a 'CAM-homology domain' of 20 amino acids has been identified in all these proteins, antibodies against which (and peptides mimicking which) inhibit CAM-stimulated axon growth *in vitro*.[206] The CAM response is blocked, moreover, in neurites of cultured PC12 cells expressing a dominant-negative form of FGFR-1 which prevents FGF receptor dimerization and subsequent receptor signalling inside the growth cone; and it is also blocked in cerebellar neurites cultured from transgenic mice expressing the dominant-negative FGF receptor.[207] FGF receptor activation via the CAM homology domain may induce a signal transduction cascade that generates arachidonic acid through sequential activation of PLCγ to generate diacylglycerol (DAG), followed by the action of DAG lipase on DAG, finally stimulating calcium ion influx through membrane calcium channels.[199]

How changes in internal ionized calcium levels alter growth cone motility is unclear. One candidate transducer is the calcium–calmodulin-dependent serine phosphatase, calcineurin; when this is laser-inactivated asymmetrically within the growth cone, filopodia show a local retraction response, and it may act through modulation of substrate proteins such as tau, a microtubule/microfilament-associated protein concentrated in growth cones, as well as GAP-43.[208] Further candidates include actin-severing proteins such as gelsolin, and calcium-activated proteases such as calpain.[200] Lastly, the modulation of cyclic AMP (cAMP) levels in the growth cone through calcium-dependent adenyl cyclase may also be important. Blockade of this signalling pathway *in vitro* by a competitive analogue of cAMP converts a turning response of growth cones *towards* a focal source of chemoattractant (netrin, BDNF or acetylcholine) into a repulsive response.[209,210] Conversely, pharmacological activation of the cAMP pathway in the same assay system can convert a repulsive response (to myelin-associated glycoprotein) into an attractive response, while activation of the cGMP pathway has the same effect on repulsion induced by sema3A.[211] Calcium is important in permitting these turning responses because they are abolished when the external calcium concentration is reduced, while straight-line growth continues unabated under these conditions. The potential importance of such calcium/cyclic nucleotide switching of the growth cone response *in vivo* has been highlighted by the finding that soluble guanylate cyclase is localized exclusively to the apical dendrites of developing cerebral cortical neurons. Since the sema3A receptor component, neuropilin-1, is expressed on both the axons and dendrites of these neurons, this could explain why apical dendrites are attracted towards sources of sema3A protein whereas axons are repelled.[177]

Another signalling route to the growth cone cytoskeleton, which may mediate the actions of cyclic nucleotides, concerns the Rho subfamily of small GTPases (Ras superfamily). These are involved in regulating cytoskeletal dynamics in a variety of non-neuronal cells,[212] and recent evidence has also implicated them in growth cone motility.[213] For example, transgenic mice expressing an activated form of Rac1 in cerebellar Purkinje cells show severe disruption of presynaptic terminals and dendritic spines,[214] while blocking Rho function prevents thrombin-induced growth cone collapse *in vitro*.[215] Gain-of-function and null alleles of a Rho family member identified in *C. elegans* also perturb axon guidance.[216] Many potential effectors of activated Rho-family members have been identified (e.g. Rho-kinase and the actin-depolymerizing protein N-WASP), and these may provide a direct link to the acto-myosin system in growth cones. There is also evidence that attractive responses involve preferential activation of one subset of Rho-like GTPases (Cdc42 and Rac), while repulsion involves activation of Rho-A, the latter being additionally regulated by the ambient level of cAMP (Fig. 9.10).[212]

By analogy with Ras signalling, Rho-based signalling in the growth cone may be controlled upstream by the balance of activity of three types of regulating molecules: guanine nucleotide exchange factors (GEFs), which convert GDP-bound (inactive) forms of the GTPases to the active GTP-bound forms, GTPase-activating proteins (which do the reverse), and guanine nucleotide dissociation inhibitors (which stabilize the inactive GDP-bound conformation).[217] How these, in turn, are regulated still further upstream is uncertain. They may interact directly with the receptors for axon guidance molecules, or indirectly via adapter proteins (e.g. Nck, see below) (Fig. 9.10).

Tyrosine phosphorylation appears to play a key role in the early transduction of external growth cone guidance signals, and the evidence comes from several sources. First, a number of transmembrane receptor tyrosine kinases (e.g. FGF receptors, Eph receptors and neurotrophin/Trk receptors) have been implicated in axon guidance decisions, for example in the retinotectal system (see Chapter 10) and in the formation of the mouse forebrain anterior commissure.[173] Second, mutations in certain transmembrane receptor tyrosine phosphatases (RTPs) expressed in the *Drosophila* nervous system generate axon pathfinding defects in subsets of motor axons.[218] Some of the phenotypes are consistent with a role for RTP activity in promoting defasciculation of axon bundles from their parent tracts at critical choice points during axon pathfinding. In this respect it is interesting that these RTPs have ectodomain structures homologous to Ig superfamily adhesion molecules (e.g. NCAM, fasciclin II), with tandem Ig domains and fibronectin type III repeats. In one phenotype, motor axons defasciculate normally but bypass their target muscles as a separate bundle, suggesting a defect in turning behaviour close to the target region rather than defasciculation.[219]

If altered tyrosine phosphorylation and GTPase activity within the growth cone are important in controlling growth cone motility, how are they linked? A clue may be provided by the finding that an adapter protein Dock, containing Src homology 3 (SH3) and SH2 domains, is necessary for the normal guidance of photoreceptor axons in the fly.[220] In its vertebrate homologue (Nck protein), the SH2 domain provides a

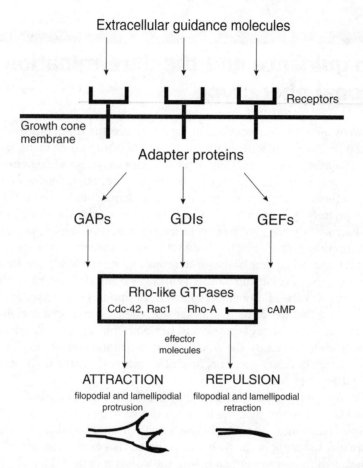

Figure 9.10 Summary of growth cone signalling via Rho-like GTPases. These are regulated upstream by the balance of activity of three types of regulating molecules: guanine nucleotide exchange factors (GEFs), GTPase-activating proteins (GAPs) and guanine nucleotide dissociation inhibitors (GDIs). The balance is determined further upstream by signalling from external guidance cues via receptors in the growth cone membrane. Cyclic nucleotide levels (e.g. cAMP) also modulate the level of Rho-like GTPase activity.

potential binding site for tyrosine phosphorylated proteins, while the SH3 domain binds Rho-family GTPases (Fig. 9.10), so proteins such as Dock and Nck may provide a direct linkage between tyrosine phosphorylation and Rho-based modulation of the growth cone cytoskeleton.

Lastly, it should be pointed out that some adhesion molecules, for example those of the L1 subset, may interact directly with the cytoskeleton of the growth cone. The intracellular domain of L1 is a conserved stretch of some 100 amino acids, and deletions or substitutions in this region can result in L1-associated neurological syndromes in humans (see above). This region contains a binding site for ankyrin, a protein that binds in turn to the membrane cytoskeleton, providing a potential route for stabilizing membrane contacts or enhancing homophilic or heterophilic L1 interactions.

Axon guidance and the determination of neuronal phenotype

An important question concerns the linkage between the mechanisms that specify the phenotype of an individual neuron and the trajectory taken by its axon. As discussed in Chapters 3 and 4, a variety of patterning mechanisms assign neurons with appropriate instructions for subsequent differentiation, but it remains unclear how these instructions are interpreted so that axon guidance cues in the environment are read appropriately by growth cones. Clues have come from the study of vertebrate motor neurons.[221] During chordate evolution the ancestral, dorsal position of motor axon exit from the neural tube has been replaced in the vertebrate spinal cord by a ventral exit point, while cranial motor neurons exiting the hindbrain have retained the ancestral dorsal exit. In the mouse, ventrally-exiting spinal cord motor neurons transiently express the LIM homeodomain transcription factors *Lhx3* and *Lhx4*, and when both genes (but not one) are knocked out, these neurons exit dorsally from the spinal cord. The importance of these transcription factors in determining motor axon trajectory is underscored by the finding that misexpression of *Lhx3* in hindbrain motor neurons, via electroporation in chick embryos, causes their axons to exit ventrally rather than dorsally.[221]

A similar function has been suggested by studies of this gene family in *Drosophila*, where the LIM homeobox gene *islet* has been shown to be necessary and sufficient to direct motor axons into the ventral muscle field of the fly embryo.[222] The study of neuromuscular targeting in the fly has also shown that expression of the homeobox gene *even-skipped* directs motor axons into the dorsal muscle field, and suggests the operation of a bimodal genetic switch that determines dorsoventral targeting in this system.[223] Presumably the products of these genes regulate the expression of neuronal target genes required for axon guidance, but the identity of these targets remains to be determined. The role of LIM and other transcription factors in determining axonal connectivity during the formation of topographic maps is discussed further in Chapter 10.

Galvanotropism

Growth cones can also be steered *in vitro* by weak electric fields. They usually grow faster towards the cathode[224] and this orientation is prevented by calcium channel blockers.[225] Local increases in internal calcium ion concentration occur on the side facing the cathode, and this is followed by local increases in filopodial production.[226] Electric fields do exist in the embryo,[227] and could in principle contribute to axon guidance, but this remains to be demonstrated *in vivo*.

Neuronal polarity and the development of differences between axons and dendrites

The two sorts of processes that grow out from a developing neuron, axon and dendrite, are functionally and structurally different from one another (see Table 9.2). Like many cell types, the neuron is therefore described as being polarized. The development of polarization has been studied in fetal hippocampal neurons grown in culture, which develop a quite normal morphology even if explanted before they have extended any cell processes.[228,229] At first, all processes grow at the same rate, but eventually one predominates and becomes the axon[230] while the others acquire typical dendritic properties. An early molecular sign of developing polarity is the distribution of GAP-43, which becomes concentrated in the axon, while expression in the dendrites falls.[231] If, however, the pioneer axon is pruned so that it is shorter than the other branches, one of these becomes the new axon.[230] Neuronal polarity is not, therefore, prespecified and this suggests that, *in vivo*, interactions with the neuronal environment are critical in generating the typical orientation of axons and dendrites. Such interactions are also involved in the development of polarity in sheets of epithelial cells.[232] In such cells the envelope glycoproteins of different viral strains have been found to be transported specifically to either the apical or basal surface once

Table 9.2 Neurons as polarized cells

Feature	Axons	Dendrites
Number	One	Many
Length	Potentially unlimited	Limited
Spines	Absent	Present
Initial segment	Specialized	Not specialized
Excitability	Conducted action potential	Usually no action potential
Synapses	Presynaptic	Usually postsynaptic
Myelin	Present on axons of >1 μm diameter	Absent
Polysomes	Absent	Present
Gap-43	Present	Little or absent
Cytoskeleton	Microtubules all with '+-end' at tip and Tau as MAP Neurofilaments	Microtubules of both polarities and MAP-2 as MAP Neurofilaments
Comparison with polarized epithelial cell	? equivalent to apical surface	? equivalent to basolateral surface

polarity has been established, but not to both. When similar tests are carried out in neurons, viral material, which in epithelial cells is directed apically, ends up in the axon, and basally-directed material in the dendrites.[229] Such directed transport probably depends on processes in the Golgi apparatus which use signal sequences to sort proteins into different trafficking streams.

It has also been suggested that the development of the differing microtubule organization in axons and dendrites (Table 9.2) may be important in initiating other differences between these processes.[233] The axon contains microtubules of a single polarity (all have the plus end situated furthest from the cell body) and this might limit what can be transported into the axon compared with dendrites, which contain microtubules of both polarities. It is possible to inhibit the development of polarity in cerebellar neurons using antisense oligonucleotides to tau protein (the microtubule-associated protein that is unique to axons).[234] Conversely, it is possible to make non-neuronal cells develop axon-like structures by transfecting the cells with a vector expressing tau protein.[235]

Nerve cell precursors are electrically inexcitable, and the expression of the appropriate ion channel membrane proteins that are essential for electrical activity probably comes about without the need for interaction with any other cells, although it may require a functioning sodium pump.[236] In some axons the earliest action potentials are of very long duration (over 100 msec) and are dependent on calcium rather than sodium currents.[237] These long calcium transients are important for maintaining further neuronal differentiation,[238] since (in spinal cord neurons of *Xenopus*) calcium spikes promote transmitter expression and ion channel maturation while slower waves are needed for neurite extension, but they disappear with the onset of expression of potassium channels capable of carrying outward repolarizing current.[239] It turns out that there is a critical period during which these potassium channels have to be expressed if they are to appear at all.[240] In other neurons even the earliest action potentials are of short duration from the start,[241] presumably due to simultaneous expression of sodium, calcium and potassium channels in the axon membrane, while in axons that become myelinated there is a later stage of rearrangement of the location of the ion channels (see Chapter 6).

Dendritic growth and nerve cell shape and size

Nerve cells of different sorts can be readily distinguished by the size of their cell bodies and the shapes of their dendritic trees. The typical sizes and branching patterns are determined both by innate factors and by interactions between the neurons and their environment. Not surprisingly perhaps, when all genetic and environmental differences between animals are minimized, as in parthenogenetically-produced crustacea or insects reared in standardized conditions, particular identifiable nerve cells in different individuals are found to be very similar and differ only in the finest terminal branch patterns.[242,243]

The presence of innate factors can be deduced from the fact that immature hippocampal neurons, when dispersed in culture, develop reasonably normal primary dendritic branches,[228] and morphological differences between neurons derived from different sources are readily detectable.[244] It seems likely that innate control of dendritic length and branching patterns is mediated by differential expression of recognition molecules on the surfaces of different nerve cell types. This could allow unique growth patterns to develop among different neurons growing on homogeneous substrata. Certainly, differences in the form of *axonal* arbors can be generated by altering the properties of the substrate on which they are growing.[245]

The effect of environment can be seen, for example, in the dendrites of Purkinje cells in the cerebellum of mice lacking parallel fibres; they are stunted and do not develop their normal fan-like shape,[246] so the parallel fibres appear to stimulate and direct the growth of the dendrites of these cells in normal mice. Another example of the importance of afferent input in controlling dendritic development is seen in the Mauthner cell of the fish. If the vestibular input is removed, the growth of the lateral dendrite is stunted.[247] Functional synaptic input in addition to simple synaptic contact may play an important part in dendrite growth. A reduction in activity in the visual cortex brought about by rearing animals in the dark reduces the number of dendritic spines on pyramidal neurons.[248] Elimination of input can cause dendritic changes even in adult animals,[249] but changes occur even without such a powerful stimulus; continuous remodelling of the dendritic tree of living neurons in auto-nomic ganglia of mice has been observed in experiments in which particular neurons were visualized on several successive occasions.[250]

Feedback signals from the target control the size of dendritic trees. For example, sympathetic neurons in the superior cervical sympathetic ganglion of the rat can develop much larger dendritic trees than normal if each cell is given the opportunity to innervate more tissue than normal, while the dendritic arbors shrink if there is less target tissue than normal.[251] The likely mediators of this target organ effect are the neurotrophins (see Chapter 12), and this may explain why large animals have neurons with more and longer dendrites and axons with more terminal branches than smaller animals of comparable type, for the greater amount of tissue present in larger animals should provide more neurotrophic support. Animals with large bodies have fewer neurons than would be expected for their size when compared with small animals, even though their brains are bigger, and the relative paucity of neurons is compensated by their larger size.[252–254]

Hormones can influence the growth of dendrites of some neurons as well. For example, neurons in one of the nuclei controlling song production in male canaries have cell bodies and dendrites that are twice the size of those in female birds. The females do not normally sing, but androgens can cause large neurons to develop in the female too.[255]

Key points

1 Axons and dendrites grow in length by adding cytoskeletal and membrane material at their ends in a specialized structure called the growth cone. Growth cones are rich in actin, vesicles, mitochondria, microtubules and growth-associated proteins, and they express cell recognition molecules on their surfaces. They throw out fine extensions called filopodia which adhere to cells, other axons or to molecules in the extracellular matrix. The exact way in which growth occurs and by which external factors influence the rate and direction of growth is not known. The level of ionized calcium in the growth cone has to be within narrow limits for growth.

2 The first processes to extend from a developing neuron grow slowly and are all alike, but eventually one accelerates its growth rate. This process becomes the axon and the rest become dendrites. The very different properties which then develop in axons and dendrites are summarized in Table 9.2. The differences probably result from regulated sorting of proteins for transport to axon or dendrites. Proteins associated with the microtubules (MAP2 in dendrites and tau in axons) are important in enabling nerve cells to develop their typical lengthy processes.

3 Both *in vivo* and *in vitro* axons can lengthen by several millimetres per day. Continued rapid growth needs the production by the cell body of cytoskeletal and growth-associated proteins, and membrane precursors. These are transported to the growth cone. The environment traversed by the growth cone also affects the rate of growth.

4 A multiplicity of molecular cues help to guide axons to the right place in the nervous system, to aid ordered (topographic) distribution within that region, and to determine the cell types that will be innervated.

5 Components in the extracellular matrix, such as laminin, laminin-related molecules in invertebrates, fibronectin, collagen and tenascin (substrate adhesion molecules or SAMs), are recognized by integrins present in the growth cone and provide good substrata for axon growth. They probably stimulate growth by activating intracellular second messenger mechanisms rather than simply providing attachment points for filopodia.

6 Growth cones are also stimulated to grow and are guided by cell adhesion molecules (CAMs). Many but by no means all CAMs in both vertebrates and invertebrates are members of the immunoglobulin superfamily, and bind homophilically or to heterophilic partners. Like the SAMs, such interactions stimulate growth by triggering molecular signalling pathways within the growth cone.

7 Growth can also be stimulated and directed by diffusible chemoattractants (chemotropism). These seem to be specific for particular classes of axons and are only produced for limited time periods during development. The structure of a chemoattractant found in the developing vertebrate spinal cord, netrin, is homologous to that of a guidance molecule that determines circumferential cell migrations in the body wall of nematode worms.

8 Chemoattractants not only direct growth of the terminal growth cone but can also stimulate the appearance of new branches on already-formed axons. This is interstitial axon growth. It can provide innervation of brain nuclei and may also help to establish topographic order within brain nuclei.

9 Growth cones can also be actively repelled by molecules which cause growth cone collapse *in vitro*. Such repulsion molecules may be diffusible or associated with cell surfaces, and prevent axon growth into particular areas during development in both vertebrates and insects. Repulsion molecules are also present in the adult mammalian CNS, where their main function may be to suppress excess sprouting.

10 Axon guidance molecules may be bifunctional, attracting some axons while repelling others. The nature of the growth cone response is dependent on the particular receptors and intracellular signalling pathways engaged by the guidance molecule.

11 For individual neurons, the overall size and branching pattern of their axon and dendrites are determined by a combination of intrinsic factors and interactions with the environment.

General reading

- Goodman, C. S. Mechanisms and molecules that control growth cone guidance. *Annu. Rev. Neurosci.* **19**, 341–77 (1996).

- Mueller, B. K. Growth cone guidance: first steps towards a deeper understanding. *Annu. Rev. Neurosci.* **22**, 351–88 (1999).

- Tessier-Lavigne, M. and Goodman, C. S. The molecular biology of axon guidance. *Science* **274**, 1123–33 (1996).

- Gordon-Weeks, P. R. *Neuronal growth cones* (Cambridge University Press, Cambridge, 2000).

References

1. Ramón y Cajal, S. Histologie du système nerveux de l'homme et des vertébrés (A. Maloine, Paris, 1909).

2. Harrison, R. G. The outgrowth of the nerve fibre as a mode of protoplasmic movement. *J. Exp. Zool.* **9**, 787–846 (1910).

3. Speidel, C. C. Studies of living nerves. VII. Growth adjustments of cutaneous terminal arborizations. *J. Comp. Neurol.* **76**, 57–69 (1942).

4. Tosney, K. W. and Landmesser, L. Growth cone morphology and trajectory in the lumbosacral region of the chick embryo. *J. Neurosci.* **5**, 2345–58 (1985).

5. Bastiani, M. J., Doe, C. Q., Helfand, S. L. and Goodman, C. S. Neuronal specificity and growth cone guidance in grasshopper. *Trends Neurosci.* **8**, 257–66 (1985).

6. Bastmeyer, M. and O'Leary, D. D. M. Dynamics of target recognition by interstitial axon branching along developing cortical axons. *J. Neurosci.* **16**, 1450–9 (1996).

7. Krystosek, A. and Seeds, N. W. Plasminogen activator release at the neuronal growth cone. *Science* **213**, 1532–4 (1981).

8. Remgard, P., Edbladh, M., Ekstroem, P. A. R. and Edstroem, A. Growth cones of regenerating

adult sciatic sensory axons release axonally transported proteins. *Brain Res.* **572**, 139–45 (1992).

9. Letourneau, P. C. Immunocytochemical evidence for colocalization in neurite growth cones of actin and myosin and their relationship to cell substratum adhesions. *Dev. Biol.* **85**, 113–22 (1981).

10. Yamada, K. M., Spooner, B. S. and Wessells, N. K. Axon growth: roles of microfilaments and microtubules. *Proc. Natl. Acad. Sci. USA* **66**, 1206–12 (1970).

11. Marsh, L. and Letourneau, P. C. Growth of neurites without filopodial or lamellipodial activity in the presence of cytochalasin B. *J. Cell Biol.* **99**, 2041–7 (1984).

12. Lamoureux, P. *et al.* Extracellular matrix allows PC12 neurite elongation in the absence of microtubules. *J. Cell Biol.* **110**, 71–9 (1990).

13. Bentley, D. and Toroian-Raymond, A. Disoriented pathfinding by pioneer neurone growth cones deprived of filopodia by cytochalasin treatment. *Nature* **323**, 712–15 (1986).

14. Chien, C. B., Rosenthal, D. E., Harris, W. A. and Holt, C. E. Navigational errors made by growth cones without filopodia in the embryonic *Xenopus* brain. *Neuron* **11**, 237–51 (1993).

15. Davenport, R. W., Dou, P., Rehder, V. and Kater, S. B. A sensory role for neuronal growth cone filopodia. *Nature* **361**, 721–4 (1993).

16. Strittmatter, S. M., Valenzuela, D., Kennedy, T. E., Neer, E. J. and Fishman, M. C. G$_0$ is a major growth cone protein subject to regulation by GAP-43. *Nature* **344**, 836–41 (1990).

17. Skene, J. H. P. *et al.* A protein induced during nerve growth (GAP-43) is a major component of growth-cone membranes. *Science* **233**, 783–6 (1986).

18. Benowitz, L. I. and Routtenberg, A. GAP-43: an intrinsic determinant of neuronal development and plasticity. *Trends Neurosci.* **20**, 84–91 (1997).

19. Zuber, M. X., Goodman, D. W., Karns, L. R. and Fishman, M. C. The neuronal growth-associated protein GAP-43 induces filopodia in non-neuronal cells. *Science* **244**, 1193–5 (1989).

20. Fishman, M. C. GAP-43: putting constraints on neuronal plasticity. *Perspect. Dev. Neurobiol.* **4**, 193–8 (1996).

21. Strittmatter, S. M., Fankhauser, C., Huang, P. L., Mashimo, H. and Fishman, M. C. Neuronal pathfinding is abnormal in mice lacking the neuronal growth cone protein GAP-43. *Cell* **80**, 445–52 (1995).

22. Aigner, L. *et al.* Overexpression of the neural growth-associated protein GAP-43 induces nerve sprouting in the adult nervous system of transgenic mice. *Cell* **83**, 269–78 (1995).

23. Bray, D. Surface movements during the growth of single explanted neurons. *Proc. Natl. Acad. Sci. USA* **65**, 905–10 (1970).

24. Popov, S., Brown, A. and Poo, M. Forward plasma membrane flow in growing nerve processes. *Science* **259**, 244–6 (1993).

25. Futerman, A. H. and Banker, G. A. The economics of neurite outgrowth—the addition of new membrane to growing axons. *Trends Neurosci.* **19**, 144–9 (1996).

26. Dai, J. W. and Sheetz, M. P. Axon membrane flows from the growth cone to the cell body. *Cell* **83**, 693–701 (1995).

27. Bretscher, M. S. Moving membrane up to the front of migrating cells. *Cell* **85**, 465–7 (1996).

28. Lockerbie, R. O., Miller, V. E. and Pfenninger, K. H. Regulated plasmalemmal expansion in nerve growth cones. *J. Cell Biol.* **112**, 1215–27 (1992).

29. Craig, A. M., Wyborski, R. J. and Banker, G. Preferential addition of newly synthesized membrane protein at axonal growth cones. *Nature* **375**, 592–4 (1995).

30. Martenson, C., Stone, K., Reedy, M. and Sheetz, M. Fast axonal transport is required for growth cone advance. *Nature* **366**, 66–9 (1993).

31. Okabe, S. and Hirokawa, N. Differential behavior of photoactivated microtubules in growing axons of mouse and frog neurons. *J. Cell Biol.* **117**, 105–20 (1992).

32. Tanaka, E. and Kirschner, M. W. Microtubule behavior in the growth cones of living neurons during axon elongation. *J. Cell Biol.* **115**, 345–3 (1991).

33. Brown, A., Slaughter, T. and Black, M. M. Newly assembled microtubules are concentrated in the proximal and distal regions of growing axons. *J. Cell Biol.* **119**, 867–82 (1992).

34. Tanaka, E., Ho, T. and Kirschner, M. W. The role of microtubule dynamics in growth cone motility and axonal growth. *J. Cell Biol.* **128**, 139–55 (1995).

35. Shaw, G. and Bray, D. Movement and extension of isolated growth cones. *Exp. Cell Res.* **104**, 56–62 (1977).

36. Harris, W. A., Holt, C. E. and Bonhoeffer, F. Retinal axons with and without their somata, growing to and arborizing in the tectum of *Xenopus* embryos: a time-lapse video study of single fibres *in vivo*. *Development* **101**, 123–33 (1987).

37. Bray, D. Cytoskeletal basis of nerve axon growth. In The nerve growth cone (ed. P. C. Letourneau, S. B. Kater and E. R. Macagno), pp. 7–18 (Raven Press, New York, 1991).

38. Sollner, T. *et al.* SNAP 25 receptors implicated in vesicle targeting and fusion. *Nature* **362**, 318–24 (1992).

39. Osen-Sand, A. *et al.* Inhibition of axonal growth by SNAP-25 antisense oligonucleotides *in vitro* and *in vivo*. *Nature* **364**, 445–8 (1993).

40. Kater, S. B., Mattson, M. P., Cohan, C. and Connor, J. Calcium regulation of the neuronal growth cone. *Trends Neurosci.* **11**, 315–21 (1988).

41. Kater, S. B. and Rehder, V. The sensory-motor role of growth cone filopodia. *Curr. Opin. Neurobiol.* **5**, 68–74 (1995).

42. Letourneau, P. C. Cell-to-substratum adhesion and guidance of axonal elongation. *Dev. Biol.* **44**, 92–101 (1975).

43. Lamoureux, P., Buxbaum, R. E. and Heidemann, S. R. Direct evidence that growth cones pull. *Nature* **340**, 159–62 (1989).

44. Letourneau, P. C. Cell to substratum adhesion and guidance of axonal elongation. *Dev. Biol.* **44**, 92–101 (1975).

45. Zheng, J., Buxbaum, R. E. and Heidemann, S. R. Measurements of growth cone adhesion to culture surfaces by micromanipulation. *J. Cell Biol.* **127**, 2049–60 (1994).

46. Campenot, R. B. The regulation of nerve fibre length by intercalated elongation and retraction. *Dev. Brain Res.* **20**, 149–84 (1985).

47. Simpson, A. H. R. W. D.M. Thesis, University of Oxford (1993).

48. Skene, J. H. P. Growth-associated proteins and the curious dichotomies of nerve regeneration. *Cell* **37**, 697–700 (1984).

49. Miller, F. D., Tetzlaff, W., Bisby, M. A., Fawcett, J. W. and Milner, R. J. Rapid induction of the major embryonic Alpha-tubulin mRNA, TAlpha1, during nerve regeneration in adult rats. *J. Neurosci.* **9**, 1452–63 (1989).

50. Tetzlaff, W., Bisby, M. A. and Kreutzberg, G. W. Changes in cytoskeletal proteins in the rat facial nucleus following axotomy. *J. Neurosci.* **8**, 3181–9 (1988).

51. Chong, M. S. *et al.* The downregulation of GAP-43 is not responsible for the failure of regeneration in freeze-killed nerve grafts in the rat. *Exp. Neurol.* **129**, 311–20 (1994).

52. Brown, M. C., Perry, V. H., Hunt, S. P. and Lapper, S. R. Further studies on motor and sensory nerve regeneration in mice with delayed Wallerian degeneration. *Eur. J. Neurosci.* **6**, 420–8 (1994).

53. Davies, A. M. Intrinsic differences in the growth rate of early nerve fibres related to target distance. *Nature* **337**, 553–5 (1989).

54. Bate, C. M. Pioneer neurones in an insect embryo. *Nature* **260**, 54–6 (1976).

55. Ho, R. K. and Goodman, C. S. Peripheral pathways are pioneered by an array of central and peripheral neurones in grasshopper embryos. *Nature* **297**, 404–6 (1982).

56. Klose, M. and Bentley, D. Transient pioneer neurons are essential for formation of an embryonic peripheral nerve. *Science* **245**, 982–4 (1989).

57. Raper, J. A., Bastiani, M. J. and Goodman, C. S. Pathfinding by neuronal growth cones in grasshopper embryos. IV. The effects of ablating the A and P axons upon the behavior of the G growth cone. *J. Neurosci.* **4**, 2329–45 (1984).

58. Hidalgo, A. and Brand, A. H. Targeted neuronal ablation: the role of pioneer neurons in guidance and fasciculation in the CNS of *Drosophila*. *Development* **124**, 3253–62 (1997).

59. Kimmel, C. B. Patterning the brain of the zebrafish embryo. *Annu. Rev. Neurosci.* **16**, 707–32 (1993).

60. Schachner, M. Neural recognition molecules and their influence on cellular functions. In The nerve growth cone (ed. P. C. Letourneau, S. B. Kater and E. R. Macagno), pp. 237–56 (Raven Press, New York, 1991).

61. Williams, A. F. Immunoglobulin-related domains for cell surface recognition. *Nature* **314**, 579–80 (1985).

62. Rao, Y., Wu, X.-F., Ganepy, J., Rutishauser, U. and Siu, C.-H. Identification of a peptide sequence involved in homophilic binding in the neural cell adhesion molecule NCAM. *J. Cell Biol.* **118**, 937–49 (1992).

63. Frei, T., von Bohlen und Halbach, F., Wille, W. and Schachner, M. Different extracellular domains of the neural cell adhesion molecule (N-CAM) are involved in different functions. *J. Cell Biol.* **118**, 177–94 (1992).

64. Bixby, J. L., Pratt, R. S., Lilien, J. and Reichardt, L. F. Neurite outgrowth on muscle cell surfaces involves matrix receptors as well as Ca^{++}-dependant and -independant cell adhesion molecules. *Proc. Natl. Acad. Sci. USA* **84**, 2555–9 (1987).

65. Whitelaw, V. A. and Cowan, J. D. Specificity and plasticity of retino-tectal connections: a computational model. *J. Neurosci.* **1**, 1369–87 (1981).

66. Goodman, C. S., Grenningloh, G. and Bieber, A. J. Guidance and steering of peripheral pioneer growth cones in grasshopper embryos. In The nerve growth cone (ed. P. C. Letourneau, S. B. Kater and E. R. Macagno), pp. 283–304 (Raven Press, New York, 1991).

67. Edelman, G. M. Cell adhesion molecules. *Science* **219**, 450–7 (1983).

68. Tosney, K. W., Watanabe, M., Landmesser, L. and Rutishauser, U. The distribution of N-CAM in the chick hindlimb during axon outgrowth and synaptogenesis. *Dev. Biol.* **114**, 468–81 (1986).

69. Rutishauser, U., Grumet, M. and Edelman, G. M. Neural cell adhesion molecule mediates

initial interactions between spinal cord neurons and muscle cells in culture. *J. Cell Biol.* **97**, 145–52 (1983).

70. Booth, C. M., Kemplay, S. and Brown, M. C. An antibody to neural cell adhesion molecule impairs motor nerve terminal sprouting in a mouse muscle locally paralysed with botulinum toxin. *Neuroscience* **35**, 85–91 (1990).

71. Thanos, S., Bonhoeffer, F. and Rutishauser, U. Fibre–fibre interaction and tectal cues influence the development of the chicken retino-tectal projection. *Proc. Natl. Acad. Sci. USA* **81**, 1906–10 (1984).

72. Martini, R. Expression and functional roles of neural cell surface molecules and extracellular matrix components during development and regeneration of peripheral nerves. *J. Neurocytol.* **23**, 1–28 (1994).

73. Martini, R., Schachner, M. and Brushart, T. M. The L2/HNK-1 carbohydrate is preferentially expressed by previously motor axon-associated Schwann cells in reinnervated peripheral nerves. *J. Neurosci.* **14**, 7180–91 (1994).

74. Rutishauser, U., Acheson, A., Hall, A. K., Mann, D. M. and Sunshine, J. The neural cell adhesion molecule (NCAM) as a regulator of cell–cell interactions. *Science* **240**, 53–7 (1988).

75. Tang, J., Landmesser, L. and Rutishauser, U. Polysialic acid influences specific pathfinding by avian motoneurons. *Neuron* **8**, 1031–44 (1992).

76. Tang, J., Rutishauser, U. and Landmesser, L. Polysialic acid regulates growth cone behavior during sorting of motor axons in the plexus region. *Neuron* **13**, 405–14 (1994).

77. Rutishauser, U. and Landmesser, L. Polysialic acid in the vertebrate nervous system: a promoter of plasticity in cell–cell interactions. *Trends Neurosci.* **19**, 422–7 (1996).

78. Tomasiewicz, H. *et al.* Genetic deletion of a neural cell adhesion molecule variant (N-CAM-180) produces distinct defects in the central nervous system. *Neuron* **11**, 1163–74 (1993).

79. Cremer, H., Chazal, G., Goridis, C. and Represa, A. NCAM is essential for axonal growth and fasciculation in the hippocampus. *Mol. Cell. Neurosci.* **8**, 323–35 (1997).

80. Ono, K., Tomasiewicz, H., Magnuson, T. and Rutishauser, U. N-CAM mutation inhibits tangential neuronal migration and is phenocopied by enzymatic removal of polysialic acid. *Neuron* **13**, 595–609 (1994).

81. Muller, D. *et al.* PSA–NCAM is required for activity-induced synaptic plasticity. *Neuron* **17**, 413–22 (1996).

82. Lin, D. M. and Goodman, C. S. Ectopic and increased expression of Fasciclin II alters moto-neuron growth cone guidance. *Neuron* **13**, 507–23 (1994).

83. Fambrough, D. and Goodman, C. S. The *Drosophila* beaten path gene encodes a novel secreted protein that regulates defasciculation at motor axon choice points. *Cell* **87**, 1049–58 (1996).

84. Chang, S., Rathjen, F. G. and Raper, J. A. Extension of neurites on axons is impaired by antibodies against specific nerve cell surface glycoproteins. *J. Cell Biol.* **104**, 355–62 (1987).

85. Appel, F., Holm, J., Conscience, J. F. and Schachner, M. Several extracellular domains of the neural cell adhesion molecule L1 are involved in neurite outgrowth and cell body adhesion. *J. Neurosci.* **13**, 4764–75 (1993).

86. Itoh, K., Stevens, B., Schachner, M. and Fields, R. D. Regulated expression of the neural cell adhesion molecule L1 by specific patterns of neural impulses. *Science* **270**, 1369–72 (1995).

87. Wong, E. V., Kenwrick, S., Willems, P. and Lemmon, V. Mutations in the cell adhesion molecule L1 cause mental retardation. *Trends Neurosci.* **18**, 168–72 (1995).

88. Kenwrick, S. and Doherty, P. Neural cell adhesion molecule L1: relating disease to function. *BioEssays* **20**, 668–75 (1998).

89. Cohen, N. R. *et al.* Errors in corticospinal axon guidance in mice lacking the neural cell adhesion molecule L1. *Curr. Biol.* **8**, 26–33 (1998).

90. Dodd, J. and Jessell, T. M. Axon guidance and the patterning of neuronal projections in vertebrates. *Science* **242**, 692–9 (1988).

91. Stoeckli, E. T. and Landmesser, L. T. Axonin-1, Nr-CAM, and Ng-CAM play different roles in the *in vivo* guidance of chick commissural neurons. *Neuron* **14**, 1165–79 (1995).

92. Takeichi, M. The cadherins: cell–cell adhesion molecules controlling animal morphogenesis. *Development* **102**, 639–55 (1988).

93. Tomaselli, K. J., Neugebauer, L. M., Bixby, J. L., Lilien, J. and Reichardt, L. F. N-cadherin and integrins: two receptor systems that mediate neuronal process outgrowth on astrocyte surfaces. *Neuron* **1**, 33–43 (1988).

94. Doherty, P. and Walsh, F. S. The contrasting roles of N-CAM and N-cadherins as neurite outgrowth-promoting molecules. *J. Cell Sci.* Suppl. **15**, 13–21 (1991).

95. Riehl, R. *et al.* Cadherin function is required for axon outgrowth in retinal ganglion cells *in vivo*. *Neuron* **17**, 837–48 (1996).

96. Adler, R., Manthorpe, M., Skaper, S. D. and Varon, S. Polyornithine-attached neurite-promoting factors (PNPFs). Culture sources and responsive neurons. *Brain Res.* **206**, 129–44 (1981).

97. Ebendal, T. and Jacobson, C. O. Tissue explants affecting extension and orientation of axons in cultured chick embryo ganglia. *Exp. Cell Res.* **105**, 379–87 (1977).

98. Lochter, A. *et al.* J1/tenascin in substrate-bound and soluble form displays contrary effects on neurite outgrowth. *J. Cell Biol.* **113**, 1159–72 (1991).

99. Rutishauser, U. and Jessell, T. M. Cell adhesion molecules in vertebrate neural development. *Physiol. Rev.* **68**, 819–57 (1988).

100. Chiu, A. Y., Matthew, W. D. and Patterson, P. H. A monoclonal antibody that blocks the activity of a neurite regeneration-promoting factor: studies on the binding site and its localization *in vivo. J. Cell Biol.* **103**, 1383–98 (1986).

101. Cole, G. J. and Glaser, L. A heparin-binding domain from N-CAM is involved in neural cell-substratum adhesion. *J. Cell Biol.* **102**, 403–12 (1986).

102. Paulsson, M. *et al.* Evidence for coiled-coil alpha-helical regions in the long arm of laminin. *EMBO J.* **4**, 309–15 (1985).

103. Carbonetto, S., Evans, D. and Cochard, P. Nerve fiber growth in culture on tissue substrates from central and peripheral nervous system. *J. Neurosci.* **7**, 610–20 (1987).

104. Rivas, R. J., Burmeister, D. W. and Goldberg, D. J. Rapid effects of laminin on the growth cone. *Neuron* **8**, 107–15 (1992).

105. Tomaselli, K. J. *et al.* Expression of Beta1 integrins in sensory neurons of the dorsal root ganglion and their functions in neurite outgrowth on two laminin isoforms. *J. Neurosci.* **13**, 4880–8 (1993).

106. Panayatou, G., End, P., Aumailley, M., Timpl, R. and Engel, J. Domains of laminin with growth factor activity. *Cell* **56**, 93–101 (1989).

107. Cornbrooks, C. J., Carey, D. L., McDonald, J. A., Timpl, R. and Bunge, R. P. *In vivo* and *in vitro* observations on laminin production by Schwann cells. *Proc. Natl. Acad. Sci. USA* **80**, 3850–4 (1983).

108. Liesi, P. and Silver, J. Is astrocyte laminin involved in axon guidance in the mammalian CNS? *Dev. Biol.* **130**, 774–85 (1988).

109. Lentz, S. I., Miner, J. H., Sanes, J. R. and Snider, W. D. Distribution of the ten known laminin chains in the pathways and targets of developing sensory axons. *J. Comp. Neurol.* **378**, 547–61 (1997).

110. Montell, D. J. and Goodman, C. S. *Drosophila* substrate adhesion molecule: sequence of laminin B1 chain reveals domains of homology with mouse. *Cell* **53**, 463–73 (1988).

111. Ishii, N., Wadsworth, W. G., Stern, B. D., Culotti, J. F. and Hedgecock, E. M. unc-6, a laminin-related protein, guides cell and pioneer axon migrations in *C. elegans. Neuron* **9**, 873–81 (1993).

112. Garcia-Alonso, L., Fetter, R. D. and Goodman, C. S. Genetic analysis of Laminin A in *Drosophila*: extracellular matrix containing laminin A is required for ocellar axon pathfinding. *Development* **122**, 2611–21 (1996).

113. Hedgecock, E. M., Culotti, J. G. and Hall, D. H. The unc-5, unc-6 and unc-40 genes guide circumferential migrations of pioneer axons and mesodermal cells on the epidermis of *C. elegans. Neuron* **4**, 61–85 (1990).

114. Reichardt, L. F. and Tomaselli, K. J. Extracellular matrix molecules and their receptors: functions in neural development. *Annu. Rev. Neurosci.* **14**, 531–70 (1991).

115. Jessell, T. M. Adhesion molecules and the hierarchy of neural development. *Neuron* **1**, 3–13 (1988).

116. Edgar, D. Neuronal laminin receptors. *Trends Neurosci.* **12**, 248–51 (1989).

117. Wang, N., Butler, J. P. and Ingber, D. E. Mechanotransduction across the cell surface and through the cytoskeleton. *Science* **260**, 1124–7 (1993).

118. Schwarz, M. A. Transmembrane signalling by integrins. *Trends Cell Biol.* **2**, 304–8 (1992).

119. Menesini Chen, M. G., Chen, J. S. and Levi Montalcini, R. Sympathetic nerve fibres ingrowth in the CNS of neonatal rodent upon intracerebral NGF injections. *Arch. Ital. Biol.* **116**, 53–84 (1978).

120. Gundersen, R. W. and Barrett, J. N. Characteristics of the turning response of dorsal root neurites towards NGF. *J. Cell Biol.* **87**, 546–54 (1980).

121. Davies, A. M. Molecular and cellular aspects of patterning sensory neuron connections in the vertebrate nervous system. *Development* **101**, 185–208 (1987).

122. Lumsden, A. G. S. and Davies, A. M. Earliest sensory nerve fibres are guided to peripheral targets by attractants other than nerve growth factor. *Nature* **306**, 786–8 (1983).

123. O'Connor, R. and Tessier-Lavigne, M. Identification of maxillary factor, a maxillary process-derived chemoattractant for developing trigeminal sensory axons. *Neuron* **24**, 165–78 (1999).

124. Tessier-Lavigne, M., Placzek, M., Lumsden, A. G. S., Dodd, J. and Jessell, T. M. Chemotropic guidance of developing axons in the mammalian central nervous system. *Nature* **336**, 775–8 (1988).

125. Guthrie, S. and Lumsden, A. Motor neuron pathfinding following rhombomere reversals in the chick embryo hindbrain. *Development* **114**, 663–73 (1992).

126. Kennedy, T. E., Serafini, T., De la Torre, J. R. and Tessier-Lavigne, M. Netrins are diffusible chemotropic factors for commissural axons in the embryonic spinal cord. *Cell* **78**, 425–35 (1994).

127. Serafini, T. *et al.* The netrins define a family of axon outgrowth-promoting proteins homologous to *C. elegans* UNC-6. *Cell* **78**, 409–24 (1994).

128. Serafini, T. *et al.* Netrin-1 is required for commissural axon guidance in the developing vertebrate nervous system. *Cell* **87**, 1001–14 (1996).

129. Keino-Masu, K. *et al.* Deleted in colorectal cancer (DCC) encodes a netrin receptor. *Cell* **87**, 175–85 (1996).

130. Keynes, R. and Cook, G. M. W. Axons turn as netrins find their receptor. *Neuron* **17**, 1031–4 (1996).

131. Fazeli, A. *et al.* Phenotype of mice lacking functional deleted in colorectal cancer (Dcc) gene. *Nature* **386**, 796–804 (1997).

132. Deiner, M. S. *et al.* Netrin-1 and DCC mediate axon guidance locally at the optic disc: loss of function leads to optic nerve hypoplasia. *Neuron* **19**, 575–89 (1997).

133. Harris, R., Sabatelli, L. M. and Seeger, M. A. Guidance cues at the *Drosophila* CNS midline: identification and characterization of two *Drosophila* Netrin/UNC-6 homologs. *Neuron* **17**, 217–28 (1996).

134. Mitchell, K. J. *et al.* Genetic analysis of netrin genes in *Drosophila*: netrins guide CNS commissural axons and peripheral motor axons. *Neuron* **17**, 203–15 (1996).

135. Kolodziej, P. A. *et al. frazzled* encodes a *Drosophila* member of the DCC immunoglobulin subfamily and is required for CNS and motor axon guidance. *Cell* **87**, 197–204 (1996).

136. Culotti, J. G. Axon guidance mechanisms in *Caenorhabditis elegans. Curr. Opin. Genet. Dev.* **4**, 587–95 (1994).

137. Ebens, A. *et al.* Hepatocyte growth factor/ scatter factor is an axonal chemoattractant and a neurotrophic factor for spinal motor neurons. *Neuron* **17**, 1157–72 (1996).

138. Cohen-Cory, S. and Fraser, S. E. Effects of brain-derived neurotrophic factor on optic axon branching and remodelling *in vivo. Nature* **378**, 192–6 (1995).

139. Tessier-Lavigne, M. and Placzek, M. Target attraction: are developing axons guided by chemotropism? *Trends Neurosci.* **14**, 303–10 (1991).

140. Patterson, P. H. On the importance of being inhibited, or saying no to growth cones. *Neuron* **1**, 263–7 (1988).

141. Keynes, R. J. and Cook, G. M. W. Axon guidance molecules. *Cell* **83**, 161–9 (1995).

142. Tessier-Lavigne, M. and Goodman, C. S. The molecular biology of axon guidance. *Science* **274**, 1123–33 (1996).

143. Pini, A. Chemorepulsion of axons in the developing mammalian central nervous system. *Science* **261**, 95–8 (1993).

144. Kapfhammer, J. P. and Raper, J. A. Collapse of growth cone structure on contact with specific neurites in culture. *J. Neurosci.* **7**, 201–12 (1987).

145. Davies, J. A., Cook, G. M., Stern, C. D. and Keynes, R. J. Isolation from chick somites of a glycoprotein fraction that causes collapse of dorsal root ganglion growth cones. *Neuron* **4**, 11–20 (1990).

146. Keynes, R. *et al.* Surround repulsion of spinal sensory axons in higher vertebrate embryos. *Neuron* **18**, 889–97 (1997).

147. Walter, J., Kern Veil, B., Huf, J., Stolze, B. and Bonhoeffer, F. Recognition of position-specific properties of tectal cell membranes by retinal axons *in vitro. Development* **101**, 685–96 (1987).

148. Schwab, M. E. and Caroni, P. Oligodendrocytes and CNS myelin are nonpermissive substrates for neurite growth and fibroblast spreading *in vitro. J. Neurosci.* **8**, 2381–93 (1988).

149. Schwab, M. E. and Schnell, L. Channeling of developing rat corticospinal tract axons by myelin-associated neurite growth inhibitors. *J. Neurosci.* **11**, 709–21 (1991).

150. Colello, R. J. and Schwab, M. E. A role for oligodendrocytes in the stabilization of optic axon numbers. *J. Neurosci.* **14**, 6446–52 (1994).

151. Schwab, M. E., Kapfhammer, J. P. and Bandtlow, C. E. Inhibitors of neurite growth. *Annu. Rev. Neurosci.* **16**, 565–95 (1993).

152. Morris, R. Thy-1, the enigmatic extrovert on the neuronal surface. *BioEssays* **14**, 715–22 (1992).

153. Fan, J. and Raper, J. A. Localized collapsing cues can steer growth cones without inducing their full collapse. *Neuron* **14**, 263–74 (1995).

154. Luo, Y., Raible, D. and Raper, J. A. Collapsin: a protein in brain that induces the collapse and paralysis of neuronal growth cones. *Cell* **75**, 217–27 (1993).

155. Kolodkin, A. L., Matthes, D. J. and Goodman, C. S. The semaphorin genes encode a family of transmembrane and secreted growth cone guidance molecules. *Cell* **75**, 1389–99 (1993).

156. Kolodkin, A. L. *et al.* Fasciclin IV: sequence, expression, and function during growth cone guidance in the grasshopper embryo. *Neuron* **9**, 831–45 (1992).

157. Matthes, D. J., Sink, H., Kolodkin, A. L. and Goodman, C. S. Semaphorin II can function as a selective inhibitor of specific synaptic arborizations. *Cell* **81**, 631–9 (1995).

158. Messersmith, E. K. *et al.* Semaphorin III can function as a selective chemorepellent to pattern sensory projections in the spinal cord. *Neuron* **14**, 949–59 (1995).

159. Shepherd, I. T., Luo, Y., Lefcort, F., Reichardt, L. F. and Raper, J. A. A sensory axon repellent secreted from ventral spinal cord explants is neutralized by antibodies raised against collapsin-1. *Development* **124**, 1377–85 (1997).

160. Bagnard, D., Lohrum, M., Uziel, D., Püschel, A. W. and Bolz, J. Semaphorins act as attractive and repulsive guidance signals during the development of cortical projections. *Development* **125**, 5043–53 (1998).

161. Raper, J. A. Semaphorins and their receptors in vertebrates and invertebrates. *Curr. Opin. Neurobiol.* **10**, 88–94 (2000).

162. Kolodkin, A. L. *et al.* Neuropilin is a semaphorin III receptor. *Cell* **90**, 753–62 (1997).

163. He, Z. and Tessier-Lavigne, M. Neuropilin is a receptor for the axonal chemorepellent Semaphorin III. *Cell* **90**, 739–51 (1997).

164. Chen, H., He, Z., Bagri, A. and Tessier-Lavigne, M. Semaphorin–neuropilin interactions underlying sympathetic axon responses to class III semaphorins. *Neuron* **21**, 1283–90 (1998).

165. Giger, R. J. *et al.* Neuropilin-2 is a receptor for semaphorin IV: insight into the structural basis of receptor function and specificity. *Neuron* **21**, 1079–92 (1998).

166. Chen, H. *et al.* Neuropilin-2 regulates the development of select cranial and sensory nerves and hippocampal mossy fiber projections. *Neuron* **25**, 43–56 (2000).

167. Feiner, L., Koppel, A. M., Kobayashi, H. and Raper, J. A. Secreted chick semaphorins bind recombinant neuropilin with similar affinities but bind different subsets of neurons *in situ*. *Neuron* **19**, 539–45 (1997).

168. Yu, H. H. and Kolodkin, A. L. Semaphorin signaling: a little less per-plexin. *Neuron* **22**, 11–14 (1999).

169. Ohta, K. *et al.* Plexin: a novel neuronal cell surface molecule that mediates cell adhesion via a homophilic binding mechanism in the presence of calcium ions. *Neuron* **14**, 1189–99 (1995).

170. Winberg, M. L. *et al.* Plexin A is a neuronal semaphorin receptor that controls axon guidance. *Cell* **95**, 903–16 (1998).

171. Tamagnone, L. *et al.* Plexins are a large family of receptors for transmembrane, secreted, and GPI-anchored semaphorins in vertebrates. *Cell* **99**, 71–80 (1999).

172. Orioli, D. and Klein, R. The Eph receptor family: axonal guidance by contact repulsion. *Trends Genet.* **13**, 354–9 (1997).

173. Henkemeyer, M. *et al.* Nuk controls pathfinding of commissural axons in the mammalian central nervous system. *Cell* **86**, 35–46 (1996).

174. Wang, H. U. and Anderson, D. J. Eph family transmembrane ligands can mediate repulsive guidance of trunk neural crest migration and motor axon outgrowth. *Neuron* **18**, 383–96 (1997).

175. Krull, C. E. *et al.* Interactions of Eph-related receptors and ligands confer rostrocaudal pattern to trunk neural crest migration. *Curr. Biol.* **7**, 571–80 (1997).

176. Nose, A., Takeichi, M. and Goodman, C. S. Ectopic expression of connectin reveals a repulsive function during growth cone guidance and synapse formation. *Neuron* **13**, 525–39 (1994).

177. Polleux, F., Morrow, T. and Ghosh, A. Semaphorin 3A is a chemoattractant for cortical apical dendrites. *Nature* **404**, 567–73 (2000).

178. Colamarino, S. A. and Tessier-Lavigne, M. The axonal chemoattractant netrin-1 is also a chemorepellent for trochlear motor axons. *Cell* **81**, 621–9 (1995).

179. Seeger, M., Tear, G., Ferres-Marco, D. and Goodman, C. S. Mutations affecting growth cone guidance in *Drosophila*: genes necessary for guidance toward or away from the midline. *Neuron* **10**, 409–26 (1993).

180. Kidd, T. *et al.* Roundabout controls axon crossing of the CNS midline and defines a novel subfamily of evolutionarily conserved guidance receptors. *Cell* **92**, 205–15 (1998).

181. Kidd, T., Bland, K. S. and Goodman, C. S. Slit is the midline repellent for the robo receptor in *Drosophila*. *Cell* **96**, 785–94 (1999).

182. Brose, K. *et al.* Slit proteins bind Robo receptors and have an evolutionarily conserved role in repulsive axon guidance. *Cell* **96**, 795–806 (1999).

183. Li, H. S. *et al.* Vertebrate slit, a secreted ligand for the transmembrane protein roundabout, is a repellent for olfactory bulb axons. *Cell* **96**, 807–18 (1999).

184. Tear, G. *et al. commissureless* controls growth cone guidance across the CNS midline in *Drosophila* and encodes a novel membrane protein. *Neuron* **16**, 501–14 (1996).

185. Kidd, T., Russell, C., Goodman, C. S. and Tear, G. Dosage-sensitive and complementary functions of roundabout and commissureless control axon crossing of the CNS midline. *Neuron* **20**, 25–33 (1998).

186. Nguyen Ba-Charvet, K. T. *et al.* Slit2-mediated chemorepulsion and collapse of developing forebrain axons. *Neuron* **22**, 463–73 (1999).

187. Guthrie, S. and Pini, A. Chemorepulsion of developing motor axons by the floor plate. *Neuron* **14**, 1117–30 (1995).

188. Harris, W. A. and Holt, C. E. Slit, the midline repellent. *Nature* **398**, 462–3 (1999).

189. Wang, K. H. *et al.* Biochemical purification of a mammalian slit protein as a positive regulator of sensory axon elongation and branching. *Cell* **96**, 771–84 (1999).

190. Brose, K. and Tessier-Lavigne, M. Slit proteins: key regulators of axon guidance, axonal branching, and cell migration. *Curr. Opin. Neurobiol.* **10**, 95–102 (2000).

191. Karlstrom, R. O. *et al.* Zebrafish mutations affecting retinotectal axon pathfinding. *Development* **123**, 427–38 (1996).

192. Karlstrom, R. O., Trowe, T. and Bonhoeffer, F. Genetic analysis of axon guidance and mapping in the zebrafish. *Trends Neurosci.* **20**, 3–8 (1997).

193. Bashaw, G. J. and Goodman, C. S. Chimeric axon guidance receptors: the cytoplasmic domains of slit and netrin receptors specify attraction versus repulsion. *Cell* **97**, 917–26 (1999).

194. Mueller, B. K. Growth cone guidance: first steps towards a deeper understanding. *Annu. Rev. Neurosci.* **22**, 351–88 (1999).

195. Silver, R. A., Lamb, A. G. and Bolsover, S. R. Calcium hotspots caused by L-channel clustering promote morphological changes in neuronal growth cones. *Nature* **343**, 751–4 (1990).

196. Zheng, J. Q., Felder, M., Connor, J. A. and Poo, M. Turning of nerve growth cones induced by neurotransmitters. *Nature* **368**, 140–4 (1994).

197. Kater, S. B. and Mills, L. R. Regulation of growth cone behavior by calcium. *J. Neurosci.* **11**, 891–9 (1991).

198. Bandtlow, C. E., Schmidt, M. F., Hassinger, T. D., Schwab, M. E. and Kater, S. B. Role of intracellular calcium in NI-35-evoked collapse of neuronal growth cones. *Science* **259**, 80–3 (1993).

199. Walsh, F. S. and Doherty, P. Neural cell adhesion molecules of the immunoglobulin superfamily: role in axon growth and guidance. *Annu. Rev. Cell Dev. Biol.* **13**, 425–56 (1997).

200. Goldberg, D. J. and Grabham, P. W. Braking news: calcium in the growth cone. *Neuron* **22**, 423–5 (1999).

201. Zheng, J. Q. Turning of nerve growth cones induced by localized increases in intracellular calcium ions. *Nature* **403**, 89–93 (2000).

202. Hong, K., Nishiyama, M., Henley, J., Tessier-Lavigne, M. and Poo, M. Calcium signalling in the guidance of nerve growth by netrin-1. *Nature* **403**, 93–8 (2000).

203. Gomez, T. M. and Spitzer, N. C. In vivo regulation of axon extension and pathfinding by growth-cone calcium transients. *Nature* **397**, 350–5 (1999).

204. Berridge, M. J. Neuronal calcium signaling. *Neuron* **21**, 13–26 (1998).

205. Mason, I. Do adhesion molecules signal via FGF receptors? *Curr. Biol.* **4**, 1158–61 (1994).

206. Doherty, P., Williams, E. and Walsh, F. S. A soluble chimeric form of the L1 glycoprotein stimulates neurite outgrowth. *Neuron* **14**, 57–66 (1995).

207. Saffell, J. L., Williams, E. J., Mason, I. J., Walsh, F. S. and Doherty, P. Expression of a dominant negative FGF receptor inhibits axonal growth and FGF receptor phosphorylation stimulated by CAMs. *Neuron* **18**, 231–42 (1997) [published erratum appears in *Neuron* **20**, 619 (1998)].

208. Chang, H. Y. *et al.* Asymmetric retraction of growth cone filopodia following focal inactivation of calcineurin. *Nature* **376**, 686–90 (1995).

209. Song, H. J., Ming, G. L. and Poo, M. M. cAMP-induced switching in turning direction of nerve growth cones. *Nature* **388**, 275–9 (1997) [published erratum appears in *Nature* **389**, 412 (1997)].

210. Ming, G. L. *et al.* cAMP-dependent growth cone guidance by netrin-1. *Neuron* **19**, 1225–35 (1997).

211. Song, H. *et al.* Conversion of neuronal growth cone responses from repulsion to attraction by cyclic nucleotides. *Science* **281**, 1515–18 (1998).

212. Hall, A. Rho GTPases and the actin cytoskeleton. *Science* **279**, 509–14 (1998).

213. Luo, L., Jan, L. Y. and Jan, Y. N. Rho family GTP-binding proteins in growth cone signalling. *Curr. Opin. Neurobiol.* **7**, 81–6 (1997).

214. Luo, L. *et al.* Differential effects of the Rac GTPase on Purkinje cell axons and dendritic trunks and spines. *Nature* **379**, 837–40 (1996).

215. Jalink, K. *et al.* Inhibition of lysophosphatidate- and thrombin-induced neurite retraction and neuronal cell rounding by ADP ribosylation of the small GTP-binding protein Rho. *J. Cell Biol.* **126**, 801–10 (1994).

216. Zipkin, I. D., Kindt, R. M. and Kenyon, C. J. Role of a new Rho family member in cell migration and axon guidance in *C. elegans*. *Cell* **90**, 883–94 (1997).

217. Van Aelst, L. and D'Souza-Schorey, C. Rho GTPases and signaling networks. *Genes Dev.* **11**, 2295–322 (1997).

218. Desai, C. J., Sun, Q. and Zinn, K. Tyrosine phosphorylation and axon guidance: of mice and flies. *Curr. Opin. Neurobiol.* **7**, 70–4 (1997).

219. Krueger, N. X. *et al.* The transmembrane tyrosine phosphatase DLAR controls motor axon guidance in *Drosophila*. *Cell* **84**, 611–22 (1996).

220. Garrity, P. A. *et al. Drosophila* photoreceptor axon guidance and targeting requires the dreadlocks SH2/SH3 adapter protein. *Cell* **85**, 639–50 (1996).

221. Sharma, K. *et al.* LIM homeodomain factors Lhx3 and Lhx4 assign subtype identities for motor neurons. *Cell* **95**, 817–28 (1998).

222. Thor, S. and Thomas, J. B. The *Drosophila* islet gene governs axon pathfinding and neurotransmitter identity. *Neuron* **18**, 397–409 (1997).

223. Landgraf, M., Roy, S., Prokop, A., Vijay Raghavan, K. and Bate, M. even-skipped determines the dorsal growth of motor axons in *Drosophila*. *Neuron* **22**, 43–52 (1999).

224. Jaffe, L. F. and Poo, M. M. Neurites grow faster towards the cathode than the anode in a steady field. *J. Exp. Zool.* **209**, 115–28 (1979).

225. McCaig, C. D. Studies on the mechanism of embryonic frog nerve orientation in a small applied electric field. *J. Cell Sci.* **93**, 723–30 (1989).

226. Davenport, R. W. and Kater, S. B. Local increases in intracellular calcium elicit local filopodial responses in helisoma neuronal growth cones. *Neuron* **9**, 405–16 (1992).

227. McCaig, C. D. and Zhao, M. Physiological electrical fields modify cell behaviour. *BioEssays* **19**, 819–26 (1997).

228. Banker, G. A. and Cowan, W. M. Further observations on hippocampal neurons in dispersed cell culture. *J. Comp. Neurol.* **187**, 469–94 (1979).

229. Craig, A. M. and Banker, G. Neuronal polarity. *Annu. Rev. Neurosci.* **17**, 267–310 (1994).

230. Goslin, K. and Banker, G. A. Experimental observations on the development of polarity by hippocampal neurones in culture. *J. Cell Biol.* **108**, 1507–16 (1989).

231. Goslin, K. and Banker, G. Rapid changes in the distribution of GAP-43 correlate with the expression of neuronal polarity during normal development and under experimental conditions. *J. Cell Biol.* **110**, 1319–31 (1990).

232. Rodriguez Boulan, E. and Nelson, W. J. Morphogenesis of the epithelial cell phenotype. *Science* **245**, 718–25 (1989).

233. Black, M. M. and Baas, P. W. The basis of polarity in neurons. *Trends Neurosci.* **12**, 211–14 (1989).

234. Caceres, A. and Kosik, K. S. Inhibition of neurite polarity by tau antisense oligonucleotides in primary cerebellar neurons. *Nature* **343**, 461–3 (1990).

235. Knops, J. *et al.* Overexpression of tau in a nonneuronal cell induces long cellular processes. *J. Cell Biol.* **114**, 725–33 (1991).

236. Messenger, E. A. and Warner, A. E. The function of the sodium pump during differentiation of amphibian embryonic neurones. *J. Physiol.* (London) **292**, 85–105 (1979).

237. Spitzer, N. C. and Lamborghini, J. E. The development of the action potential mechanism of amphibian neurons isolated in culture. *Proc. Natl. Acad. Sci. USA* **73**, 1641–50 (1976).

238. Gu, X. and Spitzer, N. C. Distinct aspects of neuronal differentiation encoded by frequency of Ca^{2+} transients. *Nature* **375**, 784–7 (1995).

239. O'Dowd, D. K., Ribera, A. B. and Spitzer, N. C. Development of voltage-dependent calcium, sodium and potassium currents in *Xenopus* spinal neurons. *J. Neurosci.* **8**, 792–805 (1988).

240. Ribera, A. B. and Spitzer, N. C. A critical period of transcription required for differentiation of the action potential mechanism of spinal neurons. *Neuron* **2**, 1055–62 (1989).

241. Ziskind-Conhaim, L. Electrical properties of motoneurons in the spinal cord of rat embryos. *Dev. Biol.* **128**, 21–9 (1988).

242. Goodman, C. S. Isogenic grasshoppers: genetic variability in the morphology of identified neurons. *J. Comp. Neurol.* **182**, 681–705 (1978).

243. Macagno, E. R., Lopresti, U. and Levinthal, C. Structure and development of neuronal connections in isogenic organisms: variations and similarities in the optic system of Daphnia magna. *Proc. Natl. Acad. Sci. USA* **70**, 57–61 (1973).

244. Banker, G. A. and Waxman, A. B. Hippocampal neurons generate natural shapes in culture. In Intrinsic determinants of neuronal form and function, vol. 37 (ed. R. J. Lasek and M. M. Black), pp. 61–82 (A. R. Liss, New York, 1988).

245. Rutishauser, U. and Landmesser, L. Polysialic acid on the surface of axons regulates patterns of normal and activity-dependent innervation. *Trends Neurosci.* **14**, 528–32 (1991).

246. Rakic, P. Role of cell interaction in development of dendritic patterns. *Adv. Neurol.* **12**, 117–34 (1975).

247. Kimmel, C. B. Development of synapses on the Mauthner neuron. *Trends Neurosci.* **5**, 47–50 (1982).

248. Valverde, F. Apical dendritic spines of the visual cortex and light deprivation in the mouse. *Exp. Brain Res.* **3**, 337–53 (1967).

249. Jones, W. H. and Thomas, D. B. Changes in the dendritic organization of neurons in the cerebral cortex following deafferentation. *J. Anat.* **96**, 375–81 (1962).

250. Purves, D. and Hadley, R. D. Changes in the dendritic branching of adult mammalian neurones revealed by repeated imaging *in vitro*. *Nature* **315**, 404–6 (1985).

251. Voyvodic, J. T. Peripheral target regulation of dendritic geometry in the rat superior cervical ganglion. *J. Neurosci.* **9**, 1997–2010 (1989).

252. Purves, D., Rubin, E., Snider, W. D. and Lichtman, J. Relation of animal size to convergence, divergence and neuronal number in peripheral sympathetic pathways. *J. Neurosci.* **6**, 158–63 (1986).

253. Purves, D., Snider, W. D. and Voyvodic, J. T. Trophic regulation of nerve cell morphology and innervation in the autonomic nervous system. *Nature* **336**, 123–8 (1988).

254. Purves, D. Body and brain (Harvard University Press, Cambridge, MA, 1988).

255. Konishi, M. and Gurney, M. E. Sexual differentiation of brain and behaviour. *Trends Neurosci.* **5**, 20–3 (1982).

256. Bastiani, M. J., Harrelson, A. L., Snow, P. M. and Goodman, C. S. Expression of fasciclin I and II glycoproteins on subsets of axon pathways during neuronal development in the grasshopper. *Cell* **48**, 745–55 (1987).

10

The Formation of Topographic Maps

Guidance mechanisms ensure that most axons reach the right area of the developing nervous system, but further levels of refinement have to be achieved as axons invade their target region and are distributed in an orderly arrangement within it. In the case of sensory projections, which terminate in topographic order within the primary sensory nuclei, an ordered mapping of connections is maintained as the projections are relayed through further nuclei to the cerebral cortex. The formation of topographic maps involves recognition by growth cones of the correct type of cell with which to make contact ('type' specificity), for example in a particular layer of cerebral cortex or midbrain tectum. But mapping also requires axons to find the appropriate subset of these cells defined by their position within the target ('place' or 'positional' specificity; see Fig. 10.1). These recognition steps give rise to a basic topographic order in neuronal connections, and maps are then refined further by the processes of cell death, branch withdrawal and synapse elimination, under the influence of functional activity and other means, as described in Chapter 14.

Target invasion

Axons often arrive at their target regions in the company of other axons destined for more distant targets, to which they may be tightly fasciculated. The first stage of target invasion may therefore involve defasciculation from other axons, but precisely how target recognition triggers defasciculation is unknown. As discussed in Chapter 9, the process of defasciculation includes the modulation of CAM-mediated inter-axonal adhesion by molecules such as Fas II, Beat and receptor tyrosine phosphatases in *Drosophila*, and polysialic acid in vertebrates, and is regulated by the overall balance of adhesive and repulsive forces acting on axons. Target invasion has been shown in some cases also to involve signalling by growth factors. Good evidence for this is

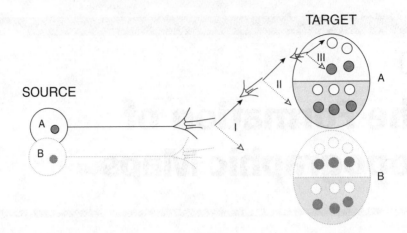

Figure 10.1 The hierarchy of guidance mechanisms for growing axons: these exist to enable neurons to target the right cells within the right area of the right part of the brain. (I) Axons are guided to the correct place within the brain using the mechanisms discussed in Chapter 9. Neurons from sources A and B respond differently to these cues. (II) Thereafter, mechanisms exist to guide axons *within* a target nucleus. Transplantation experiments show that the cues in targets A and B are potentially recognizable to neurons from a variety of sources. (III) Neurons recognize the right sort of cells to make synapses with. There is considerable choice, and decisions about which are finally chosen depends on activity during critical or sensitive periods, as described in Chapter 14.

provided by the phenotype of NT-3 knockout mice, in which postganglionic sympathetic axons reach but fail to invade two target tissues, the blood vessels and hair follicles of the external ear and the pineal gland (see also Chapter 12 for detailed discussion of the neurotrophins).[1] The production of target-derived growth factors may also explain the finding that individual muscle nerves (but not the major axon pathways) fail to appear in chick limbs depleted of muscle by focal X-irradiation of the somites in early embryos.[2] In a further example, inhibition of FGF receptor signalling in *Xenopus* retinal axons prevents them from invading the optic tectum after navigating the pathway of the optic tract.[3] In this case, however, ligand (FGF-2) levels are reduced in the target area compared with the pathway in normal embryos, so the critical requirement for target invasion seems to be a change in the ambient level of growth factor signalling between pathway and target.

Interstitial axon branching at appropriate target sites may also be triggered by target-derived chemotropic molecules, allowing axons to innervate a series of different nuclei at staggered times so that branching decisions do not always have to be made at the terminal growth cone.[4] Although the relevant chemotropic factors remain to be identified, examples where this mechanism has been suggested include the late-developing branches which sprout in the pons from cortically-originating pyramidal axons some time after the main growth cones have passed by (see also below),[5] and the development of the projections from the hippocampal formation to the mammillary bodies.[6]

Type specificity

In tissue culture it is easy to demonstrate that neurons will only form synapses with particular cell types. *In vivo* cross-innervation experiments in the peripheral nervous system have also shown that functional synaptic contacts are not established between mismatched axons and targets. Provided an axon releases a transmitter appropriate for the receptors on the target, however, synapses can usually form, but they are often not very effective.[7,8] Similar experiments have been performed to investigate the specificity of neurons for CNS targets. Cholinergic neurons were taken from different sites in fetal rats and grafted into the hippocampus of adult rats in which the normal cholinergic innervation by septal neurons had been destroyed. It was found that the most successful innervation of the hippocampus occurred when the transplanted neurons came from the septum.[9] So type specificity involves more than simply matching transmitter phenotype with appropriate receptors.

Place or positional specificity

In principle, an ordered distribution of axons within a target could arise if axons maintain their original topographical relationship with each other as they grow from their nucleus of origin to their termination site. In fact this is rarely the case, and a series of experiments, particularly those carried out on the innervation of the optic tectum in the dorsal midbrain by retinal ganglion cells in fishes and amphibia, shows that such a passive mechanism cannot account for topographic order.[10] Axons often undergo considerable positional shuffling en route, a good example being seen in the 'ribbon' optic nerve of cichlid fishes,[11] so neurons and the cells they innervate must rely on additional mechanisms to distribute connections in a topographically ordered pattern.

Origins of the concept of chemospecificity

The classical experiments which suggested that neurons might be labelled according to their position in the CNS were carried out not on developing brains but on regenerating axons in adult amphibians.[12,13] Later work on embryos has reinforced the findings of the earlier studies.[14] In some amphibia and fishes, optic axons regenerate in the adult and normal vision is restored, as judged by motor behaviour. If the eye is rotated 180°, however, the animal's behaviour after reinnervation is inverted (Fig. 10.2). This could be explained if retinal axons have an affinity for, and therefore return to, their original places in the tectum, rather than to the place appropriate to their new location in the visual field; activation of these tectal sites would trigger behaviour suitable for the original location of the ganglion cells in the retina and visual field but inappropriate for the new location (Fig. 10.2). Subsequent experiments using electrophysiological recording[15] and axon tracing have confirmed that retinal axons can recognize different parts of the tectum. For example, axons

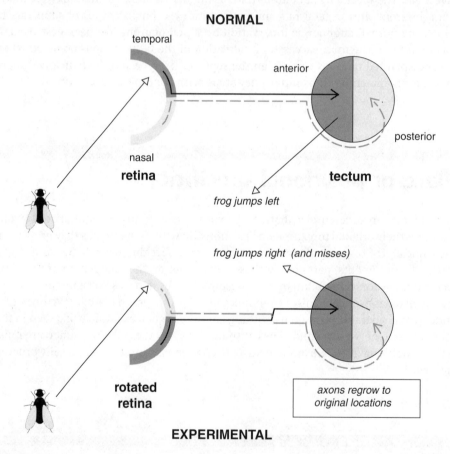

Figure 10.2 The concept of chemospecificity. The diagram shows how Sperry's eye rotation experiment, which makes frogs jump incorrectly for their prey, is evidence that neurons can regenerate back to their previous targets. If the eye (and hence the retina) is rotated 180°, the axons of the retinal ganglion cells *regrow to their original locations*, not to the location that would be appropriate for their new eye position, triggering the wrong behaviour from the frog. This classic behavioural experiment was the first to show that neurons must have labels that enable them to find their corresponding targets during the formation of the nervous system.

arising from different parts of the retina make synapses in particular parts of the optic tectum, whatever route they take to reach the tectum.[16] Even if the tectal cells are moved, the axons are able to contact them in their new location.[17] If all but part of the retina is prevented from innervating the developing tectum, the residual retinal ganglion cell axons synapse in the right place and, at least initially, do not innervate other sites that are now also available.[14] Cells isolated from different parts of the retina are also found to adhere preferentially to the area of the tectum to which they would normally project.[18]

Similar orderly projections are seen in the peripheral nervous system. Different motor pools in the ventral spinal cord innervate different muscle groups, with motor neurons placed medially projecting to nearby axial muscles, and laterally-placed neurons projecting to more distal limb muscles. In the case of the limb muscles, accurate guidance of motor axons plays an important role in the formation of neuromuscular connectivity, although the underlying molecular mechanisms are unknown (see Chapter 9). In the chick embryo, for example, axons can compensate for experimental displacement of their cell bodies along the anterior–posterior (rostrocaudal) axis by re-sorting their positions at the root of the limb, so innervating their correct muscles.[19] Other evidence suggests that place-specific labels also exist on both axons and muscle fibres within a single muscle. For example, during postnatal development in rats, there is a selective withdrawal of motor axon branches from muscle fibres in a manner that enhances the topographical projection from the motor pool to the muscle,[20] and a similar projection is re-established following reinnervation in the neonate or adult.[21,22] It is also found in amphibia that motor axons that have been made to innervate incorrect muscles lose their synaptic connections when the correct motor axons return.[23]

An important test of the presence of positional labels, and of the ability of motor axons to recognize them, has been provided by experiments on rats in which intercostal muscles from different intercostal spaces were deliberately cross-innervated by preganglionic cholinergic *sympathetic* axons originating from different spinal levels along the rostrocaudal axis. While all axons were able to innervate any muscle, muscles were innervated most successfully by motor axons originating from the same segmental level as themselves.[24,25] Mechanisms therefore seem to exist that allow neurons from different levels of the rostrocaudal axis to recognize target muscles from similar levels.

Observations like these on the visual and motor systems suggest that axons arising from neurons in particular places are programmed so that they can recognize differences between cells in different positions. While the original 'chemoaffinity' hypothesis proposed rather rigid matching of specific labels in the innervating and innervated neural populations,[13] further work has shown that axons can innervate sites that they would not innervate under normal circumstances, so it is more likely that preferences are relative. In adult fishes and amphibia, for example, regenerating axons from part of the retina will eventually spread to innervate all of the tectum if more appropriate axons have been removed,[26] and while axons can discriminate between lateral and medial tectum, inappropriate connections are made, although at a lesser synaptic density.[27] Furthermore, retinal axons must normally reposition their terminals in the tectum progressively as the eye grows, in order to accommodate the terminals of new ganglion cells that are added to the periphery of the retina.[28,29] One suggestion is that molecular labels are expressed either in gradients or in discrete compartments[30] in the tectum, and that retinal ganglion cells have complementary labels that allow them to detect the tectal signals and make optimum connections in the face of competition from other contenders for the available sites. The involvement of repulsion in the detection process is suggested by the finding that, in a membrane stripe assay, temporal retinal axons are repelled by stripes of posterior tectal membranes (the region of tectum also avoided by these axons *in vivo*), and grow preferentially on adjacent anterior membranes.[31] This phenomenon shows conservation across a variety of vertebrate species, and is complemented by the further finding that temporal growth cones collapse more readily that their nasal counterparts on exposure to posterior tectal membranes.[32]

Molecular basis of chemospecificity

To detect molecular differences in what seems otherwise to be a uniform target population of cells or neurons, one approach has been to raise monoclonal antibodies against antigens that are regionally distributed in that population. Antibodies that differentiate between different parts of the tectum,[33] chick limb buds[34] and the rostrocaudal extent of the rat sympathetic ganglionic chain[35] have been raised. Whether such antigens represent the same molecules that allow the axons to make choices is debatable,[36] but their presence does show that positional labelling of the target in a manner suitable for axons is potentially possible. The existence of positional labels has received further support from experiments on transgenic mice in which the gene for a reporter molecule, chloramphenicol acetyltransferase (CAT), is driven by the regulatory elements of the gene encoding one of the muscle myosin light chains (MLC_1). Although the relative amounts of myosin light chain do not vary systematically in muscles along the body axis, expression of the CAT reporter in these mice is a hundredfold greater in muscles towards the tail than in muscles near the head. This difference persists in culture and also in immortalized muscle cell lines derived from muscle stem cells taken from muscle in different places in the transgenic animals.[37] It has also been possible to detect antigenic differences among neurons that innervate a particular target region; these differences might allow neurons in particular locations to detect gradients of molecular labels in the target, and a good example is the gradient of one particular antigen, TOP_{DV}, in the retina (Fig. 10.3A).[38,39]

An important advance has been made recently by the identification of two multi-gene families, the Eph family of receptor tyrosine kinases and their ligands, the ephrins, members of which are expressed in topographic patterns in both source and target regions of the retinotectal projection (see also Chapter 9).[40–42] The ephrins

A

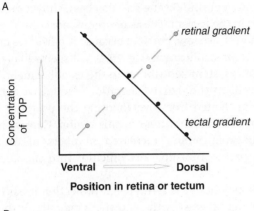

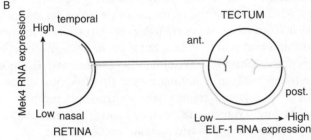

Figure 10.3 Two examples of molecular gradients that have been suggested to underlie 'chemospecificity'. (A) A glycoprotein TOP, so-called because of its *top*ographically variable distribution, is present in high amounts in the dorsal retina and low amounts in the ventral retina. The same protein is also found in the tectum, where its expression is highest in the ventral region. Axons arising in the dorsal retina project to the ventral tectum. After Trisler and Collins.[33] (B) Another example of a molecular gradient thought to underlie 'chemospecificity'. An Eph-family receptor tyrosine kinase, Mek4/EphA3, is topographically distributed across the nasotemporal axis of the chick retina while its ligand, ELF-1/ephrin-A2, is topographically distributed across the tectum, being in low concentration anteriorly and high posteriorly. This is therefore a counter gradient system. After Cheng *et al.*;[45] see also Drescher *et al.*[44]

subdivide into two main subtypes, those that are anchored to it by a glycosylphosphatidylinositol (GPI) linkage (ephrin-A) and those that span the plasma membrane (ephrin-B). The ephrin-As activate the EphA receptors while ephrin-Bs activate the EphB receptors.[43] One of the first ephrins to be identified in the retinotectal system, RAGS (repulsive axonal guidance signal, now known as ephrin-A5), was originally characterized by two-dimensional gel electrophoresis as a GPI-linked glycoprotein which causes retinal growth cone collapse, and which is expressed in a posterior (high) to anterior (low) gradient across the avian tectum.[44] A similar ligand, ELF-1/ephrin-A2, is also expressed in a gradient of this direction in the tectum, and its cognate receptor EphA3 has a reciprocal gradient in the nasotemporal axis of the retina (Fig. 10.3B).[45]

In the chick, ectopic tectal patches of retrovirally-misexpressed ELF-1 are avoided by temporal retinal axons, while nasal retinal axons are not affected.[46] Targeted deletion of the mouse RAGS/ephrin-A5 gene has also been shown to result in ectopic arbors of temporal axons in the tectum. These are found most often in regions where ELF-1/ephrinA-2 expression is also low, possibly because repulsion is now too weak in these regions to prevent their stabilization (Fig. 10.4).[47] It seems likely, then, that the ephrin/Eph ligand–receptor system contributes to the establishment of nasal versus temporal retinotectal specificity through the operation of repulsive gradients. It is also possible that axons are prevented from overshooting the posterior tectum by the increasing concentration of RAGS/ephrin-A5 in this region. Consistent with this, in the RAGS/ephrin-A5 knockout mouse increased numbers of axons transiently overshoot the posterior part of the superior colliculus into the inferior (auditory) colliculus.[47]

In modelling the development of the retinotectal projection it has been suggested that attractive gradients may coexist with repulsive gradients in the anterior–posterior and dorsoventral axes of the tectum, so that axons locate the tectal position where repulsive and attractive forces are balanced. Attractive gradients have yet to be identified for the anterior–posterior axis, but they may exist in the dorsoventral axis, where members of the ephrin-B/EphB subfamilies are expressed in retina (EphB2) and tectum (ephrin-B1 and -B2) in matching rather than reciprocal concentration gradients.[48] Although this would require that ephrin–Eph receptor interaction can promote as well as repel axon growth, such opposing ('bifunctional') actions on axon growth have a precedent in the netrin system (see Chapter 9).

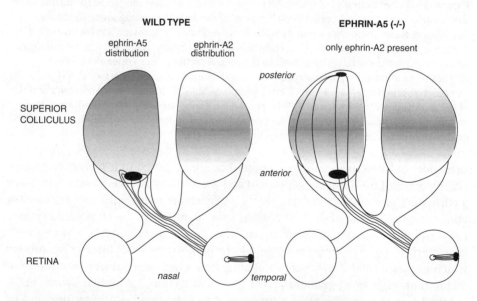

Figure 10.4 Ephrins are able to repel axons from temporal ganglion cells of the retina. In wild-type mice temporal retinal axons project to the anterior (rostral) superior colliculus only, which is the place with the lowest expression of ephrin-A5 and ephrin-A2. When ephrin-A5 is absent in knockout mice, temporal axons are no longer constrained to anterior colliculus, and can also terminate posteriorly where ephrin-A2 expression is also low. After Frisen *et al.*[47]

Additional molecular systems have been implicated in retinotectal mapping, including further cell surface repellents as well as diffusible repellents expressed by posterior tectal cells.[49] The ephrin–Eph receptor system has also been implicated in the formation of topographic maps in other parts of the vertebrate nervous system. These include the mammalian retinal axon projection to the lateral geniculate nucleus of the thalamus,[50] and the hippocampus, where reciprocal gradients of ELF-1/ ephrin-A2 and EphA5 may assist in mapping the projection from the septum onto the hippocampus.[51] Whether a role for the ephrin–Eph system in axon guidance is unique to the vertebrate nervous system is not yet clear.

One promising approach for the identification of further molecules is to characterize genes in systematic screens of zebrafish mutants with retinotectal targeting abnormalities,[52] a strategy that has been successful for invertebrate axon guidance systems such as neuromuscular connectivity and the CNS midline (see Chapter 9). Species differences also exist in the way that the maps are established, and the basis for these is unclear. For example, the development of topographic order in the retinal projection within the avian and rodent tectum (superior colliculus) seems to depend less on establishing an accurate projection from the outset, as seen in the frog or fish, than on precise, later-directed branching from the axon shafts into the correct target regions.[53-55] The topographical precision of these back-branches has been suggested to result from a combination of repulsive gradients, as already discussed, and graded attractive/branch-promoting cues expressed by target cells.[56] It is also likely that the detection of gradients of markers set up to provide specificity of placement within a target is accomplished more easily along the length of an axon rather than the smaller terminal growth cone,[46] and this mechanism may have evolved in birds and mammals (see also Chapter 9).

If the original concept of chemoaffinity based on gradients of molecular labels has now been given a firm experimental basis, much of the detail remains to be elucidated, and further confirmatory loss-of-function studies are needed *in vivo*. An important question concerns the long-term stability of ephrin gradients within the CNS. It is known, for example, that the amphibian retinotectal map can be compressed on the tectum by prior removal of half the tectum; conversely, it eventually expands after removal of half the retina. Are such results explicable in terms of anatomical realignment of molecular gradients, or do they suggest the existence of mechanisms additional to gradient matching?[57]

Olfactory mapping

A further potential source of information for axon targeting is seen in the mammalian olfactory system. Here, subsets of olfactory receptor neurons that share a unique odorant receptor protein are randomly distributed in the olfactory epithelium within one of four broad zones in the dorsoventral axis. Remarkably, they converge on just two of approximately two thousand glomeruli in the olfactory bulb, and this spatial segregation of olfactory input in the olfactory bulb underlies the encoding of odorant quality.

To account for this anatomical mapping of olfactory axons on the olfactory bulb, it has been suggested that the odorant receptor itself provides a surface marker enabling axons to find their glomerular targets during development.[58,59] This hypothesis has been tested in transgenic mice by 'knock-in' experiments, in which the promoter for one receptor is used to drive the coding sequence for another. When the substitution involves two genes expressed in the same chromosomal locus and epithelial zone, olfactory axons converge on a glomerulus adjacent to the wild-type glomerulus appropriate for the donor sequence. On the other hand, in substitutions involving sequences expressed in different loci or zones, targeting is again altered but axons converge on glomeruli sited more distantly from the 'donor' glomerulus. Lastly, deletions or nonsense mutations of an odorant receptor gene cause the related axons to wander widely within the olfactory bulb, failing to converge on the correct glomerulus.[60,61] These results argue strongly that odorant receptors do act instructively in glomerular target selection by olfactory axons, perhaps being involved in the recognition of positional cues expressed in the olfactory bulb, but precisely how is unclear at present.[56] They also suggest the existence of additional guidance factors, for example reflecting the broad epithelial zones in which the receptors are expressed. Further molecular candidates for roles in olfactory mapping include NCAM, since many olfactory axons fail to make glomerular synapses in NCAM knockout mice,[62] a galactose-binding lectin Galectin-1, in whose absence olfactory axons also make targeting errors in the caudal olfactory bulb,[62,63] and members of the semaphorin family.[64]

Setting up instructions for axon targeting

Neurons must learn their positions, and hence be able to set up appropriately specific surface labels, from instructions received during the early regionalization and diversification of the neural tube. In the neuromuscular system it has been found that, before motor cell columns form and motor neurons send their axons into the periphery in search of their targets, different populations of motor neurons can be defined by their patterns of expression of one class of homeobox multigene family (designated LIM), which encodes DNA binding proteins containing cysteine/histidine-rich domains (see also Chapter 4). These patterns define uniquely the locations of different motor neuron subtypes in the developing ventral horn of the spinal cord.[65] For example, in limb regions of the cord, the most medially placed motor neurons, which eventually innervate axial muscles, express a combination of *Islet-1*, *Islet-2* and *Lim-3*, while the most laterally placed motor neurons express *Lim-1* and *Islet-2* and innervate distal muscles on the dorsal side of the limb. It seems likely that the expression of different combinations of LIM homeobox genes may endow motor neurons with the ability to express particular sets of recognition molecules on their surfaces and hence enable them to follow particular routes and innervate particular muscles.

Individual pools of limb motor neurons, destined to innervate individual limb muscles, can be further distinguished from each other by their particular expression patterns of LIM and ETS-family transcription factors.[66] Strikingly similar patterns of ETS expression are also shown by the majority of sensory afferents and motor neurons that contact the same muscle, suggesting that these patterns may determine the specificity of the monosynaptic sensory-motor reflex circuits underlying the vertebrate stretch reflex. Their development is dependent on the presence of the muscle, which presumably provides an appropriate retrograde signal for both classes of neuron;[66] the nature of the signal and of the downstream targets of LIM/ETS genes remain to be determined.

A similar role upstream of recognition molecules may be played in the optic tectum by the genes *En-1* and *En-2*, vertebrate homologues of the *engrailed* segmental polarity gene in *Drosophila*. *En-1* and *En-2* are highly expressed in the posterior but not anterior tectum of chick embryos, a pattern established by earlier signalling from the isthmus or midbrain–hindbrain boundary (see Chapter 3). Retrovirally-induced misexpression of these genes throughout the tectum in a punctate manner is matched by ectopic expression of RAGS/ephrin-A5 and ELF-1/ephrin-A2, and causes axons from nasal retina (which normally project only to the strongly *en*-expressing posterior tectum) to terminate in patches in the anterior tectum, while temporal neurons and their axons die.[67–69]

Layer-specific axon targeting

Many target regions within the CNS, such as the cerebral and cerebellar cortex, and the midbrain tectum, are subdivided into layers of cells which are selected by appropriate afferent projections, and similar regionalized projections are made within brain nuclei such as the thalamus and amygdala. If the mechanisms discussed above ensure that axons map to the correct topographic region of the target, how do axons further refine their targeting by reaching the correct sublayer for branching and synapse formation?[70]

As discussed in Chapter 14, the development of horizontal connections within cortical layers has been examined in the cat visual cortex, where correlated neuronal activity has been shown to be an important influence on the final branching patterns. Vertical projections, on the other hand, appear to be determined at the earliest stages of axon outgrowth by targeting cues independent of patterned activity. For example, axons growing from visual cortical layers 2 and 3 extend to layer 5 and branch within it, but avoid branching within layer 4. Layer 4 neurons also preferentially innervate layers 4, 3 and 2 rather than 5 and 6. The molecular mechanisms that guide cortical axons are likely to involve contact and diffusible axon guidance cues, as discussed in Chapter 9, but these remain to be characterized in detail. Coculture experiments using cortical slices have shown that axons can make layer-specific projections from one slice to another in the absence of the appropriate pathway, suggesting the operation of diffusible targeting cues.[71] Individual cortical layers are also likely to provide non-diffusible attractive cues, for axons branch better *in vitro* on membrane preparations derived from their normal target layer *in vivo* compared with inappropriate layers. The finding that heat-inactivation of membranes derived from inappropriate layers leads to increased branching also suggests that axons may be prevented from targeting the wrong layers by repulsive mechanisms,[72] and there is evidence that members of the ephrin family and their Eph receptors (see Chapter 9) may be involved.[73] A member of the immunoglobulin superfamily, LAMP, has also been implicated in the targeting of projections within the hippocampus.[74]

A transient population of 'Cajal–Retzius' (CR) cells has been shown to mediate accurate layer-specific targeting of afferents from the entorhinal cortex to the neighbouring hippocampus. In slice cocultures of these cortical areas, entorhinal axons make the same patterns of ingrowth into hippocampal cortex that are seen *in vivo*. However, prior ablation of the CR cells within the hippocampal slice prevents this ingrowth but does not affect the ingrowth of commissural/associational afferents. Similar abnormalities are also seen after application to the cocultures of neutralizing antibody to the extracellular matrix molecule reelin, and (albeit transiently) during the development of *reeler* mutant mice. Reelin, which is normally expressed by CR cells, is therefore suggested to play some role, possibly chemoattractive, in layer-specific targeting of entorhinohippocampal afferents in addition to its known role in cortical cell migration (see Chapter 7).[75]

The role of CR cells in the formation of hippocampal connections appears to be to allow incoming entorhinal axons to arborize and make transient synapses before the arrival of their definitive targets, the dendrites of the hippocampal pyramidal neurons.[76] This is reminiscent of another transient population of neurons, the cortical subplate, which is necessary for the formation of appropriate thalamic inputs to the developing cerebral cortex, as discussed below. In both cases they appear to provide temporary choice points, or 'guidepost' cells, for subsequent axon targeting, although precisely how they function is unclear.

Topographic axon projections to the cerebral cortex

The function of the cerebral neocortex is critically dependent on the region-specific axon projections that reach it from the various thalamic nuclei. These develop in two phases. After leaving the thalamus, thalamocortical axons first traverse the internal capsule and then extend tangentially within the intermediate zone and cortical subplate (see Chapter 7) to their target area. Here they pause for a variable period (up to 2 weeks in the cat) before target invasion, when they sprout axons into the overlying cortical plate and innervate their target neurons. Fluorescent axon-labelling experiments have shown that these projections are made accurately with only occasional errors.[77]

The subplate has been shown to be essential for precise targeting of the cortex by thalamocortical axons. Its neurons are amongst the first to arise in the cortex, and they extend axons towards the thalamus and into layer 4 of the cortex. Almost all subplate cells die during the early postnatal period (in kittens at least), and the site that they occupied becomes the subcortical white matter. If the subplate cells are ablated prematurely by a localized injection of kainic acid, the development of connections between cortex and thalamus is disrupted: axons from the visual thalamus (lateral geniculate nucleus) grow aberrantly past their appropriate target areas, and the same has been shown for auditory projections from the medial geniculate nucleus.[78] The subplate is also necessary for the refinement of thalamocortical connectivity at later, postnatal stages of development, as discussed in Chapter 14.

How are thalamic axons guided by the subplate to their neocortical targets? At the cellular level, one suggestion is that the axons of subplate neurons extending towards the thalamus may form a scaffold for the fasciculation and guidance of thalamic axons extending in the opposite direction as they exit the internal capsule.[79] Other axon-labelling studies have suggested, however, that the pathways of growing thalamocortical and corticothalamic axons are physically separate rather than tightly fasciculated, arguing that the subplate-associated guidance cues reside within rather than outside the subplate.[80]

The molecular nature of such cues is uncertain. *In vitro*, thalamic neurons adhere to explants of intermediate zone and subplate, and extend axons, but avoid explants of cortical plate. These differences can be abolished both by enzymatic removal of chondroitin sulphate and by addition of soluble chondroitin sulphate, suggesting that the relevant recognition factors are regionally-localized chondroitin sulphate-binding molecules. It is possible, for example, that chondroitin sulphate proteoglycans bind guidance molecules such as semaphorins or netrins, and present them to axon growth cones.[81] Another candidate guidance factor is the immunoglobulin superfamily molecule LAMP, which has been shown to facilitate the targeting of a subset of thalamic axons to limbic (perirhinal) cortex.[82] There is also evidence that thalamic afferents to limbic cortex, which express EphA5 (see above), may be repelled from the sensorimotor cortex by ephrin-A5/RAGS.[51] Lastly, the homophilic adhesion molecule N-cadherin has been implicated in layer-specific targeting by retinal axons in the chick optic tectum,[83] raising the possibility that members of the cadherin family may be similarly involved in the mammalian cerebral cortex. Alongside such guidance cues, electrical activity is also required for thalamic axons to make the correct initial targeting decisions as they traverse the subplate. Intracranial infusion of tetrodotoxin in cats causes many lateral geniculate neurons to project aberrantly into the subplate of inappropriate cortical areas, rather than projecting to visual cortex.[84]

In summary, compared with the retinotectal system much less is known about the mechanisms that establish the initial topographic maps elsewhere in the vertebrate CNS (see reference 10 for review). Many CNS axon tracts are topographically organized, the somatosensory projections to the primary sensory cortex that serve individual rodent whiskers being a good example. Here, the mechanisms that refine the mapping of axons into organized cell groupings (barrels) within the cortex are relatively well understood, as discussed in Chapter 14, but it remains uncertain how axon order is established during the initial development of axon projections. Are there, for example, matching gradients in the relevant regions of thalamus and cortex, perhaps analogous to the retinotectal system? And if so, how are these established?

Development of efferent projections from the cerebral cortex

It is also unclear how long-distance projections from cortical layer 5 are guided to their targets. From the outset neurons take either, but not both, of two main projection pathways, one to the opposite side of the cortex across the midline corpus callosum, and one to distant subcortical targets via the internal capsule. In the latter case, an interesting finding is that all layer 5 neurons initially make a common set of collateral branches to subcortical targets in the midbrain and hindbrain as they grow towards the spinal cord, regardless of their cortical area of origin (e.g. occipital versus parietal). The mature connectivity pattern is established only later, when neurons from different cortical areas selectively consolidate different subsets of these collaterals and eliminate the remainder (Fig. 10.5). This process is a good example of the more general phenomenon of synapse elimination during development (see Chapter 14), and shows remarkable plasticity, for the final pattern of connectivity made by layer 5 neurons can be modified by their transplantation to a new cortical site.[85]

Axon targeting in the insect neuromuscular system

The experimental advantages of *Drosophila*, where identification of single axons can be combined with sophisticated molecular genetics, have been exploited to good effect in the analysis of target recognition in the neuromuscular system. Each abdominal hemisegment contains some 30 individual muscles innervated with precision by some 40 motor axons, and a number of candidate targeting molecules

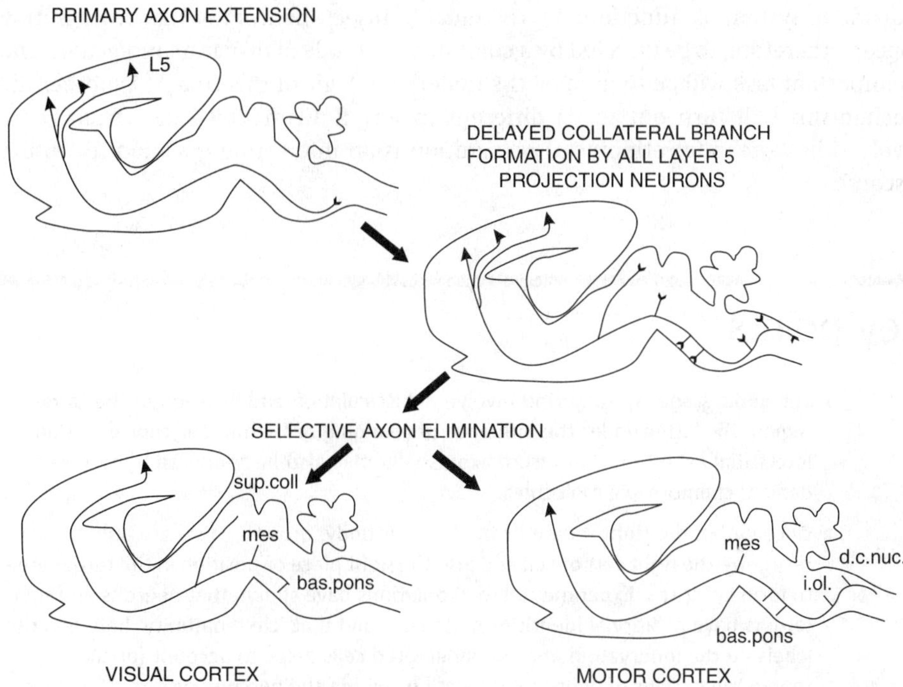

PRIMARY AXON EXTENSION

Figure 10.5 Stages in the development of specific projections by layer 5 (L5) neurons of rat neocortex. First, all cortical areas send out axons only towards the spinal cord, ignoring their correct destinations. Second, new collateral branches sprout from all axons into subcortical targets for the first time. Third, neurons placed in different cortical areas lose those new branches that are projecting inappropriately and retain only their correct projections. For neurons in the visual cortex, this means retention of connections in the superior colliculus (sup.coll.), mesencephalon (mes) and basal pons (bas.pons), while for motor cortical neurons there are no collicular connections after elimination, but branches are retained in mesencephalon, pons, inferior olive (i.ol.) and dorsal cochlear nucleus (d.c.nuc.). After O'Leary and Koester.[85]

expressed by muscles have been identified. The two *Drosophila netrin* genes are expressed in differing subsets of segmental muscles, and in *netrin* null mutants (as well in null mutations for *frazzled*, a *Drosophila* netrin receptor), the intersegmental axons that innervate these muscles often project inappropriately across segment boundaries into adjacent muscle territories. Following misexpression of either *netrin* gene in all muscles, these axons also project and branch aberrantly, sometimes stalling short of their target muscles.[86] The netrins, however, are expressed in only a minority of the segmental muscles, and in general it seems likely that targeting cues for motor axons are multiple and redundant. Further candidates are provided by the cell adhesion molecules connectin and Fasciclin III, and the secreted semaphorin semaII (see Chapter 9). As for the netrins, each gene is expressed by distinct subsets of muscles, and their ectopic expression results in innervation phenotypes consistent with attraction (connectin, FasIII) or repulsion (semaII). In each case, however, the finding that targeting is unaffected in loss-of-function mutations suggests that the individual system is functionally redundant. Insect neuromuscular recognition appears, therefore, to be directed by a combinatorial code of disparate molecules, and an important task will be to unravel the underlying logic of this code.[87] Whether the mechanisms will turn out to be different in any fundamental sense from those involved in vertebrate retinotectal recognition is an interesting question for future research.

Key points

1 The initial stages of targeting involve defasciculation and invasion of the target region, the latter under the influence of changing growth factor concentration. Interstitial axon branching from axon shafts may also be triggered by target-derived chemotropic molecules.

2 Once within the right region of the brain or body, growth cones are able to recognize the right sort of cell and also the right place or position in the target area to form synapses. Experimental manipulations have shown that neurons and their targets have positional identities or 'labels', and that 'chemoaffinity' between the labels on the innervating and the innervated cells helps to account for the topographic order of neuronal projections within the nervous system. One molecular system that may underlie this recognition is the family of Eph receptor tyrosine kinases and their ligands, the ephrins.

3 In some systems repulsive cues at the target perimeter may keep axons fenced in, preventing them from straying into inappropriate territory.

4 Target recognition may involve disparate, functionally redundant molecular recognition cues, as in the case of the insect neuromuscular system.

General reading

■ Buck, L. B. Information coding in the vertebrate olfactory system. *Annu. Rev. Neurosci.* **19**, 517–44 (1996).

■ Chenn, A., Braisted, J. E., McConnell, S. K. and O'Leary, D. D. M. Development of the cerebral cortex: mechanisms controlling cell fate, laminar and areal patterning, and axonal connectivity. In *Molecular and cellular approaches to neural development* (ed. W. M. Cowan, T. M. Jessell and S. L. Zipursky), pp. 440–73 (Oxford University Press, New York, 1997).

■ Flanagan, J. G. and Vanderhaeghen, P. The ephrins and Eph receptors in neural development. *Annu. Rev. Neurosci.* **21**, 309–45 (1998).

■ O'Leary, D. D. M. *et al.* Molecular development of sensory maps: representing sights and smells in the brain. *Cell* **96**, 255–69 (1999).

References

1. ElShamy, W. M., Linnarsson, S., Lee, K. F., Jaenisch, R. and Ernfors, P. Prenatal and postnatal requirements of NT-3 for sympathetic neuroblast survival and innervation of specific targets. *Development* **122**, 491–500 (1996).

2. Lewis, J., Chevallier, A., Kieny, M. and Wolpert, L. Muscle nerve branches do not develop in chick wings devoid of muscle. *J. Embryol. Exp. Morphol.* **64**, 211–32 (1981).

3. McFarlane, S., Cornel, E., Amaya, E. and Holt, C. E. Inhibition of FGF receptor activity in retinal ganglion cell axons causes errors in target recognition. *Neuron* **17**, 245–54 (1996).

4. Bastmeyer, M. and O'Leary, D. D. M. Dynamics of target recognition by interstitial axon branching along developing cortical axons. *J. Neurosci.* **16**, 1450–9 (1996).

5. Heffner, C. D., Lumsden, A. and O'Leary, D. D. M. Target control of collateral extension and directional axon growth in the mammalian brain. *Science* **257**, 217–20 (1990).

6. Stanfield, B. B. and O'Leary, D. D. M. Neurons in the rat subiculum with transient postmamillary collaterals during development maintain projections to the mamillary complex. *Exp. Brain Res.* **72**, 185–90 (1988).

7. Landmesser, L. Pharmacological properties, cholinesterase activity and anatomy of nerve muscle junctions in vagus innervated frog sartorius. *J. Physiol.* **220**, 243–56 (1972).

8. Ostberg, A. J., Raisman, G., Field, P. M., Iversen, L. L. and Zigmond, R. E. A quantitative comparison of the formation of synapses in the rat superior cervical ganglion by its own and by foreign nerve fibres. *Brain Res.* **107**, 445–70 (1976).

9. Nilssen, O. G., Clarke, D. J., Brundin, P. and Bjorklund, A. Comparison of growth and reinnervation properties of cholinergic neurons from different brain regions grafted to the hippocampus. *J. Comp. Neurol.* **268**, 204–22 (1988).

10. Udin, S. B. and Fawcett, J. W. Formation of topographic maps. *Annu. Rev. Neurosci.* **11**, 289–327 (1988).

11. Scholes, J. H. Nerve fibre topography in the retinal projection to the tectum. *Nature* **278**, 620–4 (1979).

12. Sperry, R. W. Effects of 180 degree rotation of the retinal field on visuomotor coordination. *J. Exp. Zool.* **92**, 263–79 (1943).

13. Sperry, R. W. Chemoaffinity in the orderly growth of nerve fibre patterns and connections. *Proc. Natl. Acad. Sci. USA* **50**, 703–10 (1963).

14. Holt, C. E. Does timing of axon outgrowth influence initial retinotectal topography in *Xenopus. J. Neurosci.* **4**, 1130–52 (1984).

15. Gaze, R. M. *The formation of nerve connections* (Academic Press, London, 1970).

16. Fujisawa, H. Retinotopic analysis of fibre pathways in the regenerating retinotectal system of the adult newt *Cynops pyrrhyogaster. Brain Res.* **206**, 27–37 (1981).

17. Hope, R. A., Hammond, B. J. and Gaze, R. M. The arrow model: retinotectal specificity and map formation in the goldfish visual system. *Proc. R. Soc. London Ser. B* **194**, 447–66 (1976).

18. Barbera, A. J., Marchase, R. B. and Roth, S. Adhesive recognition and retinotectal specificity. *Proc. Natl. Acad. Sci. USA* **70**, 2482–6 (1973).

19. Lance-Jones, C. and Landmesser, L. Motoneurone projection patterns in the chick hind limb following early partial reversals of the spinal cord. *J. Physiol. (London)* **302**, 581–602 (1980).

20. Brown, M. C. and Booth, C. M. Postnatal development of the adult pattern of motor axon distribution in rat muscle. *Nature* **304**, 741–2 (1983).

21. Hardman, V. J. and Brown, M. C. Accuracy of re-innervation of rat intercostal muscles by their own segmental nerves. *J. Neurosci.* **7**, 1031–6 (1987).

22. Laskowski, M. B. and Sanes, J. R. Topographically selective reinnervation of adult mammalian skeletal muscle. *J. Neurosci.* **8**, 3094–9 (1988).

23. Dennis, M. J. and Yip, J. W. Formation and elimination of foreign synapses on adult salamander muscle. *J. Physiol.* **274**, 299–310 (1978).

24. Wigston, D. J. and Sanes, J. R. Selective reinnervation of adult mammalian muscle by axons from different segmental levels. *Nature* **299**, 464–7 (1982).

25. Wigston, D. J. and Sanes, J. R. Selective reinnervation of intercostal muscle transplanted from different segmental levels to a common site. *J. Neurosci.* **5**, 1208–21 (1985).

26. Gaze, R. M. Neuronal specificity. *Br. Med. Bull.* **30**, 116–21 (1974).

27. Hayes, W. P. and Meyer, R. L. Retinotopically inappropriate synapses of subnormal density

formed by surgically misdirected optic fibres in goldfish tectum. *Dev. Brain Res.* **38**, 304–12 (1988).

28. Gaze, R. M., Keating, M. J., Ostberg, A. and Chung, S. H. The relationship between retinal and tectal growth in larval *Xenopus*: implications for the development of the retinotectal projection. *J. Embryol. Exp. Morphol.* **53**, 103–43 (1979).

29. Schmidt, J. T. Natural history of optic arbors on the tectum of fish and frog. *Trends Neurosci.* **7**, 358 (1984).

30. Halfter, W., Claviez, M. and Schwarz, U. Preferential adhesion of tectal membranes to anterior embryonic chick retina neurites. *Nature* **292**, 67–70 (1981).

31. Walter, J., Kern Veil, B., Huf, J., Stolze, B. and Bonhoeffer, F. Recognition of position-specific properties of tectal cell membranes by retinal axons *in vitro*. *Development* **101**, 685–96 (1987).

32. Cox, E. C., Muller, B. and Bonhoeffer, F. Axonal guidance in the chick visual system: posterior tectal membranes induce collapse of growth cones from the temporal retina. *Neuron* **4**, 31–7 (1990).

33. Trisler, D. and Collins, F. Corresponding spatial gradients of TOP molecules in the developing retina and optic tectum. *Science* **237**, 1208–9 (1987).

34. Ohsugi, K. and Ide, H. Position specific binding of a monoclonal antibody in chick limb buds. *Dev. Biol.* **117**, 676–9 (1986).

35. Suzue, T., Kaprielian, Z. and Patterson, P. H. A monoclonal antibody that defines rostrocaudal gradients in the mammalian nervous system. *Neuron* **5**, 421–31 (1990).

36. Stirling, R. V. Molecules, maps and gradients in the retinotectal projection. *Trends Neurosci.* **14**, 509–12 (1991).

37. Donoghue, M. J., Morris-Valero, R., Johnson, Y. R., Merlie, J. P. and Sanes, J. R. Mammalian muscle cells bear a cell-autonomous, heritable memory of their rostrocaudal position. *Cell* **69**, 67–77 (1992).

38. Trisler, G. D., Schneider, M. D. and Nirenberg, M. A topographic gradient of molecules in retina can be used to identify neuron position. *Proc. Natl. Acad. Sci. USA* **78**, 2145–9 (1981).

39. Kaprielian, Z. and Patterson, P. H. The molecular basis of retinotectal topography. *BioEssays* **16**, 1–11 (1994).

40. Tessier-Lavigne, M. Eph receptor tyrosine kinases, axon repulsion, and the development of topographic maps. *Cell* **82**, 345–8 (1995).

41. Orioli, D. and Klein, R. The Eph receptor family: axonal guidance by contact repulsion. *Trends Genet.* **13**, 354–9 (1997).

42. Flanagan, J. G. and Vanderhaeghen, P. The ephrins and Eph receptors in neural development. *Annu. Rev. Neurosci.* **21**, 309–45 (1998).

43. Gale, N. W. *et al.* Eph receptors and ligands comprise two major specificity subclasses and are reciprocally compartmentalized during embryogenesis. *Neuron* **17**, 9–19 (1996).

44. Drescher, U. *et al. In vitro* guidance of retinal ganglion cell axons by RAGS, a 25 kDa tectal protein related to ligands for Eph receptor tyrosine kinases. *Cell* **82**, 359–70 (1995).

45. Cheng, H. J., Nakamoto, M., Bergemann, A. D. and Flanagan, J. G. Complementary gradients in expression and binding of ELF-1 and Mek4 in development of the topographic retinotectal projection map. *Cell* **82**, 371–81 (1995).

46. Nakamoto, M. *et al.* Topographically specific effects of ELF-1 on retinal axon guidance *in vitro* and retinal axon mapping *in vivo*. *Cell* **86**, 755–66 (1996).

47. Frisen, J. *et al.* Ephrin-A5 (AL-1/RAGS) is essential for proper retinal axon guidance and topographic mapping in the mammalian visual system. *Neuron* **20**, 235–43 (1998).

48. Braisted, J. E. *et al.* Graded and lamina-specific distributions of ligands of EphB receptor tyrosine kinases in the developing retinotectal system. *Dev. Biol.* **191**, 14–28 (1997).

49. Ichijo, H. and Bonhoeffer, F. Differential withdrawal of retinal axons induced by a secreted factor. *J. Neurosci.* **18**, 5008–18 (1998).

50. Feldheim, D. A. *et al.* Topographic guidance labels in a sensory projection to the forebrain. *Neuron* **21**, 1303–13 (1998).

51. Gao, P. P. *et al.* Regulation of topographic projection in the brain: Elf-1 in the hippocamposeptal system. *Proc. Natl. Acad. Sci. USA* **93**, 11161–6 (1996).

52. Karlstrom, R. O. *et al.* Zebrafish mutations affecting retinotectal axon pathfinding. *Development* **123**, 427–38 (1996).

53. Nakamura, H. and O'Leary, D. D. M. Inaccuracies in initial growth and arborization of chick retinotectal axons followed by course corrections and axon remodelling to develop topographic order. *J. Neurosci.* **9**, 3776–95 (1989).

54. Simon, D. K. and O'Leary, D. D. M. Development of topographic order in the mammalian retinocollicular projection. *J. Neurosci.* **12**, 1212–32 (1992).

55. Roskies, A. L. and O'Leary, D. D. M. Control of topographic retinal axon branching by inhibitory membrane-bound molecules. *Science* **265**, 799–803 (1994).

56. O'Leary, D. D., Yates, P. A. and McLaughlin, T. Molecular development of sensory maps:

representing sights and smells in the brain. *Cell* **96**, 255–69 (1999).

57. Goodhill, G. J. and Richards, L. J. Retinotectal maps: molecules, models and misplaced data. *Trends Neurosci.* **22**, 529–34 (1999).

58. Buck, L. B. Information coding in the vertebrate olfactory system. *Annu. Rev. Neurosci.* **19**, 517–44 (1996).

59. Singer, M. S., Shepherd, G. M. and Greer, C. A. Olfactory receptors guide axons. *Nature* **377**, 19–20 (1995).

60. Wang, F., Nemes, A., Mendelsohn, M. and Axel, R. Odorant receptors govern the formation of a precise topographic map. *Cell* **93**, 47–60 (1998).

61. Mombaerts, P. *et al.* Visualizing an olfactory sensory map. *Cell* **87**, 675–86 (1996).

62. Treloar, H., Tomasiewicz, H., Magnuson, T. and Key, B. The central pathway of primary olfactory axons is abnormal in mice lacking the N-CAM-180 isoform. *J. Neurobiol.* **32**, 643–58 (1997).

63. Puche, A. C., Poirier, F., Hair, M., Bartlett, P. F. and Key, B. Role of galectin-1 in the developing mouse olfactory system. *Dev. Biol.* **179**, 274–87 (1996).

64. Kobayashi, H., Koppel, A. M., Luo, Y. and Raper, J. A. A role for collapsin-1 in olfactory and cranial sensory axon guidance. *J. Neurosci.* **17**, 8339–52 (1997).

65. Tsuchida, T. *et al.* Topographic organization of embryonic motor neurons defined by expression of LIM homeobox genes. *Cell* **79**, 957–70 (1994).

66. Lin, J. H. *et al.* Functionally related motor neuron pool and muscle sensory afferent subtypes defined by coordinate ETS gene expression. *Cell* **95**, 393–407 (1998).

67. Logan, C. *et al.* Rostral optic tectum acquires caudal characteristics following ectopic *Engrailed* expression. *Curr. Biol.* **6**, 1006–14 (1996).

68. Itasaki, N. and Nakamura, H. A role for gradient En expression in positional specification on the optic tectum. *Neuron* **16**, 55–62 (1996).

69. Friedman, G. C. and O'Leary, D. D. M. Retroviral misexpression of *Engrailed* genes in the chick optic tectum perturbs the topographic targeting of retinal axons. *J. Neurosci.* **16**, 5498–509 (1996).

70. Sanes, J. R. and Yamagata, M. Formation of lamina-specific synaptic connections. *Curr. Opin. Neurobiol.* **9**, 79–87 (1999).

71. Bolz, J., Novak, N., Gotz, M. and Bonhoeffer, T. Formation of target-specific neuronal projections in organotypic slice cultures from rat visual cortex. *Nature* **346**, 359–62 (1990).

72. Castellani, V. and Bolz, J. Membrane-associated molecules regulate the formation of layer-specific cortical circuits. *Proc. Natl. Acad. Sci. USA* **94**, 7030–5 (1997).

73. Castellani, V., Yue, Y., Gao, P. P., Zhou, R. and Bolz, J. Dual action of a ligand for Eph receptor tyrosine kinases on specific populations of axons during the development of cortical circuits. *J. Neurosci.* **18**, 4663–72 (1998).

74. Pimenta, A. F. *et al.* The limbic system-associated membrane protein is an Ig superfamily member that mediates selective neuronal growth and axon targeting. *Neuron* **15**, 287–97 (1995).

75. Del Rio, J. A. *et al.* A role for Cajal–Retzius cells and reelin in the development of hippocampal connections. *Nature* **385**, 70–4 (1997).

76. Super, H., Martinez, A., Del Rio, J. A. and Soriano, E. Involvement of distinct pioneer neurons in the formation of layer-specific connections in the hippocampus. *J. Neurosci.* **18**, 4616–26 (1998).

77. Chenn, A., Braisted, J. E., McConnell, S. K. and O'Leary, D. D. M. Development of the cerebral cortex: mechanisms controlling cell fate, laminar and areal patterning, and axonal connectivity. In *Molecular and cellular approaches to neural development* (ed. W. M. Cowan, T. M. Jessell and S. L. Zipursky), pp. 440–73 (Oxford University Press, New York, 1997).

78. Allendoerfer, K. L. and Shatz, C. J. The subplate, a transient neocortical structure: its role in the development of connections between thalamus and cortex. *Annu. Rev. Neurosci.* **17**, 185–218 (1994).

79. Molnar, Z., Adams, R. and Blakemore, C. Mechanisms underlying the early establishment of thalamocortical connections in the rat. *J. Neurosci.* **18**, 5723–45 (1998).

80. De Carlos, J. A. and O'Leary, D. D. M. Growth and targeting of subplate axons and establishment of major cortical pathways. *J. Neurosci.* **12**, 1194–211 (1992) [published erratum appears in *J. Neurosci.* **13** (1993)].

81. Emerling, D. E. and Lander, A. D. Inhibitors and promoters of thalamic neuron adhesion and outgrowth in embryonic neocortex: functional association with chondroitin sulfate. *Neuron* **17**, 1089–100 (1996).

82. Barbe, M. F. and Levitt, P. Attraction of specific thalamic input by cerebral grafts depends on the molecular identity of the implant. *Proc. Natl. Acad. Sci. USA* **89**, 3706–10 (1992).

83. Inoue, A. and Sanes, J. R. Lamina-specific connectivity in the brain: regulation by N-cadherin, neurotrophins, and glycoconjugates. *Science* **276**, 1428–31 (1997).

84. Catalano, S. M. and Shatz, C. J. Activity-dependent cortical target selection by thalamic axons. *Science* **281**, 559–62 (1998).

85. O'Leary, D. D. M. and Koester, S. E. Development of projection neuron types, axon pathways,

and patterned connections of the mammalian cortex. *Neuron* **10**, 991–1006 (1993).

86. Mitchell, K. J. *et al.* Genetic analysis of netrin genes in *Drosophila*: netrins guide CNS commissural axons and peripheral motor axons. *Neuron* **17**, 203–15 (1996).

87. Tessier-Lavigne, M. and Goodman, C. S. The molecular biology of axon guidance. *Science* **274**, 1123–33 (1996).

11

Synapse Formation

The previous two chapters have shown how short- and long-range signals combine to guide axons to their targets. The next developmental step is for synapses to form, and this chapter describes how the presynaptic and postsynaptic components of synapses are constructed (synaptogenesis). During synapse formation, terminal neurites stop growing and differentiate into presynaptic elements able to secrete transmitter, and the postsynaptic membrane differentiates into the mature form which can respond to transmitter molecules. These events require that instructions pass in both directions across the developing synapse. At present, detailed information about this process is available only for the developing connections between motor nerves and skeletal muscle fibres. This is largely because of ease of access to the neuromuscular junction and because each muscle fibre (at least in adult mammals—see Chapter 14) is innervated at only a single site by one type of neuron, the motor neuron. A feature of the neuromuscular junction that distinguishes it from other synapses is that chemical transmission is used to amplify the electrical signal generated by the single motor axon terminal. The amount of transmitter liberated and the number of postsynaptic receptors are much greater than at individual synapses in the CNS, ensuring that each action potential in the motor nerve is followed faithfully by one in the muscle fibre. Nonetheless, the mechanisms of synaptogenesis uncovered at the neuromuscular junction may turn out to be of wide application.[1]

Formation of the neuromuscular junction of skeletal muscle

Development of neuromuscular junctions is spread out over many days, starting in rodents at around 6 days before birth in hindlimb muscles, while myotubes are still being formed by the fusion of individual myoblast cells,[2] and not finishing until about 14 days after birth. The sequence of events is illustrated in Fig. 11.1. The first motor axon to make contact with a myotube stops growing soon after contact with the

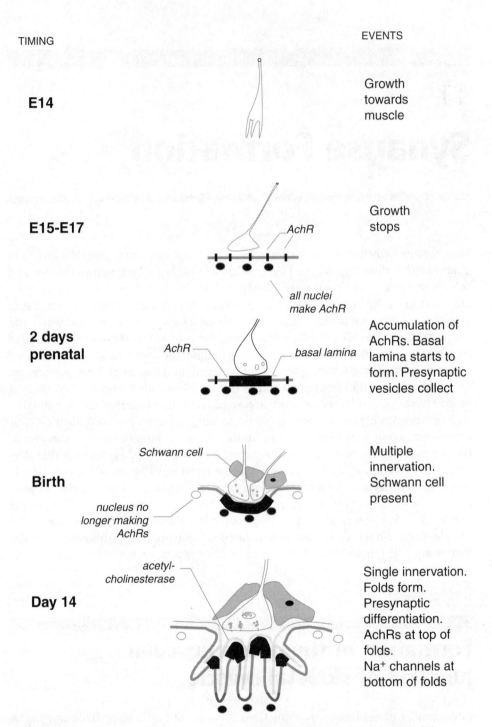

TIMING	EVENTS
E14	Growth towards muscle
E15-E17	Growth stops
2 days prenatal	Accumulation of AchRs. Basal lamina starts to form. Presynaptic vesicles collect
Birth	Multiple innervation. Schwann cell present
Day 14	Single innervation. Folds form. Presynaptic differentiation. AchRs at top of folds. Na⁺ channels at bottom of folds

AchR

all nuclei make AchR

AchR — *basal lamina*

Schwann cell

nucleus no longer making AchRs

acetyl-cholinesterase

Figure 11.1 Some of the events occurring during the formation and maturation of the neuromuscular junction between the axon of a ventral horn motor neuron and a skeletal muscle fibre. The timing of these events is given for neuromuscular junctions in the hindleg of rats and mice. See text for details.

muscle surface.[3] Junctional transmission can begin very soon thereafter[4] and is aided by several factors. First, the rapid migration within the muscle membrane of pre-existing acetylcholine receptors which accumulate under the nerve ending[5] creates a sufficient density of these to generate a large synaptic current in response to transmitter. Second, the long open times of the ionic channels of these embryonic receptors (see later) boosts the size of the current. Third, the small size and hence high input resistance of the myotubes enhances the depolarizing action of the synaptic current. Fourth, the absence of cholinesterase prolongs the synaptic action of released transmitter. The fifth and very important factor in establishing transmission rapidly is the ability of the new terminal to release acetylcholine even before the formation of special release sites.[6] Further axons accumulate at such original points of contact so that eventually each muscle fibre is multiply innervated at a single site.[7,8] This excess of innervation is later gradually removed ('synapse elimination'), a process that is discussed further in Chapter 14.

As the terminal matures, transmitter comes to be released at specialized active zones. These are in register with the clefts between the tops of secondary folds which develop in the postsynaptic membrane. It is in the top of the ridges between these clefts that the acetylcholine receptors become highly concentrated, and their turnover rate becomes much reduced as the composition of the acetylcholine receptors is changed from the non-specialized extrajunctional type to the endplate specific type. This is done by substituting an epsilon subunit for a gamma subunit in the five-ringed group of receptor subunits that together form an individual acetylcholine receptor.[9] This has the effect of decreasing the open time of the transmitter-activated ion channels but increasing their conductance (Fig. 11.2).

The acetylcholine receptors are probably anchored to the underlying cytoskeleton, a crucial part in this being played by a unique 43-kDa cytoskeletal protein, rapsyn, which may act like ankyrin in the erythrocyte membrane (Fig. 11.3).[10] Null mutant mice devoid of rapsyn die at birth. They cannot breathe because acetylcholine receptors do not form permanent tight clusters at neuromuscular junctions, despite normal synthesis, so that transmission fails.[11] Rapsyn is involved in organizing the multimolecular complex that constitutes the postsynaptic apparatus, comprising molecules such as utrophin (see below), dystroglycan and the erbB kinases; all are distributed diffusely in its absence. Other components of the apparatus, including acetylcholinesterase (which begins to accumulate in the basal lamina at the junction only after transmission begins) and MuSK (see below), remain concentrated at the junction in rapsyn-deficient mice, suggesting that different parts of the apparatus can form independently.[12]

During junctional maturation, transmitter receptors are also eliminated from the extrajunctional membrane.[13] This loss of extrajunctional receptors is due to down-regulation of synthesis of their mRNA in the myonuclei outside the immediate vicinity of the developing neuromuscular junction. This has been elegantly demonstrated using transgenic mice in which the regulatory region of the acetylcholine receptor epsilon subunit gene was made to direct the expression of the reporter gene *NlacZ*, whose product is confined within the nucleus and can be detected there histochemically. The reporter molecule accumulated only in the myonuclei lying at or

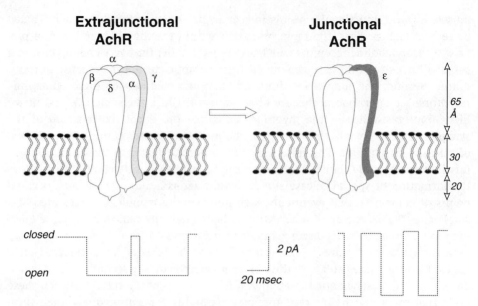

Figure 11.2 Diagram of two single pentameric acetylcholine receptors and of the electrical properties of the channel each forms when activated by acetylcholine. The channel on the left is that found in neonatal muscles and that on the right at the mature neuromuscular junction. In the mature form the substitution of the γ-subunit of the immature form with an ε-subunit changes the open channel time and the channel conductance. This change in subunit composition is a result of an inductive action of the motor nerve, the responsible factor probably being the protein ARIA/neuregulin (see text).

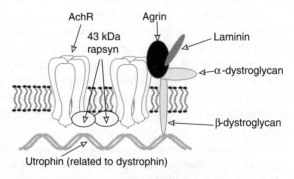

Figure 11.3 Schematic summary of some of the molecules, in addition to the acetylcholine receptor, which become localized at the neuromuscular junction during development. The junctional basal lamina also contains s-laminin, NCAM, cholinesterase and agrin, and the muscle membrane contains the agrin receptor MuSK (see text).

close to the endplate in adult mice.[14] The same technique applied to the α-subunit gene also showed that there was preferential expression of the gene in nuclei at the endplate. The loss of extrajunctional acetylcholine receptors helps to make the muscle membrane refractory to any further innervation and guarantees that all motor innervation is confined to the original synaptic site. Accompanying the downregulation of myonuclei other than those at the junction, the golgi complex becomes reorganized so that only a reduced basic structure remains extra-synaptically, while that at the neuromuscular junction remains large and active.[15]

Synapse formation in invertebrates has been studied at developing neuromuscular junctions of *Drosophila*, where a similar sequence of events to those already described for the vertebrate occurs.[16] Glutamate receptors, for example, only accumulate after the motor axon arrives. However, the mechanism of accumulation is likely to be different (see below).

Progress has been made in identifying some of the signals by which the arriving motor axons and the embryonic muscle fibres communicate to bring about the changes described above (see also reference 1 for review).

The signals used by muscle fibres to induce changes in the motor nerve

Figure 11.4 summarizes some of the factors by which muscle fibres influence motor nerves. The important tasks are to stop further elongation in the motor nerve and to promote transmitter secretion and motor neuron survival.

Halting motor axon growth

The first critical step in presynaptic differentiation is the rapid cessation of axon growth. It is still not known how this is achieved but several possibilities exist. Contact with a muscle fibre triggers a transient rise in calcium in the growth cone of motor neurons[17] and this may be triggered by a cAMP-dependent mechanism.[18] It is known that growth cone behaviour is critically dependent on the precise levels of intracellular calcium,[19,20] growth ceasing if the levels drop too low or rise too high; indeed too great a rise can trigger growth cone collapse and withdrawal (see also Chapter 9).[21] Such withdrawal would be counter-productive for synapse formation, but an appropriate rise in calcium might simply halt the advance of the growth cone. Observations on adult frog muscles killed by freezing have shown that regenerating motor axons stop growing and form normal presynaptic specializations when they regenerate onto the basal lamina of the old neuromuscular junctions, even in the complete absence of muscle cells.[22] This suggests strongly that for regenerating adult axons, axon growth-inhibition and presynaptic differentiation are under the control of molecular components of the basal lamina.[23]

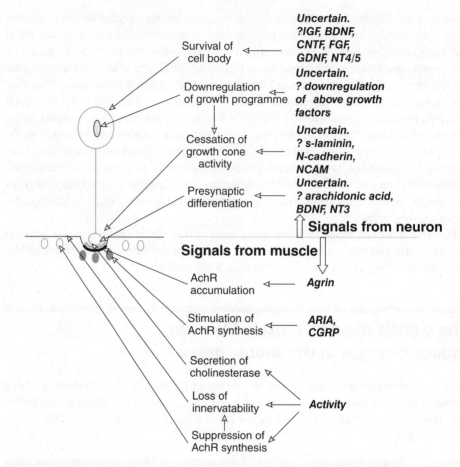

Figure 11.4 Summary of some of the events occurring during the formation of the neuromuscular junction and of some of the signals that help to bring about these developmental changes.

During development, similar or identical molecules may be present in the muscle membrane and inhibit axon growth when the axons first contact it. Possible candidates are the adhesion molecules NCAM and N-cadherin, which are present on myotubes and can interact with neurons leading to a rise in intracellular calcium;[24] in the case of NCAM, however, neuromuscular junctions show only minor abnormalities in homozygous mutant mice.[25] Another contender is a synapse-specific form of laminin (s-laminin, containing the laminin β2 chain).[26] It includes a tripeptide sequence Leu-Arg-Glu (LRE) which specifically inhibits motor axon growth[27,28] and which targets s-laminin to the synaptic region of the basal lamina.[29] Presynaptic differentiation is curtailed at neuromuscular junctions in s-laminin-deficient mice, but motor axons stop growing at them nevertheless.[30] Interestingly, junctional Schwann cells in these mutants intrude into the synaptic cleft, impairing synaptic transmission, so one function of s-laminin may be to repel Schwann cells locally at the junction.[31] Lastly, another possibility is that the protein agrin, a known function of which is to aggregate acetylcholine receptors (see below), also acts as a stop signal for axons.[32]

In *Drosophila* a protein encoded by the gene *late bloomer* is expressed transiently in motor axons at the time of synapse formation, and may play a part in recognizing or transducing stop signals provided by the muscle, for in null mutants synapse formation is delayed and there is ectopic sprouting.[33] Both cAMP and the adhesion molecule FasII (homologous to vertebrate NCAM) play essential subsequent roles in the control of synaptic stability and growth in *Drosophila*. Null mutants, with or without transgenes able to drive expression of FasII pre- or postsynaptically, have been used to show that without FasII localized to pre- and postsynaptic regions, the initial connections successfully made between motor nerves and muscle fibres break down, which is fatal.[34] A fall in the levels of FasII, which can occur either in *FasII* mutants or if activity at the junctions is increased, as it is in *Shaker* mutants, causes presynaptic sprouting but without a corresponding increase in transmitter release machinery.[35] If, however, the cAMP response element-binding protein CREB is active, the release machinery increases in parallel with the FasII-driven anatomical expansion of the terminals.[36] This machinery is likely to prove to be an important part of the mechanism controlling local synaptic growth and strength mediated by activity.[37]

During the period of synapse formation there is a gradual reduction in the supply of growth-promoting materials from the nerve cell body[38] and this must play a part in preventing further elongation of the motor axon. The exact reason for this down-regulation of expression of growth-associated genes is unclear, but it correlates at the neuromuscular junction with a fall in the output of insulin-like growth factor II (IGF-II) from the muscle fibres.[39,40] In adult mice this peptide is able to stimulate outgrowths from intact neuromuscular junctions (see Chapter 17). Even in the mature state, however, axoplasmic transport of some membrane and cytoskeletal elements continues. The supply of these materials must be controlled to prevent elongation of the axon, but the mechanisms that achieve this are not known. It has been suggested that raised levels of calcium in the terminals, associated with release of neurotransmitter, activate proteases which promote steady turnover of continually elongating microtubules and neurofilaments.[41] Alternatively, and more probably, specific recognition molecules may trigger biochemical stabilization of microtubules and neurofilaments (so-called 'capping'), so that transported precursors can no longer be incorporated at their ends and are instead returned to the cell body.[42]

Promoting transmitter release and motor neuron survival

Other retrograde signals from the muscle are needed to promote specialization of the motor nerve terminal for transmitter secretion. Simple contact with an isolated patch of muscle membrane increases secretion from growth cones,[43] and when cut motor axons reinnervate empty basal lamina tubes not only is growth brought to a halt (see above) but the presynaptic structures mature normally.[23] Mice deficient for s-laminin have poorly differentiated presynaptic terminals which lack active zones.[30] They also have poorly developed postjunctional folds and fail to express NCAM at the junction. So membrane-bound material can convey appropriate signals for differentiation. Secreted molecules are almost certainly involved also in promoting differentiation and survival. For example, muscle-derived arachidonic acid metabolites increase the frequency of spontaneous transmitter release,[44] and the neurotrophins BDNF and NT3 (see below) also assist junction formation.[45]

Contact with an appropriate muscle is vital for motor neuron survival at a critical stage of development as muscle, like other target tissues, secretes neurotrophic factors. Until recently, in spite of intensive efforts using conventional purification techniques, the identity of the neurotrophic factor(s) needed by motor neurons was unknown. There are now several plausible candidates;[46] for example, IGF 1 and 2, BDNF, CNTF, cardiotrophin-1 (a cytokine related to CNTF),[47] FGF, GDNF, NT-4 and NT-5, LIF[48] and hepatocyte growth factor[49] which are discussed more fully in Chapters 12 and 13. (NT-4, unlike most of the other factors, is upregulated by muscle activity.[50]) Why there should be so many factors is unclear.[51]

Mechanisms by which the motor axon induces changes in the muscle

Some of the signals by which motor axons are known to influence the differentiation of the muscle fibres that they innervate are given in Fig. 11.4. There are three main factors involved: electrical activity and two peptides released by motor axons, agrin and ARIA (neuregulin).

The role of electrical activity

Electrical activity is triggered by acetylcholine release and this initiates several changes in muscle fibres.[52] Those occurring at the neuromuscular junction are shown in Fig. 11.4. These effects may be mediated by the rise in calcium concentration accompanying contraction and this in turn may elevate levels of protein kinase C.[53,54] This kinase may regulate the muscle differentiation factors MyoD and myogenin,[55] a fall in whose activity reduces the output of mRNA for acetylcholine receptors from myonuclei.

The acetylcholinesterase present at the neuromuscular junction is produced by the muscle fibres, even though it is also found in the motor nerves as well. The appearance of cholinesterase at the neuromuscular junction in rat and chick muscle is one of the consequences of the onset of action potentials in the muscle,[56] although in

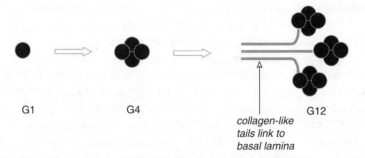

G1   G4   G12

*collagen-like
tails link to
basal lamina*

Figure 11.5 Development of different forms of cholinesterase at the neuromuscular junction.

amphibia electrical activity may not be required.[57] In muscle cell lines the rise in acetylcholinesterase which accompanies the fusion of myoblasts into myotubes is preceded by a rise in its mRNA. This is not, it turns out, a result of increased transcription (as is the case for mRNA for acetylcholine receptors) but a stabilization of the mRNA, which is otherwise rapidly degraded.[58] The pattern of electrical activity determines the composition of junctional cholinesterase. At the neuromuscular junction the basic globular protein of cholinesterase (G1) polymerizes into a range of different polymeric forms.[59] The largest polymer is the endplate-specific form (A12 with 12 globular units), which is anchored to the basal lamina in the synaptic cleft by a collagen tail (Fig. 11.5). Different proportions of high- and low-molecular-weight polymers are present in fast- and slow-twitch muscle fibres. It is possible to reproduce these characteristic differences by electrically activating denervated rat muscles with different patterns of stimulation. It is found that a pattern designed to copy the frequency of firing of motor neurons innervating fast muscle fibres induces a cholinesterase profile typical of a fast muscle. A slow rate of stimulation, on the other hand, induces a mixture of cholinesterase polymers that is characteristic of a slow muscle.[60] The transduction pathway for this frequency-dependent effect is unknown.

Agrin

Following experiments showing that synaptic basal lamina is able to direct the accumulation of acetylcholine receptors in regenerating muscle *in vivo*, the protein agrin was identified and purified from the endplate-rich electric organ of *Torpedo* (see reference 61 for review). Agrin is manufactured and secreted by motor neurons, and helps to achieve rapid transmission by its ability to aggregate pre-existing acetylcholine receptors.[62-64] Its mosaic structure, including numerous carbohydrate attachment sites, binding sites for laminin, dystroglycan and heparin, and its acetylcholine receptor aggregating activity, suggest it has several functions. The importance of agrin in synapse formation in muscle is shown by the almost total absence of endplates and immediate postnatal death of neural agrin-knockout mice.[65] Misexpression of agrin in fully innervated rat muscles can also induce ectopic acetylcholine receptor aggregates.[66] It is further possible that agrin induces clustering of the receptors for ARIA and so indirectly controls gene transcription in the nuclei at the neuromuscular junction (see next section).

Agrin signalling is mediated by a receptor tyrosine kinase MuSK (muscle specific kinase), and mice lacking MuSK also have similar, severe deficits at the neuromuscular junction.[67] Direct binding of agrin to MuSK has not been demonstrated, and agrin–MuSK interaction may require an accessory protein MASC (muscle-associated specific-component).[68] Agrin-induced clustering of acetylcholine receptors also involves a synapse-specific carbohydrate, N-acetylgalactosaminyl-terminated saccharide,[69] but its relation to MuSK or MASC is not yet clear. Lastly, an interaction between rapsyn (see above) and MuSK also appears to be required for receptor aggregation, since agrin fails to induce aggregation in cultured myotubes from rapsyn-deficient mice.[70]

Later in development, agrin is concentrated in the basal lamina at the neuromuscular junction, anchored there by glycoproteins (dystroglycans) which in turn are linked to dystrophin, a large protein (mutated in humans with Duchenne muscular dystrophy) forming a part of the subsarcolemmal cytoskeleton.[71] A dystrophin homologue, utrophin, is also concentrated in the postsynaptic cytoskeleton (Fig.11.3).[72] Together, these and associated molecules form a multimolecular complex that maintains the long-term stability of the neuromuscular junction, providing a linkage between the cytoskeleton and the extracellular matrix.

Agrin has not been detected in *Drosophila*, and glutamate receptor accumulation seems to depend on activity in the motor axons.[73] Glutamate is the excitatory transmitter, and its release may itself trigger the accumulation. In this system, moreover, the myonuclei do not reduce their production of receptor protein. This is probably because none of them is situated far from a synaptic site in these multiply-innervated muscle fibres, and so all can be considered junctional and under the influence of factors released from the motor axons.[74]

ARIA/neuregulin

Transcription of acetylcholine receptor mRNA continues at myonuclei close to the developing junction, but this is not the case in nuclei elsewhere in the muscle. The sparing of the junctional nuclei from the downregulation taking place elsewhere is mediated by factors released locally by the motor axons. One such factor is a protein synthesized by motor neurons and concentrated in the basal lamina at the neuromuscular junction, acetylcholine receptor inducing agent (ARIA), which was first isolated from chicken brain[75,76] and has turned out to be a neuregulin (see Chapter 11). Neuregulin can increase the production of acetylcholine receptors (in mice particularly the endplate specific epsilon subunit) and sodium channels in myotubes, and is likely to be an important regulator of postsynaptic differentiation. It may act directly through the nerve, but since it is also synthesized by muscle cells it could act downstream of agrin. A further possibility is that it acts indirectly via the promotion of Schwann cell development (see Chapter 6).[1]

Another factor that may influence myonuclei near to the neuromuscular junction is calcitonin-gene-related peptide (CGRP). This is present in most motor neurons and its application to myotubes in culture specifically promotes acetylcholine receptor production,[77] possibly by raising levels of cAMP.[78] Neuromuscular junctions are unaffected, however, in CGRP-deficient mice.[12]

Position of endplates

Endplates are invariably found in the middle of each skeletal muscle fibre in mammals. This is the optimum location for reducing to a minimum any delays in activation of contraction in different parts of the muscle fibre. The constancy of this position raises the possibility that the centre of each muscle fibre is a specially prepared postsynaptic site awaiting the incoming motor axons. In fact, the normal position of junctions in the middle of the long axis of muscle fibres is probably not due to any initial specialization at that point but to the short length of myotubes when first contacted by motor axons. A junction can develop at any point along the immature fibre.[3,5] The muscle fibre then grows considerably in length, but roughly equally on either side of the endplate, with the result that the junction ultimately comes to lie in the middle of the fibre.[79] In denervated adult muscles, which revert to a quasi-embryonic state (see Chapter 16), ectopic junctions can be formed at many sites along the length of a muscle fibre[80] if motor axons are prevented from reaching the already-formed endplate, which otherwise is the site at which motor axons tend to terminate.[81]

Certain muscle fibres in limb muscles of frogs and chickens and eye muscles of mammals[82] cannot generate action potentials, and rely for activation on endplate potentials occurring at motor synapses which are quite regularly spaced along their length. If transmission is impaired in developing chicks by appropriate doses of curare injected into the egg, the spacing between endplates is reduced.[83] This suggests that if depolarization during activity fails to reach a particular level at any point on a muscle fibre, additional motor innervation is not prevented. In muscle fibres with propagated action potentials only a single endplate is needed to ensure adequate depolarization throughout the muscle, but the attenuation of junction potential amplitude with distance in fibres without propagated action potentials is enough to allow new synapses to form as the fibres lengthen.

Synapse formation in the CNS

Synapse formation in the CNS is much harder to study than the formation of peripheral synapses. Apart from the difficulties of experimental access, synaptic development in the CNS seems likely to be inherently more complex than in the PNS: there are a very large number and variety of inputs, both excitatory and inhibitory, to each neuron; different inputs are often located precisely on only particular parts of the dendritic tree, and the postsynaptic cell has to generate not only appropriate transmitter receptors in the right places but even a range of receptor subtypes for a given transmitter. Although studies using autoradiography after application of radiolabelled ligands suggested that transmitter receptors might not be confined to the subsynaptic membrane,[84] immunogold electron microscopy demonstrates very precise localization of different receptor types even within one postsynaptic area, and at a considerably higher density than in non-synaptic areas.[85] Central synapses remain more modifiable in the adult than do those in the PNS, and the borderline between early synaptic development and the structural and functional plasticity underlying learning is indistinct. The important role of synaptically-induced depolarization in the development of neuromuscular junctions (see above) raises a puzzle for the development of inhibitory synapses in the CNS. Interestingly, some GABAergic synapses in the early postnatal hippocampus are initially depolarizing before converting to their more usual hyperpolarizing action.[86]

With this background it is not surprising that little is known about the signals involved in presynaptic and postsynaptic development in the central nervous system (see references 87 and 88 for reviews). It is known, however, that synaptic assembly of the brain proceeds normally in the complete absence of chemical neurotransmission.[89] The gradual structural differentiation of the synapses has been deduced from electron micrographs; presynaptic terminals, for example, can begin to form on the growth cones of elongating dendrites.[90] This suggests that, as in muscle, almost any site on the postsynaptic membrane is a potential starting point for a synapse. On the other hand, studies of the cerebellar Purkinje cells of *weaver* mice (see Chapter 7), in which most of the granule cells are absent, show that dendritic spines can form and develop postsynaptic thickenings in the absence of their major presynaptic input.[91] In the olfactory bulb, too, postsynaptic densities appear prior to innervation.[92] Continuous observation of hippocampal pyramidal cells developing in culture slices has become possible using confocal microscopy, and has shown how early filopodial protrusions on the shafts of dendrites extend and retract at first, but later are maintained as spine-like protrusions;[93] see reference 94 for review. It seems possible, then, that unlike muscle the postsynaptic cell dictates where synapses will form. This may be necessary in neurons which, unlike muscle fibres, have many and differing synaptic inputs to accommodate (see above).

The fact that ribosomal RNA is found in the dendrites of neurons, but not in their axons, may be of relevance for the correct siting of transmitter receptors, perhaps allowing their local synthesis in particular regions of the dendritic arbor and cell body.[95,96] Transmitter receptors can be restricted in the absence of innervation, as has been shown for glycine receptors, which are confined to the cell body of motor neurons developing in culture.[97] The properties of the postsynaptic cell are also known to feedback to influence the transmitter release characteristics of the presynaptic terminals. This is well illustrated by the inputs from muscle spindle afferents onto motor neurons: a given afferent may innervate several synergistic motor pools, each of which may contain a different range of motor neuron types. It is found that the transmitter release properties on a given motor neuron are all very similar from a range of spindle afferents, but each afferent develops very different properties in the terminals which innervate motor neurons of different types.[98]

While little is known about CNS synapse formation at the molecular level, it is interesting that agrin has been detected in central neurons,[99,100] and a neuregulin iso-form has been found to upregulate the expression of an NMDA-receptor subunit in the cerebellum when added to cultured cerebellar slices.[101] Moreover, several members of the cadherin family of adhesion molecule are expressed in the developing CNS, and are localized at synapses.[102] A detailed study of the expression of N- and E-cadherin in the dendritic arbor of hippocampal pyramidal neurons has shown that they are distributed in a mutually exclusive manner along dendritic shafts, raising the possibility that individual cadherin subtypes mediate synaptic specificity in the CNS.[103] This is consistent with the structural similarity between the synapse and other cadherin-based adhesive junctions between cells, namely the desmosome and the adherens junction. A further cadherin-related gene family, known as the protocadherin family, has the potential for generating wide structural diversity, with a genomic organization similar to that of the immunoglobulin and T-cell receptor gene clusters.[104] Many questions remain about the possible roles of cadherin-related proteins in the CNS, but they do provide good molecular candidates for the underpinnings of complex synaptic connectivity.[105]

In vitro studies of synapse formation between pontine explants and cerebellar granule cells have implicated two further molecular signalling systems in presynaptic differentiation. The first concerns a member of the family of secreted WNT signalling molecules, WNT7A, which is expressed *in vivo* by granule cells during the period they receive synapses from the pontine nuclei. WNT7A induces pontine axon terminals to undergo morphological changes, such as spreading and increased complexity, that resemble the initial events of presynaptic differentiation.[106] The second system concerns contact-mediated signalling between members of the neurexin protein family and the neuroligins. Presynaptic neurexin and postsynaptic neuroligin have been linked biochemically to presynaptic calcium channels,[87] and there is good evidence that neuroligins are sufficient to initiate synapse formation *in vitro*. When non-neuronal cells are transfected with neuroligin, pontine axons initiate synapse formation on them, as judged by a variety of molecular and morphological markers.[107]

Amidst all the detailed differences and added complications that are evident in CNS synapse formation, a parallel with developmental changes at the neuro-muscular junction has come to light. It concerns the subunit composition of the AMPA receptor, one of the three main classes of receptor for the principal excitatory transmitter glutamate. By using *in situ* hybridization with appropriately constructed probes, it has been found that the receptors appearing earliest in development contain only so-called 'flip' versions of the subunits. These allow more current and more calcium ions to pass through the receptor channels than the 'flop' versions, which only appear after day 8 in the neonatal rat.[108] This change in the current passing charac-teristics of the ion channel with age is reminiscent of the changes seen in the skeletal muscle nicotinic cholinergic receptor (see above) at the neuromuscular junction.

Another very important parallel with synapse formation in muscle is that the initial synaptic connections do not all survive. There is competition for survival between synapses in the neonatal and maturing CNS, leading to elimination of some synapses and retention of others. These aspects of developmental synaptic plasticity are dis-cussed further in Chapter 14.

Key points

1 Synapse formation arises when a growth cone meets a suitable synaptic partner. Both the growth cone of the axon and the membrane of the postsynaptic cell undergo crucial structural and functional alterations which depend on local inductive signals passing between the two partners. Much of the information about synapse formation has come from studies of the neuromuscular junction because of its relative simplicity and accessibility.

2 The motor nerves in vertebrates release at least two specific proteins in addition to the transmitter acetylcholine. One of these, agrin, causes pre-existing acetylcholine receptors in the muscle membrane to aggregate beneath the nerve terminal, and the second, ARIA (a neuregulin), stimulates the muscle nuclei at the endplate to synthesize the subunit components of the mature acetylcholine receptor.

3 These combined signals establish transmission and electrical activity in the muscle fibre membrane. This activity itself is important in further differentiation of the endplate and maturation of the muscle fibre. It stimulates secretion of acetylcholinesterase by the muscle at the junction and inhibits synthesis of acetylcholine receptor subunits by myonuclei outside the endplate area. This helps to render the muscle refractory to further innervation.

4 The signals present in the muscle fibre which bring the growth of the motor axons to a halt are not all known, but a synapse-specific form of laminin (s-laminin), as well as agrin, may be involved. The muscle is known to supply the motor neuron with neurotrophic support which enables it to survive, and the same agent and/or some other may assist in the differentiation of the motor nerve terminal. There are several candidate trophic agents, e.g. IGF2, BDNF and GDNF.

5 The mechanisms of synapse formation in the CNS are likely to be more complicated than those of neuromuscular junction formation. Candidate synaptic recognition molecules include cadherins and cadherin-related adhesion proteins, WNT signalling molecules and neurexin-neuroligin.

General reading

- Lee, S. H. and Sheng, M. Development of neuron–neuron synapses. *Curr. Opin. Neurobiol.* **10**, 125–31 (2000).

- Sanes, J. R. and Lichtman, J. W. Development of the vertebrate neuromuscular junction. *Annu. Rev. Neurosci.* **22**, 389–442 (1999).

- Serafini, T. Finding a partner in a crowd: neuronal diversity and synaptogenesis. *Cell* **98**, 133–6 (1999).

References

1. Sanes, J. R. and Lichtman, J. W. Development of the vertebrate neuromuscular junction. *Annu. Rev. Neurosci.* **22**, 389– 442 (1999).

2. Dennis, M. J., Ziskind Conhaim, L. and Harris, A. J. Development of neuromuscular junctions in rat embryos. *Dev. Biol.* **81**, 266–79 (1981).

3. Cohen, M. W. and Weldon, P. R. Localization of acetylcholine receptors and synaptic ultrastructure at nerve muscle contacts in culture: dependence on nerve type. *J. Cell Biol.* **86**, 388–401 (1980).

4. Chow, I. and Poo, M-m. Release of acetylcholine from embryonic neurons upon contact with muscle cell. *J. Neurosci.* **5**, 1076–82 (1985).

5. Anderson, M. J. and Cohen, M. W. Nerve-induced and spontaneous redistribution of acetylcholine receptors on cultured muscle cells. *J. Physiol. (London)* **268**, 757–73 (1977).

6. Young, S. H. and Poo, M-m. Spontaneous release of transmitter from growth cones of embryonic neurones. *Nature* **305**, 634–7 (1983).

7. Redfern, P. A. Neuromuscular transmission in newborn rats. *J. Physiol.* **209**, 701–9 (1970).

8. Brown, M. C., Jansen, J. K. S. and Van Essen, D. Polyneuronal innervation of skeletal muscle in new born rats and its elimination during maturation. *J. Physiol.* **261**, 387– 442 (1976).

9. Schuetze, S. M. and Role, L. W. Developmental regulation of the nicotinic acetylcholine receptor. *Annu. Rev. Neurosci.* **10**, 403–57 (1987).

10. Hall, Z. W. and Sanes, J. R. Synaptic structure and development: the neuromuscular junction. *Cell* **72**, 99–121 (1993).

11. Gautam, M. *et al.* Failure of postsynaptic specialization to develop at neuromuscular junctions of rapsyn-deficient mice. *Nature* **377**, 232–6 (1995).

12. Sanes, J. R. Genetic analysis of postsynaptic differentiation at the vertebrate neuromuscular junction. *Curr. Opin. Neurobiol.* **7**, 93–100 (1997).

13. Diamond, J. and Miledi, R. A study of foetal and new born rat muscle fibres. *J. Physiol.* **162**, 393–408 (1962).

14. Sanes, J. R. *et al.* Selective expression of an acetylcholine receptor-lacZ transgene in synaptic nuclei of adult muscle fibers. *Development* **113**, 1181–91 (1991).

15. Antony, C., Huchet, M., Changeux, J. P. and Cartaud, J. Developmental regulation of membrane traffic organisation during synaptogenesis in mouse diaphragm muscle. *J. Cell Biol.* **130**, 959–68 (1995).

16. Broadie, K. and Bate, M. Development of the embryonic neuromuscular synapse of *Drosophila melanogaster. J. Neurosci.* **13**, 144–66 (1993).

17. Dai, Z. and Peng, H. B. Elevation in presynaptic Ca^{2+} level accompanying initial nerve–muscle contact in tissue culture. *Neuron* **10**, 827–37 (1993).

18. Funte, L. R. and Haydon, P. G. Synaptic target contact enhances presynaptic calcium influx by activating cAMP-dependent protein kinase during synaptogenesis. *Neuron* **10**, 1069–78 (1993).

19. Kater, S. B., Mattson, M. P., Cohan, C. and Connor, J. Calcium regulation of the neuronal growth cone. *Trends Neurosci.* **11**, 315–21 (1988).

20. Kater, S. B. and Mills, L. R. Regulation of growth cone behavior by calcium. *J. Neurosci.* **11**, 891–9 (1991).

21. Bandtlow, C. E., Schmidt, M. F., Hassinger, T. D., Schwab, M. E. and Kater, S. B. Role of intracellular calcium in NI-35 evoked collapse of neuronal growth cones. *Science* **259**, 80–3 (1993).

22. Sanes, J. R., Marshall, L. M. and McMahan, U. J. Reinnervation of muscle fibre basal lamina after removal of myofibres. *J. Cell Biol.* **78**, 176–98 (1978).

23. Glicksman, M. A. and Sanes, J. R. Differentiation of motor nerve terminals formed in the absence of muscle fibres. *J. Neurocytol.* **12**, 666–77 (1983).

24. Doherty, P. and Walsh, F. S. Cell adhesion molecules, second messengers and axonal growth. *Curr. Opin. Neurobiol.* **2**, 595–601 (1992).

25. Moscoso, L. M., Cremer, H. and Sanes, J. R. Organization and reorganization of neuromuscular junctions in mice lacking neural cell adhesion molecule, tenascin-C, or fibroblast growth factor-5. *J. Neurosci.* **18**, 1465–77 (1998).

26. Hunter, D. D., Shah, V., Merlie, J. P. and Sanes, J. R. A laminin-like adhesive protein concentrated in the synaptic cleft of the neuromuscular junction. *Nature* **338**, 229–33 (1989).

27. Hunter, D. D. *et al.* An LRE (leucine-arginine-glutamate)- dependent mechanism for adhesion of neurons to S-laminin. *J. Neurosci.* **11**, 3960–71 (1991).

28. Porter, B. E., Weis, J. and Sanes, J. R. A motoneuron-selective stop signal in the synaptic protein S-laminin. *Neuron* **14**, 549–59 (1995).

29. Martin, P. T., Ettinger, A. S. and Sanes, J. R. A synaptic localisation domain in the specific cleft

protein laminin B2 (s-laminin). *Science* **269**, 413–16 (1995).

30. Noakes, P. G., Gautam, M., Mudd, J., Sanes, J. R. and Merlie, J. P. Aberrant differentiation of neuromuscular junctions in mice lacking s-laminin/laminin Beta2. *Nature* **374**, 258–62 (1995).

31. Patton, B. L., Chiu, A. Y. and Sanes, J. R. Synaptic laminin prevents glial entry into the synaptic cleft. *Nature* **393**, 698–701 (1998).

32. Campagna, J. A., Ruegg, M. A. and Bixby, J. L. Agrin is a differentiation-inducing 'stop signal' for motoneurons *in vitro*. *Neuron* **15**, 1365–74 (1995).

33. Kopozynski, C. C., Davis, G. W. and Goodman, C. S. A neural tetraspanin, encoded by late bloomer, that facilitates synapse formation. *Science* **271**, 1867–70 (1996).

34. Schuster, C. M., Davis, G. W., Fetter, R. D. and Goodman, C. S. Genetic dissection of structural and functional components of synaptic plasticity. I. Fasciclin II controls synaptic stabilization and growth. *Neuron* **17**, 641–54 (1996).

35. Schuster, C. M., Davis, G. W., Fetter, R. D. and Goodman, C. S. Genetic dissection of structural and functional components of synaptic plasticity. II. Fasciclin II controls presynaptic structural plasticity. *Neuron* **17**, 655–67 (1996).

36. Davis, G. W., Schuster, C. M. and Goodman, C. S. Genetic dissection of structural and functional components of synaptic plasticity. III. CREB is necessary for presynaptic functional plasticity. *Neuron* **17**, 669–79 (1996).

37. Martin, K. C. and Kandel, E. R. Cell adhesion molecules, CREB, and the formation of new synaptic connections. *Neuron* **17**, 567–74 (1996).

38. Tetzlaff, W., Bisby, M. A. and Kreutzberg, G. W. Changes in cytoskeletal proteins in the rat facial nucleus following axotomy. *J. Neurosci.* **8**, 3181–9 (1988).

39. Ishii, D. N. Relationship of insulin-like growth factor II gene expression in muscle to synaptogenesis. *Proc. Natl. Acad. Sci. USA* **86**, 2898–902 (1989).

40. Caroni, P. and Becker, M. The down-regulation of growth- associated proteins in motoneurons at the onset of synapse elimination is controlled by muscle activity and IGF1. *J. Neurosci.* **12**, 3849–61 (1992).

41. Lasek, R. J. and Black, M. M. How do axons stop growing? Some clues from the metabolism of the proteins in the slow component of axonal transport. In *Mechanisms of regulation and special functions of protein synthesis* (ed. S. Roberts) (Elsevier, 1977).

42. Hollenbeck, P. J. and Bray, D. Rapidly transported organelles containing membrane and cytoskeletal components: their relation to axonal growth. *J. Cell Biol.* **105**, 2827–35 (1987).

43. Xie, Z. P. and Poo, M. M. Initial events in the formation of neuromuscular synapse: rapid induction of acetylcholine release from embryonic neuron. *Proc. Natl. Acad. Sci. USA* **83**, 7069–72 (1986).

44. Harish, O. E. and Poo, M. Retrograde modulation at developing neuromuscular synapses: involvement of G protein and arachidonic acid cascade. *Neuron* **9**, 1201–9 (1992).

45. Lohof, A. M., Ip, N. Y. and Poo, M. Potentiation of developing neuromuscular synapses by the neurotrophins NT3 and BDNF. *Nature* **363**, 350–3 (1993).

46. Lindsay, R. M. Neurobiology: neuron saving schemes. *Nature* **373**, 289–90 (1995).

47. Pennica, D. *et al.* Cardiotrophin-1, a cytokine present in embryonic muscle, supports long-term survival of spinal motonoeurons. *Neuron* **17**, 63–74 (1996).

48. Sendtner, M. *et al.* Cryptic physiological trophic support of motoneurons by LIF revealed by double gene targetting of CNTF and LIF. *Curr. Biol.* **6**, 686–94 (1996).

49. Ebens, A. *et al.* Hepatocyte growth factor/scatter factor is an axonal chemoattractant and a neurotrophic factor for spinal motor neurons. *Neuron* **17**, 1157–72 (1996).

50. Funakoshi, H. *et al.* Muscle- derived neurotrophin-4 as an activity-dependent trophic signal for adult motor neurons. *Science* **268**, 1495–9 (1995).

51. Oppenheim, R. W. Neurotrophic survival molecules for motoneurons: an embarrassment of riches. *Neuron* **17**, 195–7 (1996).

52. Lomo, T. and Westgaard, R. H. Control of acetylcholine sensitivity in rat muscle fibres. *Cold Spring Harbor Symp. Quant. Biol.* **40**, 263–74 (1976).

53. Klarsfeld, A. *et al.* Regulation of muscle AChR Alpha subunit gene expression by electrical activity: involvement of protein kinase C and Ca^{2+}. *Neuron* **2**, 1229–36 (1989).

54. Huang, C. F., Tong, J. and Schmidt, J. Protein kinase C couples membrane excitation to acetylcholine receptor gene inactivation in chick skeletal muscle. *Neuron* **9**, 671–8 (1992).

55. Witzemann, V. and Sakmann, B. Differential regulation of MyoD and myogenin mRNA levels by nerve induced muscle activity. *FEBS Lett.* **282**, 259–64 (1991).

56. Lomo, T. and Slater, C. R. Control of junctional acetylcholinesterase by neural and muscular influences in the rat. *J. Physiol.* **303**, 191–202 (1980).

57. Weldon, P. R., Moody Corbett, F. and Cohen, M. W. Ultrastructure of sites of cholinesterase activity on amphibian embryonic muscle cells cultured without nerve. *Dev. Biol.* **84**, 341–50 (1981).

58. Fuentes, M. E. and Taylor, P. Control of acetylcholinesterase gene expression during myogenesis. *Neuron* **10**, 679-87 (1993).

59. Massoulie, J. and Bon, S. The molecular forms of cholinesterase in vertebrates. *Annu. Rev. Neurosci.* **5**, 57-106 (1982).

60. Lomo, T., Massoulie, J. and Vigny, M. Stimulation of denervated rat soleus muscle with fast and slow activity patterns induces different expression of acetylcholinesterase molecular forms. *J. Neurosci.* **5**, 1180-7 (1985).

61. Ruegg, M. A. and Bixby, J. L. Agrin orchestrates synaptic differentiation at the vertebrate neuromuscular junction. *Trends Neurosci.* **21**, 22-7 (1998).

62. Cohen, M. W. and Godfrey, E. W. Early appearance of and neuronal contribution to agrin-like molecules at embryonic frog nerve-muscle synapses formed in culture. *J. Neurosci.* **12**, 2982-92 (1992).

63. Kleiman, R. J. and Reichardt, L. F. Testing the agrin hypothesis. *Cell* **85**, 461-4 (1996).

64. Reist, N. E., Werle, M. J. and McMahan, U. J. Agrin released by motor neurons induces the aggregation of acetylcholine receptors at neuromuscular junctions. *Neuron* **8**, 865-8 (1992).

65. Gautam, M. *et al.* Defective neuromuscular synaptogenesis in agrin-deficient mutant mice. *Cell* **85**, 525-36 (1996).

66. Meier, T. *et al.* Neural agrin induces ectopic postsynaptic specializations in innervated muscle fibers. *J. Neurosci.* **17**, 6534-44 (1997).

67. DeChiara, T. M. *et al.* The receptor tyrosine kinase MuSK is required for neuromuscular junction formation *in vivo. Cell* **85**, 501-12 (1996).

68. Glass, D. J. *et al.* Agrin acts via a MuSK receptor complex. *Cell* **85**, 513-24 (1996).

69. Martin, P. T. and Sanes, J. R. Role for a synapse-specific carbohydrate in agrin-induced clustering of acetylcholine receptors. *Neuron* **14**, 743-54 (1995).

70. Apel, E. D., Glass, D. J., Moscoso, L. M., Yancopoulos, G. D. and Sanes, J. R. Rapsyn is required for MuSK signaling and recruits synaptic components to a MuSK-containing scaffold. *Neuron* **18**, 623-35 (1997).

71. Fallon, J. R. and Hall, Z. W. Building synapses: agrin and dystroglycan stick together. *Trends Neurosci.* **17**, 469-73 (1994).

72. Ohlendieck, K. *et al.* Dystrophin-related protein is localized to neuromuscular junctions of adult skeletal muscle. *Neuron* **7**, 499-508 (1991).

73. Broadie, K. M. and Bate, M. Activity-dependent development of the neuromuscular synapse during *Drosophila* embryogenesis. *Neuron* **11**, 607-19 (1993).

74. Keshishian, H., Broadie, K., Chiba, A. and Bate, M. The *Drosophila* neuromuscular junction: a model system for studying synaptic development and function. *Annu. Rev. Neurosci.* **19**, 545-75 (1996).

75. Falls, D. L., Rosen, K. M., Corfas, G., Lane, W. S. and Fischbach, G. D. ARIA, a protein that stimulates acetylcholine receptor synthesis, is a member of the neu ligand family. *Cell* **72**, 801-15 (1993).

76. Jo, S. A., Zhu, X., Marchionni, M. A. and Burden, S. J. Neuregulins are concentrated at nerve-muscle synapses and activate ACh-receptor gene expression. *Nature* **373**, 158-61 (1995).

77. New, H. V. and Mudge, A. W. Calcitonin gene-related peptide regulates muscle acetylcholine receptor synthesis. *Nature* **323**, 809-11 (1986).

78. Laufer, R. and Changeux, J. P. Calcitonin gene-related peptide elevates cyclic AMP levels in chick skeletal muscle: possible neurotrophic role for a coexisting neuronal messenger. *EMBO J.* **6**, 901-6 (1987).

79. Bennett, M. R. The formation of synapses in striated muscle during development. *J. Physiol.* **241**, 515-45 (1974).

80. Lomo, T. What controls the development of neuromuscular junctions? *Trends Neurosci.* **3**, 126-9 (1980).

81. Bennett, M. R., McClachlan, E. M. and Taylor, R. S. The formation of synapses in reinnervated mammalian striated muscle. *J. Physiol.* **233**, 481-500 (1973).

82. Kuffler, S. W. and Vaughan-Williams, E. M. Small-nerve junction potentials. The distribution of small motor nerves to frog skeletal muscle, and the membrane characteristics of the fibres they innervate. *J. Physiol.* **121**, 289-317 (1953).

83. Gordon, T., Perry, R., Tuffery, A. R. and Vrbova, G. Possible mechanisms determining synapse formation in developing skeletal muscles of the chick. *Cell Tissue Res.* **155**, 13-25 (1974).

84. Hunt, S. P. The development of neurotransmitter receptors. In *The making of the nervous system* (ed. J. G. Parnevalas, C. Stern and R. V. Stirling), pp. 454-72 (Oxford University Press, 1988).

85. Baude, A. *et al.* The metabotropic glutamate receptor (mGluR1 alpha) is concentrated at perisynaptic membrane of neuronal subpopulations as detected by immunogold reaction. *Neuron* **11**, 771-87 (1993).

86. Cherubini, E., Gaiarsa, J. L. and Ben-Ari, Y. GABA: an excitatory transmitter in early postnatal life. *Trends Neurosci.* **14**, 515-19 (1991).

87. Davis, G. W. The making of a synapse:target-derived signals and presynaptic differentiation. *Neuron* **26**, 551-4 (2000).

88. Lee, S. H. and Sheng, M. Development of neuron–neuron synapses. *Curr. Opin. Neurobiol.* **10**, 125–31 (2000).

89. Verhage, M. *et al.* Synaptic assembly of the brain in the absence of neurotransmitter secretion. *Science* **287**, 864–9 (2000).

90. Vaughn, J. E., Henrikson, C. K. and Grieshaber, J. A. A quantitative study of synapses on motor neuron dendritic growth cones in developing mouse spinal cord. *J. Cell Biol.* **60**, 664–72 (1974).

91. Rakic, R. and Sidman, R. L. Organization of cerebellar cortex secondary to deficit of granule cells in Weaver mutant mice. *J. Comp. Neurol.* **152**, 133–62 (1973).

92. Hinds, J. W. and Hinds, P. L. Synapse formation in the mouse olfactory bulb. II. Morphogenesis. *J. Comp. Neurol.* **169**, 41–62 (1976).

93. Dailey, M. E. and Smith, S. J. The dynamics of dendritic structure in developing hippocampal slices. *J. Neurosci.* **16**, 2983–94 (1996).

94. Wong, W. T. and Wong, R. O. L. Rapid dendritic movements during synapse formation and rearrangement. *Curr. Opin. Neurobiol.* **10**, 118–24 (2000).

95. Miyashiro, K., Dichter, M. and Eberwine, J. On the nature and differential distribution of mRNAs in hippocampal neurites: implications for neuronal functioning. *Proc. Natl. Acad. Sci. USA* **91**, 10800–4 (1994).

96. Steward, O. Targeting of mRNAs to subsynaptic microdomains in dendrites. *Curr. Opin. Neurobiol.* **5**, 55–61 (1995).

97. Srinivasan, Y., Guzikowski, A. P., Haughland, R. P. and Angelides, K. J. Distribution and lateral mobility of glycine receptors on cultured spinal cord neurons. *J. Neurosci.* **10**, 985–95 (1990).

98. Mendell, L. M., Collins, W. F. and Munson, J. B. Retrograde determination of motoneuron properties and their synaptic input. *J. Neurobiol.* **25**, 707–21 (1994).

99. Nastuk, M. A. and Fallon, J. R. Agrin and the molecular choreography of synapse formation. *Trends Neurosci.* **16**, 72–6 (1993).

100. Kroger, S., Horton, S. E. and Honig, L. S. The developing avian retina expresses agrin isoforms during synaptogenesis. *J. Neurobiol.* **29**, 165–82 (1996).

101. Ozaki, M., Sasner, M., Yano, R., Lu, H. S. and Buonanno, A. Neuregulin-beta induces expression of an NMDA-receptor subunit. *Nature* **390**, 691–4 (1997).

102. Redies, C. and Takeichi, M. Cadherins in the developing central nervous system: an adhesive code for segmental and functional subdivisions. *Dev. Biol.* **180**, 413–23 (1996).

103. Fannon, A. M. and Colman, D. R. A model for central synaptic junctional complex formation based on the differential adhesive specificities of the cadherins. *Neuron* **17**, 423–34 (1996).

104. Wu, Q. and Maniatis, T. A striking organization of a large family of human neural cadherin-like cell adhesion genes. *Cell* **97**, 779–90 (1999).

105. Serafini, T. Finding a partner in a crowd: neuronal diversity and synaptogenesis. *Cell* **98**, 133–6 (1999).

106. Hall, A. C., Lucas, F. R. and Salinas, P. C. Axonal remodeling and synaptic differentiation in the cerebellum is regulated by WNT-7a signaling. *Cell* **100**, 525–35 (2000).

107. Scheiffele, P., Fan, J., Choih, J., Fetter, R. and Serafini, T. Neuroligin expressed in nonneuronal cells triggers presynaptic development in contacting axons. *Cell* **101**, 657–69 (2000).

108. Monyer, H., Seeburg, P. H. and Wisden, W. Glutamate-operated channels: developmentally early and mature forms arise by alternative splicing. *Neuron* **6**, 799–810 (1991).

12

Neurotrophic Factors and their Receptors

For many aspects of their development and normal physiology, neurons are dependent on a small group of highly specific proteins known as neurotrophic factors, which are secreted by other neurons, glial cells and target tissues. Principal roles of neurotrophic factors include the regulation of axonal and dendritic growth, synaptic plasticity and neuronal survival. These wide-ranging functions mean that neurotrophic factors feature in many other chapters where their particular roles are described in detail. This chapter gives an overall summary of these growth factors and the receptors to which they bind to bring about their effects.

The developmental activity of neurotrophic factors was first deduced in the 1930s by Hamburger, who observed that changing the size of a target field by ablating a limb bud, or by grafting a supernumerary limb bud to the flank of a chick embryo, produced a corresponding decline or increase in the number of related dorsal root ganglion neurons and motor neurons.[1,2] It was then found that heterologous tissue, such as mouse sarcomas, could stimulate the growth of sympathetic ganglia when implanted into chick embryos.[3] These were important observations, but what led to the eventual isolation of the first neurotrophic factor was neither limb bud nor sarcoma tissue itself, which contain vanishingly small quantities, but snake venom. Used as a source of phosphodiesterase enzymes during attempts to characterize the active agent in the sarcoma, the venom turned out to have an even stronger neurotrophic action. It was then found that the mammalian homologue of the snake venom gland, the submandibular salivary gland, especially that of adult male mice, was an even richer source of activity. Although the synthesis of huge quantities of neurotrophic factor and its secretion in venom or saliva (also prostatic fluid) remains an enigma, this rich source led to purification of the protein itself, which was named the nerve growth factor or NGF.[4,5] The importance of NGF as a survival factor for sympathetic neurons was later demonstrated by making an antiserum to the purified protein and injecting it into neonatal rats. This experiment resulted in the death of all sympathetic ganglion cells; in effect an immunosympathectomy.[6]

Since the discovery of NGF half a century ago, techniques have been developed to detect the minute amounts of mRNA and protein present in the cells that synthesize NGF, and both receptors and signalling pathways have been identified, thereby elucidating the mode of action of NGF. During this time, many more proteins in addition to NGF have been shown to promote neuronal survival. These include proteins related to NGF, namely brain-derived neurotrophic factor (BDNF), neurotrophin-3 (NT-3) and neurotrophin-4 (NT-4), collectively known as the neurotrophins, and other factors unrelated to NGF. Among the latter is a family of proteins related to the glial-cell-derived neurotrophic factor (GDNF, neurturin, artemin and persephin), the neurotrophic cytokines related to interleukin-6 (IL-6, CNTF, LIF, OSM, CT-1) and hepatocyte growth factor (HGF). These individual families will now be considered in turn, followed by more general discussion of their diverse functions.

The neurotrophins

The neurotrophins are a family of structurally related, secreted proteins that have a profound influence on the development and functioning of the nervous system.[7] During development, they promote the survival of neuronal subsets of both peripheral[7-10] and central nervous systems,[11-13] and support adult neurons whose axons have been damaged.[14] In addition to their survival-promoting effects, neurotrophins regulate neuronal differentiation[15-18] and promote neurite extension and branching.[19,20] Reduced neuronal survival and deficits in morphological differentiation can lead to abnormal formation of brain regions such as the cerebellum.[13] In the mature nervous system, neurotrophins can regulate both short-term synaptic transmission and long-term potentiation, a form of synaptic plasticity that is used as a model for learning and memory.[20,21]

Neurotrophin Trk receptors

Most of the biological effects of neurotrophin signalling are thought to be mediated by the Trk family of tyrosine kinase receptors.[22] Trks are transmembrane glycoproteins that possess an intracellular region containing the catalytic tyrosine kinase (TK) domain and an extracellular, ligand-binding region with a complex subdomain organization.[23] Expression studies in cell lines have shown that TrkA is a receptor for NGF, TrkB is a receptor for BDNF and NT-4, and TrkC is a receptor for NT-3. NT-3 is also able to bind and signal less efficiently via TrkA and TrkB in cell lines[24] and developing neurons.[25] Null mutation of the *TrkA*, *TrkB* and *TrkC* genes in mice causes distinctive neuronal deficiencies that are similar to those observed in mice with null mutations in the *NGF*, *BDNF* and *NT-3* genes respectively (see below), suggesting that Trks mediate the survival-promoting actions of neurotrophins on developing neurons *in vivo*. Consistent with activation of both TrkA and TrkB receptors by NT-3, the neuronal deficiencies of $NT3^{-/-}$ mice are more severe than those of $TrkC^{-/-}$ mice.[26-28]

TrkB and TrkC variants lacking the TK domain are widely expressed by non-neu-ronal cells and by some neurons.[29-33] These non-catalytic receptors are thought to play a role in limiting the diffusion of their ligands,[31] and TK⁻ TrkB may act as a negative modulator of BDNF signalling at certain stages of sensory neuron development.[33]

Trk receptor tyrosine kinases undergo rapid transphosphorylation following ligand binding, leading to a cascade of intracellular protein phosphorylation. Although it remains uncertain how Trk receptors activate the different signalling pathways presumed necessary to mediate the diverse functions of neurotrophins, studies using the pheochromocytoma cell line PC12 have elucidated how neurotrophins, particu-larly NGF, promote neurite outgrowth and cell survival.[34-36] Upon binding NGF, TrkA receptors autophosphorylate on tyrosine residues, allowing these to become docking sites for intracellular signalling proteins. Shc adaptor proteins, ShcA, ShcB/SCK, and ShcC/N-Shc,[37,38] associate directly with a specific site in Trk receptors and activate a signalling pathway involving the small GTPase Ras, the serine/threonine kinase Raf, the dual specificity kinase mitogen- and extracellular-regulated kinase (Mek), and mitogen-activated protein kinase (MAPK), also called extracellular signal-regulated kinases (ERKs).[34] Activated ERKs and possibly other components of this pathway then activate transcription factors that regulate neurotrophin-specific gene expression. One important downstream target of neurotrophin signalling is the *bcl-2* gene family, and MAP kinase activation has been shown to upregulate expression of *bcl-2* in sympathetic neurons (via the transcription factor CREB, see below).[39] As discussed further in the next chapter, neurons (like all cells) are programmed to self-destruct through an intrinsic suicide programme, and their survival depends on the inhibition of this programme by neurotrophic signals from associated cells via regulation of *bcl-2* family genes. These play a key role in the regulation of cell death via mitochondrial release of cytochrome *c* and activation of the caspase cascade.

Neuronal survival also appears to depend on phosphatidylinositol-3 (PI-3) kinase signalling,[40] and a further important Trk effector is phospholipase Cγ1 (PLCγ1), which stimulates the release of intracellular Ca^{2+} and thereby activates the tran-scription factor CREB (cyclic AMP response element binding protein) via phosphor-ylation by calcium/calmodulin-dependent kinases.[41] CREB may be an important mediator of neurotrophin-induced synaptic changes.[20,42] PLCγ1 also induces activa-tion of MAPK and appears to cooperate with the Shc signalling pathway in inducing neurite outgrowth of PC12 cells.[43,44] Despite these several observations, the relative importance of these signalling pathways in mediating the diverse functions of neu-rotrophins *in vivo* remains unclear.

Different populations of neurons have distinctive requirements for particular neurotrophins at specific stages of their development[7,45,46] and some neurons switch their neurotrophin requirements from one ligand to another during development.[47] There is considerable evidence that the onset and changes in responsiveness to a particular neurotrophin correlate with increase in the expression of the corres-ponding Trk receptor.[33,47] Thus, elucidating what regulates neurotrophin receptor expression is a key element in understanding how trophic interactions are coordi-nated in the developing nervous system.

The low-affinity neurotrophin receptor p75^{NTR}

Besides their high-affinity Trk receptors, all neurotrophins bind to a common low-affinity neurotrophin receptor p75^{NTR}, a transmembrane glycoprotein with varied and paradoxical functions. In neurons that coexpress high-affinity Trk receptors, p75^{NTR} signalling selectively enhances responsiveness to some neurotrophins while decreasing responsiveness to others. This has emerged from in vitro studies of neurons obtained from p75^{NTR} null mutant mice and studies using mutated neurotrophins that have altered binding affinity for p75^{NTR}.[47] For example, p75^{NTR} enhances the sensitivity of TrkA-expressing neurons to the survival-promoting effects of NGF,[48,49] while decreasing their sensitivity to NT-3,[50,51] and plays a role in ligand discrimination by TrkB. Direct interaction between p75^{NTR} and Trk receptors, together with changes in ligand affinity and Trk signalling, accounts at least in part for these effects of p75^{NTR},[35] although there is some evidence that p75^{NTR}-mediated NF-κB activation plays a role in enhancing the survival response of developing sensory neurons to NGF.[52]

In the absence of Trk signalling, p75^{NTR} mediates an apoptotic response to NGF and BDNF by some neurons and other cell types.[53–56] This is discussed below.

GDNF and relatives

The TGFβ-related proteins GDNF, neurturin, persephin and artemin have neurotrophic activity on several types of peripheral and central neurons. The best characterized of these molecules is GDNF, which promotes the survival of motor neurons[57–59] and subpopulations of dopaminergic,[60] cholinergic[61] and noradrenergic CNS neurons,[62] together with subsets of sensory, sympathetic, parasympathetic and enteric neurons.[63–65] Neurturin and artemin promote the survival of a variety of PNS neurons[66,67] and persephin supports both midbrain dopaminergic neurons and motor neurons.[68] Although most neuronal survival data have come from in vitro studies, the important physiological relevance of GDNF for the survival of motor neurons has been substantiated by an appreciable reduction in the number of these cells in GDNF$^{-/-}$ mice (see also below).[69]

GDNF, neurturin, persephin and artemin act through multicomponent receptors that consist of a common signalling component, the Ret receptor tyrosine kinase,[70,71] together with one of a set of GPI-linked coreceptors (GFRα-1, -2, -3, -4), which confer ligand specificity: Ret/GFRα-1 is the preferred receptor for GDNF,[72] Ret/GFRα-2 for neurturin,[73,74] Ret/GFRα-3 for artemin[67] and Ret/GFRα-4 for persephin.[75,76]

Ret and the GFRα receptors have distinctive patterns of expression that accord with the known responses of neurons and other cells to their ligands. Although the mechanisms that regulate the regional and dynamic changes in the expression of these receptors in the developing nervous system are unclear, receptor expression and responsiveness have been linked to neural activity.[77]

CNTF and relatives

Ciliary neurotrophic factor (CNTF), leukaemia inhibitory factor (LIF), cardiotrophin-1 (CT-1) and interleukin-6 (IL-6) comprise a family of cytokines that have multiple actions on cells of the nervous system and promote the survival of various kinds of neurons during development.[78] Although there is less than 15 per cent amino acid sequence identity between these factors, they share several structural features and signal via oligomeric receptor complexes that have one or more components in common.[79] The transmembrane glycoproteins gp130 and LIFRβ are common components of the receptor complexes for CNTF, LIF, OSM and CT-1. The CNTF receptor complex has an additional GPI-linked CNTFRα subunit, and the IL-6 receptor consists of two gp130 subunits and an IL-6Rα subunit. Binding of these cytokines to their receptor complexes results in the activation of several signalling pathways, including the JAK-Stat, PI-3 kinase, Ras/MAP kinase, and PLC-γ pathways. Recent studies have shown that NF-κB activation plays a major role in mediating the survival response of some cranial sensory neurons to neurotrophic cytokines.[80] One of the key functions of CNTF is thought to be the trophic support of a subset of motor neurons whose survival is not promoted by HGF.[81,82]

HGF

Hepatocyte growth factor (HGF) is a secreted protein that exerts a variety of effects on many cell types, including neurons and glial cells, by binding to the Met receptor tyrosine kinase.[83] First known for its stimulatory effects on the dissociation and dispersal of epithelial sheets (from which it acquired the synonym 'scatter factor'), HGF is also expressed by both neural cells and neuronal target tissues[84–87] and plays a role in both axon guidance and neuronal survival.[88] Thus HGF, which is released by striated muscle, can exert a chemoattractant effect on spinal motor axons[89] and, possibly synergizing with CNTF, supports the survival of a subset of motor neurons in culture.[81] HGF also enhances survival and neurite growth of DRG neurons cultured with NGF,[85,86] and promotes the survival of both sympathetic[86] and TH-positive midbrain neurons.[90]

Although HGF uses a different receptor, it shares several downstream effectors with CNTF. Binding to the Met receptor results in the activation of signalling pathways that include STAT, JNK kinase, Src tyrosine kinase, Ras/MAP kinase, PI-3 kinase and PLC-γ. Convergence of HGF and CNTF signalling at one or more of these downstream effectors could explain an observed synergy between HGF and CNTF in the survival promotion of some neurons.[81,82]

Functions of neurotrophic factors

Each neurotrophic factor promotes the survival of a particular set of neurons during development, but it may have additional functions within the nervous system or other tissues. These may operate, moreover, not only during development but also in the adult state. As currently known, the functions of neurotrophic factors are as follows:

1. Regulating the amount of cell death in neural populations soon after their axons first make synaptic contact with their targets; this is done by preventing apoptosis in those neurons able to obtain adequate amounts of specific trophic factors, which are usually present in only limited amounts (see Chapter 13). This is the classic, first documented, function of neurotrophic factors.

2. In some neural populations, controlling the numbers of neuroblasts at an earlier stage in development, including regulation of neuroblast proliferation and triggering of apoptosis;

3. Controlling the proliferation and survival of some glial cell precursor populations (see Chapter 6);

4. Determining the phenotype of some developing sensory and autonomic neurons (see Chapter 5);

5. Regulating the growth of some axons during development (see Chapter 9);

6. Controlling the physiological sensitivity of some adult primary sensory neurons;

7. Regulating synaptic transmission and plasticity in the postnatal and adult nervous system (see Chapters 14 and 15);

8. Acting as survival factors for axotomized neurons, and as agents that promote regeneration of cut axons and trigger collateral sprouting from axons of intact neurons in partly denervated tissues (see Chapter 17).

Role of neurotrophic factors in regulating cell death

The general phenomenon of neuronal death and its molecular mechanism are discussed in more detail in Chapter 13. Following the classical approaches to investigating the function of NGF (see above), the roles of neurotrophic factors and their receptors in determining neuronal survival *in vivo* have been investigated extensively in more recent years by gene manipulation experiments in mice. These have confirmed many of the suspected trophic dependencies, particularly those of peripheral ganglionic neurons on members of the neurotrophin family (Table 12.1; see reference 46 for review). Typically, deletion of individual neurotrophin genes causes the loss of particular classes of peripheral neuron, and the degree of depletion is dependent on gene dosage. Conversely, when the same neurotrophins are overexpressed or administered exogenously, the corresponding neurons are

Table 12.1

Neurotrophic factor	Notes	Receptors	Neuronal losses in ligand- and/or receptor-deprived mice
NGF Nerve growth factor	First to be isolated by tissue extraction from mouse salivary glands as a survival factor for sympathetic neurons. Antibodies given to neonates cause immunosympathectomy	TrkA p75^{NTR}	Sympathetic neurons Pain- and temperature-sensitive DRG and trigeminal ganglion neurons
BDNF Brain-derived neurotrophic factor (NT-4 similar)	Purified from brain as a survival factor for some sensory neurons. Hard to make antibodies. Sequencing shows relationship to NGF	TrkB p75^{NTR}	Touch-sensitive DRG and trigeminal ganglion neurons Heavy sensory loss in nodose and vestibular ganglion. Some loss of cochlear neurons
NT-3 Neurotrophin-3	First to be isolated using molecular biological methods (low stringency hybridization search for mRNA related to NGFmRNA)	TrkC p75^{NTR}	Muscle proprioceptive and skin slowly adapting mechanosensitive DRG neurons. Cochlear neurons
GDNF Glial cell-derived neurotrophic factor	Extracted from brain glial cell line as a survival factor for midbrain dopaminergic neurons	GDNFR c-ret	Nodose ganglion cells Some DRG, SCG, spinal cord and enteric neurons
CNTF Ciliary neurotrophic factor	Survival factor for parasympathetic ciliary ganglion neurons	gp130 LIFR CNTFR	Some facial motor neurons Some spinal motor neurons
LIF Leukaemia inhibitory factor	Extracted cholinergic induction factor for some neural crest cells turns out to be identical to previously known haemopoietic factor	gp130 LIFR	Some facial motor neurons Some spinal motor neurons

rescued. Such studies confirm that supplies of neurotrophins can be limiting *in vivo*, at least for some neuron populations, and a good example is provided by the targeted deletion of the *NGF* or *TrkA* genes, in which approximately 80 per cent of DRG neurons are lost.[16,91] The targeted gene approach has also revealed the subtlety of the molecular details of neurotrophin signalling: both BDNF and NT-4 activate a single high-affinity receptor, TrkB, yet mutation of its Shc-binding site predominantly affects NT-4-dependent sensory neurons rather than BDNF-dependent neurons. This implies divergent, ligand-dependent signalling events downstream of TrkB activation.[92]

Critical roles for individual neurotrophic factors in the CNS have been harder to establish. This may reflect the functional complexity of CNS, where a population of neurons that appears at first sight to be anatomically homogeneous in fact comprises subpopulations with heterogeneous afferent inputs and synaptic targets. Motor neurons provide a good example here. As judged from studies of null mutant mice, no single trophic factor controls the survival of all motor neurons, but mutants for CNTF, GDNF or LIF, or their receptors, do lack significant numbers of motor neurons. In the case of GDNF,[57] for example, survival of spinal and cranial motor neurons is reduced in GDNF-deficient mice and enhanced in animals expressing increased levels of GDNF. Many motor neurons are GDNF-independent, however, and these may require other GDNF family members (e.g. neurturin, persephin, artemin), acting through different receptor combinations, or represent neurons (such as certain eye muscle motor neurons) that have an alternative trophic dependency.[93] Again, HGF is a further survival factor for somatic motor neurons in the chick embryo, but only for the lumbar population.[94]

It seems likely that there is considerable molecular redundancy in the trophic support of central neurons, even for apparently homogenous neuronal populations. Individual neurons may obtain distinct trophic molecules from different synaptic partners and from glial cells.[95] This may explain why, for example, midbrain dopaminergic neurons are present in normal numbers in GDNF-deficient mice despite the demonstrable survival-promoting action of GDNF on these neurons *in vitro*.[69] Motor neurons again provide a further example here, for the majority have been shown to die in the absence of either muscle or Schwann cells.[96] It should also be borne in mind that the consequences of gene knockout may not be straightforward to interpret because of indirect effects. Thus, small-diameter (γ) motor neurons are depleted in NT-3-deficient mice,[97] but this may result from the absence of their target muscle spindles in these animals (Table 1) rather than a direct effect NT-3 deficiency on this subclass of spinal motor neuron.

Control of neuroblast and glial cell numbers by neurotrophic factors

Several studies suggest that neurotrophic factors not only sustain a proportion of neurons after target innervation but also regulate the size of neuroblast populations at earlier stages of development. For example, mice lacking the GDNF receptor, c-RET, have early losses of neuroblasts from a subpopulation of hindbrain neural crest cells, resulting in the complete absence of intestinal enteric neurons and of neurons in the superior cervical ganglion (see also Chapter 5).[69] Similarly, sensory ganglion pre-cursor cells stop dividing prematurely in NT-3-deficient mice, implying that NT-3 acts normally to prevent precocious neuronal differentiation by maintaining presumptive neuroblasts in the cell cycle.[28] NT-3 has also been shown to increase the number of motor neurons that differentiate from progenitor cells in the developing spinal cord.[98]

As described in Chapter 13, a striking example of neuroblast regulation by a neu-rotrophin has been identified in the chick retina, where some retinal ganglion cells die before sending axons into the optic nerve. Antibodies to NGF or the low-affinity NGF receptor, p75^{NTR}, greatly attenuate this normal developmental process when delivered during the third embryonic day. The cells that die express only the p75^{NTR} and not the high-affinity Trk receptors, suggesting that NGF may trigger the death of developing neurons when acting through p75^{NTR} alone. This action is, of course, diametrically opposite to the classical survival-promoting function of neuro-trophic factors, and it has also been described *in vitro* in proprioceptive and sympa-thetic neurons and oligodendrocytes, and *in vivo* in the developing spinal cord, sympathetic ganglia and cholinergic basal forebrain nuclei.[99] The p75^{NTR} belongs to a family of molecules that includes the tumour necrosis factor receptors 1 and 2, some of which contain the short cytoplasmic 'death domain' (see Chapter 13). However, precisely how NGF triggers apoptosis via the p75^{NTR} is uncertain.[99] NRIF, a recently identified protein that interacts with the intracellular domain of p75^{NTR}, appears to be involved in transducing the death signal because the reduced cell death observed in the developing retina of *nrif*$^{-/-}$ mice is quantitatively indistinguishable from that seen in *p75*$^{NTR-/-}$ and *ngf*$^{-/-}$ mice (see Fig. 12.1).[100]

Control of the phenotype of some developing sensory and autonomic neurons

A further function of neurotrophic factors is to regulate neuronal phenotype, and this can be illustrated by diverse examples.[101] Thus, NGF diverts sympathoadrenal pre-cursor cells into the sympathetic neuronal lineage rather than adrenal chromaffin cells; anti-NGF treatment during early postnatal life in rats and mice converts high-threshold mechanoreceptors into hair afferents, and mechano/heat-sensitive neurons into pressure-sensitive neurons; LIF and CNTF can convert adrenergic sympathetic neurons into cholinergic neurons (see Chapter 5); and GABAergic cerebral cortical neurons require BDNF to coexpress neuropeptide Y. It is clear, then, that neuro-trophic factors have diverse actions during early neural development, influencing differentiation as well as survival and proliferation.

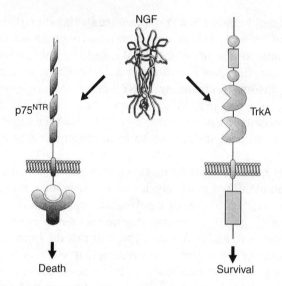

Figure 12.1 Nerve growth factor (NGF) can exert different effects on target neurons depending on the receptor to which it binds. NGF can prevent the death of neurons expressing the high-affinity receptor tyrosine kinase TrkA, whereas it can alternatively promote the death of TrkA-negative neurons that express the low-affinity pan-neurotrophin receptor p75^{NTR}. Signalling through p75^{NTR} requires the binding of cytoplasmic proteins, such as the neurotrophin receptor interacting factor (NRIF). The biologically active NGF molecule is a dimer of two identical B subunits. After Dechant and Barde.[123]

Regulation of axon growth during development

One of the most striking actions of the neurotrophins, and the property for which NGF was named and on which assays for activity have classically been based, is the promotion of neurite growth. Numerous studies of sensory and sympathetic neurons have shown that the local availability of NGF enhances neurite extension *in vitro* and influences the extent of terminal axonal branching and dendritic complexity *in vivo*.[102,103] NGF can also act as an axonal chemoattractant experimentally, both *in vitro*[104,105] and *in vivo*,[106] so the expression of neurotrophins in target areas could provide directional guidance for innervating axons. A good example, also discussed in Chapter 9, concerns the chemoattractive activity for trigeminal sensory axons secreted by the epithelium of the maxillary branchial arch, identified in part as a combination of BDNF and NT-3.[107] The initial trajectory of trigeminal axons is normal in mice deficient for both NT-3 and BDNF, so a direct role for neurotrophins in the guidance of these axons in the maxillary arch *in vivo* seems unlikely, but they might provide a supplementary growth stimulus.[107] At present there is no clear evidence that neurotrophic factors provide guidance cues for axons en route to their targets, but they may stimulate target invasion and terminal axonal branching when axons reach their target areas. One clear case is provided by the sympathetic innervation of the pineal gland, which is regulated by NT-3. In NT-3-deficient mice, sympathetic axons still approach the gland but they fail to invade it, and invasion can be restored by infusion of exogenous NT-3 (see also Chapter 10).[108]

The molecular signalling pathways that underlie neurotrophin-induced axon growth stimulation, as distinct from neuronal survival, are uncertain, although the ras–MAP kinase pathway has been implicated downstream of Trk receptor activation.[35,109] *In vitro* experiments do suggest that it is possible to distinguish these actions of neurotrophins: for example, primary sensory (DRG) neurons from mice deficient in the pro-apoptotic protein, BAX, survive in the absence of neurotrophic support *in vitro*, but only sprout axons profusely when neurotrophins are added to the medium.[110] Moreover, if mice that are null for NGF or *TrkA* are also made null for *Bax*, NGF/TrkA-dependent primary sensory neurons now survive and sprout axons, yet they fail to form a superficial cutaneous innervation.[111]

Our understanding of the molecular basis of the neurite growth-promoting effects of NGF and other neurotrophins has been further advanced by the demonstration of an interaction between p75^{NTR} and RhoA by coimmunoprecipitation, and hence of a link between neurotrophins and the cytoskeleton.[112] Rho proteins have been shown to control the organization of the actin cytoskeleton in many cell types, and have been implicated in the regulation of growth cone motility (see also Chapter 9). Like other members of the Ras superfamily of GTP-binding proteins, they cycle between active and inactive GDP-bound states. Rho activation in fibroblasts, for example, causes bundling of actin filaments into stress fibres and the clustering of integrins and associated proteins into focal adhesion complexes.[113] In neurons, p75^{NTR} constitutively activates RhoA whereas NGF, BDNF or NT-3 binding causes rapid loss of Rho activation and neurite extension.[112] This modulation of neurite growth involves a ligand-dependent interaction of p75^{NTR} with RhoA and can occur in neurons, such as those of the ciliary ganglion, which express p75^{NTR} but not Trk receptors: NGF, BDNF and NT-3 each enhance the growth of neurites from these neurons in culture, as does an enzyme, C3 transferase, which inactivates Rho. Consistent with Rho activation lying downstream of p75^{NTR} in this response to NGF, expression of a constitutively active Rho protein in ciliary neurons inhibits the neurite promoting effect of NGF.[112] That p75^{NTR} also plays a role in enhancing axonal growth *in vivo* is shown by the finding that during the early stages of axonal outgrowth, the intercostal nerves and forelimb motor axons of *p75$^{NTR\ -/-}$* mice are shorter than those of heterozygous and wild-type mice.[112]

In addition to regulating neurite growth by modulating Rho activity, a recent study suggests that NGF binding to p75^{NTR} may also enhance neurite outgrowth via the production of ceramide.[114] NGF was found to accelerate neurite formation and outgrowth from cultured hippocampal pyramidal neurons at a stage when they express p75^{NTR} but not TrkA. NGF treatment stimulated the production of ceramide, and blocking ceramide production with the sphingomyelinase inhibitor scyphostatin inhibited the neurite-promoting effects of NGF.[114]

Regulation of the physiological sensitivity of primary sensory neurons

NGF levels are increased in damaged tissues and this is partly responsible for the hyperalgesia that follows inflammation. The evidence for this is that elevation of NGF levels in adult rats causes hypersensitivity to noxious stimuli,[115,116] while NGF antibodies abolish the normal hyperalgesia of tissue damage without affecting inflammation itself. Several mechanisms have been identified through which NGF achieves this action: upregulation of levels of peptide transmitter (substance P and CGRP) in nociceptive DRG cells, release of pain-inducing compounds in the periphery by degranulating mast cells via an action on TrkA receptors, and sensitization of second-order nociceptive neurons to activation by primary nociceptive afferents.[99] Another example of regulation of primary sensation by neurotrophins concerns BDNF, which is probably required to maintain the sensitivity of slowly-adapting mechanoreceptors in the skin. These show markedly reduced sensitivity in BDNF-deficient mouse mutants, and this can be restored by exogenous BDNF.[117]

Regulation of synaptic transmission and plasticity in the postnatal and adult nervous system

As described in Chapter 14, covering up one eye during a 'critical period' of postnatal development permanently inactivates the thalamic inputs from the deprived eye in the visual cortex, so the eye is blind when uncovered later. The possible role of neurotrophins in regulating this type of developmental synaptic plasticity is discussed further in Chapter 14.

There is also evidence that neurotrophin signalling is required for normal neuronal function throughout life (see Chapter 16). Thus, application of NGF antibodies to adult sympathetic ganglia can mimic the effects of axotomy, with cell body and dendritic shrinkage resulting in reduced efficacy of preganglionic synaptic inputs.[118,119] Moreover, NGF can itself be released by electrical activity, causing transmitter release and even functioning directly as a neurotransmitter.[120,121] It has also been shown that long-term potentiation (LTP, see Chapter 15) is impaired in heterozygous BDNF mutant mice, raising a possible role for BDNF in the mechanism of LTP.[122]

Role of neurotrophic factors following nerve injury

The possible role of neurotrophic factors in promoting axon regeneration is described in Chapter 17, as is their importance for collateral sprouting from intact axons in partly denervated tissues. In addition, their presence at sites of injury may promote the survival of axotomized neurons at a time when they have been disconnected from their normal target source.

Key points

1 Neurotrophic factors are a heterogeneous group of proteins present in very small quantities in various tissues, including the brain, which play important roles at several stages of mammalian neural development and also in the adult animal.

2 The first neurotrophic factor discovered, nerve growth factor (NGF), was originally identified as an activity essential for the survival of sympathetic neurons when they innervate their peripheral targets.

3 Table 12.1 lists six of the principal neurotrophic factors known to date, their cognate receptors and the neural populations that depend on them for survival. The latter have been confirmed according to the neuronal phenotypes of mice lacking the factor and/or its receptor.

4 In addition to their classical role in promoting survival of postmitotic neurons, neurotrophic factors also control the numbers of some populations of neuroblasts at earlier development stages.

5 Later in development they may determine the phenotype of developing sensory and autonomic nerve cells, and help to determine the final pattern of terminal nerve connections during the 'critical period' (see Chapter 14).

6 In the adult they control the sensitivity of skin nociceptor and mechanoreceptor afferents, and promote regeneration and collateral sprouting after injury.

General reading

- Lewin, G. R. and Barde, Y.-A. Physiology of the neurotrophins. *Annu. Rev. Neurosci.* **19**, 289–317 (1996).

- Kaplan, D. R. and Miller, F. D. Neurotrophin signal transduction in the nervous system. *Curr. Opin. Neurobiol.* **10**, 381–91 (2000).

References

1. Hamburger, V. The effects of wing bud extirpation on the development of the central nervous system in chick embryos. *J. Exp. Zool.* **68**, 449–94 (1934).

2. Hamburger, V. Motor and sensory hyperplasia following limb-bud transplantations in chick embryos. *Physiol. Zool.* **12**, 268-84 (1939).

3. Levi-Montalcini, R. and Hamburger, V. Selective growth stimulating effects of mouse sarcoma on the sensory and sympathetic nervous system of the chick embryo. *J. Exp. Zool.* **116**, 321–62 (1951).

4. Levi-Montalcini, R. Developmental neurobiology and the natural history of nerve growth factor. *Annu. Rev. Neurosci.* **5**, 341–62 (1982).

5. Hamburger, V. The history of the discovery of the nerve growth factor. *J. Neurobiol.* **24**, 893–7 (1993).

6. Levi-Montalcini, R. and Angeletti, P. U. Immunosympathectomy. *Pharmacol. Rev.* **18**, 619–28 (1966).

7. Lewin, G. R. and Barde, Y.-A. Physiology of the neurotrophins. *Annu. Rev. Neurosci.* **19**, 289–317 (1996).

8. Henderson, C. E. Role of neurotrophic factors in neuronal development. *Curr. Opin. Neurobiol.* **6**, 64–70 (1996).

9. Fritzsch, B., Silos-Santiago, I., Bianchi, L. M. and Farinas, I. The role of neurotrophic factors in regulating the development of inner ear innervation. *Trends Neurosci.* **20**, 159–64 (1997).

10. Davies, A. M. Neurotrophin switching: where does it stand? *Curr. Opin. Neurobiol.* **1997**, 110–18 (1997).

11. Minichiello, L. and Klein, R. TrkB and TrkC neurotrophin receptors cooperate in promoting survival of hippocampal and cerebellar granule neurons. *Genes Dev.* **10**, 2849–58 (1996).

12. Alcantara, S. *et al.* TrkB signaling is required for postnatal survival of CNS neurons and protects hippocampal and motor neurons from axotomy-induced cell death. *J. Neurosci.* **17**, 3623–33 (1997).

13. Schwartz, P. M., Borghesani, P. R., Levy, R. L., Pomeroy, S. L. and Segal, R. A. Abnormal cerebellar development and foliation in BDNF$^{-/-}$ mice reveals a role for neurotrophins in CNS patterning. *Neuron* **19**, 269–81 (1997).

14. Lindvall, O., Kokaia, Z., Bengzon, J., Elmer, E. and Kokaia, M. Neurotrophins and brain insults. *Trends Neurosci.* **17**, 490–6 (1994).

15. Jones, K. R., Farinas, I., Backus, C. and Reichardt, L. F. Targeted disruption of the BDNF gene perturbs brain and sensory neuron development but not motor neuron development. *Cell* **76**, 989–99 (1994).

16. Smeyne, R. *et al.* Severe sensory and sympathetic neuropathies in mice carrying a disrupted Trk/NGF receptor gene. *Nature* **368**, 246–9 (1994).

17. Vicario-Abejon, C., Johe, K. K., Hazel, T. G., Collazo, D. and McKay, R. D. G. Functions of basic fibroblast growth factor and neurotrophins in the differentiation of hippocampal neurons. *Neuron* **15**, 105–14 (1995).

18. Altar, C. A. *et al.* Anterograde transport of brain-derived neurotrophic factor and its role in the brain. *Nature* **389**, 856–60 (1997).

19. Inoue, A. and Sanes, J. R. Lamina-specific connectivity in the brain: regulation by N-cadherin, neurotrophins, and glycoconjugates. *Science* **276**, 1428–31 (1997).

20. Shieh, P. B. and Ghosh, A. Neurotrophins: new roles for a seasoned cast. *Curr. Biol.* **7**, R627–30 (1997).

21. Thoenen, H. Neurotrophins and neuronal plasticity. Science **270**, 593–8 (1995).

22. Barbacid, M. Neurotrophic factors and their receptors. *Curr. Opin. Cell Biol.* **7**, 148–55 (1995).

23. Schneider, R. and Schweiger, M. A novel modular mosaic of cell adhesion motifs in the extracellular domains of the neurogenic trk and trkB tyrosine kinase receptors. *Oncogene* **6**, 1807–11 (1991).

24. Lamballe, F., Klein, R. and Barbacid, M. trkC, a new member of the trk family of tyrosine protein kinases, is a receptor for neurotrophin-3. *Cell* **66**, 967–79 (1991).

25. Davies, A. M., Minichiello, L. and Klein, R. Developmental changes in NT3 signalling via TrkA and TrkB in embryonic neurons. *EMBO J.* **14**, 4482–9 (1995).

26. Ernfors, P., Lee, K. F., Kucera, J. and Jaenisch, R. Lack of neurotrophin-3 leads to deficiencies in the peripheral nervous system and loss of limb proprioceptive afferents. *Cell* **77**, 503–12 (1994).

27. Klein, R. *et al.* Disruption of the neurotrophin-3 receptor gene trkC eliminates la muscle afferents and results in abnormal movements. *Nature* **368**, 249–51 (1994).

28. Farinas, I., Yoshida, C. K., Backus, C. and Reichardt, L. F. Lack of neurotrophin-3 results in death of spinal sensory neurons and premature differentiation of their precursors. *Neuron* **17**, 1065–78 (1996).

29. Tsoulfas, P. *et al.* The rat trkC locus encodes multiple neurogenic receptors that exhibit differential response to neurotrophin-3 in PC12 cells. *Neuron* **10**, 975–90 (1993).

30. Rudge, J. S. *et al.* Neurotrophic factor receptors and their signal transduction capabilities in rat astrocytes. *Eur. J. Neurosci.* **6**, 693–705 (1994).

31. Biffo, S., Offenhauser, N., Carter, B. D. and Barde, Y.-A. Selective binding and internalisation by truncated receptors restrict the availability of BDNF during development. *Development* **121**, 2461–70 (1995).

32. Armanini, M. P., McMahon, S. B., Sutherland, J., Shelton, D. L. and Phillips, H. S. Truncated and catalytic isoforms of trkB are co-expressed in

neurons of rat and mouse CNS. *Eur. J. Neurosci.* **7**, 1403–9 (1995).

33. Ninkina, N. *et al.* Expression and function of TrkB variants in developing sensory neurons. *EMBO J.* **15**, 6385–93 (1996).

34. Marshall, C. J. Specificity of receptor tyrosine kinase signaling: transient versus sustained extracellular signal-regulated kinase activation. *Cell* **80**, 179–85 (1995).

35. Kaplan, D. R. and Miller, F. D. Signal transduction by the neurotrophin receptors. *Curr. Opin. Cell Biol.* **9**, 213–21 (1997).

36. Kaplan, D. R. and Miller, F. D. Neurotrophin signal transduction in the nervous system. *Curr. Opin. Neurobiol.* **10**, 381–91 (2000).

37. Kavanaugh, W. M. and Williams, L. T. An alternative to SH2 domains for binding tyrosine-phosphorylated proteins. *Science* **266**, 1862–5 (1994).

38. O'Bryan, J. P., Songyang, Z., Cantley, L., Der, C. J. and Pawson, T. A mammalian adaptor protein with conserved Src homology 2 and phosphotyrosine-binding domains is related to Shc and is specifically expressed in the brain. *Proc. Natl. Acad. Sci. USA* **93**, 2729–34 (1996).

39. Riccio, A., Ahn, S., Davenport, C. M., Blendy, J. A. and Ginty, D. D. Mediation by a CREB family transcription factor of NGF-dependent survival of sympathetic neurons. *Science* **286**, 2358–61 (1999).

40. Franke, T. F., Kaplan, D. R. and Cantley, L. C. PI3K: downstream AKTion blocks apoptosis. *Cell* **88**, 435–7 (1997).

41. Finkbeiner, S. *et al.* CREB: a major mediator of neuronal neurotrophin responses. *Neuron* **19**, 1031–47 (1997).

42. Frank, D. A. and Greenberg, M. E. CREB: a mediator of long-term memory from mollusks to mammals. *Cell* **79**, 5–8 (1994).

43. Obermeier, A. *et al.* Neuronal differentiation signals are controlled by nerve growth factor receptor/Trk binding sites for SHC and PLCγ. *EMBO J.* **13**, 1585–90 (1994).

44. Stephens, R. M. *et al.* Trk receptors use redundant signal transduction pathways involving SHC and PLC-γ1 to mediate NGF responses. *Neuron* **12**, 691–705 (1994).

45. Davies, A. M. Role of neurotrophins in the developing nervous system. *J. Neurobiol.* **25**, 1334–48 (1994).

46. Snider, W. D. Functions of the neurotrophins during nervous system development: what the knockouts are teaching us. *Cell* **77**, 627–38 (1994).

47. Davies, A. M. The yin and yang of nerve growth factor. *Curr. Biol.* **7**, 38–40 (1997).

48. Davies, A. M., Lee, K. F. and Jaenisch, R. p75-deficient trigeminal neurons have an altered response to NGF but not to other neurotrophins. *Neuron* **11**, 565–74 (1993).

49. Horton, A. R. *et al.* NGF binding to p75 enhances the sensitivity of sensory and sympathetic neurons to NGF at different stages of development. *Mol. Cell. Neurosci.* **10**, 162–72 (1997).

50. Lee, K. F., Davies, A. M. and Jaenisch, R. p75-deficient embryonic dorsal root sensory and neonatal sympathetic neurons display a decreased sensitivity to NGF. *Development* **120**, 1027–33 (1994).

51. Clary, D. O. and Reichardt, L. F. An alternatively spliced form of the nerve growth factor receptor TrkA confers an enhanced response to neurotrophin-3. *Proc. Natl. Acad. Sci. USA* **91**, 11133–7 (1994).

52. Hamanoue, M. *et al.* p75-mediated NF-κB activation enhances the survival response of developing sensory neurons to nerve growth factor. *Mol. Cell. Neurosci.* **14**, 28–40 (1999).

53. Casaccia-Bonnefil, P., Carter, B. D., Dobrowsky, R. T. and Chao, M. V. Death of oligodendrocytes mediated by the interaction of nerve growth factor with its receptor p75. *Nature* **383**, 716–19 (1996).

54. Frade, J. M., Rodriguez-Tebar and Barde, Y.-A. Induction of cell death by endogenous nerve growth factor through its p75 receptor. *Nature* **383**, 166–8 (1996).

55. Yeo, T. T. *et al.* Absence of p75^{NTR} causes increased basal forebrain cholinergic neuron size, choline acetyltransferase activity, and target innervation. *J. Neurosci.* **17**, 7594–605 (1997).

56. Davey, F. and Davies, A. M. TrkB signalling inhibits p75-mediated apoptosis induced by NGF in embryonic proprioceptive neurons. *Curr. Biol.* **8**, 915–18 (1998).

57. Henderson, C. E. *et al.* GDNF: a potent survival factor for motoneurons present in peripheral nerve and muscle. *Science* **266**, 1062–4 (1994).

58. Zurn, A. D., Baetge, E. E., Hammang, J., Tan, S. and Aebischer, P. Glial cell line-derived neurotrophic factor (GDNF), a new neurotrophic factor for motoneurones. *NeuroReport* **6**, 113–18 (1994).

59. Oppenheim, R. W. *et al.* Developing motoneurons rescued from programmed and axotomy-induced cell death by GDNF. *Nature* **373**, 344–6 (1995).

60. Lin, L. H., Doherty, D. H., Lile, J. D., Bektesh, S. and Collins, F. GDNF: a glial cell-derived neurotrophic factor for midbrain dopaminergic neurons. *Science* **260**, 1130–2 (1993).

61. Ha, D. H., Robertson, R. T., Ribak, C. E. and Weiss, J. H. Cultured basal forebrain cholinergic neurons in contact with cortical cells display synapses, enhanced morphological features, and

decreased dependence on nerve growth factor. *J. Comp. Neurol.* **373**, 451–65.

62. Arenas, E., Trupp, M., Akerud, P. and Ibanez, C. F. GDNF prevents degeneration and promotes the phenotype of brain noradrenergic neurons *in vivo. Neuron* **15**, 1465–73 (1995).

63. Trupp, M. *et al.* Peripheral expression and biological activities of GDNF, a new neurotrophic factor for avian and mammalian peripheral neurons. *J. Cell Biol.* **130**, 137–48 (1995).

64. Buj-Bello, A., Buchman, V. L., Horton, A., Rosenthal, A. and Davies, A. M. GDNF is an age-specific survival factor for sensory and autonomic neurons. *Neuron* **15**, 821–8 (1995).

65. Heuckeroth, R. O., Lampe, P. A., Johnson, E. M. and Milbrandt, J. Neurturin and GDNF promote proliferation and survival of enteric neuron and glial progenitors *in vitro. Dev. Biol.* **200**, 116–29 (1998).

66. Kotzbauer, P. T. *et al.* Neurturin, a relative of glial-cell-line-derived neurotrophic factor. *Nature* **384**, 467–70 (1996).

67. Baloh, R. H. *et al.* Artemin, a novel member of the GDNF ligand family, supports peripheral and central neurons and signals through the GFRα3–RET receptor complex. *Neuron* **21**, 1291–302 (1998).

68. Milbrandt, J. *et al.* Persephin, a novel neurotrophic factor related to GDNF and neurturin. *Neuron* **20**, 245–53 (1998).

69. Moore, M. W. *et al.* Renal and neuronal abnormalities in mice lacking GDNF. *Nature* **382**, 76–9 (1996).

70. Durbec, P. *et al.* GDNF signalling through the Ret receptor tyrosine kinase. *Nature* **381**, 789–93 (1996).

71. Worby, C. A. *et al.* Glial cell line-derived neurotrophic factor signals through the RET receptor and activates mitogen-activated protein kinase. *J. Biol. Chem.* **271**, 23619–22 (1996).

72. Treanor, J. *et al.* Characterization of a receptor for glial cell line-derived neurotrophic factor. *Nature* **382**, 80–3 (1996).

73. Buj-Bello, A. *et al.* Neurturin responsiveness requires a GPI-linked receptor plus the Ret receptor tyrosine kinase. *Nature* **387**, 721–4 (1997).

74. Klein, R. *et al.* A GPI-linked protein that interacts with Ret to form a candidate neurturin receptor. *Nature* **387**, 717–21 (1997).

75. Enokido, Y. *et al.* GFRα-4 and the tyrosine kinase Ret form a functional receptor complex for persephin. *Curr. Biol.* **8**, 1019–22 (1998).

76. Thompson, J. *et al.* GFRα-4, a new GDNF family receptor. *Mol. Cell. Neurosci.* **11**, 117–26 (1998).

77. Doxakis, E., Wyatt, S. and Davies, A. M. Depolarization causes reciprocal changes in GFRα-1 and GFRα-2 receptor expression and shifts responsiveness to GDNF and neurturin in developing neurons. *Development* **127**, 1477–87 (2000).

78. Sendtner, M., Carroll, P., Holtmann, B., Hughes, R. and Thoenen, H. Ciliary neurotrophic factor. *J. Neurobiol.* **25**, 1436–53 (1994).

79. Stahl, N. and Yancopoulos, G. D. The tripartite CNTF receptor complex: activation and signalling involves components shared with other cytokines. *J. Neurobiol.* **25**, 1454–66 (1994).

80. Middleton, G. *et al.* Cytokine-induced nuclear factor kappa B activation promotes the survival of developing neurons. *J. Cell Biol.* **148**, 325–32 (2000).

81. Wong, V. *et al.* Hepatocyte growth factor promotes motor neuron survival and synergizes with ciliary neurotrophic factor. *J. Biol. Chem.* **272**, 5187–91 (1997).

82. Davey, F., Hilton, M. and Davies, A. M. Cooperation between HGF and CNTF in promoting the survival and growth of sensory and parasympathetic neurons. *Mol. Cell. Neurosci.* **15**, 79–87 (2000).

83. Birchmeier, C. and Gherardi, E. Developmental roles of HGF/SF and its receptor, the c-Met tyrosine kinase. *Trends Cell Biol.* **8**, 404–10 (1998).

84. Thewke, D. and Seeds, N. W. Expression of hepatocyte growth factor/scatter factor, its receptor, c-met, and tissue-type plasminogen activator during development of the murine olfactory system. *J. Neurosci.* **16**, 6933–44 (1996).

85. Maina, F., Hilton, M. C., Ponzetto, C., Davies, A. M. and Klein, R. Met receptor signalling is required for sensory nerve development. *Genes Dev.* **11**, 3341–50 (1997).

86. Maina, F. *et al.* Multiple roles for hepatocyte growth factor in sympathetic neuron development. *Neuron* **20**, 835–46 (1998).

87. Thewke, D. and Seeds, N. W. The expression of mRNAs for hepatocyte growth factor/scatter factor, its receptor c-met, and one of its activators tissue-type plasminogen activator show a systematic relationship in the developing and adult cerebral cortex and hippocampus. *Brain Res.* **821**, 356–67 (1999).

88. Maina, F. and Klein, R. Hepatocyte growth factor, a versatile signal for developing neurons. *Nat. Neurosci.* **2**, 213–17 (1999).

89. Ebens, A. *et al.* Hepatocyte growth factor/scatter factor is an axonal chemoattractant and a neurotrophic factor for spinal motor neurons. *Neuron* **17**, 1157–72 (1996).

90. Hamanoue, M. *et al.* Neurotrophic effect of hepatocyte growth factor on central nervous system neurons *in vitro. J. Neurosci. Res.* **43**, 554–64 (1966).

91. Crowley, C. *et al.* Mice lacking nerve growth factor display perinatal loss of sensory and sympathetic neurons yet develop basal forebrain cholinergic neurons. *Cell* **76**, 1001–11 (1994).

92. Minichiello, L. *et al.* Point mutation in trkB causes loss of NT4-dependent neurons without major effects on diverse BDNF responses. *Neuron* **21**, 335–45 (1998).

93. Oppenheim, R. W. *et al.* Glial cell line-derived neurotrophic factor and developing mammalian motoneurons: regulation of programmed cell death among motoneuron subtypes. *J. Neurosci.* **20**, 5001–11 (2000).

94. Novak, K. D., Prevette, D., Wang, S., Gould, T. W. and Oppenheim, R. W. Hepatocyte growth factor/scatter factor is a neurotrophic survival factor for lumbar but not for other somatic motoneurons in the chick embryo. *J. Neurosci.* **20**, 326–37 (2000).

95. Goldberg, J. L. and Barres, B. A. The relationship between neuronal survival and regeneration. *Annu. Rev. Neurosci.* **23**, 579–612 (2000).

96. Pettmann, B. and Henderson, C. E. Neuronal cell death. *Neuron* **20**, 633–47 (1998).

97. Kucera, J., Ernfors, P., Walro, J. and Jaenisch, R. Reduction in the number of spinal motor neurons in neurotrophin-3-deficient mice. *Neuroscience* **69**, 321–30 (1995).

98. Averbuch-Heller, L. *et al.* Neurotrophin 3 stimulates the differentiation of motoneurons from avian neural tube progenitor cells. *Proc. Natl. Acad. Sci. USA* **91**, 3247–51 (1994).

99. Frade, J. M. and Barde, Y.-A. Nerve growth factor: two receptors, multiple functions. *BioEssays* **20**, 137–45 (1998).

100. Casademunt, E. *et al.* The zinc finger protein NRIF interacts with the neurotrophin receptor p75(NTR) and participates in programmed cell death. *EMBO J.* **18**, 6050–1 (1999).

101. Reichardt, L. F. and Farinas, I. Neurotrophic factors and their receptors. In *Molecular and cellular approaches to neural development* (ed. W. M. Cowan, T. M. Jessell and S. L. Zipursky), pp. 220–63 (Oxford University Press, New York, 1997).

102. Purves, D., Snider, W. D. and Voyvodic, J. T. Trophic regulation of nerve cell morphology and innervation in the autonomic nervous system. *Nature* **336**, 123–8 (1988).

103. Edwards, R. H., Rutter, W. J. and Hanahan, D. Directed expression of NGF to pancreatic beta cells in transgenic mice leads to selective hyperinnervation of the islets. *Cell* **58**, 161–70 (1989).

104. Gundersen, R. W. and Barrett, J. N. Neuronal chemotaxis: chick dorsal-root axons turn toward high concentrations of nerve growth factor. *Science* **206**, 1079–80 (1979).

105. Ming, G., Lohof, A. M. and Zheng, J. Q. Acute morphogenic and chemotropic effects of neurotrophins on cultured embryonic *Xenopus* spinal neurons. *J. Neurosci.* **17**, 7860–71 (1997).

106. Menesini Chen, M. G., Chen, J. S. and Levi-Montalcini, R. Sympathetic nerve fibers ingrowth in the central nervous system of neonatal rodent upon intracerebral NGF injections. *Arch. Ital. Biol.* **116**, 53–84 (1978).

107. O'Connor, R. and Tessier-Lavigne, M. Identification of maxillary factor, a maxillary process-derived chemoattractant for developing trigeminal sensory axons. *Neuron* **24**, 165–78 (1999).

108. El Shamy, W. M., Linnarsson, S., Lee, K. F., Jaenisch, R. and Ernfors, P. Prenatal and postnatal requirements of NT-3 for sympathetic neuroblast survival and innervation of specific targets. *Development* **122**, 491–500 (1996).

109. Perron, J. C. and Bixby, J. L. Distinct neurite outgrowth signaling pathways converge on ERK activation. *Mol. Cell. Neurosci.* **13**, 362–78 (1999).

110. Lentz, S. I., Knudson, C. M., Korsmeyer, S. J. and Snider, W. D. Neurotrophins support the development of diverse sensory axon morphologies. *J. Neurosci.* **19**, 1038–48 (1999).

111. Patel, T. D., Jackman, A., Rice, F. L., Kucera, J. and Snider, W. D. Development of sensory neurons in the absence of NGF/TrkA signaling *in vivo*. *Neuron* **25**, 345–57 (2000).

112. Yamashita, T., Tucker, K. L. and Barde, Y.-A. Neurotrophin binding to the p75 receptor modulates Rho activity and axonal outgrowth. *Neuron* **24**, 585–93 (1999).

113. Mackay, D. J. and Hall, A. Rho GTPases. *J. Biol. Chem.* **273**, 20685–8 (1998).

114. Brann, A. B. *et al.* Ceramide signaling downstream of the p75 neurotrophin receptor mediates the effects of nerve growth factor on outgrowth of cultured hippocampal neurons. *J. Neurosci.* **19**, 8199–206 (1999).

115. Lewin, G. R., Ritter, A. M. and Mendell, L. M. Nerve growth factor-induced hyperalgesia in the neonatal and adult rat. *J. Neurosci.* **13**, 2136–48 (1993).

116. Romero, M. I. *et al.* Extensive sprouting of sensory afferents and hyperalgesia induced by conditional expression of nerve growth factor in the adult spinal cord. *J. Neurosci.* **20**, 4435–45 (2000).

117. Carroll, P., Lewin, G. R., Koltzenburg, M., Toyka, K. V. and Thoenen, H. A role for BDNF in mechanosensation. *Nat. Neurosci.* **1**, 42–6 (1998).

118. Nja, A. and Purves, D. The effects of nerve growth factor and its antiserum on synapses in the

superior cervical ganglion of the guinea pig. *J. Physiol.* **277**, 53–75 (1978).

119. Ruit, K. G., Osborne, P. A., Schmidt, R. E., Johnson, E. M., Jr. and Snider, W. D. Nerve growth factor regulates sympathetic ganglion cell morphology and survival in the adult mouse. *J. Neurosci.* **10**, 2412–19 (1990).

120. Blochl, A. and Thoenen, H. Characterization of nerve growth factor (NGF) release from hippocampal neurons: evidence for a constitutive and an unconventional sodium-dependent regulated pathway. *Eur. J. Neurosci.* **7**, 1220–8 (1995).

121. Blochl, A. and Sirrenberg, C. Neurotrophins stimulate the release of dopamine from rat mesencephalic neurons via Trk and p75Lntr receptors. *J. Biol. Chem.* **271**, 21100–7 (1996).

122. Patterson, S. L. *et al.* Recombinant BDNF rescues deficits in basal synaptic transmission and hippocampal LTP in BDNF knockout mice. *Neuron* **16**, 1137–45 (1996).

123. Dechant and Barde, Y.-A. Signalling through the neurotrophin receptor p75^{NTR}. *Curr. Opin. Neurobiol.* **7**, 413–18 (1997).

13

Nerve Cell Death

Despite the operation of powerful guidance systems ensuring that growing axons reach their targets, further mechanisms are needed to achieve the precision of connections that is a feature of the mature CNS. In the large brains of vertebrates there are two major phases of readjustment and they occur in sequence after synaptic connections are formed (Fig. 13.1). The first, a phase of nerve cell death, is responsible for removing redundant neurons and eliminating any neurons that have made incorrect connections. Such nerve cell death is described in this chapter, and the role of cell death in controlling the size of the vertebrate glial population is also discussed in Chapter 6. The second phase, one of pruning exuberant side branches and elimination of synapses, is coupled with stabilization and expansion of others. These processes are essential for determining the details of the synaptic connections of the neurons that survive the period of neuronal death, and are described in Chapter 14.

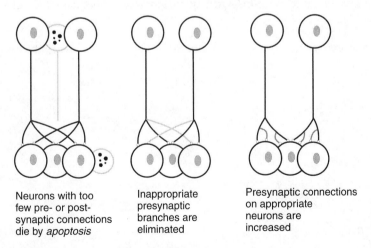

Neurons with too few pre- or post-synaptic connections die by *apoptosis*

Inappropriate presynaptic branches are eliminated

Presynaptic connections on appropriate neurons are increased

Figure 13.1 Three steps in the refinement of nerve connections: *left*, death of excess neurons or of those neurons that make wrong or inadequate connections; *middle*, elimination of many terminal branches; *right*, increase in number of branches applied to a more localized population of neurons.

The phenomenon of cell death during animal development was first observed by Vogt (1842), who studied amphibian metamorphosis, and the discovery that many neurons die during development was then made independently on more than one occasion.[1] The current awareness, however, has its origins in experiments in which limb bud primordia were removed in early chick embryos, when very few dorsal root ganglion cells and motor neurons were found at the level of the absent limb at later stages of development. These results were taken initially as evidence that the targets of the sensory and motor neurons, the skin and muscles, control the proliferation of neuronal precursor cells, but it was later realized that the deficit arose from the loss of already-generated cells which must normally depend upon their targets to supply them with vital trophic support (Fig. 13.2),[2] as discussed in Chapter 12. It was also noticed that neurons were dying in dorsal root ganglia of unoperated chicks at the same time in development that the massive losses triggered by limb removal occurred.[3] Subsequent studies have shown that cell death is a normal occurrence among many neuronal populations in the developing vertebrate nervous system (see reference 4 for review), taking place when axons begin to reach and activate their targets. The number of neurons in a given population is found to rise to a maximum as cells proliferate and settle at their final destination, and then to decline towards the constant adult number. Degenerating pyknotic nerve cell bodies can be seen as the numbers decline, although the rate at which the dying cells are removed is very fast so it is hard to estimate the extent of cell loss from the numbers of pyknotic cells seen at any one time. The proportion of cells that dies varies among different neuronal populations. Death removes only a small number of the neurons in some regions, but in others it can eliminate more than half the population.

The evidence discussed below suggests that the reason why neurons die at this stage of development is that they have to compete with one another for survival; death eliminates those neurons with quantitatively inadequate and qualitatively

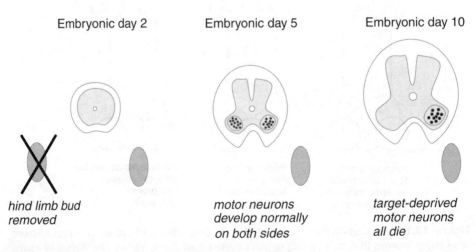

Embryonic day 2   Embryonic day 5   Embryonic day 10

hind limb bud removed

motor neurons develop normally on both sides

target-deprived motor neurons all die

Figure 13.2 Hamburger's experiment, and the origin of the idea that target-derived neurotrophic factors are needed to stop already-generated nerve cells from dying.

unsuitable pre- and postsynaptic connections. Initial surprise that neural development should involve a seemingly wasteful destructive step has given way to an appreciation of the benefits of this competitive selective process, making it unnecessary to have ultra-precise controls over the generation of neuron numbers and perfect guidance and targeting of outgrowing axons. It is also now clear that cell death occurs in many other developing systems, and that perhaps all cell types need trophic signals from other cells if they are to survive.[5] Failure to acquire specific trophic factors (Chapter 12) results in the activation of an intracellular molecular cascade that brings about self-destruction. Neurons, that is, die by an orderly sequence of events with characteristic morphological and molecular features, such as nuclear and cytoplasmic condensation and the generation of fragmented DNA 'ladders' on Southern blots. This is known as apoptosis, a process now recognized as distinguishable from necrosis.[6] Remarkably, a variety of cellular insults such as oxidative stress, ischaemia and ionizing radiation activate the same apoptotic programme, which seems to be designed to take the cell apart and have the residue rapidly phagocytosed by neighbouring cells without triggering an inflammatory reaction. This mode of death is also known as programmed cell death.

In addition to the large-scale death of developing neurons whose outcome is probably determined by competition for target-derived trophic factors, two other forms of apoptotic cell death have been discovered in the developing nervous system. The first has been described particularly clearly in the nematode worm *Caenorhabditis elegans*. In the very small nervous system of the nematode, control of cell generation can be very precise. The majority of neurons survive and, moreover, do not always seem to be dependent on target innervation to do so. Some neurons, however, do appear to be redundant, and activate the death mechanism; the process appears to be triggered cell-autonomously and independently of the environment.[7,8]

A similar form of cell death has now been recognized in the developing vertebrate CNS using sensitive morphological methods that identify fragmented nuclear DNA in dying cells. For example, large numbers (perhaps 50–70 per cent) of cells die during the development of the mammalian cerebral cortex, the majority being within proliferative rather than postmitotic regions;[9] and in the early spinal cord, death of newly-generated motor neurons, which cannot be rescued by additional supplies of neurotrophic factors, is well documented.[10] In these examples the trigger for cell death is unknown, and it is unclear to what extent cell deaths arise cell-autonomously or by cell–cell interactions. In the case of the cortex an interesting possibility is that cell death weeds out abnormal cells arising during the proliferative process, for example with errors in DNA replication. Further alternatives are that it reflects the need to generate a huge diversity of cell phenotypes, like the negative phenotype-specific selection process during development of T cells in the thymus gland, or that it arises from local trophic interactions between cells, as appears to be the case for oligodendrocytes (Chapter 6).[11] Correct spatial regulation of cell death may also be essential for ensuring the proper morphogenesis of the nervous system, as mice with targeted gene deletions of the *caspase* family (see below), in which cell death is reduced, have severe CNS malformations.[12,13]

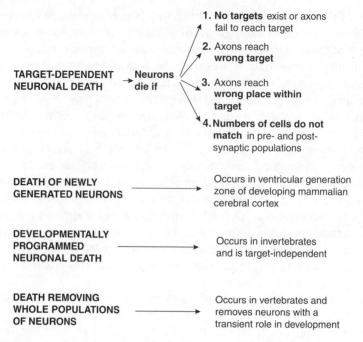

Figure 13.3 The different circumstances under which developing nerve cells can die.

An additional form of nerve cell death is seen in vertebrates, where some neuronal populations are razed after they have served a temporary role during development. A good example is the cortical subplate, a layer of cells that is critical for the normal development of cerebral cortical connectivity (see Chapter 10). A further example is provided by the Rohon–Beard cells of amphibian embryos; these are large, temporary sensory neurons in the neural tube whose sensory role is superseded by cells of the dorsal root ganglia later in development.[14]

Fig. 13.3 summarizes the situations in which neuronal death has been found, and these and the mechanisms of nerve cell death will now be discussed in more detail (see also reference 15 for review).

Target-dependent nerve cell death

Death of neurons whose axons fail to reach a target

The original limb bud extirpation experiments suggested that one role for neuronal death is elimination of those neurons that fail to reach a suitable target, and this may well account for neuronal death at some sites in the nervous system. For example, the sympathetic preganglionic motor neurons arise from a uniform column of cells (the columns of Terni) on each side of the spinal cord. At the cervical level these neurons lack a target and eventually die, but if a length of cervical spinal cord is transplanted to the thoracic level some of the neurons innervate ganglia at that level and so survive.[16]

It has, however, also been found on many occasions that long-lasting retrograde tracer injected into target tissues before cell death labels more neurons than a similar marking experiment carried out after the period of cell death.[17] As the tracer could only gain access to the nerve cell bodies by means of retrograde transport up axons from terminals that had reached the target, it follows that simply to reach a target area does not guarantee survival. Hence failure to reach a target is only one of several possible causes of cell death.

Death of neurons that make connection errors

As described above, early labelling of neurons with retrograde tracers can reveal the presence of a transient population of cells that disappears at the time of cell death. The dying cells can sometimes be located in a part of the brain which in the adult does not project axons at all to the target in question, that is, the neurons made the wrong connections. An example is seen in the efferent projection from the midbrain to the retina. In the adult chicken this arises only from cells located in the contralateral isthmo-optic nucleus. In the embryo, however, horseradish peroxidase (HRP) injected into the eye labels axons projecting to the retina not only from the appropriate contralateral isthmo-optic nucleus but also from a small number of ectopic cells around this nucleus and from some cells in the ipsilateral nucleus (Fig. 13.4A). Most of the ectopic neurons and all of the ipsilateral neurons subsequently die.[18] A second example concerns the erroneous projections in neonatal rats from retinal ganglion cells in the nasal half of the retina to the ipsilateral superior colliculus (tectum), which are removed by cell death.[19] A third example comes from the following experiment. If the outgrowing nerves from one side of the spinal cord are diverted into the developing contralateral leg in *Xenopus* tadpoles, the muscles in that leg become innervated by twice as many motor neurons as normal.[20,21] There is, however, no increase in the amount of cell death in the motor pools of the spinal cord. This suggests that provided motor neurons reach their correct muscles they can survive even if they have to share them with another equally appropriate set of motor neurons.

Neurons can, however, also die even if they project to the correct part of the brain. This may be because they project to the wrong part of the target, that is, topographic projection errors *within* a target may also be eliminated by neuronal death. Targeting errors of this sort occur in the contralateral projection from the eye to the superior colliculus and are removed during the period of retinal ganglion cell death (Fig. 13.4B).[17] Similarly the somatotopically ordered projection of motoneurons to the gluteus muscle of the toad develops during the period of motoneuron death.[22]

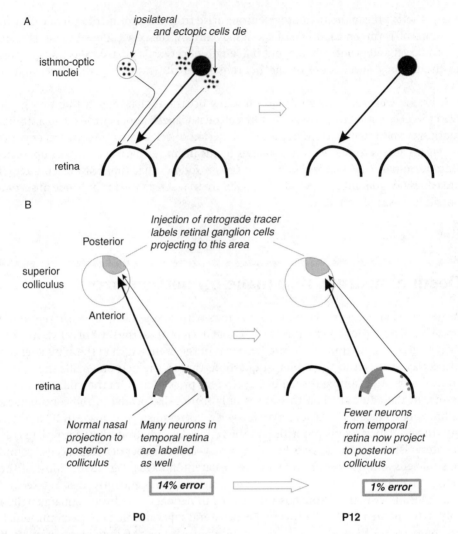

Figure 13.4 Examples of nerve cell death eliminating neurons that have made inappropriate connections. (A) Neurons projecting to the chicken retina from the ipsilateral isthmo-optic nucleus and neurons from around the contralateral isthmo-optic nucleus. (B) Neurons from the temporal retina of rats projecting to the posterior colliculus. In both cases these neurons can be labelled at early stages, but have disappeared and cannot be labelled later in development.

Matching pre- and postsynaptic numbers of neurons by neuronal death

Not all neuronal death, however, can be attributed to the elimination of neurons whose axons are incorrectly connected. In many instances axons seem to project without error to the right place and yet a proportion of the neurons dies. Similarly, neurons forced by experimental surgery to innervate the wrong target do not necessarily die.[23] Another factor that seems to matter is simply the amount of target tissue available; in the extreme, as we have seen, all innervating neurons die in the complete absence of target, a further example being the nearly total loss of all motoneurons from the lateral motor column of the mutant chick 'limbless'.[24] When there is some target, but less than usual, more death than normal occurs. This is illustrated by neuronal death in the sensory ganglia and spinal cord at different segmental levels. Death is greater at segmental levels of the trunk that do not innervate the limbs compared with those that do, presumably because in non-limb regions there is much less skin, joint and muscle tissue to be innervated. Similarly, if extra limbs are grafted onto early embryos in limb-innervating regions there is less neuronal death here than normal.[25]

These observations are consistent with the hypothesis that a given target tissue in some way supports the survival of only a limited number of the neurons that initially innervate it. Thus, cell death could be a means of matching the sizes of independently generated pre- and postsynaptic cell populations by causing the removal of any excess of presynaptic cells (Fig. 13.1).[26] Additional support for this hypothesis has come from an experiment in which chick lumbosacral cords were transplanted into quails and vice versa before the limbs became innervated.[27] Chicks are larger than quails and have bigger muscles with more muscle fibres. More quail motor neurons survived in the chick than in their native quail, and fewer chick motoneurons survived in the quail than in their own environment. There was a correlation between the number of motoneurons surviving and the number of muscle fibres available for innervation.

Quantitative loss of presynaptic neurons to match the number of postsynaptic sites also occurs in the neurons of dorsal root ganglia. If one limb bud is removed from *Xenopus* tadpoles, the single developing limb may become innervated by the motor and sensory axons of both sides, as described above. The total number of sensory dorsal root ganglion cells that survived was the same as the normal number for just one side, that is there were overall only half the normal number of dorsal root ganglion cells.[28] It seems that one limb has a limit to the number of ganglion cells it can keep alive, and this is a quite different outcome from that for motor neurons (see above).

The examples given above all point to a critical role for the postsynaptic target in determining the survival of nerve cells during the period of neuronal death. If there is not enough target, or it is incorrect, some of the neurons projecting to it die. There is good evidence that this is because the target provides neurotrophic factors which can prevent apoptosis. Historically this was shown first for postganglionic sympathetic neurons and some sensory neurons, which are dependent on nerve growth factor (NGF) (see Chapter 12). Delivery of extra supplies of NGF increases the number of these neurons that survive[29] but, even more convincingly, loss of NGF brought on by delivering antibodies to NGF can lead to the death of all postganglionic sympathetic neurons (immunosympathectomy)[30] and many sensory neurons.[31] The effects of neurotrophin deprivation have been studied more recently by generating null mutant mice lacking either the neurotrophin or its receptor, and these experiments have confirmed their vital importance (see Chapter 12).

Inadequate levels of neurotrophin for survival of any one neuron could come about during normal development because there are too many competitors, or because the neuron itself fails to gain access to the neurotrophin as a consequence of making inadequate connections. In favour of the latter possibility are experiments in which the amount of axonal branching by motor neurons in muscle was reduced by removing polysialic acid from the axons (see also Chapter 9).[32] This increased the amount of motor neuron death, possibly because of a decreased ability of motor neurons to take up neurotrophins. The expression of neurotrophin receptors is also likely to determine the ability of neurons to survive. The time during development when neurons first become dependent on neurotrophins usually coincides with the time that their axons arrive at their target. Dependence is not, however, triggered by the target but seems to be controlled by an internal clock, set so that neurons with short distances to grow switch on dependency earlier than neurons whose axons have further to grow.[33]

There is also evidence that the synaptic *input* to neurons is important for their survival (Fig. 13.1). For example, a test of whether the extent of motor neuron death (which is clearly very sensitive to the amount of postsynaptic target, muscle) is also influenced by the amount of presynaptic input has been carried out by eliminating these inputs surgically. This was done in the chick embryo by extirpating the neural crest (giving rise to sensory neurons) and removing inputs from the CNS by transecting the spinal cord,[34] a manoeuvre that brings about an increase in the amount of motor neuron death. A similar result has been obtained for motoneurons in the frog,[35] and such a partial dependency on presynaptic input for survival has also been seen in the parasympathetic ciliary ganglion of the chick.[36] Deafferentation within the CNS is also followed by death of neurons within the target nuclei, an example being the degeneration in all layers of the superior colliculus following eye removal in newborn mice.[37]

Additional factors affecting nerve cell death in vertebrates

An important matter still to be fully resolved is the role of electrical activity in nerve cell death. The extent of death of motor neurons and preganglionic sympathetic neurons can be altered by changing the electrical activity of their target tissues. Electrical stimulation of muscle fibres causes more motor neurons than normal to die,[38] while synaptic blocking agents (curare, α-bungarotoxin or botulinum toxin) can prevent motor neuron death.[39,40] Similarly, blockade of transmission reduces the amount of death in the preganglionic motor nuclei innervating sympathetic ganglia.[38] One interpretation of these results is that inactive target cells produce enough trophic support for all neurons in contact with the target, while the onset of innervation and activity sharpens competition by reducing the support available, causing some neurons to die.

Inactivity of the postsynaptic cells does not, however, always lead to less death among the innervating neurons, although it can disrupt the normal *pattern* of death. If transmission from the eye to the tectum in the rat is prevented by tetrodotoxin (TTX) injections into the eye[41] or by the N-methyl-D-aspartate (NMDA) receptor blocker MK801,[42] the overall extent of death is the same as normal but the preferential loss of retinal ganglion cells with the least appropriate connections is abolished. While it can be seen how the cells that normally die could be saved by postsynaptic inactivity, it is less easy to understand why the overall death rate should remain as high as normal.

Evidence from the autonomic nervous system suggests that while the presynaptic cells to a target may be rescued by preventing them from exciting that target, the likelihood that the silenced postsynaptic cells will die is actually increased.[43] It will be interesting to know if all neurons need to be electrically active if they are to survive the period of cell death. Clearly their activity may be needed to allow the normal amount or pattern of cell death among the neurons that innervate them.

Afferent input, which as described above is important for preventing undue amounts of nerve cell death, could influence survival *in vivo* either by promoting electrical activity or by orthograde release of trophic factors. A further potential source of trophic support is the glia, a good example being provided by Schwann cells. These express CNTF (see Chapter 12), a molecule that is able to prevent the death of axotomized neonatal motor neurons.[44] Lack of glial-derived trophic support may account for the cell death in the lateral geniculate nucleus that occurs before any afferent input has arrived or any efferent connections have been made.[45]

Sex hormones can also influence neuronal survival, for example the motor neurons innervating the bulbocavernosus muscle in rats.[46,47] This raises the possibility that other classes of neurons might be dependent on hormones for survival. A variety of endocrine influences on dendrite growth, synaptogenesis and myelination have been described, for example thyroxine, corticosteroids and growth hormone, and death of neurons following experimental manipulation in their levels is usually explicable in terms of disturbances in these processes. For example, neonatal thyroid deficiency reduces the overall growth of the mammalian cerebellar cortex, associated with increased death of granule cells, and this is probably secondary to diminished growth of Purkinje cell dendrites resulting in a smaller target available for granule cell axons. A marked growth reduction is also seen in the developing cerebral cortex in thyroid-deficient states, resulting in mental retardation in humans, although in this case it is not thought to be associated with a reduction in cell numbers. In fact there is scant evidence that hormones directly control cell death in the nervous system, a well-known exception being the effect of thyroid hormones on neuronal survival during amphibian metamorphosis (see reference 48 for review).

Problems in target-dependent neuronal death in vertebrates

From the above account it can be concluded that nerve cell death is certainly a means of correcting errors of one sort or another in the developing brain. In addition, a temporary excess of neurons, rather than representing a sign of error, might have a positive role to play. For example, muscle fibre numbers are regulated by the number of innervating motoneurons, and fewer secondary myotubes develop if there are fewer innervating motoneurons.[49] The excess of motoneurons that is generated during development may therefore be needed to ensure production of enough muscle fibres from the precursor cells in the limb. This observation is one of several perplexities posed by neuronal death, for if motor neurons allow more muscle fibres to develop, more muscle fibres should allow correspondingly more motor neurons to survive, creating a potentially unstable positive feedback mechanism. There is even *in vitro* evidence that neurotrophins may operate in an autocrine loop to promote neuronal survival,[50] providing yet more complexity. Other problems include why some motor neurons apparently die because they project incorrectly, whereas others do not, and why dorsal root ganglion cell death in *Xenopus* seems to be regulated by a number-matching process whereas motor neuron death is not (see above). It is also unclear why, when extra target tissue is provided in amounts sufficient to allow all neurons with projecting axons to survive, some cells still die.[27] Finally, although the need to regulate numbers of neurons is clear, and neuronal death could correct variations caused by variable production, in fact the extent of death is very characteristic for each region of the nervous system, implying that the production process is nevertheless accurately regulated.

Neuronal death in invertebrates

Neuronal death in invertebrates has been characterized most extensively in the nematode *C. elegans* and in insects. In *C. elegans*, stereotyped patterns of cell division generate approximately 300 adult nerve cells in each animal, and despite this small number about 20 per cent of cells in the lineage die. It seems likely that death is intrinsically programmed because the cells die even before they establish neuronal processes.[51] From the evolutionary point of view, it is presumably more effective to remove redundant cells from an initial excess than to control cell production precisely.

The high degree of anatomical reproducibility in the cells that die, the ability to observe the cells in the living worm with differential interference contrast optics, and the rapid rate of overall development have enabled screens for mutants in whom the normal pattern of death is disrupted. About a dozen cell death (*ced*) genes controlling this programmed death have been identified.[8,52] Several genes mediate late phases of the programme, such as the engulfment of already-dead cells, while three genes, *ced3*, *ced4* and *ced9*, are critical for the kill itself. Null mutations in *ced3* and *ced4* result in survival of all cells expected to die, which surprisingly seems to have no important functional consequences, and loss of *ced9* function causes extensive loss of cells over and above the number that normally die.[53] Conversely, *ced9* gain-of-function blocks cell death. The function of *ced9* is therefore antagonistic to *ced3* and *ced4*, presumably operating as a safety mechanism to protect surviving cells from accidental activation of the death programme. Studies of genetic mosaics (i.e. experimentally-manipulated animals whose genetic composition is not the same in all cells) have also shown that the cell death genes operate cell-autonomously, controlling the killing process within the cell in which their products become active.[54] Overall, this analysis has reaped impressive rewards, for it has turned out that genes closely related to *ced3*, *ced4* and *ced9* are also present in mammals and play a part in apoptotic death, as will be described later.

In insects, nerve cell death helps to generate differences in neuron numbers between segmental ganglia, and removes neurons made obsolete as development proceeds from larva to adult in holometabolous species (species such as *Drosophila* and *Manduca* that undergo a complete metamorphosis between different developmental stages).[55] Nerve cells dying by apoptosis can be stained in the developing ventral nerve cord of *Drosophila*, and the asymmetry of some of the dying cells on the two sides of the cord suggests that the process is not necessarily as rigidly specified as it is in *C. elegans*.[56]

In grasshopper embryos a stereotyped pattern of cell division in the segmental ganglia generates thoracic motor neurons which innervate the leg muscles. Homologous neurons also develop in the abdominal ganglia, but these have no tissue to innervate and die. Removal of the limb buds, however, does not cause the death of the related motor neurons in the thoracic ganglia,[57] possibly because they form other connections.[58] It therefore remains unclear whether absence of muscles is the cause of death of abdominal ganglion neurons, or whether there is some other environmental cue that determines the different fates of identical neurons in different ganglia.

During metamorphosis from pupa to adult, various neurons and muscles are made redundant and die, others change their morphology, and new neurons are generated from imaginal cells. The trigger for initiating cell death in the tobacco horn worm moth, *Manduca*, is a change in levels of the steroid moulting hormone ecdysone. During the transition from larva to pupa, an initial wave of cell death is triggered by a surge of ecdysone; on the other hand, when the level of hormone falls at the transition from pupa to adult, motor neurons that have become dependent on it die, and can be rescued by injections of steroid hormone.[59] The process that determines which neurons are vulnerable to declining hormone levels is not well understood. In the moult from pupa to adult it is possible to prevent the death in more distal segments by tying off the connectives from rostral ganglia.[55]

A factor that may be important in the control of insect neuronal death in some situations is presynaptic input. In the locust visual system a small proportion of neurons in the optic lobe normally die during development. If the retina is prevented from innervating the optic lobe there is an increased degeneration of neurons in the optic lobe. Conversely, if the projection of afferents to the lobe is increased there is less cell death.[59,60] So it is probable that some neurons in the optic lobe die during normal development because they do not become adequately innervated by retinal afferents.

Mechanisms of nerve cell death

In some circumstances neuronal death can be blocked both *in vivo* and *in vitro* by inhibitors of RNA and protein synthesis, implying that its induction involves new protein synthesis. This has been shown, for example, in the case of the apoptotic death of cultured sympathetic neurons that takes place 24 to 48 hours following the withdrawal of NGF.[61] On the other hand, cell death can occur in the absence of a nucleus, suggesting that the proteins involved in apoptosis are constitutively expressed in the cytoplasm. One possibility, therefore, is that *activation* of the death programme may require new protein synthesis, while its execution does not.

Where new protein synthesis is required, what are the inducible transcription factors that coordinate the rest of the apoptotic programme? A good candidate is the proto-oncogene *c-jun*, together with its upstream kinase JNK (Jun N-terminal kinase). Blockade of *c-jun* signalling by neutralizing antibodies prevents death of sympathetic neurons deprived of NGF.[62] A cytoplasmic protein that inhibits *c-jun* signalling by binding JNK has also been identified, and this may play an important role in the normal regulation of neuronal death induced by trophic factor deprivation.[63]

Caspases

An essential clue to the executive mechanism of neuronal death came from the structural characterization of the *ced3* gene, whose expression is essential for programmed cell death in *C. elegans* (see above). *ced3* turned out to encode a protein with homology to the mammalian cysteine protease interleukin-1β converting enzyme (ICE),[64] an enzyme needed for activation of interleukin-1 during the inflammatory response. There is good evidence that CED-3 protein also functions as a cysteine protease during programmed cell death in the worm, and the discovery suggested that ICE and/or similar proteases (collectively known as caspases as they cleave after aspartate residues) might be important in mediating cell death in mammals. This prediction has been borne out remarkably well. For example, dorsal root ganglion cells can survive NGF withdrawal in culture if ICE activity is inhibited,[65] and motor neurons similarly survive the period of normal developmental loss.[66] Several ICE homologues have now been cloned. Their importance has been confirmed by targeted deletion of *caspase-3* and *caspase-9* in mice, both of which result in ectopic masses of supernumerary cells in a variety of sites in the CNS, consistent with reduced neuronal apoptosis during CNS development.[12,13]

Events downstream of CED-3/ICE activation are thought to include cleavage of the DNA repair enzyme poly(ADP-ribose) polymerase, activation of a DNA-cleaving enzyme, and breakdown of the proteins (lamins) that maintain the nuclear envelope. Caspases function in a catalytic cascade in response to death-inducing stimuli, being synthesized as inactive precursor proteins (procaspases) that are themselves cleaved and activated by caspases, while some are also autoactivated.[67] The mitochondrion plays a key role in the regulation of caspase function and apoptosis.[68] The space between its inner and outer membranes contains several proteins involved in the execution of apoptosis, including procaspases 2, 3 and 9, cytochrome *c* and a flavoprotein (AIF) that causes chromatin condensation and large-scale fragmentation of DNA.[69] The release of such proteins through the outer membrane into the cytoplasm appears to be critical in the induction of apoptosis, although precisely how the system is activated remains unclear. It is also likely that caspase-independent mechanisms exist, an example being another class of protease, the calpains.

The *ced-9/bcl-2* family

As mentioned above, an important negative regulator of apoptosis in *C. elegans* is the product of the gene *ced9*, which prevents activation of the death programme in surviving cells. The mammalian proto-oncogene *bcl-2*, which is overexpressed in many B-cell lymphomas, has turned out to have significant structural and functional similarities to *ced9*.[70] Indeed, *bcl-2* can protect cells in *C. elegans* from programmed cell death.[71] Moreover, if *bcl-2* is overexpressed in cultured sympathetic neurons, they can survive in the absence of NGF,[72] and retinal ganglion cells are largely protected from axotomized death in adult mice overexpressing *bcl-2*.[73] The gene may also be involved in promoting axon regeneration (see Chapter 17). *bcl-2* is not always neuroprotective, however, for ciliary neurons dependent on CNTF are not rescued by overexpression,[74] and motor neurons in *bcl-2*-deficient mice are present in normal numbers at birth and can still be rescued from axotomy-induced death by BDNF or CNTF, although large numbers do die in these animals in the postnatal period.[75]

Many genes related to *ced9/bcl-2* have also been identified, such as *bax*, *bad*, *bak* and *bcl-x* in vertebrates, and these form homo- and heterodimers with each other. Several, such as *bax*, *bad* and *bak*, are pro-apoptotic and antagonize the anti-apoptotic members such as *bcl-2* and *bcl- x*, and the overall balance between their activities appears to be critical in determining whether cells are to live or die.[76] Consistent with these opposing functions, *bax* null mice possess increased numbers of motor neurons at birth,[77] while *bcl-x* knockout mice undergo massive neuronal death and die during embryonic development.[78] Interestingly, neurons rescued by *bax* deletion (or overexpression of *bcl-2*) are atrophied, suggesting that adequate trophic factor supplies are still required for full neuronal growth and expansion.

Yet further complexity in this system is provided by the analysis of the human neurodegenerative disorder spinal muscular atrophy, a condition that results in motor neuronal loss and infant mortality. The majority of cases are associated with deletion or mutation of the gene *survival of motor neuron* (*smn*), and SMN protein has been shown to interact synergistically with BCL-2, in some way promoting its anti-apoptotic action.[79]

How the products of the *bcl-2* family genes protect against apoptosis, preventing caspase activation, is still unclear. There is some evidence that reactive oxygen species may serve as a signal for the initiation of the killing process,[80] and that BCL-2 protein prevents apoptosis by enhancing an antioxidant pathway.[81] However, BCL-2 can still prevent death triggered by anaerobic conditions unlikely to produce reactive oxygen species.[82] A further possibility is that BCL-2 and its homologues regulate the release of soluble apoptotic proteins into the cytoplasm from the mitochondrial intermembrane space (e.g. cytochrome *c*, see above). Consistent with this, BCL-2 is structurally homologous to channel-forming bacterial toxins such as diphtheria toxin, and forms channels in synthetic lipid membranes.[83] Direct evidence for channel formation *in vivo* is lacking, however, and several other possible mechanisms have also been suggested.[84]

ced4 and its homologues

Another key player in the link between BCL-2 and caspase activation has been revealed by the *C. elegans* genetic analysis, namely *ced4*. CED4 protein has been shown to have intrinsic enzymatic activity, facilitating CED3 auto-activation to activate the caspase cascade, a process that requires ATP and that is blocked by CED9.[85] In one model, CED9 prevents cell death by binding to a CED3–CED4 complex, maintaining the complex in an inactive conformation, and apoptosis results when a death-inducing stimulus somehow dissociates the complex and liberates CED3 and CED4. A mammalian CED4 homologue, Apaf-1, has also been identified, and this has been shown to bind and activate caspase-9 in the presence of ATP and cytochrome *c*.[86] Many details remain to be worked out, but it is clear that the unravelling of the cell death programme in *C. elegans* has provided an outstanding example of the use of a 'simple' model organism to understand similar processes in vertebrates.

Receptor-activated death

Besides trophic factor withdrawal, death can be induced by extracellular ligand-mediated activation of cell surface receptors that trigger the apoptotic programme within the cell (see reference 87 for review). Examples of such receptors in non-neuronal cells include members of the tumour necrosis factor (TNF) and Fas receptor family. These contain a short conserved cytoplasmic segment, the 'death domain', that is necessary and sufficient for apoptosis. The *Drosophila* gene *reaper* encodes a small peptide with structural homology to the death domain, and is expressed in cells that are destined to die during normal fly development. In *reaper* mutants almost all normal cell death is prevented,[88] and the pro-apoptotic action of the peptide can be blocked by small peptide inhibitors of ICE, indicating that death results from activation of the caspase cascade.[89,90]

Strikingly, the neurotrophin NGF (see Chapter 12) has been shown to trigger death of retinal neurons through a further member of the TNF/Fas receptor family, the low-affinity NGF receptor p75, so neurotrophins do not exclusively promote neuronal survival. NGF-induced death occurs at an early stage of chick retinal development, when NGF and p75 are expressed in the retina but the high-affinity, survival-promoting receptor (TrkA) is not. Death can be prevented by administration of neutralizing antibodies to NGF or p75,[91] and is reduced in mouse embryos carrying deletions for the related genes.[92] This system has also been implicated in the death of cells in the mantle zone of the developing spinal cord,[92] and the full extent of neurotrophin-induced cell death remains to be determined.

A further example of receptor-activated cell death in the developing nervous system concerns the developing hindbrain. BMP4, a member of the TGfβ superfamily, is expressed in odd-numbered rhombomeres (r3,5) as a result of inductive interactions with the neighbouring even-numbered segments, and kills neural crest cells emanating from r3 and r5, but not r4, *in vitro*. This process presumably assists in the parcellation of migrating cranial neural crest cells into distinct streams that populate the branchial arches (see also Chapter 5).[93]

Neurotrophins and cell death

How do neurotrophins promote neuronal survival? At least two intracellular signalling pathways have been identified as critical, the ras–raf–MAP kinase pathway and the phosphatidylinositol 3'-kinase (PI-3) kinase–Akt pathway[94,95] (see Chapter 12). For example, a sustained rise in cAMP has been shown to prevent death of NGF-deprived neurons,[96] and the effectiveness of this and other survival factors can be prevented by antibodies to p21ras protein, indicating a key role for ras signalling in NGF-mediated survival.[97] The ras–raf–MAP kinase and PI-3 kinase–Akt pathways can prevent apoptosis upstream of nuclear transcription, for example by promoting sequestration of Bad protein, but they also promote survival by phosphorylating and activating nuclear transcription factors such as CREB.[94,98] The latter leads in turn to expression of Bcl-2 in neurons.[99] Other intracellular pathways almost certainly exist, and it has been shown further that neurotrophin deprivation-induced death involves activation of the Fas receptor in neurons.[87]

The degree of electrical activation of neurons is also an important influence on their survival (see above), and it has been found that NGF-deprived neurons can be rescued by chronic depolarization with high-potassium solutions. The immediate mediator of this effect may be calcium influx through voltage-gated calcium channels, which activates enzymes such as calcium-dependent adenylyl cyclases and elevates cAMP levels. Among other possible consequences, this could enhance responsiveness to neurotrophin signalling.[100]

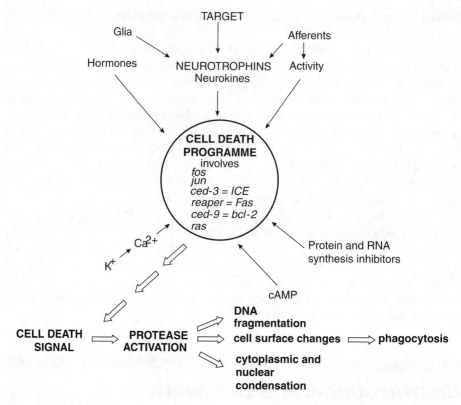

Figure 13.5 Some of the many factors that can *prevent* nerve cell death by apoptosis, presumably by interfering with the cell death programme (circle). During the development of the nervous system, the factors drawn above the circle have all been shown to influence the outcome in one system or another. Below the circle is summarized the sequence of steps that follow production of a death signal leading to apoptosis.

A diagram summarizing some of the factors described above and some others which have been found to affect nerve cell death is given in Fig. 13.5. It is likely that the rapid advances being made in understanding cell death mechanisms in a variety of systems will soon increase our knowledge of nerve cell death, for it is increasingly clear that the basic principles are shared.

Key points

1 A normal feature of the development of nervous systems is that different numbers of nerve cells die. In vertebrates up to half the neurons die. In invertebrates, whose nervous systems contain relatively small numbers of neurons, it can be seen that particular neurons invariably die.

2 Neurons die by apoptosis, a term describing a process of self-inflicted, rapid cell death in which the cell shrinks, its chromosomal material is broken up into short strands and the debris phagocytosed by neighbouring cells or tissue macrophages without initiating an inflammatory response. This is also known as programmed cell death.

3 In the nematode worm *C. elegans*, programmed cell death is controlled by several genes, some of which are related to genes controlling apoptotic cell death in vertebrate cells. *ced9* is the nematode homologue of mammalian *bcl-2*, which protects from apoptosis, and *ced3* is the equivalent of mammalian interleukin-1 converting enzyme (ICE), required for activation of the death programme. The genetic studies in the worm have clarified the molecular details of programmed cell death in all animal cells.

4 In the vertebrate nervous system most neuronal death is not preordained, as the amount of death can be changed experimentally. Death usually occurs after the axons of neurons have reached their synaptic targets.

5 Apoptotic death during development of vertebrate neurons is probably caused by a failure to obtain adequate trophic supplies. This occurs (i) when too many neurons attempt to innervate a target population, (ii) if the wrong target, or wrong place within an otherwise correct target, is innervated or (iii) if there is inadequate incoming innervation.

6 Target-dependent neuronal death provides an element of plasticity that is lacking in invertebrate neural development, and serves to match population numbers and eliminate projection errors.

7 In certain regions of the developing CNS, whole populations of neurons are removed when the function they serve is no longer needed, e.g. amphibian Rohon–Beard cells and neurons of the mammalian cortical subplate.

8 During rapid generation of nerve cells, as in the ventricular zone of the developing mammalian cerebral cortex, many neurons may die too, a process that may serve to eliminate abnormal cells formed during mitosis.

General reading

- Oppenheim, R. W. Cell death during development of the nervous system. *Annu. Rev. Neurosci.* 14, 453–501 (1991).

- Pettmann, B. and Henderson, C. E. Neuronal cell death. *Neuron* 20, 633–47 (1998).

References

1. Clarke, P. and Clarke, S. Nineteenth century research on naturally occurring cell death and related phenomena. *Anat. Embryol.* **193**, 81–99 (1996).

2. Hamburger, V. Regression versus peripheral control of differentiation in motor hypoplasia. *Am. J. Anat.* **102**, 365–409 (1958).

3. Hamburger, V. and Levi Montalcini, R. Proliferation, differentiation and degeneration in the spinal ganglia of the chick embryo under normal and experimental conditions. *J. Exp. Zool.* **111**, 457–507 (1949).

4. Oppenheim, R. W. Cell death during development of the nervous system. *Annu. Rev. Neurosci.* **14**, 453–501 (1991).

5. Jacobson, M. D., Weil, M. and Raff, M. C. Programmed cell death in animal development. *Cell* **88**, 347–54 (1997).

6. Wyllie, A. H., Kerr, J. F. R. and Currie, A. R. Cell death: the significance of apoptosis. *Int. Rev. Cytol.* **68**, 251–306 (1980).

7. Ellis, R. E., Yuan, J. Y. and Horvitz, H. R. Mechanisms and functions of cell death. *Annu. Rev. Cell Biol.* **7**, 663–98 (1991).

8. Hengartner, M. O. Programmed cell death in invertebrates. *Curr. Opin. Genet. Dev.* **6**, 34–8 (1996).

9. Blaschke, A. S., Staley, K. and Chun, J. Widespread programmed cell death in proliferative and postmitotic regions of the fetal cerebral cortex. *Development* **122**, 1165–74 (1996).

10. Yaginuma, H. *et al.* A novel type of programmed neuronal death in the cervical spinal cord of the chick embryo. *J. Neurosci.* **16**, 3685–703 (1996).

11. Voyvodic, J. T. Cell death in cortical development. How much? Why? So what? *Neuron* **16**, 690–93 (1996).

12. Kuida, K. *et al.* Decreased apoptosis in the brain and premature lethality in CPP32-deficient mice. *Nature* **384**, 368–72 (1996).

13. Kuida, K. *et al.* Reduced apoptosis and cytochrome *c*-mediated caspase activation in mice lacking caspase 9. *Cell* **94**, 325–37 (1998).

14. Lamborghini, J. E. Disappearance of Rohon-Beard neurons from the spinal cord of larval *Xenopus laevis*. *J. Comp. Neurol.* **264**, 47–55 (1987).

15. Pettmann, B. and Henderson, C. E. Neuronal cell death. *Neuron* **20**, 633–47 (1998).

16. Shieh, P. The neoformation of cells of preganglionic type in the cervical spinal cord of the chick embryo following its transplantation to the thoracic level. *J. Exp. Zool.* **117**, 354–95 (1951).

17. O'Leary, D. D. M., Fawcett, J. W. and Cowan, W. M. Topographic targeting errors in the retinocollicular projection and their elimination by selective ganglion cell death. *J. Neurosci.* **6**, 3692–705 (1986).

18. Clarke, P. G. H. and Cowan, W. M. The development of the isthmo optic tract in the chick, with special reference to the occurrence and correction of developmental errors in the location and connections of isthmo optic neurons. *J. Comp. Neurol.* **167**, 143–64 (1976).

19. Jeffery, G. and Perry, V. H. Evidence for ganglia cell death during development of the ipsilateral retinal projection in the rat. *Dev. Brain Res.* **2**, 176–80 (1982).

20. Lamb, A. H. Motoneurone counts in *Xenopus* frogs reared with one bilaterally innervated hind limb. *Nature* **284**, 347–50 (1980).

21. Lamb, A. H. Selective bilateral motor innervation in *Xenopus* tadpoles with one hindlimb. *J. Embryol. Exp. Morphol.* **65**, 149–63 (1981).

22. Bennett, M. R. and Lavidis, N. A. Development of the topographical projection of motoneurons to amphibian muscle accompanies motoneuron death. *Dev. Brain Res.* **2**, 448–52 (1982).

23. Landmesser, L. T. and O'Donovan, M. J. The activation patterns of embryonic chick motoneurones projecting to inappropriate muscles. *J. Physiol.* **347**, 205–24 (1984).

24. Lanser, M. E. and Fallon, J. F. Development of the brachial lateral motor column in the wingless mutant chick embryo. *J. Neurosci.* **4**, 2043–50 (1984).

25. Hollyday, M. and Hamburger, V. Reduction in naturally occurring motor neuron loss by enlargement of the periphery. *J. Comp. Neurol.* **170**, 311–20 (1976).

26. Cowan, W. M. Neuronal death as a regulative mechanism in the control of cell number in the nervous system. In *Development and aging in the nervous system* (ed. M. Rockstein) (Academic Press, New York, 1973).

27. Tanaka, H. and Landmesser, L. M. Cell death of lumbosacral motoneurons in chick, quail and chick–quail chimera embryos. *J. Neurosci.* **6**, 2889–99 (1986).

28. Lamb, A. H., Ferns, M. J. and Klose, K. Peripheral competition in the control of sensory neuron numbers in *Xenopus* frogs reared with a singly bilaterally innervated hindlimb. *Dev. Brain Res.* **45**, 149–53 (1989).

29. Hamburger, V., Brunso Bechtold, J. L. and Yip, J. W. Neuronal death in the spinal ganglia of the chick embryo and its reduction by nerve growth factor. *J. Neurosci.* **1**, 60–71 (1981).

30. Levi Montalcini, R. and Cohen, S. Effects of the extract of the mouse submaxillary salivary glands on the sympathetic system of mammals. *Ann. New York Acad. Sci.* **85**, 324–41 (1960).

31. Johnson, E. M., Gorin, P. D., Brandeis, L. D. and Pearson, J. Dorsal root ganglion neurons are destroyed by exposure *in utero* to maternal antibody to nerve growth factor. *Science* **210**, 916–18 (1980).

32. Tang, J. and Landmesser, L. Reduction of intramuscular nerve branching and synaptogenesis is correlated with decreased motoneuron survival. *J. Neurosci.* **13**, 3095–103 (1993).

33. Davies, A. Intrinsic programmes of growth and survival in developing vertebrate neurons. *Trends Neurosci.* **17**, 195–9 (1994).

34. Okada, N. and Oppenheim, R. W. Cell death of motoneurons in the chick embryo spinal cord. IX. The loss of motoneurons following removal of afferent input. *J. Neurosci.* **4**, 1639–52 (1984).

35. Davis, M. R., Constantine Paton, M. and Schorr, D. Dorsal root ganglion removal in Rana pipiens produces fewer motoneurons. *Brain Res.* **265**, 282–8 (1983).

36. Furber, S., Oppenheim, R. W. and Prevette, D. Naturally-occurring neuron death in the ciliary ganglion of the chick embryo following removal of preganglionic input: evidence for the role of afferents in ganglion cell survival. *J. Neurosci.* **7**, 1816–32 (1987).

37. DeLong, G. R. and Sidman, R. L. Effect of eye removal at birth on histogenesis of the mouse superior colliculus: an autoradiographic analysis with tritiated thymidine. *J. Comp. Neurol.* **118**, 205–19 (1962).

38. Oppenheim, R. W., Maderdrut, J. L. and Wells, D. J. Reduction of naturally occurring cell death in the thoraco lumbar preganglionic cell column of the chick embryo by nerve growth factor and hemicholinum 3. *Dev. Brain Res.* **3**, 134–9 (1982).

39. Pittman, R. H. and Oppenheim, R. W. Neuromuscular blockade increases motoneuron survival during normal cell death in chick embryo. *Nature* **271**, 364–6 (1978).

40. Laing, N. G. and Prestige, M. C. Prevention of spontaneous motoneurone death in chick embryos. *J. Physiol.* **282**, 33P (1978).

41. O'Leary, D. D. M., Crespo, D., Fawcett, J. W. and Cowan, W. M. The effect of intraocular tetrodotoxin on the postnatal reduction in the numbers of optic nerve axons in the rat. *Dev. Brain Res.* **30**, 96–103 (1986).

42. Bunch, S. T. and Fawcett, J. W. NMDA receptor blockade alters the topography of naturally occurring ganglion cell death in the rat retina. *Dev. Biol.* **160**, 434–42 (1993).

43. Maderut, J. L., Oppenheim, R. W. and Prevette, D. Enhancement of naturally occurring cell death in the sympathetic and parasympathetic ganglia of the chicken embryo following blockade of ganglionic transmission. *Brain Res.* **444**, 189–94 (1988).

44. Sendtner, M., Kreutzberg, G. W. and Thoenen, H. Ciliary neurotrophic factor prevents the degeneration of motor neurons after axotomy. *Nature* **345**, 440–1 (1990).

45. Williams, R. F. and Rakic, P. Elimination of neurons from the Rhesus monkey's lateral geniculate nucleus during development. *J. Comp. Neurol.* **272**, 424–36 (1988).

46. Breedlove, S. M. and Arnold, A. P. Hormonal control of a developing neuromuscular system. I. Complete demasculinization of the male rat spinal nucleus of bulbocavernosus using the anti-androgen flutamide. *J. Neurosci.* **3**, 417–23 (1983).

47. Breedlove, S. M. and Arnold, A. P. Hormonal control of a developing neuromuscular system. II. Sensitive periods for the androgen-induced masculinization of the rat spinal nucleus of the bulbocavernosus. *J. Neurosci.* **3**, 424–32 (1983).

48. Jacobson, M. *Developmental neurobiology* (Plenum Press, London, 1991).

49. Ross, J. J., Duxson, M. J. and Harris, A. J. Neural determination of muscle fibre number in embryonic rat lumbrical muscles. *Development* **100**, 395–410 (1987).

50. Acheson, A. *et al.* A BDNF autocrine loop in adult sensory neurons prevents cell death. *Nature* **374**, 450–3 (1995).

51. Sulston, J. E. and Horvitz, H. R. Post embryonic cell lineages of the nematode *Caenorhabditis elegans*. *Dev. Biol.* **56**, 110–56 (1977).

52. Ellis, H. M. and Horvitz, H. R. Genetic control of programmed cell death in the nematode *C. elegans*. *Cell* **44**, 817–29 (1986).

53. Hengartner, M. O., Ellis, R. E. and Horvitz, H. R. *Caenorhabditis elegans* gene *ced*-9 protects cells from programmed cell death. *Nature* **356**, 494–9 (1992).

54. Yuan, J. and Horvitz, H. R. The *Caenorhabditis elegans* genes *ced*-3 and *ced*-4 act cell autonomously to cause programmed cell death. *Dev. Biol.* **138**, 33–41 (1990).

55. Truman, J. W., Thorn, R. S. and Robinow, S. Programmed neuronal death in insect development. *J. Neurobiol.* **23**, 1295–311 (1992).

56. Abrams, J. M., White, K. and Fessler, H. Programmed cell death during *Drosophila* embryogenesis. *Development* **117**, 29–43 (1992).

57. Goodman, C. S. and Bate, M. Neuronal development of the grasshopper. *Trends Neurosci.* **4**, 163–9 (1981).

58. Whitington, P. M. Functional connections with foreign muscles made by a target-deprived insect motorneuron. *Dev. Biol.* **107**, 537–40 (1985).

59. Truman, J. W. Cell death in invertebrate nervous systems. *Annu. Rev. Neurosci.* **7**, 171–88 (1984).

60. Anderson, H., Edwards, J. S. and Palka, J. Developmental neurobiology of invertebrates. *Annu. Rev. Neurosci.* **3**, 97–139 (1980).

61. Martin, D. P. *et al.* Inhibitors of protein synthesis and RNA synthesis prevent neuronal

death caused by nerve growth factor deprivation. *J. Cell Biol.* **106**, 829–44 (1988).

62. Estus, S. *et al.* Altered gene expression in neurons during programmed cell death: identification of c-jun as necessary for neuronal apoptosis. *J. Cell Biol.* **127**, 1717–27 (1994).

63. Dickens, M. *et al.* A cytoplasmic inhibitor of the JNK signal transduction pathway. *Science* **277**, 693–6 (1997).

64. Yuan, J., Shaham, S., Ledoux, S., Ellis, H. M. and Horvitz, H. R. The *C. elegans* cell death gene *ced-3* encodes a protein similar to mammalian interleukin-1 beta-converting enzyme. *Cell* **75**, 641–52 (1993).

65. Gagliardini, V. *et al.* Prevention of vertebrate neuronal death by the *crmA* gene. *Science* **263**, 826–8 (1994).

66. Milligan, C. E. *et al.* Peptide inhibitors of the ICE protease family arrest programmed cell death of motoneurons *in vivo* and *in vitro. Neuron* **15**, 385–93 (1995).

67. Nicholson, D. W. and Thornberry, N. A. Caspases: killer proteases. *Trends Biochem. Sci.* **22**, 299–306 (1997).

68. Green, D. R. and Reed, J. C. Mitochondria and apoptosis. *Science* **281**, 1309–12 (1998).

69. Susin, S. A. *et al.* Molecular characterization of mitochondrial apoptosis-inducing factor. *Nature* **397**, 441–6 (1999).

70. Hengartner, M. O. and Horvitz, H. R. *C. elegans* cell survival gene ced-9 encodes a functional homolog of the mammalian proto-oncogene *bcl-2. Cell* **76**, 665–76 (1994).

71. Vaux, D. L., Weissman, I. L. and Kim, S. K. Prevention of programmed cell death in *Caenorhabditis elegans* by human bcl-2. *Science* **258**, 1955–7 (1992).

72. Garcia, I., Martinou, I., Tsujimoto, Y. and Martinou, J.-C. Prevention of programmed cell death of sympathetic neurons by the bcl-2 proto-oncogene. *Science* **258**, 302–4 (1992).

73. Cenni, M. L. *et al.* Long-term survival of retinal ganglion cells following optic nerve section in adult bcl-2 transgenic mice. *Eur. J. Neurosci.* **8**, 1735–45 (1996).

74. Allsopp, T. E., Wyatt, S., Paterson, H. F. and Davies, A. M. The proto-oncogene bcl-2 can selectively rescue neurotrophic factor-dependent neurons from apoptosis. *Cell* **73**, 295–307 (1993).

75. Michaelidis, T. M. *et al.* Inactivation of Bcl-2 results in progressive degeneration of motoneurons, sympathetic and sensory neurons during early postnatal development. *Neuron* **17**, 75–89 (1996).

76. Kuan, C.-Y., Roth, K. A., Flavell, R. A. and Rakic, P. Mechanisms of programmed cell death in the developing brain. *Trends Neurosci.* **23**, 291–7 (2000).

77. Deckwerth, T. L. *et al.* BAX is required for neuronal death after trophic factor deprivation and during development. *Neuron* **17**, 401–11 (1997).

78. Motoyama, N. *et al.* Massive cell death of immature hematopoietic cells and neurons in Bcl-x-deficient mice. *Science* **267**, 1506–10 (1995).

79. Iwahashi, H. *et al.* Synergistic anti-apoptopic activity between Bcl-2 and SMN implicated in spinal muscular atrophy. *Nature* **390**, 413–17 (1997).

80. Greenlund, L. J. S., Deckwerth, T. L. and Johnson, E. M. Superoxide dismutase delays neuronal apoptosis: a role for reactive oxygen species in programmed neuronal death. *Neuron* **14**, 303–15 (1995).

81. Hockenbery, D. M., Oltvai, Z. N., Yin, X.-M., Milliman, C. L. and Korsmeyer, S. J. Bcl-2 functions in an antioxidant pathway to prevent apoptosis. *Cell* **75**, 241–51 (1993).

82. Jacobson, M. D. and Raff, M. C. Programmed cell death and Bcl-2 protection in very low oxygen. *Nature* **374**, 814–16 (1995).

83. Minn, A. J. *et al.* Bcl-x(L) forms an ion channel in synthetic lipid membranes. *Nature* **385**, 353–7 (1997).

84. Reed, J. C. Double identity for proteins of the Bcl-2 family. *Nature* **387**, 773–6 (1997).

85. Chinnaiyan, A. M., Chaudhary, D., O'Rourke, K., Koonin, E. V. and Dixit, V. M. Role of CED-4 in the activation of CED-3. *Nature* **388**, 728–9 (1997).

86. Zou, H., Henzel, W. J., Liu, X., Lutschg, A. and Wang, X. Apaf-1, a human protein homologous to *C. elegans* CED-4, participates in cytochrome *c*-dependent activation of caspase-3. *Cell* **90**, 405–13 (1997).

87. Raoul, C., Pettemann, B. and Henderson, C. E. Active killing of neurons during development and following stress: a role for p75NTR and Fas? *Curr. Opin. Neurobiol.* **10**, 111–17 (2000).

88. White, K. *et al.* Genetic control of programmed cell death in *Drosophila. Science* **264**, 677–83 (1994).

89. White, K., Tahaoglu, E. and Steller, H. Cell killing by the *Drosophila* gene *reaper. Science* **271**, 805–7 (1996).

90. Pronk, G. J., Ramer, K., Amiri, P. and Williams, L. T. Requirement of an ICE-like protease for induction of apoptosis and ceramide generation by reaper. *Science* **271**, 808–10 (1996).

91. Frade, J. M., Rodriguez-Tebar, A. and Barde, Y. A. Induction of cell death by endogenous nerve growth factor through its p75 receptor. *Nature* **383**, 166–8 (1996).

92. Frade, J. M. and Barde, Y. A. Genetic evidence for cell death mediated by nerve growth factor and the neurotrophin receptor p75 in the developing mouse retina and spinal cord. *Development* **126**, 683–90 (1999).

93. Graham, A., Francis-West, P., Brickell, P. and Lumsden, A. The signalling molecule BMP4 mediates apoptosis in the rhombencephalic neural crest. *Nature* **372**, 684–6 (1994).

94. Grewal, S. S., York, R. D. and Strok, P. J. S. Extracellular-signal-related kinase signalling in neurons. *Curr. Opin. Neurobiol.* **9**, 544–53 (1999).

95. Nunez, G. and del Peso, L. Linking extracellular survival signals and the apoptotic machinery. *Curr. Opin. Neurobiol.* **8**, 613–18 (1998).

96. Rydel, R. E. and Greene, L. A. cAMP analogs promote survival and neurite outgrowth in cultures of rat sympathetic and sensory neurons independently of nerve growth factor. *Proc. Natl. Acad. Sci. USA* **85**, 1257–61 (1988).

97. Nobes, C. D. and Tolkovsky, A. M. Neutralizing anti-p21ras Fabs suppress rat sympathetic neuron survival induced by NGF, LIF, CNTF and cAMP. *Eur. J. Neurosci.* **7**, 344–50 (1995).

98. Datta, S. R., Brunet, A. and Greenberg, M. E. Cellular survival: a play in three Akts. *Genes Dev.* **13**, 2905–27 (1999).

99. Riccio, A., Ahn, S., Davenport, C. M., Blendy, J. A. and Ginty, D. D. Mediation by a CREB family transcription factor of NGF-dependent survival of sympathetic neurons. *Science* **286**, 2358–61 (1999).

100. Goldberg, J. L. and Barres, B. A. The relationship between neuronal survival and regeneration. *Annu. Rev. Neurosci.* **23**, 579–612 (2000).

14

Rearrangement and Stabilization of Synaptic Connections

Even after axons have found the correct region of brain or the right tissue in the periphery (Chapter 9), and neuron numbers have been adjusted to their adult levels (Chapter 13), substantial modifications have still to be made to the connections that have been formed (see Fig. 13.1). This is necessary because the initial distribution of the terminal branches of each axon within the target territory is wider than in the adult and lacks its precision. For each neuron a selective loss of some of these pioneer synaptic terminals and terminal branches occurs, while its other synaptic connections are expanded and consolidated. One of the key factors in the CNS determining which branches are maintained and which are lost is the relative activity patterns in the various neurons with inputs converging onto a postsynaptic cell. Those inputs which act together to drive the cell to fire action potentials tend to be stabilized, whereas those with weak inputs, out of synchrony with the majority, tend to be lost. In this way functionally effective terminals of a neuron are kept while ineffective ones are removed. Progress has been made recently in discovering possible molecular mechanisms to account for these effects. Terminal connections can be modified in a major way for only a limited time period during development, the so-called critical or sensitive period. Unusual activity patterns during the critical period can have profound, permanent effects on connectivity. There is, however, also good evidence that a lesser degree of adaptability remains in the adult nervous system. The adaptability in the adult was revealed first following injury and so it is described later (see Chapter 17), although it is now clear that adult plasticity of connections is a normal physiological mechanism and is not simply a response triggered by pathology.

The discovery of a remodelling–expansion phase of neural connectivity was as much of a surprise to neuroscientists as the discovery of the phase of nerve cell death, and the outline picture given above has emerged only fitfully, principally from experiments on the innervation of skeletal muscles and autonomic ganglia of neonatal rats, and the visual pathways of *Xenopus* toads, kittens, ferrets and infant monkeys. These will be described below. With hindsight, however, it is possible to see that some sort of synaptic connection refinement based on functional need would be essential. First, far too many neurons exist for each to be controlled by a unique genetic programme designed to determine the last detail of its branching pattern. Second, it would be impossible to harmonize connections between neurons if each independently determined the fine detail of its branches. Third, in some animals continued growth changes the geometry of the peripheral sensory map and this needs to be remapped in the central nervous system.[1] The adopted strategy, as described above, is for each neuron to use genetically programmed guidance mechanisms to generate an initial array of connections in which gross topographic order is developed. Neurons then lose some connections while retaining and expanding others, especially those whose input combines synchronously with the input of other neurons and so generates activity. In this way the brain becomes as well-tuned as possible to fit the uses required of it.

Multiple innervation at the neonatal neuromuscular junction and its elimination

The motor innervation of skeletal muscle provides the clearest demonstration that neurons make more extensive synaptic connections in the neonate than in the adult, because its innervation is so simple. In the adult each endplate is innervated by a single axon but in the newborn several axons can be seen converging on each end-plate (Fig. 14.1). This was first noticed in 1917,[2] but these histological results were forgotten and the phenomenon was rediscovered by chance, using physiological methods, some 50 years later.[3] It came to light when the maturation of transmitter release in neonatal rat diaphragm was being investigated by recording *in vitro* from muscle fibres in which the endplate potentials had been reduced to subthreshold levels with curare. Under such conditions the endplate potential of an adult muscle fibre has a constant amplitude, independent of the stimulus size, once the excitation threshold for the single axon innervating it has been exceeded. In the neonate, however, it was found that the endplate potentials of individual muscle fibres varied in size in a stepwise manner, depending on the stimulus strength and hence on the number of axons in the muscle nerve that were being stimulated (Fig. 14.1).

It was subsequently found that individual motor neurons in newborn rats and in kittens each innervated more muscle fibres than in the adult because the fraction of the muscle's total tension that each motor axon could activate in the newborn animals was several times greater than in the adult,[4,5] even in muscles which already contained the full adult number of muscle fibres. Examination of nerve terminals in light and electron microscopes[4-7] revealed the multiple innervation seen 50 years previously.

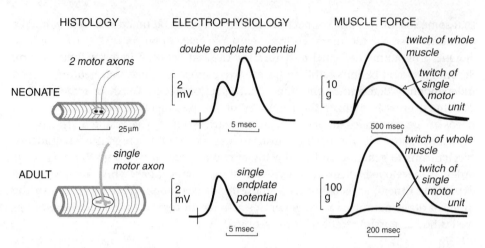

Figure 14.1 Polyneuronal innervation of neonatal skeletal muscle fibres can be revealed by histology and electrophysiology. By recording the strength of individual motor units in relation to the strength of the whole muscle, and by counting the number of motor neurons, it is clear that the polyneuronal innervation is caused by each neonatal motor neuron innervating many more muscle fibres than in the adult. The findings in neonatal muscle contrast with those from normal adult muscles, in which each endplate is innervated by a single motor axon and each motor neuron innervates far fewer muscle fibres, so that the relative strength of each motor unit compared to the total muscle strength is much less. These simple experiments were the first to show unequivocally that nerve cells made major modifications to their terminal branches during development. After Brown et al.[5]

During the second and third weeks after birth, all but one axon is withdrawn from each endplate and the motor units gradually shrink in size towards their adult values (Fig. 14.1).[5] It is unusual in mammals for any skeletal muscle with a propagated action potential to have fibres with endplates that are multiply innervated. An exception is the rat levator ani muscle, which has a low proportion (20 per cent) of multiply innervated fibres. Here, the presence of multiple innervation is determined by the level of circulating androgens. Castration lowers the amount of polyinnervation, an effect which can be overridden by androgen administration. The amount of poly-innervation remains high if androgens are withdrawn once the animal is adult, so the dependence on sex hormones is limited to a brief developmental period.[8,9]

Mechanisms of synapse elimination in skeletal muscle

In most skeletal muscles motor terminals are eliminated until only one axon remains in contact with each muscle fibre. The cellular mechanisms that bring this about are not yet clear but certain facts are well established. The eliminated terminal branches retract backwards towards their point of origin from a parent axon, and do not degenerate simultaneously along their length. Swollen nerve terminals not in contact with an endplate can be seen by light microscopy during the elimination period[10] and it is possible that structural components are broken down in and reabsorbed from these so-called 'retraction bulbs'.[11] Protease inhibitors delay the withdrawal of branches.[12] The remaining motor terminal left at the endplate enlarges as the muscle fibre grows but it does not expand into the endplate territory of the loser. This has been shown by some technically demanding experiments in which endplates in living mice were examined using fluorescent dyes that stain the nerve terminals or the acetylcholine receptors in the postsynaptic membrane. The same endplate is visualized on several occasions during the time of terminal branch withdrawal and it is found that the acetylcholine receptors may become redistributed. This leaves one axon whose terminal branches have no underlying transmitter receptors and this is the axon that later retracts (Fig. 14.2A).[13,14] Even more strikingly, it has been possible to block just one or two terminal branches of a *single* axon by puffing a directed stream of α-bungarotoxin at them. The nerve terminals overlying the blocked receptors are withdrawn, a step which is again preceded by loss of the postsynaptic receptors (Fig. 14.2B).[15] Blockade of all the receptors at the endplate simultaneously does not lead to the loss of any terminal branches of the axon.

It thus appears that a motor terminal that cannot activate the muscle when another input is doing so is unable to survive. This is borne out by experiments on *Xenopus* muscle *in vitro*. When a muscle is repetitively depolarized by iontophoretically applied acetylcholine, the motor axon becomes less able to excite the muscle.[16] The depression of an inactive terminal on an active muscle fibre is dependent on a rise in calcium concentration in the muscle, and possibly on a retrograde signal transmitted from the muscle to the nerve. This may be nitric oxide (NO),[17] which is interesting since NO may act as a retrograde messenger mediating presynaptic changes during learning in the adult (see Chapter 15). The ability of the axon to excite the muscle can be protected if the motor neuron is stimulated at the same time as the acetylcholine is applied.

A long-standing suggestion is that each terminal needs access to a survival factor (possibly the same factors needed for survival of the motor neurons earlier in development) that is released from the junctional membrane and that, it is presumed, is normally obtained by the motor nerve terminal only if it is active during endplate activation. A precedent for this possibility is the sympathetic neuron: nerve growth factor (NGF) applied locally to individual sympathetic nerve branches in tissue culture can promote their survival.[18] It is known that systemic application of basic fibroblast growth factor (FGF) and ciliary neurotrophic factor (CNTF) can prolong the period of polyneuronal innervation in skeletal muscle,[19] and the neurotrophins NT-3 and brain-derived neurotrophic factor (BDNF), the calcitonin-gene-related peptide (CGRP) and the cytokine leukaemia inhibitory factor (LIF) have also been implicated.[20] A further candidate is the neurotrophic factor, glial cell-derived neurotrophic factor (GDNF) (see Chapter 12); overexpression of this molecule in transgenic mice results in hyperinnervation of the neuromuscular junctions, and the extent of hyperinnervation correlates with the level of overexpression.[21]

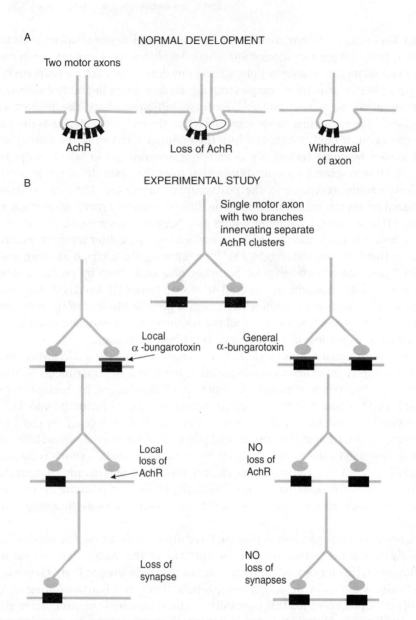

A NORMAL DEVELOPMENT

Two motor axons

AchR

Loss of AchR

Withdrawal
of axon

B EXPERIMENTAL STUDY

Single motor axon
with two branches
innervating separate
AchR clusters

Local
α-bungarotoxin

General
α-bungarotoxin

Local
loss of
AchR

NO
loss of
AchR

Loss of
synapse

NO
loss of
synapses

Figure 14.2 What determines which nerve terminal is lost at a multiply innervated motor endplate during the neonatal phase of synapse withdrawal? (A) The first step in branch withdrawal is the localized loss of acetylcholine receptors (AchRs) beneath one of the axons. It is after this that the affected axon invariably withdraws. (B) Local blockade of just one branch of a single motor axon by highly focal application of bungarotoxin is followed by loss of the inactivated receptors and then by withdrawal of the overlying axon. If all receptors are blocked, however, no receptors are lost and no branches withdrawn. So it is the relative ability of axons to activate their postsynaptic receptors that determines the outcome of synaptic competition; once synaptic transmission becomes impossible after transmitter receptors have been removed, the branch cannot survive if other inputs are successfully activating the postsynaptic membrane. After Balice-Gordon and Lichtman.[14,15]

In summary, it is possible that branches of a neuron active in synchrony with the muscle receive a positive survival signal from the muscle (possibly a neurotrophic factor), which may enable them to resist a rejection signal, while inactive branches or branches not strong enough always to excite a muscle action potential receive, and are unable to counteract, a rejection signal (possibly NO or a protease such as thrombin).[20] Such a scheme would clearly lead to single innervation but is still unfortunately vague about how the signals might affect nerve terminals.

Role of changes in the motor neuron cell body

During the postnatal period motor neurons themselves seem to become less able to sustain their initial complement of branches.[5,22] Coinciding with this, in the 2- or 3-week period when motor neurons are losing terminal branches, it has been found that there is a profound fall within the motor nerve cell bodies of the synthesis of some proteins that are associated with nerve growth, for example Gap-43 and Tα1 tubulin, and the level of Gap-43 protein in the nerve terminal also falls.[23] Such a reduction in growth potential could be responsible for the tendency of motor neurons to lose branches at this stage of development (although it might also be a *consequence* of the loss of branches). Another overall change during the early postnatal weeks is an increase in electrical activity in motor neurons. This will accelerate branch elimination because it is known that the rate of synapse elimination is increased if activity is increased artificially by stimulating the motor nerves or the muscle fibres directly, especially if the activity occurs in high-frequency bursts.[24,25] Conversely, if the muscle is made inactive, no or little terminal withdrawal occurs[26-28] and the levels of Gap-43 stop falling in the cell bodies of motor neurons.[23]

Selection of which branch to lose

None of the above observations throws light on how it is that, during normal development, one terminal gains an initial advantage over others so that it alone is able to survive. It might simply be chance, but three possible factors that could tip the balance are considered below:

1. Some terminal branches of motor neurons might be inappropriately placed in the muscle and such branches might be uncompetitive. These could be synapses made on muscle fibres of a type that did not match the motor neuron's type, or synapses made on fibres in regions within the muscle that did not correspond to the motor neuron's somatotopic order. Some synapse elimination may be decided by such factors but the effects are not large, as most motor units are nearly homogeneous in fibre type before synapse elimination is complete,[29,30] and the degree of somatotopic order is never very great; any improvement achieved by elimination is small.[31-34]

2. The outcome of a competition between individual terminals may depend on how many other branches the parent neurons have. A mechanism which puts terminals of motor neurons with fewer branches at an advantage and terminals of motor neurons with more branches at a disadvantage during synapse elimination is needed to achieve a balance in the final sizes of motor units in developing muscles. There is only indirect evidence for this idea. For example, extra motor axons can be forced to grow into a normally innervated muscle and if they can reach an already innervated endplate (which is not often) they are able to evict the normal terminal whose parent neuron has many branches to supply,[35] unlike the neurons supplying the invading axons which have not yet formed any terminals. The nerve terminals at endplates formed by collateral sprouts in a partially denervated muscle (see Chapter 17) appear to be at a similar disadvantage, as most of them withdraw when the original axons regenerate to their endplates.[36] Finally, experiments on reinnervated adult muscles have shown that the safety factor for transmission is lower in large motor units and higher in smaller units;[37,38] during the period of synapse elimination such a difference would favour survival of the terminals of the smaller units.

3. The relative rates of electrical impulse activity of different motor neurons may play a part in selective terminal withdrawal, although it cannot be the overriding factor as motor neurons with very different firing patterns coexist in most muscles; no one pattern is clearly superior to another as far as terminal survival is concerned. In fact, *in vivo* experiments to decide whether active or inactive motor neurons are more likely to retain terminal branches have yielded conflicting results.[39,40] More clear-cut results have come, however, from experiments on motor neurons of *Xenopus* toads in culture. If a myotube is innervated by two motor neurons whose axons can be stimulated independently, it is found that a burst of impulses in one nerve will reduce the amount of transmitter liberated by the other unless it too is given the same stimuli at the same time.[41]

Although skeletal muscle's simple innervation provides clear evidence for multiple innervation and later elimination of all but one nerve branch, it should be remembered that this situation is unique because most vertebrate skeletal muscle fibres can propagate action potentials and only one motor axon suffices to trigger this. Additional innervation would not only be unnecessary but a handicap, as the steady generation of tension driven by the rhythmic firing of a single motor neuron would be disrupted by the asynchronous addition of input from another motor neuron. In all other cases in the nervous system the postsynaptic cell has many physically separate input sites, and it is rare for one input on it own to be able to make the neuron reach threshold and fire an action potential. Instead, it is necessary for many inputs to coexist, and mechanisms must have evolved to allow this to happen during the process of synaptic rearrangement.

Synaptic reorganization in autonomic ganglia

One of the simplest of all neuronal systems in which to study the postnatal rearrangement of nerve terminal branches is the parasympathetic submandibular ganglion. In the adult rat there is usually only one axonal input per ganglion cell, and the synapses are all located on small elevations on the globular cell body, there being no dendrites. Unlike skeletal muscle, however, there are many synaptic sites on each cell in the adult, although it has been argued that the endplate of an adult skeletal muscle fibre is composed of a collection of independent sites not dissimilar to those on a submandibular ganglion cell.[42] Graded stimulation of preganglionic axons, while making intracellular recordings from ganglion cells, has revealed that in the neonatal rat the cells of the submandibular ganglion are innervated by up to five preganglionic fibres. All but one of these is then lost, so that by 40 days of age the adult state of one axonal input per ganglion cell is established. When the preganglionic axons and the synaptic boutons are stained and counted in the light microscope, it is found that as the number of axons within the whole ganglion decreases, the total number of boutons on each neuron actually increases (Fig. 14.3). It follows that each preganglionic cell withdraws inputs from many neurons, but simultaneously places additional synapses on the few remaining cells which it still innervates.[43]

A slightly more complex situation is provided by the superior cervical ganglion of the guinea-pig. Adult neurons in this ganglion are innervated by six to seven separate preganglionic axons, arising from less than three segmental levels of the spinal cord, while in the immature animal each neuron has nearly twice as many inputs, arising from an average of four segmental levels.[44] It is possible, therefore, that segmental labels play a part in the competitive removal of excess inputs from ganglion cells. This view is strengthened by experiments on the pattern of connections formed on reinnervation or partial denervation of ganglia of adult guinea-pigs.[45] These have revealed preferential affinities between terminals of different preganglionic fibres and particular neurons in the superior cervical ganglion and, as for motor neurons, terminal branches of preganglionic neurons which make many connections are at a competitive disadvantage compared with those with fewer connections.

One of the factors enabling multiple synaptic inputs to survive the period of branch elimination has been uncovered in studies of another autonomic ganglion, the rabbit ciliary ganglion. At birth all the postsynaptic cells are contacted by four to five axons, but in the adult this is reduced to a range of one to five. There is then a strong correlation between the number of afferent axons innervating each neuron and the number of dendrites it possesses.[46] This suggested that the separate inputs might become confined to separate dendrites during development. Afferent terminals

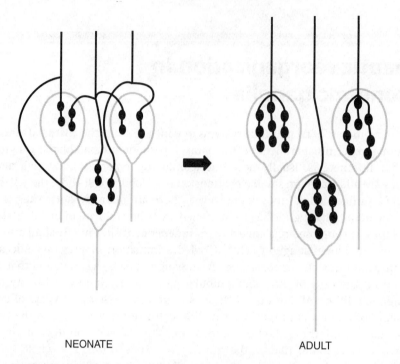

NEONATE   ADULT

Figure 14.3 Synaptic rearrangement in the submandibular ganglion of the rat after birth. Each afferent axon makes synapses with fewer neurons but increases the number of synaptic boutons on those neurons that it still innervates. After Lichtman.[43]

labelled with horseradish peroxidase (HRP) were indeed found to be confined to parts of the dendritic tree rather than being randomly dispersed over several dendrites.[47] Thus the presence of separate dendrites upon which inputs from different neurons can become segregated may help to allow multiple inputs to survive on adult nerve cells.

In general, it seems that elimination and rearrangement of branches in autonomic ganglia are controlled by factors similar to those at the neuromuscular junction. Success in competition for synaptic sites may be determined by the relative sizes of terminal tree supported by the competing neurons and the degree of 'chemoaffinity' between various possible synaptic partners. Preganglionic sympathetic neurons do seem to be labelled according to position as they are organized into discrete segmental units, each with a rostrocaudal polarity which determines the direction in which the axons in the sympathetic chain will run.[48] As in skeletal muscle the rate of synapse rearrangement is determined by the degree of electrical activity. Decreases in the amount of activity in the pathways to the rabbit ciliary ganglion slow the rate of removal of excess branches.[49] Unlike the situation in muscle, however, multiple inputs can persist in the adult when afferent terminals can be segregated at separate locations.

Synaptic reorganization in the CNS

The complexity and density of connections in the brain have made it less easy to identify the developmental changes that occur, but evidence for extensive synaptic rearrangement in the CNS during development has come from the use of several techniques. In the cerebellum, extra inputs can be demonstrated on immature Purkinje cells using the same simple stimulation and recording technique that was applied to muscle fibres and autonomic ganglia. Physiological recording has been particularly useful in the developing sensory pathways, especially the visual pathway, as it has shown the gradual refinement of receptive fields with age, and the dramatic effects that functional deprivation can have on these fields as they mature. These recording methods have more recently been supplemented by visualizing the changes in terminal branches of axons at several sites in the optic pathway at different ages by labelling axon terminals with a variety of tracers. Anatomical techniques have also uncovered the existence of branches that travel considerable distances to wholly abnormal sites in neonatal brains and which are later removed. The changes that occur in most, if not all, of these connections during development are dependent upon the electrical activity in the pathways and, as in the examples given already from the peripheral nervous system, competition between the terminals of different neurons determines which ones survive and expand.

The visual pathway: normal synaptic development, critical periods, electrical activity and competition

The ease with which the development of a normal adult visual system can be disrupted by brief periods of abnormal vision in early life gave one of the clearest hints that developing neural pathways are malleable and rely on activity to dictate how they mature. The changes in synaptic connections underlying normal and abnormal maturation could not be seen until the development of modern tracing techniques, and the earliest evidence was obtained from physiological recording. If one eye was permanently covered in kittens by suturing the lids together, or covering it with a patch, for a few critical weeks (the critical/sensitive period), starting at the normal time of eye opening and extending over the next four or so weeks, it was found impossible at the end of this time to excite cells in the visual cortex by stimulating the deprived eye. Stimuli to both eyes, however, could activate cells in the cortex of newborn kittens, and monocular deprivation had no such effect in adult cats.[50] If the deprived eye was opened during the sensitive period, only a limited degree of functional recovery occurred, but if the previously open eye was also closed (so-called reverse suture) the deprived eye recovered much more successfully.[51,52] It was shown later that restricting visual experience to a limited range of contours during the same critical period resulted in cortical neurons being able only to detect visual stimuli of the orientation to which the animal had been exposed.[53-55] The refinement in tuning of receptive fields in normal animals during the sensitive period has also been documented.

Since these pioneering experiments, several histological methods based on axonal transport have been used to display the distribution of axon terminals in the visual pathways. These methods have shown that the physiological changes of normal maturation, and the grossly abnormal responses following deprivation experiments, are accompanied by changes in the pattern of nerve terminal branches. A radioactively labelled amino acid can be injected into one eye, from where it is transported along the axons of the retinal ganglion cells to their terminals in the lateral geniculate nucleus (LGN) and superior colliculus; subsequent autoradiography of sections of the brain can then reveal the gross distribution of the terminals from one eye in the LGN and superior colliculus. Some label is also transferred to the cells in the LGN and thence to the terminals of these cells in layer IV of the visual cortex, where it can also be detected by so-called 'transneuronal' autoradiography. In addition, small deposits of HRP or fluorescently labelled tracers can be injected near terminals for retrograde transport, or on the visual pathways for anterograde transport, to outline the terminal arbors at different stages of development with and without various experimental manipulations.

Together with the electrophysiological recording methods, these techniques have shown that, at all levels in the visual pathway, the initial terminal distributions of afferent axons are more widespread but generally more sparse than in the adult (Fig. 14.4). The main change during normal development is for terminals to become considerably more restricted in distribution, but to become much more densely

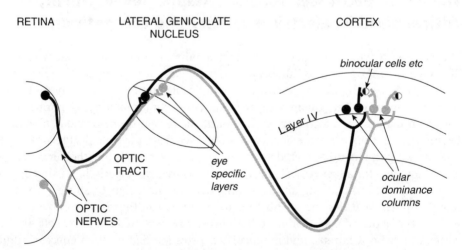

Figure 14.4 Simplified diagram of the pathway from retinal ganglion cells to the visual cortex of a mature mammal. Note the separation of the pathways from the two eyes up to layer IV of the visual cortex, where eye-specific ocular dominance bands occur. Binocular inputs to cortical cells occur in other cortical layers.

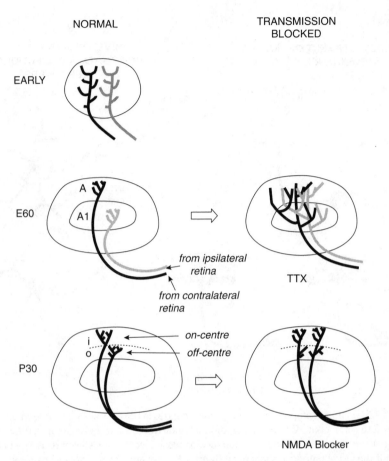

NORMAL

TRANSMISSION
BLOCKED

EARLY

E60

A

A1

from ipsilateral
retina

from contralateral
retina

TTX

P30

i

o

on-centre

off-centre

NMDA Blocker

Figure 14.5 Eye-specific layers in the kitten lateral geniculate nucleus arise as side-branches are pruned away from the axons, leaving the terminals from the two eyes in different regions of the nucleus. By embryonic day 60, layers A and A1 have formed and layer A is subsequently divided by separation of terminals of on-centre and off-centre axons. If transmission is blocked at any stage, the tidy separation of specific terminals does not occur. After Sretavan et al.[59] and Hahm et al.[67]

packed in these more limited areas (Figs 14.5 and 14.6). At all sites, the normal process is prevented if impulse activity is stopped. Many of these changes take place before birth in the LGN, and after birth in the cortex, so the activity that guides the earliest changes in the LGN is generated spontaneously in the retina while normal visual experience provides the activity after birth.

Lateral geniculate nucleus

The layered structure of the LGN in cats and primates, which separates the input from each eye into separate bands, is not laid down from the start. Transport of

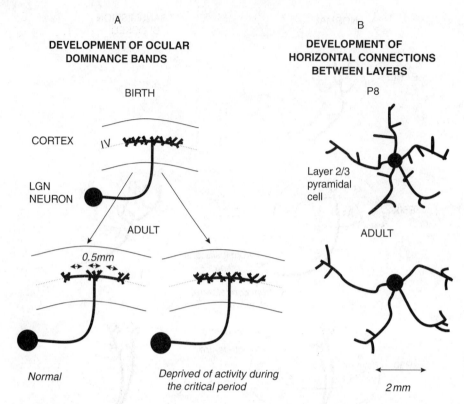

A
DEVELOPMENT OF OCULAR
DOMINANCE BANDS

B
DEVELOPMENT OF
HORIZONTAL CONNECTIONS
BETWEEN LAYERS

BIRTH

P8

CORTEX   IV

LGN
NEURON

Layer 2/3
pyramidal
cell

ADULT

ADULT

0.5mm

Normal

*Deprived of activity during
the critical period*

2 mm

Figure 14.6 Further examples of axon terminal changes in the CNS during development. In the cortex, diffuse connections are lost and additional branches form at more circumscribed specific regions. (A) This gives rise to ocular dominance bands in layer IV of visual cortex. The bands do not form if the visual pathway is inactivated. After Ferster and LeVay.[75] (B) Horizontal connections between layers also become localized between day 8 and adulthood. After Callaway and Katz.[111]

radiolabelled amino acids injected into one eye well before birth shows that the ganglion cell terminals initially project to all layers of the nucleus, while the same injection given just before birth shows them now to be confined to their appropriate layers as in the adult.[56] While some of this rearrangement may follow from death of retinal ganglion cells,[57] it cannot occur without additional major pruning of retinal ganglion cell arbors in the LGN. If HRP is applied to ganglion cell axons in the optic tract of fetal cats at different embryonic ages (between day 40 and birth at day 63) to stain the terminal arbors within the LGN, it can be seen that major changes occur over this time (Fig. 14.5).[58] The earliest terminals in the LGN stretch throughout the depth of the nucleus and have a few sparse side-branches in many layers. With time the distribution becomes limited to a single layer, but within that layer the terminals are much more dense.

This prenatal confinement and concentration of terminals to a single layer is prevented by infusion of tetrodotoxin (TTX) into the eye.[59] This blocks spontaneous waves of impulse activity that travel across the ganglion cell layer of the retina prenatally from reaching the terminals in the geniculate.[60-63] These waves can be detected by simultaneous recording from hundreds of ganglion cells, and are probably generated by cholinergic amacrine cells under the modulation of adenosine.[64,65] Under electrically silent conditions the terminals continue to expand but do not become confined to eye-specific layers (Fig. 14.5).[59,66] Postnatally, further separation of retinal ganglion cell afferent terminals subdivides the eye-specific layers into on-centre and off-centre compartments, and this separation is prevented by antagonists of the N-methyl-d-aspartate (NMDA) subtype of glutamate receptor (Fig. 14.5).[67] This effect of NMDA receptor blockade will be discussed later.

Cortical layer IV

The transneuronal labelling technique shows that at birth, when the retinal ganglion cell axon terminals in the LGN have already become separated into eye-specific bands, the terminals derived from neurons in these eye-specific bands are intermingled with one another in cortical layer IV. The terminals gradually segregate into eye-specific bands by several weeks of age.[68] Recording from neurons in layer IV reveals that there is a correlated functional segregation of the inputs from each eye into 'ocular dominance columns'.[69]

The segregation into bands is dependent on competition between terminals from the left and right eyes. If one eye is removed in monkeys before birth, the terminals in the cortex belonging to the pathway from the remaining eye do not condense into bands.[70] Activity is important for segregation to occur: if both eyes are sutured at birth, the separation of the geniculate afferents into bands in layer IV is reduced,[71] and it is abolished if TTX is used to block impulses which may arise spontaneously in the two eyes.[72] It is also possible to control the relative activity patterns in the visual pathways from the two eyes in kittens, using TTX to block impulse activity from one retina; a significant ocular dominance shift in favour of the active eye is found.[73] Moreover, if one eye is sutured shut at birth, its bands in layer IV shrink while those of the open eye remain expanded, providing evidence that the pathway from the open, active eye has a competitive advantage.[69] If deprivation is sufficiently prolonged, inputs from a deprived eye lose all functional connections in the cortex, presumably because connections are either permanently suppressed or withdrawn.[74]

Staining of terminal arborizations of individual geniculate afferents in the cortex of adult cats by anterograde labelling with HRP has shown a branching pattern in which areas of dense projection, approximately 0.5 mm in width (the same width as ocular dominance columns), are separated by similar-sized areas largely devoid of branches.[75] The development of this pattern has been followed by anterograde labelling of geniculate terminals in the cortex at different ages. As for retinal afferents in the geniculate, the cortical arbors change gradually from being sparse but widely dispersed to being less dispersed and patchily concentrated, with local sprouting and synapse formation in the selected cortical region. If impulse activity is blocked, the arbors continue to grow but do not show regions of high branch density separated by ones of low density.[76] Ocular dominance columns fail to develop if the subplate neurons (which form a transient population of neurons which make connections to layer IV and the LGN, see Chapter 7) are destroyed by exposing them to the excitotoxin kainic acid in the first postnatal week,[77] but it is unknown how subplate cells interact with the geniculate afferent terminals to influence the development of the dominance columns.

While experiments on the plasticity of ocular dominance columns have emphasized the importance of visual experience in instructing the development of cortical circuitry, more recent work has also shown the operation of other factors. Ocular dominance columns in non-human primates are in fact fully formed at birth,[78] and it is possible that they are generated *in utero* by correlated patterns of LGN neuronal activity driven by the spontaneous waves of retinal activity discussed above.[79] The degree to which activity-*independent* mechanisms are also involved in their development is uncertain.

Eye-dominance stripes in the tectum of three-eyed frogs

A further example of competitive interaction between pathways from different eyes has come from experiments in which bands of tectal innervation alternately dominated by one of two eyes have been created experimentally in amphibia. In normal amphibia the decussation of axons from each eye is complete, so each tectum is normally the territory of only one eye. However, bands remarkably similar to those in the mammalian visual cortex can be induced in the tectum if it is made to receive innervation from two eyes, either the two normal ones[80] or from a transplanted third eye in addition to the normal eye.[81] The recognition mechanisms which distribute terminals across the tectum in a retinotopic fashion (Chapter 10) will operate for axons from each eye, and it has been suggested that some 'nearest neighbour' interaction between axons groups together terminals from the same eye within any one retinotopically labelled territory.[82] It is probably the approximately synchronous electrical activity of neighbouring retinal ganglion cells from one eye which constitutes the driving force for segregation of terminals from different eyes, as bands do not form in a tectum receiving projections from eyes whose retinae are made unable to fire action potentials by injections of TTX.[83,84] It is also known that optic nerve terminals vacate a small area of tectum that has been blocked postsynaptically with α-bungarotoxin and make new connections nearby.[85] The basis of the nearest-neighbour interaction may therefore be synchronous activity in axon terminals and postsynaptic tectal cells, producing stabilization of connections in localized bands. Thus the pattern of ocular dominance stripes in the tectum of three-eyed frogs could develop in the same way as in the cortex of mammals. In the LGN, where the bands are always in the same places, some additional mechanisms are probably needed.[86] This may indicate that there are differences in the sorting mechanisms employed when afferents project to sheets of cells arranged in layers (cortex or tectum) and when they project to collections of neurons in nuclei (LGN).

Receptive fields of neurons within the visual cortex

As we have seen, visual information is conducted to the neurons of layer IV of the visual cortex by the geniculate afferents and is distributed within the cortex by local intracortical connections (Fig. 14.4). The pattern of these connections and the changes that occur in them during development determine the receptive field properties of cortical neurons and these are considered now.

The properties of neurons in the visual cortex of normal kittens immediately after eye opening are not unlike those of adult cats, suggesting that these properties are innately determined.[87,88] It is clear, however, that the properties are only partly specified in visually naive animals. Receptive field sizes are larger in newborn kittens than in the adult, orientation specificities are found in only a minority of cells and these are crudely tuned,[89] and in binocular cells there is poor matching between the receptive field properties for each eye.[90] Furthermore, dark rearing prevents much of the normal maturation of receptive field properties of cortical neurons, with binocular neurons especially affected.[91] In the monkey, certain properties may be more accurately prespecified than in kittens,[92] but a careful study of spatial resolution and contrast sensitivity of cortical neurons in monkeys deprived of vision since birth shows that these are seriously impaired.[93] This cortical impairment is not due to deterioration at the level of the LGN.[94] The postnatal period is thus a time when connections within the cortex are easily modified and the electrophysiological properties resulting from the connections can be tuned or refined by visual experience. Little activity is needed to produce tuning of cortical neurons. Kittens reared in the dark and then exposed to a restricted visual environment for as little as an hour during the critical period develop restricted responses in visual cortical cells.[95] Responses can be modified in an anaesthetized, visually naive kitten in several minutes of testing of a neuron's receptive field.[96] In kittens the critical period is, as we have seen, quite short.

In humans the critical period during which binocular vision can be impaired by untreated strabismus (see below) extends up to about the age of 5.[97] Further studies on children born with congenital cataracts (the equivalent of lid suture in kittens) who have then been treated have shown that several other aspects of visual performance, especially acuity, are severely impaired by early deprivation. Improvements, but not to normality, are achieved by cataract removal if this is carried out before 5 years of age, and they are greater the earlier surgery is carried out. While rearrangement of intracortical connections is very important for the improvement of visual processing after birth, it should also be noted that much of the improvement is due to changes occurring in the retina (eye enlargement and receptor density packing)[98] and in the optics of the eye, and substantial improvements go on for up to 4 months after eye opening in kittens, that is for longer than the classical critical period.[99]

Development of binocular receptive fields

The first property of visual cortical neurons found to be modified by experience was the binocular field. Closing one eye of kittens for a few days or more during weeks 4–8 after birth reduced the number of cells in the cortex which could be activated by both eyes.[100] Closure of one eye also causes shrinkage of geniculate afferent terminals conveying information from it, as we have seen, so it was not clear whether the loss of binocularity of higher-order neurons was a consequence of this shrinkage or a direct effect on intracortical connections. Loss of binocular cells was, however, also detected in cats that had been raised with an artificial squint (strabismus). A loss of binocular cells was also found when kittens were reared with alternate daily occlusion of each eye throughout the critical period,[101] or if raised in an environment lit only intermittently and briefly by stroboscopic flashes.[102] This means that the loss of binocularity is likely to be an effect of the experimental manipulations on connections within the cortex from the eye-specific neurons of layer IV, because none of them, unlike eye suture throughout the critical period, has an effect on development of the LGN.

All the manipulations preventing the development of binocularly driven cells have in common the fact that they reduce the probability of visual inputs from the two eyes synchronously activating cells in layer IV whose outputs converge onto neurons in other layers. A role for synchronous activity in the development of binocular cells in the tectum of normal frogs was proposed independently many years ago.[103] Frogs have polysynaptic connections linking points on the two tecta which receive input from the same point in space. As the animals metamorphose the eyes migrate more dorsally, so to continue to link visually equivalent points on each tectum the intertectal connections must move, which they normally do. They do not succeed in doing so if the animals are reared in the dark.[104]

Development of orientation selectivity

The orientation preference of cortical neurons has also been shown to be modified by experience. If kittens are reared in a variety of ways that restrict their vision to contours of only one orientation, single neurons recorded in the visual cortex are found to respond predominantly to lines and bars of that orientation.[53–55]

This limitation of performance can be induced only during the critical period (e.g. reference 95), and the finding has been confirmed using optical recording, which eliminates any sampling bias.[105]

When vision is restricted to such a limited range of orientations, more cortical cells than normal respond to that orientation; the corresponding orientation columns on the cortical surface are also wider and there are few non-responsive cells.[106] Exposure to a single orientation therefore tunes not only the receptive fields of neurons that would respond to that orientation in the normal adult but also those of additional neurons to that orientation. This is possible, presumably, because the receptive fields in the neonate are broadly tuned: the cells receive many inputs, most of which are normally eliminated but which can be stabilized by exceptional overuse in unusual environments.

While the development of normal orientation-tuned receptive fields needs visual experience, there is also evidence that the overall layout of orientation preference maps in the right and left visual cortices may be innate and develops without the two eyes having common visual experience.[107] This allows alignment of the input from the two eyes and binocular interactions. The finding that orientation-selective neurons are detectable at birth in the visual cortex of cats and monkeys also supports a degree of innate prespecification. As for the segregation *in utero* of primate LGN axons into ocular dominance columns, this could arise from spontaneous activity within the developing visual pathway as much as from activity-independent mechanisms. For example, groups of neurons in the developing cortex have been shown to undergo spontaneous, coordinated fluctuations in intracellular calcium concentration, propagated via gap junctions and elicited by metabotropic glutamate receptors, and these could provide correlated patterns of activity to guide cortical circuit formation in the absence of environmental stimulation.[79,108] The importance of neuronal activity in shaping orientation selectivity at an early stage is also shown by the reduced selectivity that results from synchronous activation of retinal axons in the optic nerve in the developing ferret, an animal whose visual system is accessible experimentally at a younger maturational phase than the cat or monkey.[109]

Anatomical changes during intracortical remodelling

The precise details of intracortical wiring that account for the various sorts of receptive field found in the visual cortex are not known, and so it is not possible to visualize the changing patterns of connections that presumably underlie the normal maturation of properties, and also the development of abnormal properties under unusual conditions, although interesting theoretical models have been proposed.[110] Developmental changes in the branch pattern of some intracortical connections have been seen, however, by labelling the horizontal connections of layer 2/3 pyramidal cells by microinjections of non-diffusing microspheres. These are taken up by terminals in the vicinity and label these and all other parts of the neurons by retrograde transport.[111] The results are illustrated in Fig. 14.6. It has also been shown that these intrinsic horizontal connections are selected by correlated neuronal activity.[112] Another method used to visualize the development of intracortical circuits is optical recording of cortical slices with voltage-sensitive dyes. This has shown that neurons making horizontal connections in the developing visual cortex add large numbers of new branches and synapses to local, selected cortical regions.[113] Cortical maturation, in other words, does not exclusively involve selecting and stabilizing pre-existing synapses.

Further examples of synaptic reorganization in the developing brain

Multiple climbing fibre inputs on Purkinje cells

Purkinje cells are large output neurons of the cerebellar cortex. In the adult mammalian cerebellum each Purkinje cell is innervated by a single climbing fibre which originates from one of the neurons in the inferior olive. In the newborn rat two to three climbing fibre inputs project onto each Purkinje cell, and these can be detected by recording from the Purkinje cells with a microelectrode and applying graded stimulation to the inferior olive.[114] These multiple climbing fibre inputs are normally lost over the first few postnatal weeks but persist in some mouse mutants with cerebellar disorders in which there is a failure in the formation of parallel fibre synapses on the Purkinje dendrites. It is possible that parallel fibre synapses increase the competitive interaction among the climbing fibres by also competing for a shared trophic factor.[115] Blockade of NMDA receptors by D-2-amino-5-phosphonovalerate (APV) has been found to prevent the elimination of multiple climbing fibre inputs on Purkinje cells,[116] and the role of NMDA receptors is described later. Elimination of multiple climbing fibre inputs is also incomplete in mice with targeted deletions of the type 1 metabotropic glutamate receptor (mGluR1)[117] and protein kinase A.[118]

Auditory system

Behavioural adaptations which can come about only during early postnatal life, and whose basis is presumably the stabilization of the most utilized neuronal circuits, have been described in the auditory system of birds. Particularly precise localization of sounds is important for a nocturnal hunter like the owl and depends on analysis of input from the two ears. Adult barn owls not surprisingly lose the ability to localize sound accurately whenever binaural input is distorted with an earplug. Young birds, however, can learn to compensate for an earplug,[119] presumably by adjusting central connections to allow for the weaker sound intensity in the plugged ear. Normal maps of auditory space also need normal binaural inputs in mammals, and do not develop in ferrets if NMDA receptors in the superior colliculus are blocked during early life.[120]

Most birds which can sing learn their repertoire of songs during their first year of life. The birds have innate calls of their own but learn during this period to match these to the calls of adults or other environmental sounds (not necessarily even bird-calls). The connections underlying the innate calls provide a rough template which can be modified in the light of experience. As the birds age it eventually becomes impossible for them to learn to make any new sounds.[121]

A third example providing evidence for a limited period of neuronal plasticity in the auditory system is given by an experiment analogous to the restricted vision experiments carried out on the visual pathways. If the normal range of sound patterns is prevented from reaching the auditory pathways of mice by entraining all primary auditory neurons to fire together, the tuning curves of cells in the inferior colliculus of young mice can never become as sharply tuned as normal.[122]

Somatosensory system

Three examples of developmental changes in nerve terminal distribution in the somatosensory system will be given, one at the level of the spinal cord and the other two in the somatosensory cortex.

In the adult, large-diameter cutaneous sensory afferents and small-diameter sensory afferents project to different laminae in the spinal grey matter. In particular, the large afferents avoid lamina II, the substantia gelatinosa. Specific labelling of large-diameter afferents with HRP conjugated to cholera toxin has shown that up to the third postnatal week in rats they project throughout laminae I to V, and only later become confined largely to lamina III.[123]

The somatosensory cortex in rodents can undergo major neural modifications only during a critical neonatal period. Sensory axons innervating the snout whiskers (vibrissae) relay via the trigeminal nucleus in the medulla and the thalamus to layer 4 of the somatosensory cortex, where they occupy a large proportion of the available territory. Axons from each whisker project to a corresponding cluster of cells in the cortex, known as a barrel. Barrels are visible in sections of the cortex made parallel to the surface of normal adult animals, and the barrel pattern matches precisely the layout of whiskers on the snout.[124] The projection develops in a peripheral-to-central direction, with the trigeminal nucleus receiving innervation from the periphery *in utero*, while thalamocortical projections are not established until after birth. Destruction of an individual vibrissa in animals a few days old halts the development of the cortical barrel corresponding to the deleted whisker, but the same injury in the adult has no effect.[125] It appears that NMDA receptors are critically involved in refining the barrel map, as discussed below.

In children and young animals, section of a peripheral nerve is followed by much less sensory disability than in adults. It is probable that the success of peripheral nerve regeneration is not very different at the two ages, but topographic maps can be restored much more successfully in the somatosensory cortex of the young. This is possible because at the time of injury there still exist widespread as yet unrefined connections in the cortex. These provide an innervation density great enough to re-establish somatotopic maps by favouring preservation of synapses which successfully correlate their patterns of activity with other inputs, and this is most likely between inputs innervating neighbouring skin areas.[126] In other words, in the young a jumbled innervation at the periphery can be compensated by appropriate modification at the cortical level.

Temperature regulation circuits

The ability of animals to regulate their temperature depends on circuitry which has to be activated during development. If animals are not exposed to cool temperatures during rearing then the ability of animals to maintain their body temperature in a cool environment is impaired thereafter.[127,128] This effect is not caused by changes in the sensitivity of peripheral thermoreceptors, so it probably depends on development of central regulatory pathways.

Aberrant collaterals

A further sort of rearrangement of axon branches occurs in the CNS during development. The branch rearrangements described above all occur within the normal terminal territory of the axons concerned. There is also a wholesale loss of axons which have grown to unusual (aberrant) sites in the brain. The presence of these transient aberrant projections is perhaps surprising given the guidance systems that have been described (Chapter 9), but they might arise because of the presence in the developing brain of several non-discriminatory pathways which can be followed by a range of growing axons.[129] The aberrant branches have been detected by finding that dyes injected into a given part of the brain of neonates are retrogradely transported and label cell bodies at places within the brain which in the adult never send branches to the dye-injection site. The axon collaterals that pick up the dye in the neonate eventually disappear, but not because the parent neurons themselves die. This is made clear from the fact that the cell bodies retrogradely labelled in the neonate are still detectable weeks or months later even though their aberrant branches have by now gone.

For example, an injection of dye into the pyramidal tract projecting down the spinal cord labels neurons right across the cortex of newborn rats, including the visual cortex, while the same injections made three weeks later fail to label any neurons in the visual cortex.[130] Another example is revealed by injections of dye into any part of the cortex of newborn rats. These label cells in the corresponding region of the contralateral cortex, having been picked up by collaterals running to the other side of the brain in the corpus callosum. In the adult the callosal connections are only found in the somatosensory areas[131] and the visual areas which represent the midline of visual space.[132] Large numbers of the axons in the developing corpus callosum appear to be of this aberrant type.[133] It is interesting that in cats with a squint, there are considerably more connections between the visual areas.[134] This suggests that those axon branches in the corpus callosum that join together areas sharing the same region of visual space are retained because they are activated synchronously by visual stimuli.

Possible mechanisms underlying changes in neural connections

It is clear from the previous sections that electrical activity and competition between inputs are both important in determining the pattern of neural connectivity. The competitive mechanism seems to involve stabilization of only those inputs where there is synchrony of pre- and postsynaptic activity, with other inputs being lost—the so-called 'fire together, wire together' rule, or Hebbian synapse. In some situations there is even electrical coupling between neurons present during the critical period, for example certain cortical units with a common function, so that their firing patterns are inevitably synchronized and connections harmonized.[135]

It was first suggested over 50 years ago[136] that modifications of synaptic effectiveness based on the 'fire together, wire together' idea underlie the processes of learning and memory in the adult, and the same now appears to apply to stabilization of developing synapses. An important part of the cellular mechanism for learning is the NMDA subtype of glutamate receptor in the postsynaptic membrane, which is known to be involved in the initiation of long-term potentiation (LTP) in many regions of the cerebral cortex (Chapter 15). A possible role for the NMDA receptor in the modification of connections in the developing visual cortex was originally indicated by two observations. If these receptors are blocked with a specific antagonist during monocular occlusion in kittens, the development of dominance by the open eye does not occur.[137] Conversely, iontophoretic application of specific receptor agonists during presentation of visual stimuli to kittens induces receptive fields tuned to the form of the stimulus.[138] Furthermore, the specific antagonist APV causes the ocular dominance stripes formed in the tectum of three-eyed frogs to disappear[139] and, as noted earlier, it also prevents the subdivision of the ocular bands in the LGN of kittens.

The endogenous ligand for the NMDA receptor is glutamate, but it only succeeds in opening the ionic channels and allowing depolarizing calcium current to pass if there is sufficient overall depolarization of the cell (Chapter 15). This could explain why simultaneously active inputs may be stabilized, for the overall depolarization will then be greater. The NMDA receptor acts as a coincidence detector and each active input tends to assist others active at the same time. The degree of synchrony in the timing of activity in convergent inputs needed to mutually reinforce their connections is probably of the order of a few hundreds of milliseconds.[140] This is a long time compared to the duration of conventional postsynaptic potentials. Synaptic potentials may, however, last longer in dendrites, and there is evidence that action potentials propagate retrogradely back into the dendritic tree when cortical neurons are discharging impulses and these antidromic potentials are accompanied by a sustained rise in calcium concentration. Cortical plasticity can be blocked if non-specific excitatory noradrenergic[141] and cholinergic[142] inputs are inactivated. This may be because the visual inputs on their own may not produce enough depolarization to open the NMDA-coupled Ca^{2+} channels. Similarly, the extra depolarization produced by iontophoretic application of acetylcholine or noradrenaline may explain the induction of receptive fields specific to visual stimuli given at the same time as the transmitters are applied.[138]

A study of the developing retinotectal projection in *Xenopus* embryos has shown just how tightly correlated electrical activity needs to be in the pre- and postsynaptic elements of this system for the presynaptic element to be potentiated. If an individual input to a target tectal neuron is below threshold for initiating an action potential, it can be potentiated (in an NMDA-receptor-dependent manner) by the other pre-synaptic inputs provided it is itself active within a critical 20-ms time window before the action potential. If input activity arises within a 20-ms window *after* the tectal spike it is further depressed, and this depressive effect also applies to late-arriving suprathreshold inputs.[143]

There is an attractive parsimony in the idea that the same biophysical mechanism underlies memory storage in the adult hippocampus and synaptic stabilization during the critical period. However, in the mammalian cortex it remains unclear whether the result of NMDA receptor blockade is a specific effect or a non-specific consequence of transmission failure, and the relationship of LTP to critical periods is still tentative.[79] This is particularly clear from experiments using knockout mice: animals lacking some forms of cortical LTP (for example following protein kinase A knockout) may show, nonetheless, robust ocular dominance shifts in response to monocular deprivation. Conversely, animals lacking such ocular dominance shifts (for example following knockout of an isoform of the synthetic enzyme for the inhibitory transmitter GABA) may show normal LTP.[144] Even if the NMDA receptor is involved, the mechanism by which its activation causes retention of active pre-synaptic synapses and the loss of inactive ones is unclear; one speculation is that activation of NMDA receptors is coupled to release of neurotrophic factors needed for survival—see below. Another cellular element, however, provides a further parallel between adult learning and developmental plasticity. It is the calcium-sensitive enzyme CamKII (calcium/calmodulin protein kinase II), which is important in the generation of LTP in the hippocampus (see Chapter 15). Overexpression of a truncated version of CamKII, by exposure of cells of the developing *Xenopus* tectum to engineered vaccinia virus, causes retinal axon terminals to lose branches and become less elaborate, probably by promoting the early retraction of new synapses.[145]

The relation between LTP and developmental plasticity has also been investigated in the development of whisker barrels in the rodent somatosensory cortex. Robust LTP can be demonstrated between thalamic inputs and layer 4 cells of the sensory cortex in slice preparations of thalamus and cortex, but only during early postnatal life,[146] a finding at least consistent with a role for LTP in barrel development. A role for NMDA receptors has also been suggested by experiments designed to block them pharmacologically, for example by local application of the NMDA receptor antagonist AP5 to the neocortex in postnatal rats. In this case the barrel pattern is unperturbed, but the one-to-one functional relation between whiskers and barrels is disrupted.[147] In general, though, the results of different pharmacological studies have been conflicting, and a more recent approach has been to exploit the advantages of the rodent system in creating targeted gene deletions that disrupt LTP during development. In knockouts of the NMDA R1 subunit, in which the NMDA receptor is rendered functionally inactive, whisker-related innervation territories in the trigeminal nucleus fail to appear, but the early postnatal death of these animals precludes assessment of the consequences for cortical barrel development.[148] The life of these animals can be prolonged, however, by ectopic expression of an NMDAR1 transgene: while barrels develop normally in the presence of high levels of transgene, they fail to develop in the presence of low levels, despite a normal density of axon projections. This result argues strongly that NMDA receptor-mediated events are critical in refining the pattern of somatosensory projections.[149]

Role of neurotrophins in synaptic plasticity

There is evidence that neurotrophins (Chapter 12) may also have a part to play in cortical synaptic plasticity (see reference 150 for review). Infusions of NGF into rat and kitten cerebral ventricles during the critical period prevent the effects of monocular deprivation,[151,152] and infusions of NT-4 or -5 or BDNF prevent the formation of ocular dominance columns in the region of visual cortex exposed to these factors.[153] Local cortical injections of NT-4 also reduce the shrinkage of LGN cell bodies that receive input from a visually-deprived eye during the critical period.[154] Such results suggest that terminals that would otherwise be eliminated may be rescued by exogenous supplies of trophic support, and a similar hypothesis has been discussed in the section on synapse elimination at the neuromuscular junction. It is conceivable that all types of pre- and postsynaptic contact are maintained by synchronous activity, partly because it provides optimal provision of trophic factors; for example, the activated postsynaptic cell might release neurotrophins which would be effective only on simultaneously activated presynaptic inputs. Even developmental changes in inhibitory synapses are disrupted if they are not activated.[155]

A diagram of the sort of positive feedback mechanism that may be present is given in Fig. 14.7. In such a scheme, exogenous supplies of appropriate growth factors could

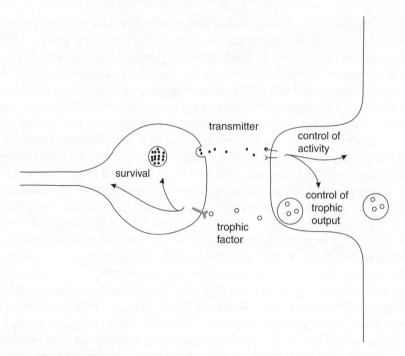

Figure 14.7 Hypothetical linkage between successful presynaptic activation of a postsynaptic site and retrograde support for presynaptic survival mediated by neurotrophin release. Whether target neurons do release neurotrophins locally in response to local synaptic activity is unknown, as is the way in which neurotrophins promote local terminal survival.

compensate neurons and their terminals for lack of activity-stimulated supplies. It remains important to determine whether endogenous supplies of the appropriate neurotrophins are expressed in localized regions of cortex as required by the model, and whether neural activity is able to regulate local neurotrophin signalling with sufficient rapidity. In support of the model, it has been shown both *in vivo* and *in vitro* that levels of neuronal NGF mRNA are increased following activation of excitatory inputs to hippocampus and cerebral neocortex, and NGF release has also been shown to be regulated by electrical activity in hippocampal neurons *in vitro*.[156] A further question is how neurotrophins might work to modulate synaptic efficacy: is their role at the synapse directly instructive, or are they just permissive in setting the threshold for activity-dependent synaptic rearrangements?

An alternative model for the action of neurotrophins is suggested by the consequences of a genetic manipulation in mice in which BDNF is overexpressed in excitatory cortical neurons. The model just discussed predicts that such an excess of BDNF, available to all presynaptic terminals, would abolish the advantages of correlated activity. Instead, however, the surprising result is an *acceleration* of the critical period: monocular closure continues to exert its effects on ocular dominance, but these are seen several days earlier than normal. This appears to be the result of an accelerated maturation of cortical inhibitory interneurons, which express abundant receptors for BDNF, and the implication is that such inhibitory circuits are also critically involved in the regulation of the critical period.[144,157]

Expansion of synaptic circuitry during the critical period

Several examples of expansion of nerve branches and connections during the critical period have been given above, and a much greater emphasis has been put on this aspect of synaptic rearrangement in recent years. Indeed, it has been argued that the brain is constructed more by the 'gradual accretion of circuitry' rather than by selection and elimination of initial excess connections.[158] The driving force for this selective expansion is not known, but it has been proposed that it is driven in unknown ways by activity, the so-called 'glow and grow' hypothesis.[158] In keeping with this there is evidence that the level of expression of mRNA for neurotrophic factors is higher in active than inactive neurons,[159,160] and that the more exercise an adult rat takes the higher are the levels of neurotrophin mRNAs![161] There is also evidence that neurons can respond better to sprout-inducing stimuli if they are active.[162]

What controls the duration of the critical period?

There is at present no clear explanation for the limited time span of the postnatal critical period during which major changes in synaptic connectivity in many parts of the nervous system can be made in mammals. It is unclear too how the major plasticity evident during the critical period relates to the lesser degree of adaptability present in the adult (to be described in Chapter 17). Are the mechanisms different, or is the adult plasticity a quantitatively scaled-down version of the same processes, and does adaptability really change rather less suddenly than is usually described? It is also necessary to be aware that *maintenance* of already fully refined circuits may need active help for some time after their formation and this period may extend beyond the classical critical period. In children, for example, visual acuity improves to adult levels by around 5 years of age, but vision can be seriously impaired by damage to the optics of the eye at any time up to the late-teenage years but not thereafter.

In fishes and amphibians, in which new neurons are continuously added in parts of the brain and their axons can grow, 'neonatal'-like plasticity is a permanent feature and terminals can become modified extensively at all ages.[163,164] Regeneration of severed axons is also possible. It may be that the loss of plasticity amongst the terminal branches of neurons in older mammals parallels the inability of severed axons to regrow, and possible reasons for this are discussed in Chapter 17. It is also possible that there is downregulation of neurotrophic factors postnatally in the brain, as has been seen in skeletal muscle during the time of synapse elimination, and that there is also downregulation of growth-associated genes in nerve cell bodies.[23,165] If supplies of NGF are kept at low levels for all neurons in the developing rat cerebral cortex, by implanting hybridoma cells secreting antibodies to NGF into the cerebral ventricles for the duration of the normal critical period, subsequent monocular deprivation results in amblyopia in the deprived eye showing that the critical period can be prolonged;[166] it is as if all weapons of competition had been temporarily removed and so no branches could lose. In songbirds such as the zebrafinch the limited time span over which their singing matures coincides with a reduction in expression of a specific protein (synelfin) in one particular nucleus.[167] There may also be age-related changes in NMDA receptor subunits which could affect their possible role in plasticity.[168]

Synaptic reorganization that occurs prenatally is driven by spontaneous waves of activity and the time course of this activity presumably partly determines the duration of the reorganization process. The electrical activity in the developing retina has been described earlier; such spontaneous activity occurs elsewhere, for example in the developing spinal cord of the chick.[169]

Conclusions

There are two main features of the stage of development in which synaptic connections are being reorganized: withdrawal of many connections and stabilization and expansion of others. Branches which fail to activate the postsynaptic cell, either alone or when acting in concert with other inputs, fail to survive and are usually withdrawn, although some may persist as 'silent' synapses (Fig. 14.8, see also Chapter 17). There is evidence that the NMDA glutamate receptor, which is involved in learning in the adult brain (Chapter 15), plays a part in stabilizing active synapses and also that levels of neurotrophins affect the amount of rearrangement that occurs. Before birth, patterns of correlated activity arise spontaneously from the intrinsic design of developing circuits and are vital for laying out basic connections. Activity driven by behaviour provides the patterns at later times, allowing environmental influences to shape circuitry.

The mechanism of expansion of branches in the surviving regions of the network is less clear, but activity again may be important. The factors that determine the duration of the sensitive critical period, when such extensive reorganization of functional connections occurs, remain uncertain. After this period the amount of residual plasticity is considerably less, although limited readjustments do occur following injury or other situations in the adult in which particular inputs are made relatively much less or much more active than others (Chapter 17).

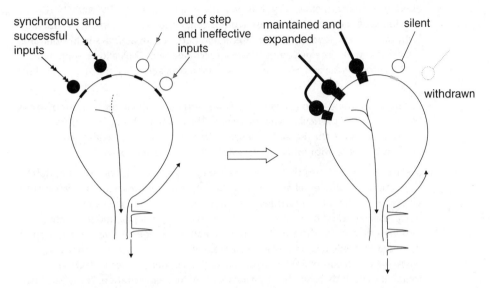

DURING CRITICAL PERIOD   AFTER CRITICAL PERIOD

synchronous and successful inputs

out of step and ineffective inputs

maintained and expanded

silent

withdrawn

Figure 14.8 Summary of possible events during synapse stabilization. Synchronous inputs succeed in activating the postsynaptic neuron. They receive positive 'trophic' feedback and their postsynaptic receptors are increased and new branches grow. Inputs out of step with the majority do not succeed in activating the cell and get no or negative reinforcement. Some are maintained as 'silent' synapses, capable of reactivation under circumstances more favourable to them (Chapter 15), while other inputs are withdrawn.

Key points

1 Following the phase of nerve cell death, further modifications occur in the developing nervous system as the branching pattern of axon terminals and the detailed distribution of synaptic connections made by each neuron gradually evolve from the initial array that formed when axons first reached their synaptic targets.

2 It is usual for the initial connections of each neuron to be spread over a large area but nowhere to be very dense. The maturation process typically reduces the overall spread of the axonal tree but increases the density of branches in the remaining areas. Some parts of the first-formed axonal tree are therefore eliminated while other parts are stabilized and enlarged, thus concentrating the connections of neurons onto fewer postsynaptic cells.

3 The major changes occur over a limited time period, the critical or sensitive period, the onset of which varies in different parts of the nervous system. In the visual pathways, for example, many of the changes in the lateral geniculate nucleus take place before birth, but in the visual cortex they occur after birth.

4 Normal patterns of impulse activity are needed for the formation of typical normal branching and connectivity patterns; by preventing impulse activity, or otherwise altering the pattern of activity, it is possible to alter connectivity. Activity is developed at early times by spontaneously generated waves of impulses, but after birth the activity depends on the interaction between an animal's behaviour and the environment. The period of synapse rearrangement thus allows epigenetic (e.g. environmental and behavioural) factors to play a part in determining the final shape of neural circuits.

5 The most profound changes come from preventing activity in one of a set of axons that projects to a particular synaptic region. The inactive neurons lose all functional connections, while the remaining neurons have larger terminal fields than usual. So neurons compete with others to establish their connection patterns.

6 In skeletal muscle fibres that have only a single synaptic site, the motor endplate, competition eliminates all but the branches of a single motor neuron. Postsynaptic blockade of even a few branches of a single axon at an endplate causes the synaptically blocked branches to be withdrawn. It seems possible that active terminals that excite the endplate to an adequate degree receive trophic support from neurotrophic factors passed retrogradely from the muscle. In contrast, postsynaptic receptors are lost from the regions underlying less-effective terminals, which therefore become incapable of further excitation. These terminals probably also receive a retrograde message but one which triggers withdrawal.

7 On most neurons very large numbers of synaptic sites coexist. The synaptic terminals that survive competition are probably those whose activity pattern coincides with that of a substantial number of other inputs and succeed in activating the postsynaptic cell. There is evidence that successful activation of NMDA glutamate receptors is needed for synapses to survive during the critical period at many places in the CNS, and that acquisition of neurotrophic factors is important for survival of terminals.

8 It is not known what determines the limited time span of the critical period, but it may be associated with an intrinsic downregulation of growth-associated genes, changes in NMDA receptor subunits with age, and the onset of an environment which is inhibitory to growth.

9 It is also unknown what drives the expansion of successful parts of the axonal tree, but it has been suggested that impulse activity is needed.

General reading

- Berardi, N. *et al.* Critical periods during sensory development. *Curr. Opin. Neurobiol.* **10**, 138–45 (2000).

- Sanes, J. R. and Lichtman, J. W. Can molecules explain long-term potentiation? *Nat. Neurosci.* **2**, 597–604 (1999).

- Katz, L. C. What's critical for the critical period in visual cortex? *Cell* **99**, 673–6 (1999).

References

1. Gaze, R. M., Chung, S. and Keating, M. J. Development of the retinotectal projection in *Xenopus. Nature (New Biology)* **236**, 133–5 (1972).

2. Tello, J. F. Genesis de los terminaciones nerviosas motrices y sensitivas. I. En el sistema locomotor de los vertebrados superiores. Histogenesis muscular. *Trab. Lab. Invest. Biol. Univ. Madrid* **15**, 101–99 (1917).

3. Redfern, P. A. Neuromuscular transmission in newborn rats. *J. Physiol.* **209**, 701–9 (1970).

4. Bagust, J., Lewis, D. M. and Westerman, R. A. Polyneuronal innervation of kitten skeletal muscle. *J. Physiol.* **229**, 241–55 (1973).

5. Brown, M. C., Jansen, J. K. S. and Van Essen, D. Polyneuronal innervation of skeletal muscle in new born rats and its elimination during maturation. *J. Physiol.* **261**, 387–442 (1976).

6. Korneliussen, H. and Jansen, J. K. S. Morphological aspects of the elimination of polyneuronal innervation of skeletal muscle fibres in newborn rats. *J. Neurocytol.* **5**, 591–604 (1976).

7. Riley, D. A. Multiple axon branches innervating single endplates of kitten soleus myofibres. *Brain Res.* **110**, 158–61 (1976).

8. Jordan, C. L., Letinsky, M. S. and Arnold, A. P. The role of gonadal hormones in neuromuscular synapse elimination in rats. I. Androgen delays the loss of multiple innervation in the levator ani muscle. *J. Neurosci.* **9**, 229–38 (1989).

9. Jordan, C. L., Letinsky, M. S. and Arnold, A. P. The role of gonadal hormones in neuromuscular synapse elimination in rats. II. Multiple innervation persists in the adult levator ani muscle after juvenile androgen treatment. *J. Neurosci.* **9**, 239–47 (1989).

10. Riley, D. A. Spontaneous elimination of nerve terminals from the endplates of developing skeletal myofibres. *Brain Res.* **134**, 279–85 (1977).

11. Riley, D. A. Ultrastructural evidence for axon retraction during the spontaneous elimination of polyneuronal innervation of the rat soleus muscle. *J. Neurocytol.* **10**, 425–40 (1981).

12. Connold, A. L., Evers, J. V. and Vrbova, G. Effect of low calcium and protease inhibitors on synapse elimination during postnatal development in the rat soleus muscle. *Dev. Brain Res.* **28**, 99–107 (1986).

13. Rich, M. M. and Lichtman, J. W. *In vivo* visualization of pre- and post-synaptic changes during synapse elimination in reinnervated mouse muscle. *J. Neurosci.* **9**, 1781–805 (1989).

14. Balice-Gordon, R. J. and Lichtman, J. W. *In vivo* observations of pre- and postsynaptic changes during the transition from multiple to single innervation at developing neuromuscular junctions. *J. Neurosci.* **13**, 834–55 (1993).

15. Balice-Gordon, R. J. and Lichtman, J. W. Long-term synapse loss induced by focal blockade of postsynaptic receptors. *Nature* **372**, 519–24 (1994).

16. Dan, Y. and Poo, M. Hebbian depression of isolated neuromuscular synapses *in vitro. Science* **256**, 1570–3 (1992).

17. Wang, T., Xie, Z. and Lu, B. Nitric oxide mediates activity-dependent synaptic suppression at developing neuromuscular synapses. *Nature* **374**, 262–6 (1995).

18. Campenot, R. B. Local control of neurite development by nerve growth factor. *Proc. Natl. Acad. Sci. USA* **74**, 4516–19 (1977).

19. English, A. W. and Schwartz, G. Both basic fibroblast growth factor and ciliary neurotrophic factor promote the retention of polyneuronal innervation of developing skeletal muscle fibers. *Dev. Biol.* **169**, 57–64 (1995).

20. Chang, Q. and Balice-Gordon, R. J. Nip and tuck at the neuromuscular junction: a role for proteases in developmental synapse elimination. *BioEssays* **19**, 271–5 (1997).

21. Nguyen, Q. T., Parsadanian, A. S., Snider, W. D. and Lichtman, J. W. Hyperinnervation of neuromuscular junctions caused by GDNF overexpression in muscle. *Science* **279**, 1725–9 (1998).

22. Jansen, J. K. S. and Fladby, T. The perinatal reorganization of the innervation of skeletal muscle in mammals. *Prog. Neurobiol.* **34**, 39–90 (1990).

23. Caroni, P. and Becker, M. The downregulation of growth-associated proteins in motoneurons at the onset of synapse elimination is controlled by muscle activity and IGF1. *J. Neurosci.* **12**, 3849–61 (1992).

24. O'Brien, R. A., Ostberg, A. J. and Vrbova, G. Observations on the elimination of polyneuronal innervation in developing mammalian skeletal muscle. *J. Physiol. (London)* **282**, 571–82 (1978).

25. Thompson, W. Synapse elimination in neonatal rat muscles is sensitive to the pattern of use. *Nature* **302**, 614–16 (1983).

26. Benoit, P. and Changeux, J. P. Consequences of tenotomy on the evolution of multi innervation

in developing rat soleus muscle. *Brain Res.* **99**, 345–58 (1975).

27. Thompson, W., Kuffler, D. P. and Jansen, J. K. S. The effect of prolonged reversible block of nerve impulses on the elimination of polyneuronal innervation of new-born rat skeletal muscle fibres. *Neuroscience* **4**, 271–81 (1979).

28. Brown, M. C., Holland, R. L. and Hopkins, W. G. Restoration of focal multiple innervation in rat muscles by transmission block during a critical stage of development. *J. Physiol.* **318**, 355–64 (1981).

29. Thompson, W. J., Sutton, L. A. and Riley, D. A. Fibre type composition of single motor units during synapse elimination in neonatal rat soleus muscle. *Nature* **309**, 709–11 (1984).

30. Gordon, H. and Van Essen, D. C. Specific innervation of muscle fibre types in a developmentally polyinnervated muscle. *Dev. Biol.* **111**, 42–50 (1985).

31. Brown, M. C. and Booth, C. M. Postnatal development of the adult pattern of motor axon distribution in rat muscle. *Nature* **304**, 741–2 (1983).

32. Bennett, M. R. and Lavidis, N. Development of the topographical projection of motor neurons to a rat muscle accompanies loss of polyneuronal innervation. *J. Neurosci.* **4**, 2204–12 (1984).

33. Laskowski, M. B. and Sanes, J. R. Topographically selective reinnervation of adult mammalian skeletal muscle. *J. Neurosci.* **8**, 3094–9 (1988).

34. Laskowski, M. B. and High, J. A. Expression of nerve–muscle topography during development. *J. Neurosci.* **9**, 175–82 (1989).

35. Bixby, J. L. and Van Essen, D. C. Competition between foreign and original nerves in adult mammalian skeletal muscle. *Nature* **282**, 726–8 (1979).

36. Brown, M. C. and Ironton, R. Sprouting and regression of neuromuscular synapses in partially denervated mammalian muscles. *J. Physiol.* **278**, 325–8 (1978).

37. Slack, J. R. and Hopkins, W. G. Neuromuscular transmission at terminals of sprouted mammalian motoneurons. *Brain Res.* **237**, 121–35 (1982).

38. Pockett, S. and Slack, J. R. Ability of motoneurons to regulate quantal release and terminal growth after reduction in motor unit size. *Brain Res.* **258**, 296–8 (1983).

39. Ridge, R. M. A. P. and Betz, W. J. The effect of selective chronic stimulation on motor unit size in developing rat muscle. *J. Neurosci.* **4**, 2614–20 (1984).

40. Callaway, E. M., Soha, J. M. and Van Essen, D. C. Competition favouring inactive over active motor neurons during synapse elimination. *Nature* **328**, 422–6 (1987).

41. Lo, Y. J. and Poo, M. M. Activity-dependent synaptic competition *in vitro*: heterosynaptic suppression of developing synapses. *Science* **254**, 1019–22 (1991).

42. Purves, D. and Lichtman, J. W. *Principles of neural development* (Sinauer, 1985).

43. Lichtman, J. W. The organisation of synaptic connections in the rat submandibular ganglion during post natal development. *J. Physiol.* **273**, 155–78 (1977).

44. Lichtman, J. W. and Purves, D. The elimination of redundant preganglionic innervation to hamster sympathetic ganglion cells in early postnatal life. *J. Physiol.* **301**, 213–28 (1980).

45. Leistol, I. L., Maehlen, J. and Nja, A. Selective synaptic connections: significance of recognition and competition in mature sympathetic ganglion. *Trends Neurosci.* **9**, 21–4 (1986).

46. Hume, R. I. and Purves, D. Geometry of neonatal neurones and the regulation of synapse elimination. *Nature* **293**, 469–71 (1981).

47. Forehand, C. J. and Purves, D. Regional innervation of rabbit ciliary ganglion cells by the terminals of preganglion axons. *J. Neurosci.* **4**, 1–12 (1984).

48. Forehand, C. J., Ezerman, E. B., Rubin, E. and Glover, J. C. Segmental patterning of rat and chicken sympathetic preganglionic neurons: correlation between soma position and axon projection pathway. *J. Neurosci.* **14**, 231–41 (1994).

49. Jackson, P. C. Reduced activity during development delays the normal rearrangement of synapses in the rabbit ciliary ganglion. *J. Physiol.*, **345**, 319–27 (1983).

50. Wiesel, T. N. and Hubel, D. H. Single cell responses in striate cortex of kittens deprived of vision in one eye. *J. Neurophysiol.* **26**, 1003–17 (1963).

51. Chow, K. L. and Stewart, D. L. Reversal of structural and functional effects of long-standing visual deprivation in cats. *Exp. Neurol.* **34**, 409–33 (1972).

52. Blakemore, C. Development of functional connexions in the mammalian visual system. *Br. Med. Bull.* **30**, 152–7 (1974).

53. Blakemore, C. and Cooper, G. F. Development of the brain depends on the visual environment. *Nature* **228**, 477–8 (1970).

54. Hirsch, V. B. and Spinelli, D. N. Modification of the distribution of receptive field orientation in cats by selective visual exposure during development. *Exp. Brain Res.* **12**, 509–27 (1971).

55. Stryker, M. P. and Sherk, H. Modification of cortical orientation selectivity in the cat by restricted visual experience: a re-examination. *Science* **190**, 904–5 (1975).

56. Rakic, P. Genesis of the dorsal lateral geniculate nucleus in the rhesus monkey. *J. Comp. Neurol.* **176**, 23–52 (1977).

57. Rakic, P. Mechanisms of ocular dominance segregation in the lateral geniculate nucleus: competitive elimination hypothesis. *Trends Neurosci.* **9**, 11–15 (1986).

58. Sretavan, D. W. and Shatz, C. J. Prenatal development of retinal ganglion cell axons: segregation into eye-specific layers within the cat's lateral geniculate nucleus. *J. Neurosci.* **6**, 234–51 (1986).

59. Sretavan, D. W., Shatz, C. J. and Stryker, M. P. Modification of retinal ganglion cell axon morphology by prenatal infusion of tetrodotoxin. *Nature* **336**, 468–71 (1988).

60. Galli, L. and Maffei, L. Spontaneous impulse activity of rat retinal ganglion cells in prenatal life. *Science* **242**, 90–1 (1988).

61. Wong, R. O. L., Meister, M. and Shatz, C. J. Transient period of correlated bursting activity during development of the mammalian retina. *Neuron* **11**, 923–38 (1993).

62. Wong, R. O., Chernjavsky, A., Smith, S. J. and Shatz, C. J. Early functional neural networks in the developing retina. *Nature* **374**, 716–18 (1995).

63. Wong, R. O. Retinal waves and visual system development. *Annu. Rev. Neurosci.* **22**, 29–47 (1999).

64. Feller, M. B., Wellis, D. P., Stellwagen, D., Werblin, F. S. and Shatz, C. J. Requirement for cholinergic synaptic transmission in the propagation of spontaneous retinal waves. *Science* **272**, 1182–7 (1996).

65. Stellwagen, D., Shatz, C. J. and Feller, M. B. Dynamics of retinal waves are controlled by cyclic AMP. *Neuron* **24**, 673–85 (1999).

66. Dubin, M. W., Stark, L. A. and Archer, S. M. A role for action-potential activity in the development of neuronal connections in the kitten retinogeniculate pathway. *J. Neurosci.* **6**, 1021–36 (1986).

67. Hahm, J. O., Langdon, R. B. and Sur, M. Disruption of retinogeniculate afferent segregation by antagonists to NMDA receptors. *Nature* **351**, 568–70 (1991).

68. Rakic, P. Prenatal development of the visual system in Rhesus monkey. *Philos. Trans. R. Soc. London Ser. B* **278**, 245–60 (1977).

69. Hubel, D. H., Wiesel, T. N. and Le Vay, S. Plasticity of ocular dominance columns in monkey striate cortex. *Philos. Trans. R. Soc. London Ser. B* **278**, 377–404 (1977).

70. Rakic, P. Development of visual centres in the primate brain depends on binocular competition before birth. *Science* **214**, 928–31 (1981).

71. Swindale, N. V. Absence of ocular dominance patches in dark reared cats. *Nature* **290**, 332–3 (1981).

72. Stryker, M. P. and Harris, W. A. Binocular impulse traffic blockade prevents the formation of ocular dominance columns in cat visual cortex. *J. Neurosci.* **6**, 2117–33 (1986).

73. Chapman, B., Jacobson, M. D., Reiter, H. O. and Stryker, M. P. Ocular dominance shift in kitten visual cortex caused by imbalance in retinal electrical activity. *Nature* **324**, 154–6 (1986).

74. Freeman, R. D. and Ohzawa, I. Monocularly deprived cats: binocular tests of cortical cells reveal functional connections from the deprived eye. *J. Neurosci.* **8**, 2491–506 (1988).

75. Ferster, D. and LeVay, S. The axonal arborizations of the lateral geniculate neurons in the striate cortex of the cat. *J. Comp. Neurol.* **182**, 923–44 (1978).

76. Antonini, A. and Stryker, M. P. Development of individual geniculocortical arbors in the cat striate cortex and effects of binocular impulse blockade. *J. Neurosci.* **13**, 3549–73 (1993).

77. Ghosh, A. and Shatz, C. J. Involvement of subplate neurons in the formation of ocular dominance columns. *Science* **255**, 1441–3 (1992).

78. Horton, J. C. and Hocking, D. R. An adult-like pattern of ocular dominance columns in striate cortex of newborn monkeys prior to visual experience. *J. Neurosci.* **16**, 1791–807 (1996).

79. Katz, L. C. and Shatz, C. J. Synaptic activity and the construction of cortical circuits. *Science* **274**, 1133–8 (1996).

80. Levine, R. L. and Jacobson, M. Discontinuous mapping of retina onto tectum innervated by both eyes. *Brain Res.* **98**, 172–6 (1975).

81. Law, M. I. and Constantine Paton, M. Anatomy and physiology of experimentally induced striped tecta. *J. Neurosci.* **1**, 741–59 (1981).

82. Fawcett, J. W. and Willshaw, D. J. Compound eyes project stripes on the optic tectum in *Xenopus*. *Nature* **296**, 350–2 (1982).

83. Meyer, R. L. Tetrodotoxin blocks the formation of ocular dominance columns in goldfish. *Science* **218**, 589–91 (1982).

84. Reh, T. A. and Constantine-Paton, M. Eye specific segregation requires neural activity in three-eyed *R. pipiens*. *J. Neurosci.* **5**, 1132–43 (1985).

85. Freeman, J. A. Possible regulatory function of acetylcholine receptor in maintenance of retinotectal synapses. *Nature* **269**, 218–22 (1977).

86. Lee, D. and Malpeli, J. G. Global form and singularity: modeling the blind spot's role in lateral geniculate morphogenesis. *Science* **263**, 1292–4 (1994).

87. Hubel, D. H. and Wiesel, T. N. Receptive fields in striate cortex of very young, visually inexperienced kittens. *J. Neurophysiol.* **26**, 994–1002 (1963).

88. Wiesel, T. N. Postnatal development of the visual cortex and the influence of the environment. *Nature* **299**, 583–91 (1982).

89. Blakemore, C. and Van Sluyters, R. C. Innate and environmental factors in the development of the kitten's visual cortex. *J. Physiol.* **248**, 663–716 (1975).

90. Pettigrew, J. D. The effect of visual experience on the development of stimulus specificity by kitten cortical neurons. *J. Physiol.* **237**, 49–74 (1974).

91. Fregnac, Y. and Imbert, M. Development of neuronal selectivity in primary visual cortex of cat. *Physiol. Rev.* **64**, 325–434 (1984).

92. Wiesel, T. N. and Hubel, D. H. Ordered arrangement of orientation columns in monkeys lacking visual experience. *J. Comp. Neurol.* **158**, 307–18 (1974).

93. Blakemore, C. and Vital Durand, F. Visual deprivation prevents the postnatal maturation of spatial resolution and contrast sensitivity for neurons of the monkey's striate cortex. *J. Physiol.* **345**, 40P (1983).

94. Blakemore, C. and Vital Durand, F. Effects of visual deprivation on the development of the monkey's lateral geniculate nucleus. *J. Physiol.* **380**, 493–511 (1986).

95. Blakemore, C. and Mitchell, D. E. Environmental modification of the visual cortex and the neural basis of learning and memory. *Nature* **241**, 467–8 (1973).

96. Pettigrew, J., Olson, C. and Barlow, H. B. Kitten visual cortex: short term, stimulus induced changes in connectivity. *Science* **180**, 1202–3 (1973).

97. Banks, M. S., Aslin, R. N. and Letson, R. D. Sensitive period for the development of human binocular vision. *Science* **190**, 675–7 (1975).

98. Jacobs, D. S. and Blakemore, C. Factors limiting the postnatal development of visual acuity in the monkey. *Vision Res.* **28**, 947–58 (1988).

99. Teller, D. Y. and Movshon, J. A. Visual development. *Vision Res.* **26**, 1483–506 (1986).

100. Hubel, D. H. and Wiesel, T. N. The period of susceptibility to the physiological effects of unilateral eye closure in kittens. *J. Physiol.* **206**, 419–36 (1970).

101. Hubel, D. H. and Wiesel, T. N. Binocular interaction in striate cortex of kittens reared with artificial squint. *J. Neurophysiol.* **28**, 1041–59 (1965).

102. Kennedy, H. and Orban, G. A. Response properties of visual cortical neurons in cats reared in stroboscopic illumination. *J. Neurophysiol.* **49**, 686–704 (1983).

103. Keating, M. J. The role of visual function in the patterning of binocular visual connections. *Br. Med. Bull.* **30**, 145–51 (1974).

104. Keating, M. J. and Kennard, C. Visual experience and the maturation of the ipsilateral visuotectal projection in *Xenopus laevis*. *Neuroscience* **21**, 519–28 (1987).

105. Sengpiel, F., Stawinski, P. and Bonhoeffer, T. Influence of experience on orientation maps in cat visual cortex. *Nat. Neurosci.* **2**, 727–32 (1999).

106. Rauschecker, J. P. and Singer, W. The effects of early visual experience on the cat's visual cortex and their possible explanation by Hebb synapses. *J. Physiol.* **310**, 215–39 (1981).

107. Goedecke, I. and Bonhoeffer, T. Development of identical orientation maps for two eyes without common visual experience. *Nature* **379**, 251–4 (1996).

108. Kandler, K. and Katz, L. C. Coordination of neuronal activity in developing visual cortex by gap junction-mediated biochemical communication. *J. Neurosci.* **18**, 1419–27 (1998).

109. Weliky, M. and Katz, L. C. Disruption of orientation tuning in visual cortex by artificially correlated neuronal activity. *Nature* **386**, 680–5 (1997).

110. Miller, K. D. A model for the development of simple cell receptive fields and the ordered arrangement of orientation columns through activity-dependent competition between on- and off-center inputs. *J. Neurosci.* **14**, 409–41 (1994).

111. Callaway, E. M. and Katz, L. C. Emergence and refinement of clustered horizontal connection in cat striate cortex. *J. Neurosci.* **10**, 1134–53 (1990).

112. Lowel, S. and Singer, W. Selection of intrinsic horizontal connections in the visual cortex by correlated neuronal activity. *Science* **255**, 209–12 (1992).

113. Nelson, D. A. and Katz, L. C. Emergence of functional circuits in ferret visual cortex visualized by optical imaging. *Neuron* **15**, 23–34 (1995).

114. Crepel, F., Mariani, J. and Delhaye Bouchaud, N. Evidence for a multiple innervation of Purkinje cells by climbing fibres in the immature rat cerebellum. *J. Neurobiol.* **7**, 567–78 (1976).

115. Crepel, F. Regression of functional synapses in the immature mammalian cerebellum. *Trends Neurosci.* **5**, 266–70 (1982).

116. Rabacchi, S., Bailly, Y., Delhaye-Bouchaud, N. and Mariani, J. Involvement of the N-methyl-D-aspartate (NMDA) receptor in synapse elimination during cerebellar development. *Science* **256**, 1823–5 (1992).

117. Kano, M. *et al.* Persistent multiple climbing fibre innervation of cerebellar Purkinje cells in mice lacking mGluR1. *Neuron* **18**, 71–9 (1997).

118. Kano, M. *et al.* Impaired synapse elimination during cerebellar development in PKC gamma mutant mice. *Cell* **83**, 1223–31 (1995).

119. Knudsen, E. I., Knudsen, P. F. and Esterly, S. D. Early auditory experience modifies sound localisation in barn owls. *Nature* **295**, 238–40 (1982).

120. Schnupp, J. W. H., King, A. J., Smith, A. L. and Thompson, I. D. NMDA-receptor antagonists disrupt the formation of the auditory space map in the mammalian superior colliculus. *J. Neurosci.* **15**, 1516–31 (1995).

121. Nottebohm, F. Ontogeny of bird song. *Science* **167**, 950–6 (1970).

122. Sanes, D. H. and Constantine Paton, M. Altered activity patterns during development reduce neural tuning. *Science* **221**, 1183–4 (1983).

123. Fitzgerald, M., Butcher, T. and Shortland, P. Developmental changes in the laminar termination of A fibre cutaneous sensory afferents in the rat spinal cord dorsal horn. *J. Comp. Neurol.* **348**, 225–33 (1994).

124. Woolsey, T. A. and Van der Loos, H. The structural organization of layer IV in the somatosensory region (SI) of mouse cerebral cortex. The description of a cortical field composed of discrete cytoarchitectonic units. *Brain Res.* **17**, 205–42 (1970).

125. Van der Loos, H. and Woolsey, T. A. Somatosensory cortex: structural alterations following early injury to sense organs. *Science* **179**, 395–8 (1973).

126. Florence, S. L. *et al.* Central reorganisation of sensory pathways following peripheral nerve regeneration in fetal monkeys. *Nature* **381**, 69–71 (1996).

127. Cooper, K. E., Ferguson, A. V. and Veale, W. L. Modification of thermoregulatory responses in rabbits reared at elevated environmental temperatures. *J. Physiol.* **303**, 165–72 (1980).

128. Dawson, N. J., Hellon, R. F., Herington, J. G. and Young, A. A. Facial thermal input in the caudal trigeminal nucleus of rats reared at 30°C. *J. Physiol.* **333**, 545–54 (1982).

129. Katz, M. J., Lasek, R. J. and Nauta, H. J. W. Ontogeny of substrate pathways and the origin of the neural circuit pattern. *Neuroscience* **5**, 821–33 (1980).

130. Stanfield, B. B., O'Leary, D. D. M. and Fricks, C. Selective collateral elimination in early postnatal development restricts cortical distribution of rat pyramidal tract neurones. *Nature* **298**, 371–3 (1982).

131. O'Leary, D. D. M., Stanfield, B. B. and Cowan, W. M. Evidence that the early postnatal restriction of the cells of origin of the callosal projection is due to the elimination of axon collaterals rather than to the death of neurons. *Dev. Brain Res.* **1**, 607–17 (1981).

132. Innocenti, G. M. Growth and reshaping of axons in the establishment of visual callosal connections. *Science* **212**, 824–7 (1981).

133. Koppel, H. and Innocenti, G. M. Is there a genuine exuberancy of callosal projections in development? A quantitative EM study in the cat. *Neurosci. Lett.* **41**, 33–40 (1983).

134. Lund, R. D., Mitchell, D. E. and Henry, G. H. Squint induced modification of callosal connections in cats. *Brain Res.* **144**, 169–72 (1978).

135. Kandler, K. and Katz, L. C. Neuronal coupling and uncoupling in the developing nervous system. *Curr. Opin. Neurobiol.* **5**, 98–105 (1995).

136. Hebb, D. O. *The organisation of behaviour* (Wiley, New York, 1949).

137. Kleinschmidt, A., Bear, M. F. and Singer, W. Blockade of 'NMDA' receptors disrupts experience dependent plasticity of kitten striate cortex. *Science* **238**, 355–8 (1987).

138. Greuel, J. M., Luhmann, H. J. and Singer, W. Pharmacological induction of use-dependent receptive field modifications in the visual cortex. *Science* **242**, 74–7 (1988).

139. Cline, H. T., Debski, E. A. and Constantine-Paton, M. N-methyl-D-aspartate receptor antagonist desegregates eye-specific stripes. *Proc. Natl. Acad. Sci. USA* **84**, 4342–5 (1987).

140. Von der Malsburg, C. and Singer, W. Principles of cortical network organization. In *Neurobiology of neocortex* (ed. P. Rakic and W. Singer), pp. 69–99 (Wiley, Chichester, 1988).

141. Kasamatsu, T. and Pettigrew, J. D. Depletion of brain catecholamines: failure of ocular dominance shift after monocular occlusion in kittens. *Science* **194**, 206–9 (1976).

142. Bear, M. F. and Singer, W. Modulation of visual cortical plasticity by acetylcholine and noradrenaline. *Nature* **320**, 172–6 (1986).

143. Zhang, L. I., Tao, H. W., Holt, C. E., Harris, W. A. and Poo, M. A critical window for cooperation and competition among developing retinotectal synapses. *Nature* **395**, 37–44 (1998).

144. Katz, L. C. What's critical for the critical period in visual cortex? *Cell* **99**, 673–6 (1999).

145. Zou, D.-J. and Cline, H. T. Expression of constitutively active CaMKII in target tissue modifies presynaptic axon arbour growth. *Neuron* **16**, 529–39 (1996).

146. Crair, M. C. and Malenka, R. C. A critical period for long-term potentiation at thalamocortical synapses. *Nature* **375**, 325–8 (1995).

147. Fox, K., Schlaggar, B. L., Glazewski, S. and O'Leary, D. D. Glutamate receptor blockade at cortical synapses disrupts development of thalamocortical and columnar organization in

somatosensory cortex. *Proc. Natl. Acad. Sci. USA* **93**, 5584–9 (1996).

148. Li, Y., Erzurumlu, R. S., Chen, C., Jhaveri, S. and Tonegawa, S. Whisker-related neuronal patterns fail to develop in the trigeminal brainstem nuclei of NMDAR1 knockout mice. *Cell* **76**, 427–37 (1994).

149. Iwasato, T. *et al.* NMDA receptor-dependent refinement of somatotopic maps. *Neuron* **19**, 1201–10 (1997).

150. McAllister, A. K., Katz, L. C. and Lo, D. C. Neurotrophins and synaptic plasticity. *Annu. Rev. Neurosci.* **22**, 295–318 (1999).

151. Maffei, L., Berardi, N., Domenici, L., Parisi, V. and Pizzorusso, T. Nerve growth factor (NGF) prevents the shift in ocular dominance distribution of visual cortical neurons in monocularly deprived rats. *J. Neurosci.* **12**, 4651–62 (1992).

152. Carmignoto, G., Canella, R., Candeo, P., Comelli, M. C. and Maffei, L. Effects of nerve growth factor on neuronal plasticity of the kitten visual cortex. *J. Physiol. (London)* **464**, 343–60 (1993).

153. Cabelli, R. J., Hohn, A. and Shatz, C. J. Inhibition of ocular dominance column formation by infusion of NT-4/5 or BDNF. *Science* **267**, 1662–6 (1995).

154. Riddle, D. R., Lo, D. C. and Katz, L. C. NT-4-mediated rescue of lateral geniculate neurons from effects of monocular deprivation. *Nature* **378**, 189–91 (1995).

155. Sanes, D. H. and Takacs, C. Activity-dependent refinement of inhibitory connections. *Eur. J. Neurosci.* **5**, 570–4 (1993).

156. Blochl, A. and Thoenen, H. Characterization of nerve growth factor (NGF) release from hippocampal neurons: evidence for a constitutive and an unconventional sodium-dependent pathway. *Eur. J. Neurosci.* **7**, 1220–8 (1995).

157. Huang, Z. J. *et al.* BDNF regulates the maturation of inhibition and the critical period of plasticity in mouse visual cortex. *Cell* **98**, 739–55 (1999).

158. Purves, D. *Neural activity and the growth of the brain* (Cambridge University Press, 1994).

159. Zafra, F., Castren, E., Thoenen, H. and Lindholm, D. Interplay between glutamate and gamma-aminobutyric acid transmitter systems in the physiological regulation of brain-derived neurotrophic factor and nerve growth factor synthesis in hippocampal neurons. *Proc. Natl. Acad. Sci. USA* **88**, 10037–9 (1991).

160. Castren, E., Zafra, F., Thoenen, H. and Lindholm, D. Light regulates expression of brain-derived neurotrophic factor mRNA in rat visual cortex. *Proc. Natl. Acad. Sci. USA* **89**, 9444–8 (1992).

161. Neeper, S. A., Gomez-Pinilla, F., Choi, J. and Cotman, C. Exercise and brain neurotrophins. *Nature* **373**, 109 (1995).

162. Diamond, J., Holmes, M. and Coughlin, M. Endogenous NGF and nerve impulses regulate the collateral sprouting of sensory axons in the skin of the adult rat. *J. Neurosci.* **12**, 1454–66 (1992).

163. Gaze, R. M., Keating, M. J., Ostberg, A. and Chung, S. H. The relationship between retinal and tectal growth in larval *Xenopus*: implications for the development of the retinotectal projection. *J. Embryol. Exp. Morphol.* **53**, 103–43 (1979).

164. Schmidt, J. T. Natural history of optic arbors on the tectum of fish and frog. *Trends Neurosci.* **7**, 358–60 (1984).

165. Kapfhammer, J. P. and Schwab, M. E. Inverse patterns of myelination and GAP-43 expression in the adult CNS: neurite growth inhibitors as regulators of neuronal plasticity. *J. Comp. Neurol.* **340**, 194–206 (1995).

166. Domenici, L., Cellerino, A., Berardi, N., Cattaneo, A. and Maffei, L. Antibodies to nerve growth factor (NGF) prolong the sensitive period for monocular deprivation in the rat. *NeuroReport* **5**, 2041–4 (1996).

167. George, J. M., Jin, H., Woods, W. S. and Clayton, D. F. Characterization of a novel protein regulated during the critical period for song learning in the Zebra finch. *Neuron* **15**, 361–72 (1995).

168. Fox, K. and Zahs, K. Critical period control in sensory cortex. *Curr. Opin. Neurobiol.* **4**, 112–19 (1994).

169. Bekoff, A. Embryonic development of chick motor behaviour. *Trends Neurosci.* **4**, 181–4 (1981).

15

The Synaptic Basis of Learning

Animals of all ages are able to learn from experience. In order to be translated into altered electrical activity, learning must involve long-term changes in the effectiveness of synaptic transmission. Mechanisms for bringing about long-lasting changes in synaptic efficacy must, therefore, be present in adults long after the completion of the major synaptic rearrangements described in Chapter 14. Several different long-lasting physiological, biochemical and structural changes in synapses have been discovered in both invertebrates and vertebrates, and these usually come about after repetitive activation of neural pathways. This chapter will describe a few prominent examples.

As well as having mechanisms that allow synaptic transmission to be potentiated or depressed for long periods of time during the course of normal activity, the mature brain can also undergo changes in synaptic efficacy and connectivity as a result of damage or grossly altered patterns of activity. An account of these responses is postponed until Chapter 17. It is possible that future work will find links between the mechanisms of synaptic learning, responses to injury and the synaptic reorganization during development described in the last chapter.

Habituation, sensitization and associative learning in *Aplysia*

Even though much of their behaviour is preprogrammed, invertebrates can learn to adapt to changed circumstances. As their nervous systems have far fewer nerve cells than vertebrates, they offer the simplest systems in which the synaptic mechanisms involved in learning can be studied. The withdrawal reflex of the marine mollusc *Aplysia californica* (the sea hare) is one in which the synapses involved can undergo long-term changes in effectiveness, and these have been investigated intensively.[1,2] The reflex is monosynaptic and consists of a brief withdrawal of the gills and the siphon (a small respiratory spout near the head) when the siphon is lightly touched or electrically stimulated (Fig. 15.1).

Repeated stimulation of the siphon reduces the vigour of the withdrawal and this reduction can last for several weeks. This phenomenon is known as habituation and is a simple form of learning. By contrast, long-lasting enhancement of the gill-withdrawal reflex can be caused by strong electric shocks applied to the head (which themselves produce a massive withdrawal response). This is known as sensitization. Both habituation and sensitization are forms of non-associative learning, in which the animal learns about the properties of a single stimulus. A shock to the tail may also cause sensitization of the gill-withdrawal reflex but, more importantly, if a touch to the siphon is given at the same time as a shock to the tail on several successive occasions, there is a clear extra enhancement of the withdrawal triggered by a touch to the siphon alone. This lasts for several weeks[3] and shows that associative learning of the withdrawal response has occurred, for the marked response to tail shock (the unconditioned stimulus) has now also become associated with a light touch to the

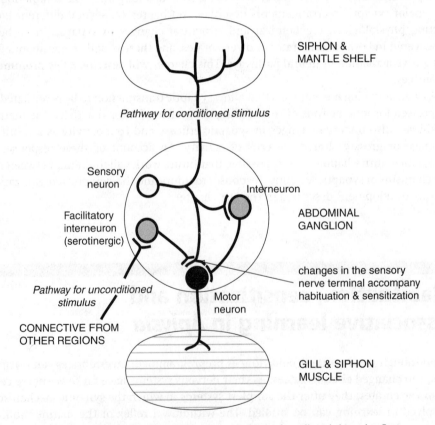

Figure 15.1 The neuronal pathways underlying the gill-withdrawal reflex.

siphon alone (the conditioned stimulus). This form of associative learning, in which the animal learns about the relationship between two stimuli, is also known as classical conditioning, after the famous training experiments of Pavlov; it is distinguished from operant conditioning, which involves learning the relation between a stimulus and a response.

The synaptic mechanism of habituation has been studied in detail. It is due to depression of transmission at the synapse between the sensory neurons innervating the siphon skin and the gill motor neurons. This is a consequence of a fall in the number of calcium channels in the presynaptic terminal, possibly triggered by the rise in intracellular calcium ion concentration in the terminals which follows repeated activation of the pathway.[4] The consequence of having fewer functioning calcium channels is that less calcium enters the terminal per nerve impulse and so less transmitter is released. There is also a fall in the number of active zones for transmitter release in the terminals of the sensory neuron.[5]

The basis of both short- and long-term sensitization has also been intensively investigated. Enhancement of the withdrawal response is caused by an increase in the amount of transmitter released from the terminals of the sensory neurons.[1,6] Serotonin (5-hydroxytryptamine, 5-HT) released from interneurons onto the sensory nerve's synapses on motoneurons brings about this increase in release directly[7-9] and so this is known as presynaptic facilitation. Serotonin produces its effects on the sensory neuron terminals by G-protein-mediated activation of adenylate cyclase, which increases the intracellular concentration of cyclic AMP (cAMP) in the terminal. The immediate short-term effect is phosphorylation of potassium channels by cAMP-dependent protein kinase A. This reduces the number of functional potassium channels in the sensory nerve terminal membrane so that repolarization is slower, the action potential is longer and there is time for a greater influx of calcium ions through N-type voltage-gated calcium channels. This increases transmitter release, as summarized in Fig. 15.2.

More recently, it has proved possible to reconstitute circuits between isolated sensory neurons and motor neurons in culture. The action of presynaptic facilitatory pathways can be simulated by applying serotonin to the preparation.[10] This has been of considerable use in further unravelling the sequence of events underlying long-term changes in transmitter release from the sensory nerve terminal. Brief single applications of serotonin generate a short-term facilitation which cannot be prevented by inhibitors of protein or RNA synthesis, but repeated application of serotonin causes long-term facilitation and this is blocked by inhibitors of protein synthesis provided they are present while serotonin is being applied. Short-term facilitation therefore probably modifies existing structures in the sensory terminals, such as potassium channels, but longer-term changes can only occur after synthesis of new proteins. If, moreover, a single bifurcated sensory neuron is cultured with two separate motor neurons, local serotonin application at the synapses on one motor neuron leads to long-term facilitation exclusively at those synapses, and the process requires local protein synthesis in the presynaptic but not the postsynaptic cell. Synthesis can take place even in the absence of the presynaptic cell body, raising the possibility that the mRNAs and ribosomes found at the base of dendritic spines in

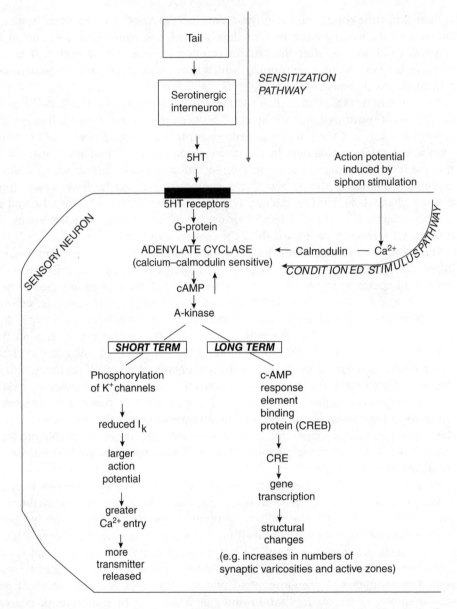

Figure 15.2 The pathways for short- and long-term sensitization of the gill-withdrawal reflex. Changes occur in the sensory nerve to produce short-term increases in transmitter release, and longer term there are changes in synaptic structure. The enzyme adenylate cyclase plays a part in both these events and, because of its dual sensitivity to G protein and calmodulin, provides a molecular site for associative learning.

the vertebrate brain might be involved similarly in locally-regulated synaptic plasticity.[11]

Administration of cAMP on its own *in vitro* can also bring about both short-term and long-term sensitization,[12] and the latter is again blocked by protein synthesis inhibitors. It is also blocked if the transcription factor CREB (cAMP response element binding protein), which is phosphorylated by cAMP-dependent protein kinase (PKA), is short-circuited by injecting CREB oligonucleotides into the sensory neuron before endogenous activated CREB can reach the chromosomes (Fig. 15.2).[13] It has been further shown that mice and fruit flies with targeted CREB deletions have a deficiency in long-term memory. CREB knockout mice, for example, show defects in fear conditioning and water-maze conditioning (see below).[14,15] In an olfactory discrimination task in flies, expression of a CREB activator converts the need for multiple training trials to a single trial, and this phenotype is abolished by mutation of the phosphorylation site for activated CREB. CREB activation, therefore, is sufficient for conversion of a form of short-term memory to long-term memory.[16] A CREB repressor protein has also been identified.[17]

The genes regulated by CREB are not well characterized, but include a set of immediate-early genes. It should be noted, however, that CREB is not a memory-specific protein; hippocampal CREB, for example, can be phosphorylated and activated by any stimulus (such as traumatic injury or seizure) that increases cellular cAMP levels. CREB can also be activated by calcium ions acting through calmodulin-dependent protein kinase CaM kinase II (see also below), providing another potential route for its regulation via electrical activity.

Long-term maintenance of *Aplysia* sensitization *in vivo* is accompanied by increases in the number of active transmitter release zones and there are also increases in the numbers of varicosities that each sensory terminal makes on a motoneuron.[18] The same is true *in vitro*, where it has been shown that the growth of sensory nerve terminals only occurs after application of 5-HT if the motor neuron is present in the culture too.[19] This growth may be partly a consequence of endocytosis and down-regulation of an NCAM-related adhesion molecule (apCAM) on the terminal of the sensory neuron.[20] A similar mechanism has been identified at the fly neuromuscular junction, where CREB activation in the *dunce* mutation (see below) is associated with the downregulation of the NCAM homologue FasII and increased synaptic growth. In this case, though, CREB activation can be dissociated from synaptic growth, suggesting that the two processes operate in parallel rather than in series in response to increased levels of cAMP.[21] An important feature of both these studies is the demonstration that long-term changes in synaptic efficacy are also likely to involve the regulation of cell adhesion and the removal of restraints on cell growth.

A possible explanation at a molecular level of the classical conditioning of the withdrawal reflex has also been put forward.[2,22] The adenylate cyclase activated by serotonin is also modulated by calcium–calmodulin. Calcium ions enter the sensory nerve terminal during an action potential. Therefore, if sensory nerve stimulation is paired with activation of the serotinergic neuron, two stimulatory effects (calcium and serotonin) will converge on the adenylate cyclase (Fig. 15.2). In this way, more cAMP could be generated than by either input alone. It is unlikely, however, that changes occurring in the presynaptic terminals of the sensory neuron are the only ones accompanying the associative learning, and there is evidence that the synapses between motor neurons and the gill muscles are also facilitated.[23]

Associative learning in *Hermissenda*

Whereas studies in *Aplysia* have tended to emphasize the involvement of cAMP-dependent signalling in learning mechanisms, those in its smaller relative, *Hermissenda crassicornis*, have highlighted the importance of calcium-based events. Mechanical stimuli, such as waves, cause *Hermissenda* to contract its foot to cling more tightly, while light stimuli alter its foot contraction so that it moves towards the light. If the animal is repeatedly exposed to a light stimulus paired with mechanical agitation, foot contraction is eventually triggered by light alone, another example of Pavlovian associative conditioning. Its basis includes a reduction in the voltage-dependent potassium currents that are involved in repolarization of the action potential. This drop in potassium conductance may be mediated by calexcitin, a cytosolic calcium- and GTP-binding protein that is phosphorylated and activated by protein kinase C, in turn activated by calcium influx during the action potential. Calexcitin also appears to activate the type II ryanodine receptor to stimulate further calcium release from the endoplasmic reticulum. The increase in cytosolic calcium has many consequences within the cell, including activation of enzymes such as CaM kinase II which could alter gene regulation within the nucleus.[24]

Parallels with findings in *Drosophila*

Over a dozen mutations have been discovered in *Drosophila* which impair learning in olfactory discrimination tasks, and the related genes and their products have been identified.[25] These are expressed preferentially in the mushroom bodies, regions of the insect neuropil that are known to mediate olfactory learning. Perhaps not surprisingly, many of these genes encode cellular components that are very similar to those involved in *Aplysia* learning mechanisms, working through the cAMP–PKA pathway: in addition to the *CREB* gene discussed above, the *dunce* gene codes for a cyclic AMP phosphodiesterase (see also above),[26] *rutabaga* codes for a calcium/calmodulin-responsive adenylyl cyclase,[27] *DCO* encodes a catalytic subunit of protein kinase A,[28] and the *amnesiac* product is homologous to a peptide transmitter (PACAP) that activates adenylyl cyclase.[29] In a further mutant, *radish*, a distinct type of long-term, consolidated memory (anaesthesia-resistant memory, ARM) is abolished; ARM also differs from other forms of consolidated memory in being independent of protein synthesis.[30] Lastly, the *Volado* locus mediates short-term olfactory memory, and encodes two isoforms of an alpha-integrin; although its exact role in learning is unclear, the involvement of an integrin again suggests that modulation of adhesion at the synapse may contribute to synaptic efficacy.[31]

Long-term potentiation and depression in the hippocampus

The hippocampus, sited in the temporal lobe, is phylogenetically the oldest part of the cerebral cortex and functionally part of the limbic system, a collection of brain centres concerned with emotion, behaviour and memory. That the hippocampus is important in both acquiring memories and retaining them is clearly shown by the fact that damage to it impairs memory in humans. Rats also lose the memory of how best to negotiate a path through a maze to get a reward of food, and they cannot relearn following hippocampal lesions.[32] Many of the neurons in the hippocampus of conscious rats alter their firing patterns in a way that is specific to the animal's position in a familiar environment.[33,34] In primates, the hippocampus appears to be involved particularly in the initial storage of declarative memory (i.e. memory for people, places and things) for a period of days to weeks, before the memory is finally consolidated elsewhere in the cerebral cortex.[35]

Electrophysiological studies carried out on the hippocampus have shown that synaptic transmission can be both enhanced and depressed for long periods of time by particular patterns of stimulation. Transmission was first studied in anaesthetized rabbits in response to direct stimulation of one of its main afferent tracts, the perforant path (Fig. 15.3),[36] although most experiments nowadays are carried out on 400–500-μm slices of rat or guinea-pig hippocampus maintained for some hours in special perfusion chambers. The perforant path originates in the entorhinal cortex and ends on dendrites of the granule cells of the dentate gyrus of the hippocampus. The excitatory post-synaptic potentials activated in the granule cells by stimulation of the perforant path generate a flow of current into the dendrites which can be recorded with an extra-cellular electrode. When enough fibres are activated there may also be a spike super-imposed on the slow wave. This is caused by the synchronous firing of action potentials in a group of granule cells. Single stimuli delivered to the perforant path every few seconds produce a constant-sized depolarization of the granule cells. If, however, an extra train of stimuli at a frequency of 10–100 Hz is applied for 10 or more seconds, substantial changes in transmission occur both in the short and long term. During the train there is a potentiation of transmission, as shown by increases in the amplitude of the wave and spike potentials. Immediately after the train there is a period lasting for up to a minute during which there is depression in the size of the slow wave, but this is followed by a return of potentiation which can last for hours in anaesthetized animals and for over a week in conscious animals. This long-lasting potentiation of the excitatory postsynaptic potential is known as long-term potentiation (LTP).

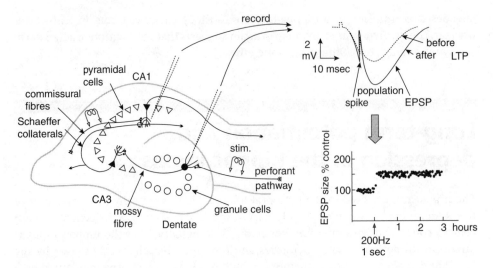

Figure 15.3 Hippocampal pathways used in the study of long-term potentiation (LTP) and long-term depression (LTD). To the right are examples of typical responses recorded before and after LTP.

LTP has been observed in several pathways within the hippocampus. In the dentate gyrus (as described above) and CA1, the high-frequency stimulation has to be above a certain threshold level of intensity to generate LTP ('cooperativity'); when weak stimulation of one input pathway, itself insufficient to produce LTP, is combined with strong stimulation to another input pathway that can produce LTP, the weak input also undergoes LTP ('associative LTP'). LTP in CA3, by contrast, is non-associative.

Whereas high-frequency stimulation gives rise to LTP, low-frequency stimulation at 1 Hz for a minute or so depresses transmission to test stimuli for long periods. This has become known as long-term depression (LTD). As LTP was discovered first, and as it is often assumed that the most active pathways will be the ones carrying the information that needs to be stored, LTP has received the lion's share of experimental attention. It is perfectly possible, however, to store information by reducing synaptic traffic, and a system that continually wound itself up by continued potentiation might saturate its ability to store new information. So LTD is probably as important a mechanism as LTP. In the cerebellum, a brain centre involved in the learning of various motor tasks, there is good evidence that LTD takes part in the learning process (see below).[37]

LTP and long-term changes in synaptic strength elsewhere in the brain

Elsewhere in the nervous system potentiation can also be produced by trains of stimuli, but it is usually harder to induce very long-term effects. For example, transmission between the layers of neocortex from layer IV to layer III can be both potentiated and depressed for long periods using the same stimulation patterns that are successful in the hippocampus,[38] but there may only be a limited time period during development when such results can be obtained.[39] As described in Chapter 14, there is also evidence that unusual activation or lack of activity of sensory pathways alters the balance among synapses, increasing the effectiveness of the active over the less active. The same factors which play a part in LTP (see next section) can influence this phenomenon. It is conceivable that LTP-like mechanisms are widespread in the brain but exaggerated in the hippocampus because of its role in general memory acquisition and storage; such a function may be different to the formation of circuits adapted to sensory processing following specific environmental changes or learning particular motor tasks.

One non-hippocampal area where it has been possible to associate the induction of LTP with a learned behaviour is the amygdala, a nucleus at the tip of the temporal lobe. This has been shown to be important in fear conditioning, a form of Pavlovian conditioning where a neutral stimulus such as a tone is followed by an unconditioned stimulus such as a foot shock. After several pairings the tone alone can elicit the full behavioural response (the conditioned stimulus). During the acquisition of fear conditioning in rats, the extracellular potential that can be recorded in the lateral amygdala in response to the tone is enhanced, returning to the baseline as further presentations of the tone alone extinguish the response (i.e. memory disappears).[40] This enhancement is identical to that elicited by electrical induction of LTP in the auditory–amygdala pathway, and is accompanied by enhanced synaptic responses of amygdala neurons to stimulation of afferents from the auditory thalamus in brain slices prepared from fear-conditioned rats.[41] It remains to be seen whether the experimental induction of LTP in the auditory inputs to the amygdala causes animals to attach fear to auditory stimuli.[42]

Induction and maintenance of LTP

LTP does not normally occur unless enough axons are activated by a train of conditioning stimuli, and there is evidence that induction of LTP only follows if presynaptic firing coincides with adequate depolarization of the postsynaptic membrane, the key characteristic of the Hebbian synapse (see Chapter 14). Consistent with this is the fact that a single presynaptic volley can cause LTP if the postsynaptic cell is simultaneously depolarized by passing current through an intracellular electrode; conversely, hyperpolarization of the cell prevents LTP.[43] LTP also appears to have at least two major phases, an early phase elicited by a weak stimulus, and a late phase induced by strong stimuli (see below).

There has been intense debate about how LTP is induced and maintained, and matters have been made no easier by the discovery that detailed mechanisms differ in different parts of the hippocampus.[44] In the most studied pathway, that to the CA1 area (see Fig. 15.3), it is now clear that a critical element may be the unique properties of the NMDA receptor (cf. Chapter 14), although it may not be involved in other pathways such as CA3.[45] Considerably less is known about the other mechanisms so this account will concentrate on the NMDA-dependent type of LTP.

The NMDA receptor, which is present in high density in CA1, is specifically activated by the synthetic compound N-methyl-D-aspartate, and is activated *in vivo* by the naturally occurring excitatory transmitter glutamate which can also bind to the non-NMDA receptors (AMPA receptors) and the metabotropic receptors. Binding of glutamate does not open the ionophore associated with the NMDA receptor unless the postsynaptic membrane is also sufficiently depolarized. This depolarization removes magnesium ions which block the channel. This ligand *and* voltage gating is the key to NMDA receptor function, and explains plausibly why several pathways have to cooperate to induce LTP. It is one reason why the NMDA receptor is theoretically such an attractive candidate for playing an important role in the induction of LTP. A second reason is the receptor's ability to allow calcium ions into the postsynaptic cell once its ionophore has been opened. There is much evidence to show that a rise in postsynaptic calcium ion concentration is necessary for LTP to be induced. For example, in one sophisticated experiment calcium was released inside a postsynaptic pyramidal cell in the CA1 region by UV irradiation of a UV-sensitive calcium ion chelator and this induced potentiation of synaptic inputs.[46] Conversely if calcium ions were buffered in the postsynaptic cell by activation of a different calcium chelator, LTP induced by tetanization was blocked.[47] It was also possible to show that allowing a rise in calcium for less than 1 s was too short to induce LTP, but a rise for 2 s or more was sufficient. Rises of between 1 and 2 s could induce a short-lasting potentiation (STP).

Given that a rise in postsynaptic calcium ion concentration results in LTP and that preventing that rise does not, the obvious site for the changes accompanying long-term maintenance of enhanced transmission is in the postsynaptic cell. In keeping with this it has been found that excitatory current passed by the non-NMDA receptors in the postsynaptic cell is increased during LTP.[48] There is, indeed, evidence that many AMPA glutamate receptors pass no current prior to LTP and that their activation is an important part of the synaptic enhancement that LTP brings.[49]

There is, however, evidence that long-term changes also occur on the presynaptic side of tetanized pathways, and it has therefore been postulated that some form of signal must pass retrogradely from the postsynaptic side of the synapse, where the rise in calcium ion concentration induces LTP, to the presynaptic side. The need for a retrograde messenger to bring about presynaptic changes can be demonstrated by showing that high-frequency activity confined to the presynaptic terminals by specifically blocking the postsynaptic NMDA receptors cannot induce LTP.[50] Possible retrograde messengers will be discussed below.

Early evidence for presynaptic changes during LTP was the finding that following potentiation of the perforant pathway, a perfusate collected from the dentate area after a standard stimulation of this pathway contained more glutamate than a perfusate collected before LTP had been induced.[51] More recently, whole-cell patch clamping of CA1 pyramidal cells has been used to show that after LTP induced by coupling postsynaptic depolarization with presynaptic stimulation (see earlier) there is a reduction in the number of occasions in which single presynaptic inputs fail to release transmitter quanta; in other words, the probability of transmitter release, which is determined presynaptically, is increased.[52] Further experiments have used quantal analysis of transmitter release following LTP, which is not straightforward in the CNS because of the small size of the unitary depolarizations caused by each quantum of transmitter and the amount of background noise. This has shown that LTP involves increases in transmitter release probability and increases in the depolarization produced by individual transmitter quanta, the latter being a postsynaptic change. Interestingly, the main change during LTP is likely to be presynaptic if the release probability is initially low at a synapse, and postsynaptic if it is high.[53] An increase in presynaptic vesicle recycling after LTP at synapses between hippocampal neurons in culture has also been detected by using antibodies specific to intraluminal vesicle antigens. Here too, presynaptic changes were greater at synapses which started with low quantal contents.[54]

Overall, the main conclusion from these experiments is that both postsynaptic and presynaptic modifications can occur during LTP, and the initial state of the synapse determines whether the changes will be mainly pre- or postsynaptic. Further information on presynaptic and postsynaptic changes has come from anatomical studies of the hippocampus following the induction of LTP. A significant increase in the diameters of dendritic spines in the region of perforant path termination has been found following perforant pathway stimulation.[55] Significant changes in spine diameters and lengths after induction of LTP have also been described.[56] An increased conductance between the dendritic spines and the dendritic shaft accompanying this structural change should increase the depolarization of dendrites by synapses situated on those spines. A rise in the number of synapses made on the shafts of dendrites has also been found after high-frequency stimulation.[57,58] GAP-43, a protein found in growing axons (see Chapter 9), and protein kinase C, which is known to phosphorylate it, are both present in high concentrations in the hippocampus.[59] It seems reasonable that they might participate in some way in producing the long-term structural changes.

It also seems likely that the synaptic changes accompanying LTP might involve parallel changes in adhesion between the pre- and postsynaptic components. Members of the immunoglobulin superfamily of adhesion molecules (e.g. NCAM) have been implicated in the induction of LTP,[60] and this view is also supported by experiments investigating the role of members of the cadherin family (see Chapter 9) of calcium-dependent cell adhesion molecules.[61] Both N- and E-cadherin are expressed in the dendritic arbor of hippocampal pyramidal neurons, and pretreatment of hippocampal slices with antibodies raised against the extracellular domain of either molecule reduces LTP. Infusion of peptides containing the HAV consensus sequence of cadherin dimerization also reduces LTP, and these effects can be counteracted by raising the extracellular calcium concentration.[62] Whether cadherins directly regulate the signalling pathways required for LTP is unclear, but such results do implicate adhesion molecules in the process in some way.

Biochemical pathways involved in LTP

The experimental dissection of the biochemical signalling pathways leading from a rise in postsynaptic calcium ion concentration to the pre- and postsynaptic changes accompanying LTP has relied heavily on pharmacological tools, and more recently on genetic manipulation experiments in mice.[63] In fact, more than 100 molecules have now been implicated in the phenomenon, many of which may modulate it rather than mediate it directly, and a clear consensus view has proved elusive.[64] A simplified summary is shown in Fig. 15.4. There is evidence for the involvement of CaM kinase II (cf. *Aplysia* and *Drosophila* above), protein kinase C (PKC),[65,66] and the cAMP-dependent protein kinase A (PKA).[67] For example, injection of calmodulin antagonists into the soma of hippocampal pyramidal cells blocks LTP,[68] and a PKC inhibitor (H-7) applied extracellularly does the same.[69] If injected into the postsynaptic cell after LTP has

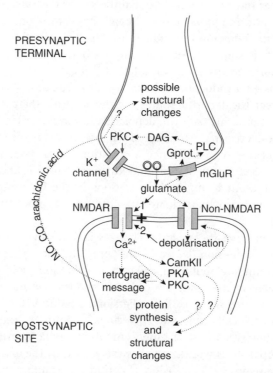

Figure 15.4 Possible routes by which pre- and postsynaptic changes may be brought about during LTP. Note that the NMDA receptor (NMDAR) only permits influx of calcium ions (a key element in triggering LTP) if glutamate is bound *and* the postsynaptic cell is depolarized. This may account for the need for several afferents to be active simultaneously if LTP is to be induced. The presynaptic changes are dependent upon a retrograde signal from the postsynaptic side of the synapse (possibly NO, CO or arachidonic acid). These may interact with signals generated by activation of presynaptic metabotropic glutamate receptors (mGluR).

been induced, H-7 has no action,[70] so it is possible that kinases located pre-synaptically are important too. It has also been shown that late LTP (see above) is dependent on both PKA and new protein synthesis, while early LTP is not, although mutant mice deficient in the cAMP pathway have yet to provide a clear picture of the role of cAMP and CREB in LTP.

One role of PKA may be to gate LTP by suppressing a phosphatase cascade that acts as an inhibitory constraint on the induction of LTP, and that can lead to LTD (see below). Calcium influx through the NMDA receptor is known to initiate a phospha-tase cascade, and the first step in this cascade is thought to be activation of calci-neurin, a calcium-sensitive serine/threonine phosphatase expressed at high levels in hippocampal synapses. If calcineurin is overexpressed genetically in the hippo-campus, LTP is suppressed and mice show defective spatial and visual long-term memory.[71]

The consequences of CaM kinase II activation are multiple; one outcome is phos-phorylation of the postsynaptic glutamate receptors, which enhances the current flowing through non-NMDA channels some threefold.[72] Overexpression of CaM kinase II, by injection of a recombinant vaccinia virus expressing a constitutively active form of the enzyme, increases transmission in the hippocampus and saturates the system so that further potentiation can no longer occur.[73]

It seems likely that any retrograde signal(s) involved in LTP can diffuse widely: presynaptic facilitation has been detected at synapses on postsynaptic cells that did not participate in the experimental induction of hippocampal LTP.[74] There are at least three candidates for the role of retrograde messenger, namely arachidonic acid, nitric oxide (NO) and carbon monoxide (CO).[44] Arachidonic acid is released into the extracellular medium by the activation of NMDA receptors, and inhibitors of phos-pholipase A_2, an enzyme needed to liberate arachidonic acid from membrane phos-pholipids, block the induction of LTP. One way that arachidonic acid could potentiate transmitter release is by a synergistic action on metabotropic glutamate receptors in the presynaptic membrane.[75] There is evidence that this unique class of glutamate receptor, operating by means of second messenger mechanisms triggered by gluta-mate binding rather than passing ionic current, is needed to initiate LTP.[76,77] Indeed mice with an induced mutation in the metabotropic mGluR1 receptor gene have impaired LTP and perform poorly in context-specific learning tasks.[78]

The candidacy of NO and CO is intriguing as both are toxic gases. NO has in recent years turned out to be a mediator of a diverse range of physiological effects. It can act, for example, as a relaxant of smooth muscle and as a bactericidal agent in macro-phages. Nitric oxide synthase is present in the CNS and if this enzyme is inhibited, LTP cannot be induced.[79] It has also been found that exogenously delivered NO (and CO) can potentiate the LTP induced by a traditional course of tetanic nerve stimula-tion.[80] However, unequivocal evidence that NO is synthesized in postsynaptic cells undergoing LTP is lacking: for example, mice with targeted deletion of the neuronal NO synthase gene do not show impaired LTP, although NO inhibition still blocks LTP in these animals, suggesting the involvement of other enzyme isoforms.[81] Nor is it clear how these gaseous messengers bring about their effects on LTP. Further complexity is added by evidence that the neurotrophins BDNF and NT-3 cause long-lasting enhancement of transmission when infused into the adult rat hippocampus, although this potentiation does not occlude a further enhancement by LTP.[82] Neurotrophins, then, can have local effects on synaptic transmission in the adult as well as at developing synapses in the cerebral cortex and at the neuromuscular junction (see also Chapter 14).

It should also be remembered that LTP in some brain regions may be induced independently of NMDA receptor activation. In the basolateral amygdala, for example, muscarinic receptors appear to play a critical role in the induction of LTP, and may work through the Ras signalling pathway. When Ras signalling is impaired in mice by targeted gene deletion of a neuronal specific guanine-nucleotide-exchange factor, memory consolidation for several emotional conditioning tasks involving the amygdala is defective, along with LTP induction in the amygdala, but spatial learning and NMDA-receptor-dependent LTP in the hippocampus are unaffected.[83] Fear conditioning in the lateral amygdala, on the other hand, is dependent on NMDA receptors (see above).

Mechanism of LTD

The mechanism of LTD has also been investigated. In area CA1 of the hippocampus it too requires NMDA receptor activation, and probably changes in internal calcium concentration, for intracellular chelators prevent its appearance.[84] Inhibitors of phosphatases also prevent LTD.[85] A possible scenario is that LTD and LTP produce antagonistic effects on the phosphorylation of several proteins, for example postsynaptic glutamate receptors: LTD may be a consequence of their dephosphorylation and LTP of their phosphorylation. The balance between the two processes may be determined by the level of postsynaptic calcium ions, a high level favouring kinase activation and LTP, and a low level favouring calcineurin/phosphatase activation and LTD (Fig. 15.5).

LTD of the parallel fibre input to Purkinje cells has been intensively studied in the cerebellum. Conjoint stimulation of parallel and climbing fibres is followed by a depression in parallel fibre synaptic transmission that can last as long as the recording from the Purkinje cell can be maintained (up to 1 h). Stimulation of climbing fibres and simultaneous iontophoretic application of glutamate lead to a decreased sensitivity of the Purkinje cells to the transmitter. This is strong evidence that the change in transmission of the parallel fibre synapses is postsynaptic in origin. Other studies have implicated a subtype of metabotropic glutamate receptor that is abundant in Purkinje cells, mGluR1, as cerebellar LTD is deficient in two independent lines of mGluR1 knockout mice.[78,86] One possible mechanism is a desensitization of glutamate receptors activated during the period of raised intradendritic calcium levels following climbing fibre stimulation,[37] although it has been suggested that activation of PKC rather than calcium release is the critical event following mGluR1 activation.[78]

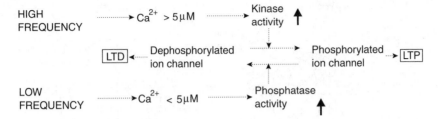

Figure 15.5 Possible relationship between LTP and LTD. High-frequency activity, raising calcium ion levels above $5\,\mu M$, activates protein kinases and leads to phosphorylation of ion channels and LTP. Low-frequency activity maintains intracellular calcium below $5\,\mu M$, which activates phosphatases and leads to ion channel dephosphorylation and LTD.

Effects of interfering with LTP and LTD mechanisms on learning in the whole animal

The relevance of the NMDA receptor to learning in the intact animal has been tested by examining the effect of a specific NMDA blocker, AP5, on the ability of rats to learn their whereabouts and find a particular place.[87] Intraventricular infusion of AP5 selectively impaired the ability to learn the necessary spatial cues, an ability that is highly sensitive to hippocampal damage. Rats were trained to swim and find an underwater platform placed in one of the four quadrants of a pool filled with water (made opaque so that the location of the platform had to be remembered by its association with objects around the pool). Rats normally quickly learned after a few trials to get to the correct quadrant, but AP5-treated animals would spend equal times in all four quadrants, usually swimming around the pool edge even after many trials (Fig. 15.6). In monkeys, however, application of a systemic NMDA receptor antagonist at a dose large enough to protect against the NMDA-induced neurotoxicity did not interfere with memory acquisition.[88]

A variety of targeted gene knockouts in mice have been studied for correlated changes in LTP, hippocampal plasticity and spatial learning. Their interpretation is complicated by the usual caveats in such animals: the possibility of functional compensation by other genes during development, and lack of anatomical selectivity in the knockout. The latter problem has been avoided in a knockout mouse in which deletion of the *NMDAR1* gene was restricted to the pyramidal cells of the CA1 region of the hippocampus. The mutant mice grew normally without obvious abnormality, but LTP in the CA1 synapses was absent and spatial memory, but not other forms of memory, was impaired.[89]

Other proposed links in the biochemical chain from tetanization to LTP to learning have been examined to see if their disruption also interferes with learning ability.

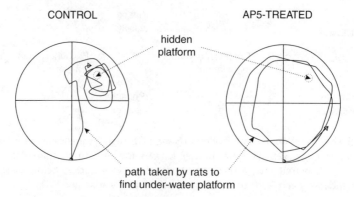

CONTROL   AP5-TREATED

hidden
platform

path taken by rats to
find under-water platform

Figure 15.6 Effects of an NMDA channel blocker (AP5) on spatial learning in the Morris water maze. *Left*: control rats learn where the underwater invisible platform is after a training session which allows them to pinpoint the site by reference to landmarks around the pool; when retested they swim immediately to the spot and circle it. *Right*: AP5-treated rats cannot learn the necessary landmarks and, when retested, swim round and round the whole pool. After Morris *et al.*[87]

CaM kinase II knockout mice have impaired learning in the water-maze test as well as poor LTP in CA1.[90] Mice with a targeted deletion of a PKC subtype can generate LTP, although the stimulation protocol needed is unusual and their ability to learn in the water maze is only slightly impaired.[91] A further conclusion from such studies is that CA1 LTP is the primary synaptic mechanism for hippocampal-dependent spatial learning, and that LTP in other areas of the hippocampus is less critical.

The role of LTD in cerebellar motor learning has also been tested through the use of knockout mice, although the caveats mentioned above have caused continuing difficulty in interpreting the results.[92] Two relatively simple forms of motor learning which are known to involve the cerebellum have been studied. The first is a form of associative conditioning, eyeblink conditioning. The conditioned stimulus, a neutral tone, is paired with the unconditioned stimulus, a periorbital airpuff which evokes an eyeblink, so that after a number of trials the tone alone evokes the eyeblink. The tone signal enters the cerebellum via its mossy fibre input while the airpuff signal enters via the climbing fibres, both inputs converging on the Purkinje cells and one of the deep cerebellar nuclei. During conditioning it appears that LTD at the Purkinje cells and LTP at the deep nuclear neurons combine to increase the excitability of the deep nuclear neurons, the latter providing an increased output to the periorbital musculature. In mGluR1 knockout mice, in which cerebellar LTD is deficient (see above), the amplitude of the conditioned response is reduced.[78]

The second form of cerebellar learning concerns the adaptive plasticity of the vestibular–ocular reflex, where head turning is compensated by eye movement in the opposite direction.[93] This also involves LTD: selective inhibition of PKC in Purkinje cells in transgenic mice abolishes both plasticity and Purkinje cell LTD.[94]

Conclusions

The complexity of the mechanisms of LTP and LTD in the hippocampus will be evident from even this brief account, and the uncertainty about the details of both processes is still considerable. They are both very striking phenomena and it is likely, given the evidence discussed in the last paragraph, that they do play a part in memory storage in intact brains. That the same transmitter receptor (the NMDA receptor) should turn out to be important in both LTP and LTD, and in synaptic stabilization during development (Chapter 14), is not, with hindsight, surprising, as all these processes are designed to alter the strength of synaptic connections. The structural effects of intense stimulation are much less striking in the adult than in the neonate, presumably because the overall ability of the nerve cells to grow is so much diminished. In the future, improvements in 'conditional' targeted gene manipulation, so that gene expression can be altered in specific regions of the CNS at specific times, are likely to yield important advances in our understanding of the mechanisms of learning and memory in mammals. This is particularly important in the analysis of complex, learned behaviour in the mammalian brain, where the detailed operation of neural circuits underlying even seemingly simple reflexes, such as the vestibular–ocular reflex, is poorly understood.

Key points

1 After the critical period of major synaptic rearrangements is over, less dramatic but vitally important long-term changes in synaptic effectiveness can be induced in the adult nervous systems of both invertebrates and vertebrates. Transmission may be facilitated or depressed for long periods of time.

2 Usually, high-frequency stimulation causes facilitation and low-frequency stimulation depression of the active pathway. Cooperation between two active pathways can give rise to associative long-term changes in synaptic effectiveness.

3 In the nervous system of *Aplysia* long-term synaptic depression (habituation) is a consequence of a fall in the number of calcium channels in the presynaptic membrane and this reduces the amount of transmitter released.

4 Sensitization in *Aplysia* is also a result of changes in presynaptic transmitter release mechanisms. 5-HT acting on the terminals raises the level of cAMP and activates a cAMP-dependent protein kinase. In the short term, potassium channels are phosphorylated and made less effective so that presynaptic depolarization and hence transmitter liberation is prolonged. In the long term, gene transcription is altered via the cAMP transcription factor (CREB). Structural changes in synapses can be seen after induction of long-term sensitization.

5 In the mammalian hippocampus long-term potentiation (LTP) is accompanied by both pre- and postsynaptic changes. Activation of both the NMDA receptor in

the postsynaptic membrane and metabotropic glutamate receptors in the presynaptic membrane is usually required. Raised levels of postsynaptic calcium ions, a consequence most probably of NMDA receptor activation, are essential for both the pre- and postsynaptic changes.

6 Calcium achieves its effects by activation of both calcium/calmodulin-dependent kinase II and protein kinase C, and cAMP-mediated protein kinase A activation as well as *de novo* protein synthesis are also necessary for prolonged effects of LTP. The non-NMDA glutamate receptors in the postsynaptic membrane are activated by phosphorylation, and presynaptic changes are brought about by generation of a retrograde message (possibly arachidonic acid, NO or CO) which could activate the metabotropic glutamate receptors. Structural changes in synapses following LTP have also been seen.

7 Long-term depression (LTD) in the hippocampus may result from a lower level of calcium signalling than that needed for LTP, resulting in phosphatase activation rather than the kinase activation characteristic of LTP.

8 A drug that blocks NMDA receptors, AP5, selectively impairs the spatial learning ability of rats; mice with targeted deletion of NMDAR1 receptors in the CA1 region of the hippocampus also have difficulties in learning spatial cues, and LTP is absent in CA1. In monkeys, on the other hand, NMDA receptor blockade does not interfere with spatial learning, and LTP in brain areas other than hippocampal CA1 may not be dependent exclusively on NMDA receptors.

9 Neurotrophins may modulate synaptic efficacy in the adult.

10 Chapter 14 describes synaptic modifications induced in sensory pathways by excess over- or under-use and the possible links with LTP mechanisms.

General reading

- Bliss, T. V. P. and Collingridge, G. L. A synaptic model of memory: long-term potentiation in the hippocampus. *Nature* **361**, 31–9 (1993).

- Kandel, E. R. and Pittenger, C. The past, the future and the biology of memory storage. *Philos. Trans. R. Soc. London Ser. B Biol. Sci.* **354**, 2027–52 (1999).

- Sanes, J. R. and Lichtman, J. W. Can molecules explain long-term potentiation? *Nat. Neurosci.* **2**, 597–604 (1999).

- Stevens, C. F. A million dollar question: does LTP = memory? *Neuron* **20**, 1–2 (1998).

References

1. Kandel, E. R. and Schwartz, J. H. Molecular biology of an elementary form of learning: modulation of transmitter release through cyclic AMP-dependent protein kinase. *Science* **218**, 433–43 (1982).

2. Hawkins, R. D., Kandel, E. R. and Siegelbaum, S. A. Learning to modulate transmitter release: themes and variations in synaptic plasticity. *Annu. Rev. Neurosci.* **16**, 625–65 (1993).

3. Carew, T. J., Walters, E. T. and Kandel, E. R. Classical conditioning in a simple withdrawal reflex in *Aplysia californica*. *J. Neurosci.* **1**, 1426–37 (1981).

4. Klein, M., Shapiro, E. and Kandel, E. R. Synaptic plasticity and the modulation of the Ca^{++} current. *J. Exp. Biol.* **89**, 117–57 (1980).

5. Bailey, C. H. and Chen, M. Morphological basis of long-term habituation and sensitization in *Aplysia*. *Science* **220**, 91–3 (1983).

6. Dale, N., Schachner, S. and Kandel, E. R. Long-term facilitation in *Aplysia* involves increase in transmitter release. *Science* **239**, 282–5 (1988).

7. Castellucci, V. and Kandel, E. R. Pre-synaptic facilitation as a mechanism for behavioural sensitization in *Aplysia*. *Science* **194**, 1176–8 (1976).

8. Brunelli, M., Castellucci, V. and Kandel, E. R. Synaptic facilitation and behavioural sensitization in *Aplysia*: possible role of serotonin and cyclic AMP. *Science* **194**, 1178–81 (1976).

9. Hawkins, R. D., Castellucci, V. F. and Kandel, E. R. Interneurons involved in mediation and modulation of the gill-withdrawal reflex in *Aplysia*. II. Identified neurons produce heterosynaptic facilitation contributing to behavioural sensitization. *J. Neurophysiol.* **45**, 315–26 (1981).

10. Montarolo, P. G. *et al.* A critical period for macromolecular synthesis in long-term heterosynaptic facilitation in *Aplysia*. *Science* **234**, 1249–54 (1986).

11. Martin, K. C. *et al.* Synapse-specific, long-term facilitation of *Aplysia* sensory to motor synapses: a function for local protein synthesis in memory storage. *Cell* **91**, 927–38 (1997).

12. Schacher, S., Castellucci, V. F. and Kandel, E. R. cAMP evokes long-term facilitation in *Aplysia* sensory neurons that requires new protein synthesis. *Science* **240**, 1667–9 (1988).

13. Dash, P. K., Hochner, B. and Kandel, E. R. Injection of the cAMP-responsive element into the nucleus of *Aplysia* sensory neurons blocks long-term facilitation. *Nature* **345**, 718–21 (1990).

14. Bourtchuladze, R. *et al.* Deficient long-term memory in mice with a targeted mutation of the cAMP-responsive element-binding protein. *Cell* **79**, 59–68 (1994).

15. Yin, J. C. P. *et al.* Induction of a dominant negative CREB transgene specifically blocks long-term memory in *Drosophila*. *Cell* **79**, 49–58 (1994).

16. Yin, J. C., Del Vecchio, M., Zhou, H. and Tully, T. CREB as a memory modulator: induced expression of a dCREB2 activator isoform enhances long-term memory in *Drosophila*. *Cell* **81**, 107–15 (1995).

17. Bartsch, D. *et al. Aplysia* CREB2 represses long-term facilitation: relief of repression converts transient facilitation into long-term functional and structural change. *Cell* **83**, 979–92 (1995).

18. Bailey, C. H. and Chen, M. Time course of structural changes at identified sensory neuron synapses during long-term sensitization in *Aplysia*. *J. Neurosci.* **9**, 1774–80 (1989).

19. Glanzman, D. L., Kandel, E. R. and Schacher, S. Target- dependent structural changes accompanying long-term synaptic facilitation in *Aplysia* neurons. *Science* **249**, 799–802 (1990).

20. Bailey, C. H., Chen, M., Keller, F. and Kandel, E. R. Serotonin-mediated endocytosis of apCAM: an early step of learning-related synaptic growth in *Aplysia*. *Science* **256**, 645–9 (1992).

21. Davis, G. W., Schuster, C. M. and Goodman, C. S. Genetic dissection of structural and functional components of synaptic plasticity. III. CREB is necessary for presynaptic functional plasticity. *Neuron* **17**, 669–79 (1996).

22. Abrams, T. W. and Kandel, E. R. Is contiguity detection in classical conditioning a system or a cellular property? Learning in *Aplysia* suggests a possible molecular site. *Trends Neurosci.* **11**, 128–35 (1988).

23. Lukowiak, K. and Colebrook, E. Classical conditioning alters the efficacy of identified gill motor neurones in producing gill withdrawal movements in *Aplysia*. *J. Exp. Biol.* **140**, 273–85 (1988).

24. Nelson, T. J. and Alkon, D. L. Biochemistry of molluscan learning and memory. *BioEssays* **19**, 1045–53 (1997).

25. Belvin, M. P. and Yin, J. C. *Drosophila* learning and memory: recent progress and new approaches. *BioEssays* **19**, 1083–9 (1997).

26. Byers, D., Davis, R. L. and Kiger, J. A. Defect in cyclic-AMP phosphodiesterase due to the *dunce* mutation of learning in *Drosophila melanogaster*. *Nature* **289**, 79–81 (1981).

27. Levin, L. R. *et al.* The *Drosophila* learning and memory gene *rutabaga* encodes a Ca^{2+}/calmodulin-responsive adenylyl cyclase. *Cell* **68**, 479–89 (1992).

28. Skoulakis, E. M., Kalderon, D. and Davis, R. L. Preferential expression in mushroom bodies of the catalytic subunit of protein kinase A and its role in learning and memory. *Neuron* **11**, 197–208 (1993).

29. Feany, M. B. and Quinn, W. G. A neuropeptide gene defined by the *Drosophila* memory mutant amnesiac. *Science* **268**, 869–73 (1995).

30. Folkers, E., Drain, P. and Quinn, W. G. *Radish*, a *Drosophila* mutant deficient in consolidated memory. *Proc. Natl. Acad. Sci. USA* **90**, 8123–7 (1993).

31. Grotewiel, M. S., Beck, C. D., Wu, K. H., Zhu, X. R. and Davis, R. L. Integrin-mediated short-term memory in *Drosophila*. *Nature* **391**, 455–60 (1998).

32. Olton, D. S., Walker, J. A. and Gage, F. H. Hippocampal connections in spatial discrimination. *Brain Res.* **139**, 295-308 (1978).

33. O'Keefe, J. and Dostrovsky, J. The hippocampus as a spatial map. Preliminary evidence from unit activity in the freely-moving rat. *Brain Res.* **34**, 171-5 (1971).

34. O'Keefe, J. Place units in the hippocampus of the freely-moving rat. *Exp. Neurol.* **51**, 78-109 (1976).

35. Zola-Morgan, S. M. and Squire, L. R. The primate hippocampal formation: evidence for a time-limited role in memory storage. *Science* **250**, 288-90 (1990).

36. Bliss, T. V. P. and Lomo, T. Long-lasting potentiation of synaptic transmission in the dentate area of the anaesthetised rabbit following stimulation of the perforant path. *J. Physiol.* **232**, 331-6 (1973).

37. Ito, M. Long-term depression. *Annu. Rev. Neurosci.* **12**, 85-102 (1989).

38. Kirkwood, A., Dudek, S. M., Gold, J. T., Aizenman, C. D. and Bear, M. F. Common forms of synaptic plasticity in the hippocampus and neocortex *in vitro. Science* **260**, 1518-21 (1993).

39. Fox, K. The critical period for long-term potentiation in primary sensory cortex. *Neuron* **15**, 485-8 (1995).

40. Rogan, M. T., Staubli, U. V. and LeDoux, J. E. Fear conditioning induces associative long-term potentiation in the amygdala. *Nature* **390**, 604-7 (1997).

41. McKernan, M. G. and Shinnick-Gallagher, P. Fear conditioning induces a lasting potentiation of synaptic currents *in vitro. Nature* **390**, 607-11 (1997).

42. Stevens, C. F. A million dollar question: does LTP = memory? *Neuron* **20**, 1-2 (1998).

43. Gustafsson, B. and Wigstrom, H. Physiological mechanisms underlying long-term potentiation. *Trends Neurosci.* **11**, 156-62 (1988).

44. Bliss, T. V. P. and Collingridge, G. L. A synaptic model of memory: long-term potentiation in the hippocampus. *Nature* **361**, 31-9 (1993).

45. Zalutsky, R. A. and Nicoll, R. A. Comparison of two forms of long-term potentiation in single hippocampal neurons. *Science* **248**, 1619-24 (1990).

46. Malenka, R. C., Kauer, J. A., Zucker, R. S. and Nicoll, R. A. Postsynaptic calcium is sufficient for potentiation of hippocampal synaptic transmission. *Science* **242**, 81-4 (1988).

47. Malenka, R. C., Lancaster, B. and Zucker, R. S. Temporal limits on the rise in postsynaptic calcium required for the induction of long-term potentiation. *Neuron* **9**, 121-8 (1992).

48. Kauer, J. A., Malenka, R. C. and Nicoll, R. A. A persistent postsynaptic modification mediates long-term potentiation in the hippocampus. *Neuron* **1**, 911-17 (1988).

49. Isaac, T. R., Nicoll, R. A. and Malenka, R. C. Evidence for silent synapses: implications for the expression of LTP. *Neuron* **15**, 427-34 (1995).

50. Collingridge, G. L. and Bliss, T. V. P. NMDA receptors—their role in long-term potentiation. *Trends Neurosci.* **10**, 228-9 (1987).

51. Dolphin, A. C., Errington, M. L. and Bliss, R. V. P. Long-term potentiation of the perforant path *in vivo* is associated with increased glutamate release. *Nature* **297**, 496-8 (1982).

52. Malinow, R. and Tsien, R. W. Presynaptic enhancement shown by whole-cell recordings of long-term potentiation in hippocampal slices. *Nature* **346**, 177-80 (1990).

53. Larkman, A., Hannay, T., Stratford, K. and Jack, J. Presynaptic release probability influences the locus of long-term potentiation. *Nature* **360**, 70-3 (1992).

54. Malgaroli, A. *et al.* Presynaptic component of long-term potentiation visualised at individual hippocampal synapses. *Science* **268**, 1624-8 (1995).

55. Fifkova, E. and Van Harreveld, A. Long-lasting morphological changes in dendritic spines of dentate granular cells following stimulation of the entorhinal area. *J. Neurocytol.* **6**, 211-30 (1977).

56. Andersen, P., Blackstad, T., Hulleberg, G., Trommald, M. and Vaaland, J. L. Dimensions of dendritic spines of rat dentate granule cells during long-term potentiation. *J. Physiol.* **390**, 264P (1987).

57. Lee, K. S., Schotter, F., Oliver, M. and Lynch, G. Brief bursts of high-frequency stimulation produce two types of structural changes in rat hippocampus. *J. Neurophysiol.* **44**, 247-58 (1980).

58. Chang, F. L. and Greenhough, W. T. Transient and enduring morphological correlates of synaptic activity and efficacy change in the rat hippocampal slice. *Brain Res.* **309**, 35-46 (1984).

59. Nelson, R. B., Linden, D. J., Hyman, C., Pfenninger, K. H. and Routtenberg, A. The two major phosphoproteins in growth cones are probably identical to two protein kinase C substrates correlated with persistence of long-term potentiation. *J. Neurosci.* **9**, 381-9 (1989).

60. Muller, D. *et al.* PSA–NCAM is required for activity-induced synaptic plasticity. *Neuron* **17**, 413-22 (1996).

61. Hagler, D. J., Jr. and Goda, Y. Synaptic adhesion: the building blocks of memory? *Neuron* **20**, 1059-62 (1998).

62. Tang, L., Hung, C. P. and Schuman, E. M. A role for the cadherin family of cell adhesion

molecules in hippocampal long-term potentiation. *Neuron* **20**, 1165–75 (1998).

63. Chen, C. and Tonegawa, S. Molecular genetic analysis of synaptic plasticity, activity-dependent neural development, learning, and memory in the mammalian brain. *Annu. Rev. Neurosci.* **20**, 157–84 (1997).

64. Sanes, J. R. and Lichtman, J. W. Can molecules explain long-term potentiation? *Nat. Neurosci.* **2**, 597–604 (1999).

65. Brown, T. H., Chapman, P. F., Kairiss, E. W. and Keenan, C. L. Long-term synaptic potentiation. *Science* **242**, 724–8 (1988).

66. Anwyl, R. Protein kinase C and long-term potentiation. *Trends Pharmacol. Sci.* **10**, 236–8 (1989).

67. Winder, D. G., Mansuy, I. M., Osman, M., Moallem, T. M. and Kandel, E. R. Genetic and pharmacological evidence for a novel, intermediate phase of long-term potentiation suppressed by calcineurin. *Cell* **92**, 25–37 (1998).

68. Malenka, R. C. *et al.* An essential role for postsynaptic calmodulin and protein kinase activity in long-term potentiation. *Nature* **340**, 554–6 (1989).

69. Malinow, R., Madison, D. V. and Tsien, R. W. Persistent protein kinase activity underlying long-term potentiation. *Nature* **335**, 820–4 (1988).

70. Malinow, R., Schulman, H. and Tsien, R. W. Inhibition of postsynaptic PKC or CaMKII blocks induction but not expression of LTP. *Science* **245**, 862–6 (1989).

71. Mansuy, I. M., Mayford, M., Jacob, B., Kandel, E. R. and Bach, M. E. Restricted regulated overexpression reveals calcineurin as a key component in the transition from short-term to long-term memory. *Cell* **92**, 39–49 (1998).

72. McGlade-McCulloh, E., Yamamoto, H., Tan, S. E., Brickey, D. A. and Soderling, T. R. Phosphorylation and regulation of glutamate receptors by calcium/calmodulin-dependent protein kinase II. *Nature* **362**, 640–2 (1993).

73. Pettit, D. L., Perlman, S. and Malinow, R. Potentiated transmission and prevention of further LTP by increased CaMKII activity in postsynaptic hippocampal slice. *Science* **266**, 1881–5 (1994).

74. Bonhoeffer, T., Staiger, V. and Aertsen, A. Synaptic plasticity in rat hippocampal slice cultures: local 'Hebbian' conjunction of pre- and postsynaptic stimulation leads to distributed synaptic enhancement. *Proc. Natl. Acad. Sci. USA* **86**, 8113–17 (1989).

75. Herrero, I., Miras-Portugal, M. T. and Sanchez-Prieto, J. Positive feedback of glutamate exocytosis by metabotropic presynaptic receptor stimulation. *Nature* **360**, 163–6 (1992).

76. Bashir, Z. I. *et al.* Induction of LTP in the hippocampus needs synaptic activation of glutamate metabotropic receptors. *Nature* **363**, 347–50 (1993).

77. Bartolotto, Z. A., Bashir, Z. I., Davies, C. H. and Collingridge, G. L. A molecular switch activated by metabotropic glutamate receptors regulates induction of long-term potentiation. *Nature* **368**, 740–3 (1994).

78. Aiba, A. *et al.* Reduced hippocampal long-term potentiation and context-specific deficit in associative learning in mGluR1 mutant mice. *Cell* **79**, 365–75 (1994).

79. Schuman, E. M. and Madison, D. V. A requirement for the intercellular messenger nitric oxide in long-term potentiation. *Science* **254**, 1503–6 (1991).

80. Zhuo, M., Small, S. A., Kandel, E. R. and Hawkins, R. P. Nitric oxide and carbon monoxide produce activity-dependent long-term synaptic enhancement in hippocampus. *Science* **260**, 1946–50 (1993).

81. O'Dell, T. J. *et al.* Endothelial NOS and the blockade of LTP by NOS inhibitors in mice lacking neuronal NOS. *Science* **265**, 542–6 (1994).

82. Kang, H. and Schuman, E. M. Long-lasting neurotrophin-induced enhancement of synaptic transmission in the adult rat hippocampus. *Science* **267**, 1658–62 (1995).

83. Brambilla, R. *et al.* A role for the Ras signalling pathway in synaptic transmission and long-term memory. *Nature* **390**, 281–6 (1997).

84. Mulkey, R. M. and Malenka, R. C. Mechanisms underlying induction of homosynaptic long-term depression in area CA1 of the hippocampus. *Neuron* **9**, 967–75 (1992).

85. Mulkey, R. M., Herron, C. E. and Malenka, R. C. An essential role for protein phosphatases in hippocampal long-term depression. *Science* **261**, 1051–5 (1993).

86. Conquet, F. *et al.* Motor deficit and impairment of synaptic plasticity in mice lacking mGluR1. *Nature* **372**, 237–43 (1994).

87. Morris, R. G., Anderson, B., Lynch, G. S. and Baudry, M. Selective impairment of learning and blockade of long-term potentiation by an N-methyl-D-aspartate receptor antagonist, AP5. *Nature* **319**, 774–6 (1986).

88. Gutnikov, S. A. and Gaffan, D. Systemic NMDA receptor antagonist CGP-40116 does not impair memory acquisition but protects against NMDA neurotoxicity in Rhesus monkeys. *J. Neurosci.* **16**, 4041–5 (1996).

89. Tsien, J. Z. *et al.* Subregion and cell type-restricted gene knockout in mouse brain. *Cell* **87**, 1317–26 (1996).

90. Silva, A. J., Paylor, R., Wehner, J. M. and Tonegawa, S. Impaired spatial learning in alpha-calcium-calmodulin kinase II in mutant mice. *Science* **257**, 206–11 (1992).

91. Abeliovich, A. *et al.* PKC gamma mutant mice exhibit mild deficits in spatial and contextual learning. *Cell* **75**, 1263–71 (1993).

92. Mauk, M. D., Garcia, K. S., Medina, J. F. and Steele, P. M. Does cerebellar LTD mediate motor learning? Toward a resolution without a smoking gun. *Neuron* **20**, 359–62 (1998).

93. Lisberger, S. G. Cerebellar LTD: a molecular mechanism of behavioral learning? *Cell* **92**, 701–4 (1998).

94. De Zeeuw, C. I. *et al.* Expression of a protein kinase C inhibitor in Purkinje cells blocks cerebellar LTD and adaptation of the vestibulo-ocular reflex. *Neuron* **20**, 495–508 (1998).

16

Trophic Interactions between Neurons in the Adult Nervous System

The normal morphology, biochemistry and physiology of nerve cells are maintained by their synaptic connections, which allow continuous exchange of chemical and electrical signals across the synaptic cleft. This mutual maintenance by synaptic partners is known as the *trophic* effect of neurons. Trophic interactions begin when synaptic relationships are first established, and some of the effects particular to the embryonic and neonatal period have been described in Chapter 11. At that stage in development the cellular interactions are usually described as *inductive*, because they induce a change in the properties of the interacting tissues. Many of the properties induced need continuous signalling for their upkeep, and so changes in the structure and function of neurons occur even in the adult when synaptic connections are broken. The nature of the positive trophic effects can be deduced by seeing what happens when trophic interactions can no longer occur (see Fig. 16.1). The classical example is the dramatic wasting of skeletal muscle in denervated limbs. Muscle bulk and power can be restored if the muscle is successfully reinnervated. This influence of the nerve, in this case the spinal motor neuron, on its target is called the *orthograde* trophic effect, because the direction in which the trophic signal flows is the same as that of impulse conduction and synaptic transmission. Orthograde effects of axotomy can spread distally along a chain of neurons, producing transneuronal effects (Fig. 16.1).

There also exist *retrograde* trophic effects, so-called because they occur in the opposite direction to that of impulse conduction and synaptic transmission. The observation is that neurons that have been disconnected from their postsynaptic targets, for example by section of their axons, undergo a variety of changes. The morphological changes have been termed *chromatolysis* (see later), and there are additional changes in physiological and biochemical properties. The glial cells around axotomized neurons also change. The retrograde effects of axotomy are probably mediated in part by the interruption of the supply of trophic factors (see Chapter 12)

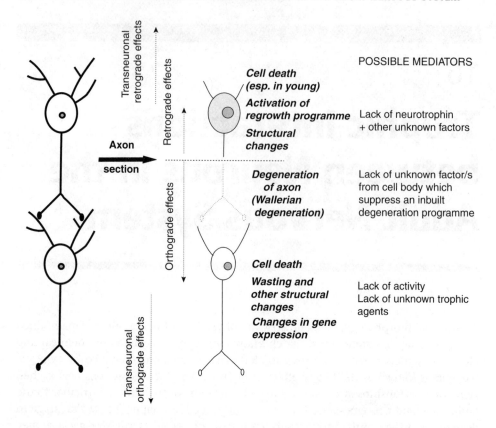

Figure 16.1 Neurotrophic interactions in the adult. If communication is broken in a neuronal network, most simply by cutting the axon(s) at some point, not only does the disconnected axon(s) degenerate (Wallerian degeneration) but there are also changes in properties in: (1) the axotomized nerve cell (a retrograde change); (2) the neurons that synapse on it (transneuronal retrograde changes); (3) the neurons downstream with which the axotomized neuron synapsed (orthograde change); and (4) neurons further downstream of this (transneuronal orthograde changes). The molecular signals that bring these effects about are still being sought, but changes in neurotrophin levels are almost certainly involved. So too may be changes in the levels of impulse activity and the reactions of glial cells and recruited and resident macrophages.

released by target tissues, and possibly also by glial cells, which are normally taken up by the axons and retrogradely transported to the cell body (Fig. 16.1). The reaction of axotomized neurons can in turn influence the neurons that innervate them, so-called *transneuronal*, retrograde reactions.

Many of the properties that the nerve, target and glial cells develop after they have been disconnected from each other are not simply degenerative, but are similar to those which the cells possessed during early stages of development before they were innervated. The changes may therefore help to promote the regrowth of axons, and thus the re-establishment of connections, leading finally to the redevelopment of the normal differentiated adult state.

The following account first describes orthograde trophic effects. These could theoretically be mediated by electrical events triggered by the synaptic input or by molecules liberated by the innervating axons. Retrograde trophic effects, which, because of the one-way nature of synaptic transmission, can only be mediated by chemical means, are then described.

Orthograde trophic effects on peripheral nerve

A special case of trophic dependence is that of a nerve cell's own processes, in particular the axon, which is often very long and is easily damaged by cutting, crushing and stretching. The axon contains no machinery to manufacture the large number of proteins that it contains, so when isolated from its cell body it is fated eventually to degenerate as structural proteins are broken down and cannot be replaced. The first description of axonal degeneration after nerve section was made by the English physician Waller (1816–70), and henceforth this type of nerve degeneration has been called Wallerian degeneration to distinguish it from degeneration of the nerve cells themselves. In fact, the rate of axon degeneration is much faster than would occur by a gradual process of repair failure, and degeneration is probably carried out by activation of a specific programme of degradative enzymes. This is known from the discovery of a genetic strain of mouse whose axons degenerate very much more slowly than normal after separation from the cell body. The axons of such mice can last in good structural and functional order for up to 3 weeks after being isolated from the cell body,[1-3] compared with the normal survival time of axons from other genetic strains of 1 or 2 days. The identity of the degenerative programme is unknown, and appears to be distinct from the caspase family of cysteine proteases that mediates apoptosis (see Chapter 13); caspase 3 is not activated in Wallerian degeneration and caspase inhibition does not affect the degenerative process.[4]

Very soon after transection, within about half an hour, the open ends of both proximal and distal nerve stumps seal over,[5,6] and for a day or two in mammals the axons in the distal stump are capable of conducting action potentials if stimulated. The earliest changes in the distal nerve stump of an axotomized motor neuron occur at the neuromuscular junction after 12 hours or so. The spontaneous and evoked release of transmitter cease, and this is followed by degeneration of the nerve terminal. These changes are slower to develop if the nerve is cut some distance away from the muscle. It seems that there is a signal travelling distally from the site of nerve transection at the rate of fast axoplasmic transport which triggers transmission failure.[7] The degeneration probably begins because there is a drop in the level of some critical factor supplied by the cell body, but its nature remains obscure. The entry of substances into the axon at the site of injury is probably not responsible, because the proximal stump of the axon (still connected to the cell body) does not usually degenerate. It is also unclear why the terminals degenerate before the rest of the axon; perhaps they are more metabolically active and so more rapidly depleted of the crucial factor transported from the cell body. During degeneration of the axon the levels of sodium and calcium in its cytoplasm rise;[8] eventually the membrane becomes leaky and the neurofilaments and microtubules disintegrate, probably by means of calcium-activated proteases.[9,10] Degeneration spreads rapidly backwards from the terminals[11,12] and may also spread distally from the site of injury.

The myelinating Schwann cells respond to the changes in the axon by extensive changes in gene expression. There is downregulation of genes transcribing myelin-associated proteins,[13] as well as upregulation of genes for NGF, p75NTR (the low-affinity NGF receptor), IGFs, BDNF, NCAM and L1 (see Chapter 6 for discussion of the reverse process during myelin formation). NGF binding to p75NTR receptor activates the nuclear transcription factor nuclear factor kappa B (NF-κB), and this could be the cause of the upregulation of the adhesion molecules NCAM and L1.[14] The breakdown of myelin is heralded by the separation of myelin lamellae from one another at the intraperiod line close to the incisures of Schmidt–Lantermann.[15,16] The paranodal myelin is then withdrawn, and lipid droplets appear in the Schwann cell cytoplasm. Within 12 hours of axotomy proteases appear in the distal nerve, and these attack the proteins binding the myelin layers together.[17] The nerve is invaded by macrophages some 3 days after nerve section, and these cells become laden with myelin debris and thus speed the later stages of its removal,[18] although some myelin is completely removed without their help.

The breakdown and removal of the myelin is accompanied by mitosis of the Schwann cells, and adjacent Schwann cells may become coupled by gap junctions.[19] Glial growth factor (GGF/neuregulin) expressed by axons is an important Schwann cell mitogen during embryonic development (see Chapter 6), and following axotomy it is upregulated transiently by Schwann cells, together with erbB2 and erbB3 receptors. This suggests that neuregulin may contribute to Schwann cell mitosis during Wallerian degeneration, probably through autocrine or paracrine signalling.[14] There is also evidence that transforming growth factors TGFβ1 and β2 from macrophages, and fibroblast growth factor (FGF) from degenerating axons, are mitogens for Schwann cells.[20-22] Lastly, a secreted signalling molecule, Reg-2, is expressed by regenerating (and developing) rodent motor and sensory neurons, and may also stimulate Schwann cell mitosis.[23] The result of all these changes is the production of large numbers of dedifferentiated Schwann cells lying within their basal lamina sheaths, forming the so-called bands of Büngner, which provide an attractive environment for regrowing axons and provide them with an ideal pathway for regeneration (see Chapter 17). The main events of Wallerian degeneration are summarized in Fig. 16.2 and Table 16.1.

In the CNS, the degeneration of cut axons occurs a little more slowly than in the PNS, but the degeneration of myelin is very much slower.[24,25] This is probably a result of the inability of the oligodendroglia to reprogramme themselves in the same way as Schwann cells. They continue to make myelin-associated proteins[26] and may not be

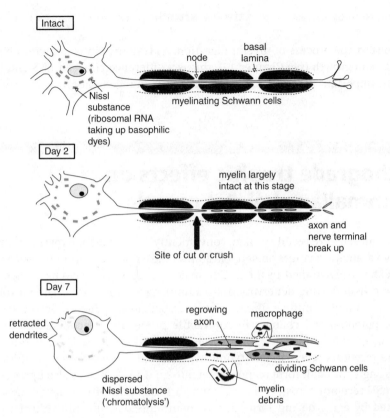

Figure 16.2 Effects of axotomy on a motor neuron: 'chromatolysis' of the cell body and dendritic retraction, degeneration of the axon (called 'Wallerian' degeneration after the man who first described the phenomenon), loss of myelin, mitosis of Schwann cells, and invasion by monocytes which become macrophages loaded with myelin debris.

Table 16.1 Some biochemical events following axotomy

Cell body	Axon	Schwann cell	Fibroblasts and macrophages
Upregulation of:	*Activation of self-*	*Upregulation of:*	*Upregulation of:*
c-Jun	*destruct programme*	NCAM	NGF
Gap-43	*normally held in*	L1	Il-1
Tα1-tubulin-subunit	*check by factors from*	IGFs	Il-6
Actin	*the cell body.*	NGF and LNGFR	TGFα and β
CGRP (in motor	*Result:*	BDNF	Proteases
neurons)	Ca^{2+} entry, calpain	LIF	? Lipases
GGF	activation and	Proteases (MMPS)	
	Wallerian	? Lipases	
	degeneration		
Downregulation of:	*Release of factors*	*Downregulation of:*	
Neurofilaments	*from axon:*	Myelin-associated	
LNGFR (in sensory axons)	e.g. FGFs	proteins	
In some cases:		CNTF	
Apoptosis			

able to start the process of myelin digestion. As CNS myelin is known to be able to inhibit axon growth (see Chapter 17), this is a difference between CNS and PNS glia that has important practical consequences for axon regeneration.

Orthograde trophic effects on mammalian skeletal muscle

Skeletal muscles are readily visible, conveniently accessible for experimentation and undergo dramatic changes on denervation, so the trophic effects of nerves have been most extensively studied in them. The major changes that have been identified in muscle cells following denervation are summarized in Fig. 16.3. The most striking effect is atrophy of muscle fibres; there is also a small reduction in the size of the resting potential and changes in contractile properties, junctional and extrajunctional membrane properties, and in the composition of the basal lamina. Acetylcholine receptors revert to embryonic type (α2,β,d,y, see Chapter 11) initially, but interestingly the adult form reappears later (α2,β,d,Σ).[27] There is also upregulation of the MuSK receptor tyrosine kinase,[28] which forms part of the signalling sequence activated by agrin during formation of neuromuscular junctions during embryogenesis (see Chapter 11).

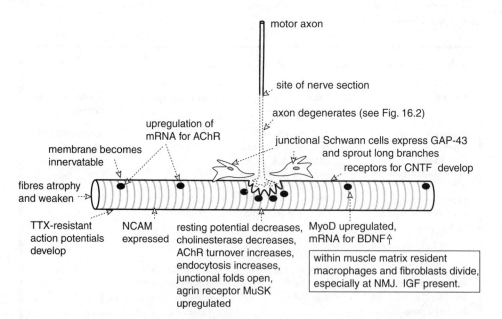

Figure 16.3 Effects of denervation on skeletal muscle fibres.

In muscle, as in other innervated tissue, the effects of denervation could be mediated either by lack of postsynaptic electrical activity or by lack of molecules synthesized in the nerve cell body, transported along the axons and released onto the target cells (Fig. 16.1). The neurotransmitter itself could also have a direct trophic effect quite apart from any effect of the electrical activity it causes. In mammalian skeletal muscle, the trophic effect of motor nerves in preventing muscle atrophy and associated changes is found to be mediated predominantly by the muscle fibre action potentials. Because of the small size and very localized distribution of motor nerve terminals, molecules released by them might be expected to affect mainly the properties of the synaptic region of the muscle fibres. There is indeed evidence that motor nerves do release several factors which are important during endplate·formation (see Chapter 11).

The dominant role of activity in maintaining normal muscle properties was shown conclusively when it was found that increases in acetylcholine sensitivity associated with denervation (the result of synthesis of acetylcholine receptors by myonuclei all along the length of each fibre and their incorporation into the membrane)[29] did not occur in denervated muscles kept active by direct stimulation through implanted electrodes. It also became clear that muscles with intact innervation developed changes very like those of denervated muscles if they were prevented from being active by applying small cuffs containing local anaesthetic to their nerves.[30] It was further discovered that other properties of the muscle membrane, and the form of cholinesterase at the neuromuscular junction, are controlled by activity.[31,32]

While any form of electrical activity, provided it is given reasonably frequently, can reduce muscle wasting, it turns out that the *pattern* of electrical activity determines the details of several muscle properties. Since the 1960s it has been known that major changes in the contractile properties of skeletal muscles can be brought about by exchanging nerves between slow muscles (composed mostly of slow, type I motor units) and fast muscles (composed mostly of fast, type II motor units).[33] The muscle receiving the foreign nerve changes its properties to resemble those of the muscle from which the nerve originated. It is now clear that an appropriate pattern of electrical activity can also bring about changes. Continuous, low-frequency stimulation, used to mimic the firing pattern of motor neurons innervating slow oxidative motor units, slows the contraction time of fast glycolytic muscles and causes them to develop more mitochondria and capillaries. On the other hand, the same number of stimuli delivered in high-frequency bursts separated by long pauses, that is, in a pattern characteristic of fast, fatiguable motor units, converts slow muscles into fast muscles by changing both myofibrillar proteins and proteins involved in excitation–contraction coupling. A particular pattern is equally effective whether delivered through electrodes directly to denervated muscles[34] or to muscles with their nerves intact.[35]

The changes in muscle contractile properties brought about by nerve exchange or stimulation pattern are based on the synthesis of different isoforms of the protein subunits used in the construction of myosin, tropomyosin and troponin.[36] The extent of conversion from slow to fast properties is not perfect, because slow isoforms continue to be synthesized, and the new fast isoforms are not identical to those of a genuine fast muscle.[37] It does not seem possible, therefore, to turn a fibre developmentally destined to be slow into a true fast fibre by means of patterned electrical activity.[38] Each intrinsic type has, however, an adaptive range,[39] which allows considerable overlap of functional properties between the basic types if an appropriate pattern of stimulation is applied. Slow fibres have a greater adaptive range than fast fibres. The intracellular mechanisms of the control of contractile proteins by pattern of activity remain uncertain.

Can motor nerves influence muscle contractile and membrane properties outside the junctional region by means other than activity?

The question also remains whether there is an additional trophic effect, independent of muscle activity, on regions of the muscle outside the immediate vicinity of the neuromuscular junction. Attempts to answer this question have been made as follows.

First, the effects of blockade of axoplasmic transport with colchicine while nerve electrical activity is maintained for a period have been examined. It is found that denervation-like changes develop in muscles before the nerves degenerate and cease to activate the muscle. Colchicine, however, causes similar changes when it reaches the muscle fibres directly via the circulation.[40]

Second, careful comparison of the magnitude of the changes in muscle brought about by denervation with those caused by nerve impulse blockade alone has shown that many denervation-like changes in inactive muscles are less well developed than in the denervated muscles. Some of the changes seen after denervation, however, are caused additionally by factors associated with the degeneration of the cut axons,[34,41-43] as denervated, but not paralysed, muscles contain large numbers of dividing fibroblasts and other cell types,[44,45] and these could produce effects on muscle. For example, tumour necrosis factor, a product of activated macrophages, is known to cause depolarization of skeletal muscle fibres.[46]

Third, nerve extracts have been applied to see if they can partially reverse the effects of denervation, usually by adding them to cultures of embryonic muscle *in vitro*. The findings are open to the criticism, however, that additions of tissue extracts simply improve the nutritional conditions. Furthermore, the added material is provided all over the fibres, whereas *in vivo* nerve-derived material is applied to a highly restricted part of the muscle. An example of these difficulties was a protein extracted from chicken sciatic nerves, which induced morphological maturation in cultured embryonic muscle.[47] This protein, originally called sciatin, was later found to be transferrin, a protein needed to make iron available to tissues around the body. Extracts of various tissues, including nerve, can stimulate the synthesis of cholinesterase in organ-cultured muscles,[48] and an extract of spinal cord can change the properties of both the action potential and the acetylcholine receptors of denervated muscles, making them more like those found in innervated muscle fibres.[49] Whether motor nerves release these substances *in vivo* remains to be seen, and this qualification also applies to the trophic effect demonstrated by another nerve extract which was applied daily to denervated rat muscles *in vivo*.[50]

More recently, it has been shown that denervated muscle upregulates CNTF receptors (see Chapter 12), and that daily injections of CNTF slow the rate at which muscle weight and contractile force are lost after denervation.[51] Although these findings have therapeutic possibilities, it is unclear whether CNTF plays a trophic role in normal muscle, or if there is release of CNTF from endogenous supplies only following denervation (a built-in measure to slow muscle atrophy), or if these effects are only obtained by giving large exogenous doses.

In short, none of these approaches has provided unequivocal proof of a motor nerve-derived trophic factor with actions on contractile and other properties throughout the muscle, although all have hinted that there is indeed an effect.

Frog slow muscle

Some muscles in the frog contain fibres that cannot generate action potentials. They are depolarized instead by acetylcholine released from terminals distributed at regular intervals along the fibres that generate local endplate potentials. Action potentials can be propagated, however, in denervated fibres, and this capability is lost when the nerve regenerates.[52] Paralysis with α-bungarotoxin also induces the action potential mechanism. This suggests that acetylcholine itself may be the agent which maintains the normal state of electrical inexcitability of the muscle.[53]

Orthograde trophic effects in other tissues

Some examples of orthograde trophic effects in neurons

Intravenous infusions of neurotransmitters demonstrated earlier this century that denervated sympathetic ganglia became abnormally sensitive to acetylcholine. At least some of this rise in sensitivity is caused by a decrease in cholinesterase activity rather than a rise in the number of postsynaptic transmitter receptors such as occurs in skeletal muscle fibres.[54] Supersensitivity in denervated parasympathetic ganglion cells in the heart was, however, detected by recording intracellular responses to iontophoretically-applied acetylcholine,[55] and this was interpreted to be a consequence of increased postsynaptic sensitivity to the drug. More recent studies show that no supersensitivity develops to carbachol, the non-hydrolysable analogue of acetylcholine, so it is clear that in these parasympathetic ganglia too, super-sensitivity to acetylcholine is a result of the loss of cholinesterase.[56] If the pregan-glionic nerve regenerates into the cardiac ganglion, supersensitivity is reduced in many ganglion cells before the regenerated axons can activate an electrical response in the cells. This suggests that a trophic agent may be responsible for maintaining the normal sensitivity of the cells independently of activity.[57]

The regulation of the enzyme tyrosine hydroxylase, essential for the synthesis of noradrenaline, has been much studied in the superior cervical ganglion. Section of the preganglionic afferent axons produces a gradual decline in the level of tyrosine hydroxylase in the ganglion cells.[58] As in other systems, there have been attempts to discover the relative roles of activity and of trophic factors in controlling the level of the enzyme. Activity in the presynaptic terminals appears to be important, because a short period of intense preganglionic stimulation produces a significant increase in tyrosine hydroxylase activity in the ganglion within 3 days, whereas the same amount of electrical activity in the ganglion cells generated by stimulating the postsynaptic nerve, and so resulting in antidromic activity in the cells, is ineffective.[59] The effect of presynaptic stimulation is prevented by the ganglion blocking drug hexamethonium, so the responsible trophic factor could be the transmitter itself.[59] There are two mechanisms by which tyrosine hydroxylase activity is increased. The first involves phosphorylation of enzyme already present in the cell. This occurs rapidly and can be induced by a variety of peptide and other transmitters, all of which act via protein kinases.[60] A slower mechanism occurs over a period of days and involves an increase in the amount of mRNA coding for tyrosine hydroxylase.[61]

The transmitter noradrenaline is the trophic agent responsible for maintenance of the pineal gland. Denervation of the gland, or a period of inactivity, causes super-sensitivity to noradrenaline, while increases in presynaptic activity reduce the sen-sitivity to transmitter and increase the synthesis of the enzyme needed for melatonin production in the gland. The initial step by which noradrenaline acts is by hyper-polarizing the gland cells.[62]

Much less is known about trophic interactions within the CNS, but it is clear that neurons that are denervated (deafferented) often shrink in size and may sometimes die. For example, cells in the lateral geniculate nucleus degenerate when the optic nerve is cut even in adult animals.[63] On the other hand, while the survival during development of rat cholinergic basal forebrain neurons is dependent on neuro-trophins derived from their hippocampal target neurons, this dependence appears not be retained into maturity, and similar results have been reported for dopami-nergic neurons of the substantia nigra. It is possible that target-derived trophic factors predominantly regulate sprouting rather than survival in the adult CNS.[64]

Sensory end organs

Sensory neurons exert trophic effects on their end organs. Taste buds, for example, atrophy after section of the gustatory nerves and are restored to normal after rein-nervation. Sensory nerves other than true taste-bud afferent axons are able to restore taste buds to normal, but motor nerves will not.[65] Little is known about the nature of the trophic support supplied by afferent nerve fibres. It is possible that peptide or other transmitter substances released by sensory nerves at central terminals are also released in the periphery and maintain end organs. This idea has been raised by experiments showing that calcitonin-gene-related peptide released from sensory cells of the olfactory epithelium can make periglomerular cells of the olfactory bulb become dopaminergic.[66]

Effects of nerves on limb regeneration

A curious but well-known trophic action of nerves is to support the regrowth of amputated limbs in Urodeles and Crustacea. This action depends on the number of axons present rather than the type of axons (reviewed in reference 67). Regrowth of the amputated limb is due to mitosis of mesenchymal cells at the stump tip, and mitosis is stimulated by glial growth factor present in both motor and sensory axons (see also Chapter 6).[68] The amputated limbs of mammals and birds do not regenerate, even at the embryonic limb bud stage, although basic FGF, which is present in nerve tissue, can stimulate experimentally the regrowth of amputated embryonic avian limb buds.[69]

Trophic effects in invertebrates

Fewer observations of trophic effects have been made in invertebrates, although it is known that there are both similarities and differences compared with vertebrates. The peripheral stump of a severed nerve degenerates as in vertebrates, but in some cases degeneration occurs very slowly and action potentials can be conducted for several months. Remarkably, in some instances the severed ends can fuse together again.[70] While crustacean leg muscles atrophy following denervation, their fibres do not develop supersensitivity to the excitatory transmitter glutamate.[71] A small increase in sensitivity can, however, be detected in denervated insect leg muscles.[72] The role of activity has been investigated, and shown to be important for trans-forming a particular type of fast muscle into a slow muscle in lobsters during development.[73] It is probably also important for maintaining muscle properties in the adult. The pattern of activity has been found to determine the different properties of motoneurons innervating the crusher and cutter claws in lobsters.[74]

Conclusions about orthograde trophic effects

It is clear that electrical activity arising in the postsynaptic cell as a result of its synaptic input provides a very important trophic action in most situations. In the presence of this effect, it is usually harder to establish whether there are additional, chemically-mediated trophic effects. They have not yet been excluded, but their molecular nature remains largely unknown.

Retrograde trophic effects

Neurons whose axons have been cut undergo a great variety of changes, grouped collectively under the cell-body reaction to injury. The most obvious structural change is dispersion of the aggregates of ribosomes and endoplasmic reticulum in the cell body. This was originally seen in the light microscope as a disappearance of the basophilic staining Nissl substance, and so the term chromatolysis was used to describe it. In addition to these changes, it was found that some cells are killed by axotomy. It seems, then, that axotomy triggers two alternative sequences of events: one which helps to restore the lost axon, and one which removes the damaged neuron permanently. It is unclear what determines which sequence is followed, but it is known that nerve cell death induced by axotomy is much commoner when axons are cut in very young animals (see below).[75] It has also been found that retrograde changes occur more rapidly, and are more pronounced, when lesions are made close to the cell body. Changes are also more intense when a nerve is cut or tied off (ligated) compared with when it is crushed and so able to reinnervate the distal stump and thence the target tissue.

Many techniques have been used to analyse the changes that occur in and around axotomized neurons. Biophysical and biochemical methods have uncovered transient increases in RNA and protein synthesis, and turnover rates in the nerve cell body, and also in the surrounding glial cells. Some of these glial cells divide.[76] There is a rapid increase in metabolic activity which can be detected autoradiographically with 2-deoxyglucose.[77] The synthesis of c-jun protein, actin, the embryonic $T\alpha$-1 subunit of tubulin and GAP-43 all rise during the course of the first week after axotomy;[78-80] the first changes can be detected within a few hours of axotomy by *in situ* hybridization for mRNA.[81] Conversely, the synthesis of neurofilament proteins falls,[78] and so does the mRNA for glutamate receptors.[82] These molecular changes are summarized in Table 16.1. Physiological techniques have shown alterations in the waveform of the action potential recorded in the cell body and a loss of the effectiveness of synaptic inputs. This correlates with the shedding of synaptic boutons and retraction of the dendrites.[83]

Cell death following axotomy

Many of the changes described above assist the process of regeneration of the lost axon (see Chapter 17), but this can only occur if the neuron itself does not die. The number of neurons that die depends critically on the age at which axotomy is carried out, death being universal if axotomy is done at birth but less likely if the lesion is made a week or two later.[84] Death is also more frequent in the adult mammalian CNS than PNS. It is generally held that the neurons die for the same reasons, and by the same apoptotic process,[57] as do embryonic neurons deprived of access to neurotrophins from their targets, and that this target dependency diminishes with age. The amount of death among motor neurons after axotomy may also depend on the reactions of Schwann cells in the distal nerve stump, as Schwann cells may provide an alternative source of neurotrophic support (see later). In support of this, in a mutant strain of mice in which axons degenerate very slowly, and hence whose Schwann cells react very slowly, many motor neurons die after axotomy even if this is carried out in fully mature mice.[85]

Neuronal cell death is discussed in Chapter 13. Additional factors that may play a part in axotomy-induced death are the induction of nitric oxide synthase and an interferon-like molecule. The number of cells dying after axotomy seems to be related to the extent and persistence of such inductions.[86,87] Nitric oxide, in addition to its proposed role in long-term potentiation (LTP; see Chapter 15), has been implicated as a neurotoxin.[88] A further finding is that axotomized neonatal motor neurons become very susceptible to glutamate, an excess of which in the adult brain is believed to be responsible for killing nerve cells after excessive activity or under partially ischaemic conditions.[89] Blockade of NMDA glutamate receptors with the compound MK-801 can prevent motor neurons, whose axons are cut at birth, from dying.[90]

Possible causes of the cell-body reaction to injury

Several possible reasons for the retrograde reactions in neurons have been suggested.[91] They are: first, early return and accumulation in the cell body of substances normally transported to the end of the axonal tree and not returned; second, entry into the axon at the site of injury of a substance or substances derived either from the circulation or generated locally; third, generation of antidromic action potentials at the axotomy site; fourth, interruption of a retrograde trophic signal from the tissue that the neurons innervate; and fifth, interruption of supply of signals/factors from glial cells around the axon.

Many experimental results favour the fourth reason above, namely the interruption of the supply of a retrograde trophic factor from the target (see also Chapter 12). The evidence is very convincing for sympathetic and sensory neurons, which are trophically dependent on NGF. They express specific, high-affinity receptors for NGF and take up NGF from their terminals and deliver it to the cell body by the fast component of axonal transport.[92] It has been found that the effects of postganglionic axotomy can be prevented in an adult sympathetic ganglion if a pellet releasing NGF is implanted next to the ganglion.[93] Even more significant is the demonstration that antibodies to NGF produce some of the changes which follow axotomy. For example, if the supply of NGF is interrupted for long periods by immunizing animals to NGF, sympathetic neurons atrophy and die.[94] Sensory neurons in these same animals do not die, although there is a loss of substance P from their central terminals,[95] an effect which also occurs after peripheral nerve section.[96] Transcription of mRNA for peptide transmitters is also reduced in sensory neurons deprived of NGF.[97] Antibodies to NGF can in addition cause sensory nerve terminals in the skin of adult rats to retract.[98,99]

From all these studies it is clear that NGF is essential for normal sympathetic and sensory nerve cell function in adult mammals. When colchicine, a drug that disrupts microtubules, is applied locally to the axons of a variety of neurons, the same retrograde changes result, presumably because the drug interrupts the transport of retrograde trophic factors.[83] Transport can also be blocked by prolonged cooling of a length of nerve, and this causes a cell-body reaction which is as great as after axotomy.[100] It is possible to measure low levels of NGF mRNA in tissues innervated by the sympathetic nervous system, and to show that blockade of axonal transport leads to a rise in NGF in the tissue and to a fall in the nerve cells innervating it.[101] In the case of spinal motor neurons, BDNF and NT4/5 administration can reverse some of the changes brought about by axotomy,[102] although neonatal motor neurons are only temporarily rescued from death by administering of these factors.[103]

In invertebrates too, neurons can undergo changes after axotomy that suggest retrograde trophic influences exist whose withdrawal can trigger a reaction in the cell body. For example, nerve section, or interruption of axonal transport with colchicine, is followed by the development of a sodium-sensitive action potential in insect motoneuron cell bodies.[104] There is also evidence that the branches of a single neuron can be influenced independently by the type of muscle fibres they innervate, as it has been shown that branches of a single lobster motor neuron innervating different types of muscle fibre have subtle differences in the way transmitter release is affected by repetitive activation.[105]

Despite all this evidence, it is unlikely that lack of target-derived material is the sole contributor to the onset and maintenance of the cell-body reaction. In the first place, the reaction is very much less when the nerve is cut a long way from the cell body than close to it,[106,107] yet both lesions should deprive the nerve cell body of target material equally effectively. In dorsal root ganglion cells, it is interesting that only section of the peripherally projecting axons evokes a reaction in the cell body, there being no reaction to section of the axons in the dorsal roots unless the section is made extremely close to the ganglion.[108] Second, a further lesion made soon after the first not only accelerates axon regrowth, which is partly dependent on the cell-body reaction (see Chapter 17), but may also precipitate the death of some neurons. This would not happen after a single operation.[109] Third, application of NGF does not reverse all the biochemical consequences of axotomy in dorsal root ganglion cells, many of which are NGF sensitive,[110] and neonatal motor neurons are only temporarily rescued from death by the application of NT3, BDNF and NT4.[111] Finally, the cell-body reaction can subside before axons have regenerated as far as their targets,[112] and this is particularly clear in axotomized neurons within the CNS.

It is likely, therefore, that several different stimuli can trigger a cell-body response in neurons, and that once it is initiated it may be modified by a variety of factors. The above discussion has also implicitly assumed that the reaction is an all-or-none phenomenon, but it is quite possible that hitherto undetectable differences in the quality or quantity of the reaction exist under different circumstances, and there is still no clear explanation for the death of some neurons and the survival of others. A major influence may be the reaction of glial cells. Schwann cells, for example, manufacture several neurotrophic factors (Table 16.1), the levels of each depending on the state of the axon. Changes in these levels could increase or decrease the cell-body reaction of neurons. This may explain why the cell-body reaction to injury can begin to subside before regenerating axons reach their peripheral targets. The susceptibility of neonatal motor neurons to death following axotomy might be a consequence of the low levels of CNTF in neonatal Schwann cells compared with mature myelinating Schwann cells.[113] It is known that exogenous supplies of CNTF can reduce to some extent the number of neonatal motor neurons that die after axotomy,[114] and motor neurons gradually die in a mutant unable to make CNTF.[115] IGF-1, generated locally at the lesion site to the axon may also influence the magnitude of the cell-body reaction.[116]

Conclusions

The normal adult state of neurons is maintained by continuous interactions between the neurons and their target cells and glia. The innervated cells, whether other neurons or a peripheral tissue such as muscle, are maintained by being kept electrically active and also by means of trophic molecules, many of which have not yet been identified. The trophic effect of motor nerves on muscle, for example, is mediated largely by postsynaptic activity, but the endplate region is probably influenced directly by molecular factors as well. Target and glial cells in turn maintain their neurons by means of retrograde trophic factors which are usually the same molecules required for neuronal survival during development.

Interruption of trophic interactions results in changes in the properties of the cells. Some of the changes recall properties present during early development. For example, muscle fibres become supersensitive to transmitter, Schwann cells re-express various adhesion molecules and axotomized neurons lose their presynaptic contacts and dendritic complexity. A conservative hypothesis is that the interactions that occur during development to cause the maturation of neuronal properties continue to operate in the adult, and these are the trophic interactions that maintain the normal physiological state of the nervous system.

Key points

1 When synaptic contact between neurons is broken in adult animals, changes occur in the properties of both the innervated cells and the innervating neurons. Classical examples are the wasting of denervated skeletal muscles and the chromatolytic reaction of neurons which have had their axons cut.

2 The maintenance by neurons of normal properties in the cells that they innervate is known as the orthograde trophic effect, and may be mediated by synaptically-triggered electrical activity or by chemical means. The maintenance of normal properties in the innervating neurons by the cells they innervate is known as the retrograde trophic effect and, because of the one-way nature of synaptic excitation, must be mediated by chemical means.

3 Trophic effects have been most intensively studied in the peripheral nervous system. The trophic action of motor nerves on skeletal muscle is exerted largely by electrical activity. There is also good evidence that the motor nerves liberate molecules that are trophically active at the endplate region of muscle (see Chapter 11), but the evidence for chemically-mediated trophic effects outside the endplate zone is weaker.

4 Many of the retrograde changes following axotomy may be due to a lack of target-derived neurotrophins (Chapter 12), but not all the results of axotomy can be explained in this way.

5 The effect of axotomy on neurons is to activate either a phase of synthesis of proteins needed for axon regrowth or to trigger apoptosis. The latter course is more likely in neurons of young animals or if the axon is cut very close to the cell body.

6 An axon which is detached from its cell body usually degenerates very fast (Wallerian degeneration), and this is followed by the breakdown of the myelin made by associated glial cells. This is a result of proteolytic activity by Schwann cells and later by macrophages. Myelin in the CNS disintegrates much more slowly than myelin in the peripheral nervous system.

General reading

■ Lomo, T. and Westgaard, R. H. Control of acetylcholine sensitivity in rat muscle fibres. *Cold Spring Harbor Symp. Quant. Biol.* **40**, 263–74 (1976).

■ Raivich, G. *et al.* Neuroglial activation repertoire in the injured brain: graded response, molecular mechanisms and cues to physiological function. *Brain Res. Brain Res. Rev.* **30**, 77–105 (1999).

■ Svendsen, C. N. and Sofroniew, M. V. Do central nervous system neurons require target-derived neurotrophic support for survival throughout adult life and aging? *Perspect. Dev. Neurobiol.* **3**, 133–42 (1996).

References

1. Lunn, E. R., Perry, V. H., Brown, M. C., Rosen, H. and Gordon, S. (1989) Absence of Wallerian degeneration does not hinder regeneration in peripheral nerve. *Eur. J. Neurosci.* **1**, 27–33 (1989).

2. Perry, V. H., Lunn, E. R., Brown, M. C., Cahusac, S. and Gordon, S. Evidence that the rate of Wallerian degeneration is controlled by a single autosomal dominant gene. *Eur. J. Neurosci.* **2**, 408–13 (1990).

3. Perry, V. H., Brown, M. C., Lunn, E. R., Tree, P. and Gordon, S. Evidence that very slow Wallerian degeneration in C57BL/Ola mice is an intrinsic property of the peripheral nerve. *Eur. J. Neurosci.* **2**, 802–8 (1990).

4. Finn, J. T. *et al.* Evidence that Wallerian degeneration and localized axon degeneration induced by local neurotrophin deprivation do not involve caspases. *J. Neurosci.* **20**, 1333–41 (2000).

5. Yawo, H. and Kuno, M. How a nerve repairs its cut end: involvement of phospholipase A2. *Science* **222**, 1351–3 (1983).

6. Spira, M. E., Benbassat, D. and Dormann, A. Resealing of the proximal and distal cut ends of transected axons: electrophysiological and ultrastructural analysis. *J. Neurobiol.* **24**, 300–16 (1993).

7. Miledi, R. and Slater, C. R. On the degeneration of rat neuromuscular junctions after nerve section. *J. Physiol.* **207**, 507–28 (1970).

8. LoPachin, R. M., LoPachin, V. R. and Saubermann, A. J. Effects of axotomy on distribution and concentration of elements in rat sciatic nerve. *J. Neurochem.* **54**, 320–32 (1990).

9. Schlaepfer, W. W. Calcium-induced degeneration of axoplasm in isolated segments of rats peripheral nerve. *Brain Res.* **69**, 203–15 (1974).

10. George, E. B., Glass, J. D. and Griffin, J. W. Axotomy-induced axonal degeneration is mediated by calcium influx through ion-specific channels. *J. Neurosci.* **15**, 6445–52 (1995).

11. Brown, M. C., Hopkins, W. G. and Keynes, R. J. Importance of pathway formation for nodal sprout production in partly denervated muscles. *Brain Res.* **243**, 345–9 (1982).

12. Lunn, E. R., Brown, M. C. and Perry, V. H. The pattern of axonal degeneration in the peripheral nervous system varies with different types of lesion. *Neuroscience* **35**, 157–65 (1990).

13. Lemke, G. Myelin and myelination. In *An introduction to molecular neurobiology* (ed. Z. Hall) (Sinauer, 1991).

14. Carter, B. D. *et al.* Selective activation of NF-kappa B by nerve growth factor through the neurotrophin receptor p75. *Science* **272**, 542–5 (1996).

15. Williams, P. L. and Hall, S. M. Prolonged *in vivo* observations of normal peripheral nerve fibres and their acute reactions to crush and deliberate trauma. *J. Anat.* **108**, 397–408 (1971).

16. Stoll, G., Griffin, J. W., Li, C. Y. and Trapp, B. D. Wallerian degeneration in the peripheral nervous system: participation of both Schwann cells and macrophages in myelin degradation. *J. Neurocytol.* **18**, 671–83 (1989).

17. Hallpike, J. F. and Adams, C. W. M. Proteolysis and myelin breakdown: a review of recent histochemical and biochemical studies. *Histochem. J.* **1**, 559–78 (1969).

18. Perry, V. H., Tsao, J. W., Fearn, S. and Brown, M. C. Radiation-induced reductions in macrophage recruitment have only slight effects on myelin degeneration in sectioned peripheral nerves of mice. *Eur. J. Neurosci.* **7**, 271–80 (1995).

19. Tetzlaff, W. Tight junction contact events and temporary gap junctions in the sciatic nerve fibres of the chicken during Wallerian degeneration and subsequent regeneration. *J. Neurocytol.* **11**, 839–58 (1982).

20. Ridley, A. J., Davis, J. B., Stroobant, P. and Land, H. Transforming growth factors b1 and b2

are mitogens for rat Schwann cells. *J. Cell Biol.* **109**, 3419–24 (1989).

21. Davis, J. B. and Stroobant, P. Platelet-derived growth factors and fibroblast growth factors are mitogens for rat Schwann cells. *J. Cell Biol.* **110**, 1353–60 (1990).

22. Fernandez-Valle, C., Bunge, R. P. and Bunge, M. B. Schwann cells degrade myelin and proliferate in the absence of macrophages: evidence from *in vitro* studies of Wallerian degeneration. *J. Neurocytol.* **24**, 667–79 (1995).

23. Livesey, F. J. *et al.* A Schwann cell mitogen accompanying regeneration of motor neurons. *Nature* **390**, 614–18 (1997).

24. Bignami, A. and Ralston, H. J. The cellular reaction to Wallerian degeneration in the central nervous system of the cat. *Brain Res.* **13**, 444–61 (1969).

25. Cook, R. D. and Wisniewski, H. M. The role of oligodendroglia and astroglia in Wallerian degeneration of the optic nerve. *Brain Res.* **61**, 191–206 (1973).

26. Lemke, G. Unwrapping the genes of myelin. *Neuron* **1**, 535–43 (1988).

27. Adams, L., Carlson, B. M., Henderson, L. and Goldman, D. Adaptation of nicotinic acetylcholine receptor, myogenin, and MRF4 gene expression to long-term muscle denervation. *J. Cell Biol.* **131**, 1341–9 (1995).

28. Valenzuela, D. M. *et al.* Receptor tyrosine kinase specific for the skeletal muscle lineage: expression in embryonic muscle, at the neuromuscular junction, and after injury. *Neuron* **15**, 573–84 (1995).

29. Axelsson, J. and Thesleff, S. (1959) A study of supersensitivity in denervated mammalian skeletal muscle. *J. Physiol.* **147**, 178–93 (1959).

30. Lomo, T. and Rosenthal, J. Control of acetylcholine sensitivity by muscle activity in the rat. *J. Physiol.* **221**, 493–513 (1972).

31. Westgaard, R. H. Influence of activity on the passive electrical properties of denervated soleus muscle fibres in the rat. *J. Physiol. (London)* **251**, 683–97 (1975).

32. Weinberg, C. B. and Hall, Z. W. Junctional form of acetylcholinesterase restored at nerve free endplates. *Dev. Biol.* **68**, 631–5 (1979).

33. Buller, A. J., Eccles, J. C. and Eccles, R. M. Interaction between motoneurones and muscles in respect of the characteristic speeds of their responses. *J. Physiol.* **150**, 417–39 (1960).

34. Lomo, T. and Westgaard, R. H. Control of acetylcholine sensitivity in rat muscle fibres. *Cold Spring Harbor Symp. Quant. Biol.* **40**, 263–74 (1976).

35. Salmons, S. and Sreter, F. A. Significance of impulse activity in the transformation of skeletal muscle types. *Nature* **263**, 30–4 (1976).

36. Pette, D. and Staron, R. S. Molecular basis of the phenotypic characteristics of mammalian muscle fibres. *Ciba Symp.* **138**, 22–34 (1988).

37. Gorza, L., Gundersen, K., Lomo, T., Schiaffino, S. and Westgaard, R. H. Slow-to-fast transformation of denervated soleus muscles by chronic high-frequency stimulation in the rat. *J. Physiol.* **402**, 627–49 (1988).

38. Miller, J. B. and Stockdale, F. E. Developmental regulation of the multiple myogenic cell lineages of the avian embryo. *J. Cell Biol.* **103**, 2197–208 (1986).

39. Westgaard, R. H. and Lomo, T. Control of contractile properties within adaptive ranges by patterns of impulse activity in the rat. *J. Neurosci.* **8**, 4415–26 (1988).

40. Lomo, T. Neurotrophic control of colchicine effects on muscle? *Nature* **249**, 473–4 (1974).

41. Jones, R. and Vrbova, G. Two factors responsible for the development of denervation hypersensitivity. *J. Physiol.* **236**, 517P (1974).

42. Cangiano, A. and Lutzemberger, L. Partial denervation in inactive muscle affects innervated and denervated fibres equally. *Nature* **285**, 233–5 (1980).

43. Cangiano, A. Denervation supersensitivity as a model for the neural control of muscle. *Neuroscience* **14**, 963–71 (1985).

44. Murray, M. A. and Robbins, N. Cell proliferation in denervated muscle: identity and origin of dividing cells. *Neuroscience* **7**, 1823–33 (1982).

45. Murray, M. A. and Robbins, N. Cell proliferation in denervated muscle: time course, distribution and relation to disease. *Neuroscience* **7**, 1817–22 (1982).

46. Tracey, K. J. *et al.* Cachectin/tumor necrosis factor mediates changes of skeletal muscle membrane potential. *J. Exp. Med.* **164**, 1368–73 (1986).

47. Markelonis, G. J. and Oh, T. H. A sciatic nerve protein has a trophic effect on development and maintenance of skeletal muscle cells in culture. *Proc. Natl. Acad. Sci. USA* **76**, 2470–4 (1979).

48. Davey, B., Younkin, L. H. and Younkin, S. G. Neural control of skeletal muscle cholinesterase: a study using organ cultured rat muscle. *J. Physiol.* **289**, 501–15 (1979).

49. Kuromi, H., Gonoi, T. and Hosegawa, S. Partial purification and characterisation of neurotrophic substance affecting tetrodotoxin sensitivity of organ cultured mouse muscle. *Brain Res.* **175**, 109–18 (1979).

50. Davis, H. L. and Heinicke, E. A. Prevention of denervation atrophy in muscle : mammalian neurotrophic factor is not transferrin. *Brain Res.* **309**, 293–8 (1984).

51. Helgren, M. E. *et al.* Trophic effect of ciliary neurotrophic factor on denervated skeletal muscle. *Cell* **76**, 493–504 (1994).

52. Schmidt, H. and Stefani, E. Action potentials in slow muscle fibres of the frog during regeneration of motor nerves. *J. Physiol.* **270**, 507–17 (1977).

53. Miledi, R. and Uchitel, O. D. Induction of action potentials in frog slow muscle fibres paralysed by alpha bungarotoxin. *Proc. R. Soc. London Ser. B* **213**, 243–8 (1981).

54. Dunn, P. M. and Marshall, L. M. Lack of nicotine supersensitivity in frog sympathetic neurones following denervation. *J. Physiol.* **363**, 211–25 (1985).

55. Kuffler, S. W., Dennis, M. J. and Harris, A. J. The development of chemosensitivity in extra synaptic areas of the neuronal surface after denervation of parasympathetic ganglion cells in the heart of the frog. *Proc. R. Soc. London Ser. B* **177**, 555–63 (1971).

56. Streichert, L. C. and Sargent, P. B. The role of acetylcholinesterase in denervation supersensitivity in the frog cardiac ganglion. *J. Physiol. (London)* **445**, 249–60 (1992).

57. Dennis, M. J. and Sargent, P. B. Loss of extrasynaptic acetylcholine sensitivity upon reinnervation of parasympathetic ganglion cells. *J. Physiol. (London)* **289**, 263–75 (1979).

58. Hendry, I. H., Iversen, L. L. and Black, I. B. A comparison of the neural regulation of tyrosine hydroxylase activity in sympathetic ganglia of adult mice and rats. *J. Neurochem.* **20**, 1683–9 (1973).

59. Chalazonitis, A. and Zigmond, R. E. Effects of synaptic and antidromic stimulation on tyrosine hydroxylase activity in the rat superior cervical ganglion. *J. Physiol.* **300**, 525–38 (1980).

60. Zigmond, R. E., Schwarzschild, A. and Rittenhouse, A. R. Acute regulation of tyrosine hydroxylase by nerve activity and by neurotransmitters via phosphorylation. *Annu. Rev. Neurosci.* **12**, 415–61 (1989).

61. Black, I. B., Chikaraishi, D. M. and Lewis, E. J. Trans-synaptic increase in RNA coding for tyrosine hydroxylase in a rat sympathetic ganglion. *Brain Res.* **339**, 151–3 (1985).

62. Zigmond, R. E. and Bowers, C. W. Influence of nerve activity on the macromolecular content of neurons and their effector organs. *Annu. Rev. Physiol.* **43**, 673–87 (1981).

63. Matthews, M. R., Cowan, W. M. and Powell, T. P. S. Transneuronal cell degeneration in the lateral geniculate nucleus of the macaque monkey. *J. Physiol.* **94**, 145–69 (1960).

64. Svendsen, C. N. and Sofroniew, M. V. Do central nervous system neurons require target-derived neurotrophic support for survival throughout adult life and aging? *Perspect. Dev. Neurobiol.* **3**, 133–42 (1996).

65. Zalewski, A. A. Combined effects of testosterone and motor, sensory or gustatory nerve reinnervation on the regeneration of taste buds. *Exp. Neurol.* **24**, 285–97 (1969).

66. Denis Donini, S. Expression of dopaminergic phenotypes in the mouse olfactory bulb induced by the calcitonin gene-related peptide. *Nature* **339**, 701–3 (1989).

67. Singer, M. Neurotrophic control of limb regeneration in the newt. *Ann. New York Acad. Sci.* **228**, 308–22 (1974).

68. Brockes, J. P. and Kintner, C. R. Glial growth factor and nerve-dependant proliferation in the regeneration blastema of urodele amphibious. *Cell* **45**, 301–6 (1986).

69. Taylor, G. P., Anderson, R., Reginelli, A. D. and Muneoka, K. FGF-2 induces regeneration of the chick limb bud. *Dev. Biol.* **163**, 282–4 (1994).

70. Hoy, R. R., Bittner, G. D. and Kennedy, D. Regeneration in crustacean motoneurons: evidence for axonal fusion. *Science* **156**, 251–3 (1967).

71. Frank, E. The sensitivity to glutamate of denervated muscles of the crayfish. *J. Physiol.* **242**, 371–82 (1974).

72. Usherwood, P. N. R. Glutamate sensitivity of denervated insect muscle fibres. *Nature* **223**, 411–13 (1969).

73. Govind, C. K. and Kent, K. S. Transformation of fast fibres to slow prevented by lack of activity in developing lobster muscle. *Nature* **298**, 755–7 (1982).

74. Luenicka, G. A., Blundon, J. A. and Govind, C. K. Early experience influences the development of bilateral asymmetry in a lobster motoneuron. *Dev. Biol.* **129**, 84–90 (1988).

75. Lieberman, A. R. Some factors affecting retrograde neuronal responses to axonal lesions. In *Essays on the nervous system* (ed. R. Bellairs and E. R. Gray), pp. 71–105 (Clarendon Press, Oxford, 1974).

76. Watson, W. E. Cellular responses to axotomy and to related procedures. *Br. Med. Bull.* **30**, 112–15 (1974).

77. Singer, P. A. and Mehler, S. 2-Deoxy ^{14}C glucose uptake in rat hypoglossal nucleus after nerve transection. *Exp. Neurol.* **69**, 617–26 (1980).

78. Tetzlaff, W., Bisby, M. A. and Kreutzberg, G. W. Changes in cytoskeletal proteins in the rat facial nucleus following axotomy. *J. Neurosci.* **8**, 3181–9 (1988).

79. Skene, J. H. P. Axonal growth-associated proteins. *Annu. Rev. Neurosci.* **12**, 127–56 (1989).

80. Jenkins, R. and Hunt, S. P. Long-term increase in the levels of c-jun mRNA and Jun protein-like immunoreactivity in motor and sensory neurons following axon damage. *Neurosci. Lett.* **129**, 107–10 (1991).

81. Miller, F. D., Tetzlaff, W., Bisby, M. A., Fawcett, J. W. and Milner, R. J. Rapid induction of the major embryonic Alpha-tubulin mRNA, TAlpha1, during nerve regeneration in adult rats. *J. Neurosci.* **9**, 1452–63 (1989).

82. Piehl, F., Tabar, G. and Cullheim, S. Expression of NMDA receptor mRNAs in rat motoneurons is down-regulated after axotomy. *Eur. J. Neurosci.* **7**, 2101–10 (1995).

83. Purves, D. Functional and structural changes in mammalian sympathetic neurons following colchicine application to postganglionic nerves. *J. Physiol.* **259**, 159–75 (1975).

84. Pollin, M. M., McHanwell, S. and Slater, C. R. The effect of age on motor neurone death following axotomy in the mouse. *Development* **112**, 83–9 (1991).

85. Chen, S. and Bisby, M. A. Long-term consequences of impaired regeneration on facial motoneurons in the C57BL/Ola mouse. *J. Comp. Neurol.* **335**, 576–85 (1993).

86. Clowry, G. J. Axotomy induces NADPH diaphorase activity in neonatal but not in adult motoneurons. *NeuroReport* **5**, 361–3 (1993).

87. Kristensson, K. *et al.* Co-induction of neuronal interferon-gamma and nitric oxide synthase in rat motor neurons after axotomy: a role in nerve repair or death? *J. Neurocytol.* **23**, 453–9 (1994).

88. Zhang, J., Dawson, V. L., Dawson, T. M. and Snyder, S. H. Nitric oxide activation of poly(ADP-ribose) synthetase in neurotoxicity. *Science* **263**, 687–9 (1994).

89. Choi, D. W. Glutamate neurotoxicity and diseases of the nervous system. *Neuron* **1**, 623–34 (1988).

90. Mentis, G. Z., Greensmith, L. and Vrbova, G. Motoneurons destined to die are rescued by blocking N-methyl-d-aspartate receptors by MK-801. *Neuroscience* **54**, 283–5 (1993).

91. Ambron, R. T. and Walters, E. T. Priming events and retrograde injury signals. A new perspective on the cellular and molecular biology of nerve regeneration. *Mol. Neurobiol.* **13**, 61–79 (1996).

92. Stockel, K., Paravicini, U. and Thoenen, H. Specificity of the retrograde axonal transport of nerve growth factor. *Brain Res.* **76**, 413–21 (1974).

93. Nja, A. and Purves, D. The effects of nerve growth factor and its antiserum on synapses in the superior cervical ganglion of the guinea pig. *J. Physiol.* **277**, 53–75 (1978).

94. Gorin, P. D. and Johnson, E. M. Effects of long term NGF deprivation on the nervous system of the adult rat: an experimental autoimmune approach. *Brain Res.* **198**, 27–42 (1980).

95. Schwarz, J. P., Pearson, J. and Johnson, E. M. Effects of exposure to anti NGF on sensory neurons of adult rats and guinea pigs. *Brain Res.* **244**, 378–81 (1982).

96. Barbut, D., Polak, J. and Wall, P. D. Substance P in spinal cord dorsal horn decreases following peripheral nerve injury. *Brain Res.* **205**, 289–98 (1981).

97. Lindsay, R. M. and Harman, A. J. Nerve growth factor regulates expression of neuropeptide genes in adult sensory neurons. *Nature* **337**, 362–4 (1989).

98. Diamond, J., Holmes, M. and Coughlin, M. Endogenous NGF and nerve impulses regulate the collateral sprouting of sensory axons in the skin of the adult rat. *J. Neurosci.* **12**, 1454–66 (1992).

99. Diamond, J., Foerster, A., Holmes, M. and Coughlin, M. Sensory nerves in adult rats regenerate and restore sensory function to the skin independently of endogenous NGF. *J. Neurosci.* **12**, 1467–76 (1992).

100. Wu, W., Mathew, T. C. and Miller, F. D. Evidence that the loss of homeostatic signals induces regeneration-associated alterations in neuronal gene expression. *Dev. Biol.* **158**, 456–66 (1993).

101. Heumann, R. Regulation of the synthesis of nerve growth factor. *J. Exp. Biol.* **132**, 133–50 (1987).

102. Friedman, B. *et al.* BDNF and NT-4/5 exert neurotrophic influences on injured adult spinal motor neurons. *J. Neurosci.* **15**, 1044–56 (1995).

103. Vejsada, R., Sagot, Y. and Kato, A. C. Quantitative comparison of the transient rescue effects of neurotrophic factors on axotomised motoneurons *in vivo. Eur. J. Neurosci.* **7**, 108–15 (1995).

104. Pitman, R. M. The ionic dependence of action potentials induced by colchicine in an insect motoneuron cell body. *J. Physiol.* **247**, 511–20 (1975).

105. Frank, E. Matching of facilitation at the neuromuscular junction of the lobsters: a possible case for influence of muscle on nerve. *J. Physiol.* **223**, 635–58 (1973).

106. Jenkins, R., McMahon, S. B., Bond, A. B. and Hunt, S. P. Expression of c-Jun as a response to dorsal root and peripheral nerve section in damaged and adjacent intact primary sensory neurons in the rat. *Eur. J. Neurosci.* **5**, 751–9 (1993).

107. Mathew, T. C. and Miller, F. D. Induction of TAlpha1 Alpha-tubulin mRNA during neuronal regeneration is a function of the amount of axon lost. *Dev. Biol.* **158**, 467–74 (1993).

108. Chong, M. S. *et al.* GAP-43 expression in primary sensory neurons following central axotomy. *J. Neurosci.* **14**, 4375–84 (1994).

109. Arvidsson, J. and Aldskogius, H. Effect of repeated hypoglossal nerve lesions on the number of neurons in the hypoglossal nucleus of adult rats. *Exp. Neurol.* **75**, 520–4 (1982).

110. Verge, V. M. K. *et al.* Colocalization of NGF binding sites, trk mRNA, and low-affinity NGF receptor mRNA in primary sensory neurons: responses to injury and infusion of NGF. *J. Neurosci.* **12**, 4011–22 (1992).

111. Vejsada, R., Sagot, Y. and Kato, A. C. Quantitative comparison of the transient rescue effects of neurotrophic factors on axotomized motoneurons *in vivo*. *Eur. J. Neurosci.* **7**, 108–15 (1995).

112. Tetzlaff, W., Alexander, S. W., Miller, F. D. and Bisby, M. A. Response of facial and rubrospinal neurons to axotomy: changes in mRNA expression for cytoskeletal proteins and GAP-43. *J. Neurosci.* **11**, 2528–44 (1991).

113. Stockli, K. A. *et al.* Molecular cloning, expression and regional distribution of rat ciliary neurotrophic factor. *Nature* **342**, 920–3 (1989).

114. Sendtner, M., Kreutzberg, G. W. and Thoenen, H. Ciliary neurotrophic factor prevents the degeneration of motor neurons after axotomy. *Nature* **345**, 440–1 (1990).

115. Masu, Y. *et al.* Disruption of the CNTF gene results in motor neuron degeneration. *Nature* **365**, 27–32 (1993).

116. Kanje, M., Skottner, A., Lundborg, G. and Sjoeberg, J. Does insulin-like growth factor I (IGF-1) trigger the cell body reaction in the rat sciatic nerve? *Brain Res.* **563**, 285–7 (1991).

17

Repair and Plasticity in the Adult Vertebrate Nervous System

It has been emphasized in earlier chapters that the nervous system is constructed of very long-lived cells, most of which are born during early development. With some notable exceptions (see below), no new neurons are generated in the adult nervous systems of amphibians, reptiles, birds or mammals, nor can new neurons be generated if any are killed by injury, ischaemia, toxicity or degeneration. When axons degenerate, however, attempts at repair occur naturally, and these take two forms (see Fig. 17.1). First, in the peripheral nervous system (PNS) of nearly all species, and in the central nervous system (CNS) of many lower vertebrates,[1] regeneration of axons from the proximal stumps usually occurs. The new outgrowths can sometimes grow back to their original target cells if guided by the structures in the degenerating distal nerve segment. Such regeneration does not occur naturally in the CNS of mammals. Second, both in the PNS and in the CNS, new growths can develop from any intact axons left within a partly denervated target. These are called *collateral sprouts*. They originate at or close to the nerve terminals and can reinnervate nearby vacant post-synaptic sites.

The axotomy-induced changes described in Chapter 16 in the cell body, distal degenerated nerve stump and denervated tissue are each important for nerve regeneration and collateral sprouting. The local changes provide factors that stimulate axonal growth and an environment to guide the new growth cones. The nerve cell body plays its part in regrowth by switching its synthetic capacity to provide materials needed for axonal elongation and growth cone function. Both local changes *and* central metabolic changes are needed for regeneration to be successful. In the case of the adult mammalian CNS it turns out that the local environment is positively hostile to growth cones, and the cell body reaction can be weak, transient or non-existent so that no successful regeneration occurs.

Nerve injury has also been found to lead to almost immediate or very rapid (within hours) changes in central connectivity of uninjured pathways. This time scale is too

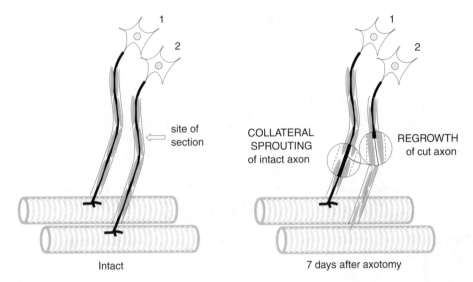

Figure 17.1 Two forms of reinnervation triggered by axotomy, *regrowth* of the cut axon and *collateral sprouting* of intact axons with terminals in the vicinity of those of the cut axon. In the diagram, only two motor neurons are drawn for simplicity. Motor neuron 1 remains intact and grows collateral sprouts after the axon of motor neuron 2 has been cut. Motor neuron 2 regenerates its cut axon.

short to be explained by collateral sprouting, and it is believed that synapses that are functionally ineffective in the normal animal become 'unmasked' by disinhibition as tonic activity in the damaged pathway is withdrawn. These findings have been followed by others showing that changes in receptive fields can be readily induced simply by altering the balance of activity in pathways converging on neighbouring nuclear or cortical areas.

Axon regeneration

Outgrowths from the proximal stump of a severed mammalian peripheral axon can be seen within a few hours of injury.[2] In myelinated fibres they usually emerge from nodes of Ranvier in parts of the axon just proximal to the lesion. They grow between the Schwann cell basal lamina and the myelin until they reach the lesion site, at which point they may branch profusely.[3] The rate of regrowth in a peripheral nerve is at first slow, but after a few days rates of up to 8 mm/day are possible, although rates of 3 or 4 mm/day are more usual.[4] The increase in the rate of regrowth is probably determined by the development in the degenerating nerve of an environment more suitable for growth, and by changes in the synthetic programme in the cell body (see below).

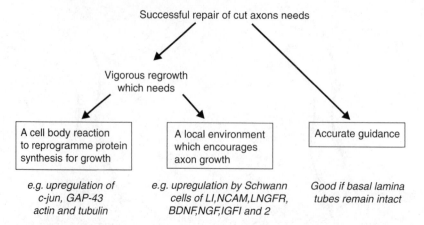

Figure 17.2 The three factors needed to bring about successful functional recovery by axon regeneration.

If recovery of function is to be optimal after axotomy, axon regeneration must be vigorous and it must be directed to the denervated target (Fig. 17.2). It has become clear that if growth is to be vigorous, (i) the cell body of the axotomized neuron must reprogramme for growth; (ii) the tissues through which the regenerating sprouts have to grow must be at least permissive; and (iii) if long distances have to be covered by the regrowing axons, the local tissue must be more than simply permissive; it must be actively supportive, and growth factors (as yet unidentified) must be available in the vicinity of the regrowing axons. Dedifferentiated Schwann cells seem to be critical for regeneration because they are a good source of these factors. There is considerable evidence for all of these statements, and just a few examples of typical experiments upon which they are based are given below.

The importance of the local environment can be illustrated by the behaviour of motor axons. After axotomy these usually regrow robustly into the degenerated distal nerve stump, but if they are confronted with a piece of nerve which has not degenerated they fail to advance.[5,6] When, however, the distal stump starts to degenerate, regeneration proceeds.[7] Again, dorsal root ganglion cell axons from adult mice will not grow *in vitro* on thin sections of normal peripheral nerve but they will on sections of degenerated nerve.[8] Similarly, retinal ganglion cell axons, which regrow very poorly into their own (optic) nerve, will grow into a segment of implanted degenerating peripheral sciatic nerve.[9] Further study of this optic nerve–sciatic nerve system has provided an example of the importance of the cell body reaction (see Chapter 16). It is found that the percentage of retinal ganglion cells that succeed in sending axons into the transplanted sciatic nerve depends critically on where the optic nerve has been cut. When it is cut close to the eye, near to the cell bodies of the ganglion cells, success is much greater and it is only such close axotomies that evoke a large cell body response in the retinal ganglion cells (it is interesting that nerve section close to the cell body is also more likely to trigger cell death).[9-12] The need for something more than a passive permissive growth surface for regeneration distances of more than 5 to 10 mm is shown by comparing regeneration along a long length of transplanted sciatic nerve, in which Schwann cells remain alive, with regeneration along a similar length of sciatic nerve, in which all living cells have been killed by repeated freezing and thawing. Only in the nerve with living cells do axons grow regularly right to the end of the transplant.[13] The failure to grow to the end of the frozen graft is not due to downregulation of GAP-43 protein production in the cell bodies of the motor neurons.[14] Hence high levels of growth-associated proteins cannot alone guarantee sustained growth.

Changes in the distal nerve stump of possible importance for regeneration

The ability of a degenerated peripheral nerve stump to attract regenerating axons towards it has been documented many times since Cajal first observed the phenomenon over 70 years ago (for one example see reference 15), and it is generally agreed that Schwann cells are the most important source of these and other factors that stimulate regrowth. It has already been noted that regeneration is limited to short distances if cells in the distal nerve stump are killed, and it has been shown that regeneration is abnormal in the *Eur* mutation, which gives rise to Schwann cell defects.[16] It is also well known that the basal lamina components provide a permissive surface for regenerating axon growth cones.[17-19] The identities of the relevant cell surface and extracellular matrix molecules, and secreted trophic and tropic factors, are still being actively investigated.

Both collagen and laminin in the Schwann cell basal lamina are known from *in vitro* studies to be good substrates for growth cones. NCAM, L1 (Ng-CAM) and N-cadherin (see Chapter 9), which are present on Schwann cells that are not making myelin,[20,21] are also all known from *in vitro* blocking experiments to play a role in axon growth on Schwann cell surfaces.[22] There seems to be considerable redundancy, as only when all these factors are inhibited does all growth cease *in vitro*. Levels of the neurotrophic factors NGF, IGF and BDNF also rise in degenerated nerve stumps (see Chapter 16). NGF may play a role in the regeneration of peripheral adrenergic axons, and regeneration of newt retinal ganglion cell axons is enhanced by injections of NGF and inhibited by injections of neutralizing antibodies to NGF.[23-25] One suggestion is that NGF is maintained at high concentrations within the distal nerve stump by binding to low affinity receptors on the Schwann cell surface, from where it could transfer to high-affinity (Trk) receptors on the growth cone surface.[26] The role of NGF in regeneration of other axon types is, however, less clear. Sensory axons regenerate normally in rats treated with NGF antibodies given at a concentration that completely inhibits collateral sprouting of the same axons.[27] Injections of IGF-1, however, stimulate axon regrowth in the rat sciatic nerve.[28] The same is true for IGF-2 and antibodies to it impair regrowth.[29] BDNF levels rise in the distal nerve stump, and could theoretically be available to motor axons via the low-affinity neurotrophin receptors,[30] but the time course of its appearance is very slow compared with the normal rate of motor nerve regeneration. Other evidence for a role for the low-affinity neurotrophin receptor in regeneration has come from experiments showing that inhibition of a metalloprotease in the distal nerve improves nerve regeneration, probably by preventing the metalloprotease from degrading these receptors.[31]

Further support for regrowth, and eventually remyelination, might come from other cells in the distal stump. Macrophage-derived apolipoprotein E, scavenged from degenerating axons, may serve as a source of lipid for regenerating axons.[32] Regeneration is, however, normal in a mutant mouse which completely lacks apolipoprotein E,[33] and there is no clear evidence that the presence of macrophages is important in other ways for axonal regeneration.

The cell body reaction and 'conditioning' of axon regeneration

The rate of axon advance can be increased by a 'conditioning' lesion, namely a nerve crush applied some days before the eventual test crush. There is indirect evidence that the increased rate of regrowth is partly a result of an enhanced activation of the cell body reaction to injury; as explained in Chapter 16, this alters the balance of protein synthesis from material needed for 'housekeeping' functions and synaptic transmission to material needed for growth. Of particular importance may be upregulated expression of GAP-43. Mice constitutively overexpressing chicken GAP-43 have spontaneous sprouts at motor nerve endings, and axon regrowth is considerably enhanced after axotomy.[34]

A conditioning lesion in peripheral nerves produces a significant enhancement of growth of sensory and motor axons after the test lesion.[35] The growth rate after a single lesion never matches the rates achieved when a conditioning lesion has also been given,[36] so it appears that something extra has been triggered in the axotomized neurons by the conditioning lesion. Enhancement is slightly greater when the conditioning and test lesions are made at the same site, but is also apparent when the test lesion is made proximal to the conditioning lesion so that the regrowing axons are initially confronted with a pathway in the same state of degeneration as following a single lesion.[37] These results indicate that the conditioning lesion enhances changes which are conducive for regrowth in both the cell body and the distal nerve stump. The conditioning effect is prevented if the nerve is treated at the site of the conditioning lesion with agents that inhibit protein synthesis. This inhibition is overcome if the treated nerve is perfused with IGF-1.[38] A possibility, then, is that locally synthesized IGF-1 is able to enhance the cell body reaction in some way.

Regeneration of the optic nerve in amphibia is also enhanced by a conditioning injury. This may be because retinal ganglion cells become more responsive to NGF; if the retina is cultured in the presence of NGF, axon outgrowth is enhanced if the optic nerve is lesioned before isolation.[39] However, not all axon regeneration is improved by a conditioning lesion; regeneration of adrenergic axons, for example, is inhibited.[35]

Accuracy of peripheral nerve regeneration

If the lesion to a nerve does not disrupt the continuity of the basal lamina and collagenous sheath (together comprising the endoneurial sheath) that encloses the intact axon and its Schwann cells, regenerating axons are often guided back to their original target cells, for most of them seem to remain within their own sheath. When a nerve is cut, however, and even if the cut ends are sutured together, many axons may grow down inappropriate sheaths and restoration of function is poor. Less disability is therefore likely after crush lesions. In very young mammals, however, regrowth following motor nerve section must be guided to some extent, as reinnervation, although not perfect, is not random.[40,41] There is also evidence that motor axons in young adult rats can discriminate between motor and sensory pathways. They do this by extending branches indiscriminately down both types of pathway and then withdrawing branches from the sensory pathway.[42] Proprioceptive sensory axons also preferentially reinnervate muscle rather than skin.[43] The molecular basis for these example of guided regeneration is unknown.

If the cut proximal and distal nerve stumps are not sutured together, glial cells usually migrate from both nerve ends and can create a bridge between the two stumps along which axons may grow into the distal stump. A wide range of materials has been used clinically to help bridge gaps between those proximal and distal nerve stumps which are too large to allow direct surgical union. These include silicon tubes, grafts of muscle-derived basal lamina,[44] and pieces of peripheral nerve taken either from the patient (typically from the sural nerve in the calf) or from cadavers. There seem to be no important functional differences between them,[45] although the individual graft types may offer distinct practical advantages to the surgeon.

A particular difficulty for nerve repair in humans is the very long distances that axons may have to grow. When lesions are made close to the target so that regeneration distances are short, regeneration may also be poor because the cell body reaction may not be adequate (see above).

Unwanted side-effects of peripheral nerve lesions

In mammals, axons that fail to find the distal stump grow for a time among each other in a random way until eventually growth stops. This creates a swelling known as a neuroma. Sensory neurons whose axons fail to find a target have a high chance of dying.[46] In lower vertebrates, however, axons are capable of continued growth through adjacent tissues and may often eventually reach and reinnervate their targets.[47]

Sensory loss and motor paralysis are the obvious consequences of peripheral nerve lesions, but they are also often accompanied by pain which can arise spontaneously or be triggered by stimuli that would normally be innocuous. Spontaneous discharges arise from nerve endings in neuromas and probably contribute to this.[48] A second factor is the sprouting of branches from non-nociceptive, large-diameter afferent terminals into the superficial layers of the spinal cord that are usually innervated by terminals of unmyelinated nociceptive afferents.[49] This sprouting is probably set in motion by the upregulation of growth-associated proteins in the cell bodies of the dorsal root ganglion (DRG) cells and also by withdrawal of nociceptive terminals from the dorsal horn which follows the death of small DRG cells. Both of these reactions are initiated by the original lesion to the peripheral nerve. Inflammatory lesions also give rise to pain, some of which is due to the release of peptides that excite nociceptive C fibres. In addition, levels of NGF are raised in inflamed tissue; as NGF antibodies reduce the hyperalgesia arising in inflamed tissue, this neurotrophin may contribute to the mechanisms generating pain.[50,51]

Regeneration in the mammalian CNS

Most axons in the adult mammalian CNS regenerate very poorly if they are sectioned. Central neurons, however, are not all intrinsically unable to regrow their axons; if a segment of peripheral nerve is inserted into the brain, axons of some central neurons will invade and grow along it.[52] Moreover, following section of primary sensory axons outside the spinal cord, but proximal to their cell bodies in the dorsal root ganglion (rhizotomy), axons are able to regenerate towards the spinal cord within their Schwann cell-lined endoneurial sheaths, but growth stops when they encounter the CNS glia at the dorsal root entry zone of the cord.[53]

The cell body reaction of some axotomized neurons in the CNS can be quite vigorous, and not dissimilar to that of neurons whose axons project into the periphery, but it is usually not sustained.[54] On the other hand, cells which grow well in culture find it difficult to extend long axonal processes in the adult brain. For example, embryonic monoaminergic and cholinergic neurons transplanted to the adult brain cannot reinnervate and restore function to denervated target neurons unless they are transplanted into or very near to the target area.[55] It seems probable, therefore, that the environment of the adult mammalian CNS does not support axon growth for one or more of the following reasons.

Absence of growth stimuli for sustained regeneration

Endoneurial sheaths exist only in the periphery, where they guide regenerating axons and localize dividing Schwann cells. CNS glia (astrocytes and oligodendroglia) are not equivalent to Schwann cells, and may not provide sufficient levels of neurotrophic factors that maintain the cell body during regeneration and stimulate growth cone motility. Unlike Schwann cells, they do not appear to reprogramme their synthetic repertoire when their associated axons degenerate.

It is also clear that the survival response of many types of cultured CNS neuron to neurotrophic factors is critically dependent on the intraneuronal levels of cAMP, while adult PNS neurons have less stringent requirements and can survive even in the absence of neurotrophic support. Elevation of cAMP levels significantly enhances the trophic responsiveness of cultured CNS neurons, and this can also be achieved by depolarization (via activation of calcium-dependent adenyl cyclase). If this is similarly true for adult CNS neurons *in vivo*, a further reason for the differing responses of CNS and PNS neurons to injury could be that injured CNS neurons become less sensitive to the limited neurotrophic support available, perhaps as a result of diminished electrical activity.[56]

Presence of axon growth inhibitors

Factors that are directly inhibitory to growth are produced by astrocytes, oligodendrocytes and CNS myelin,[57,58] and molecules that induce growth cone collapse are also present in normal grey matter.[59] These could act by suppressing the cell body reaction or inhibiting growth cone movement. Liposomes incorporating the inhibitory material from rat oligodendroglia induce growth cone collapse *in vitro* by raising levels of calcium ions which are released from internal stores (see also Chapter 9).[60] On the other hand, the myelin present in fish, in whose brains axons can grow at all ages, does not contain factors that inhibit growth cone motility.[61] Myelin-derived factors therefore appear to be responsible for at least some of the poor regeneration in the mammalian CNS, especially since a monoclonal antibody (IN-1) against a myelin-associated inhibitory protein (Nogo-A)[58] allows long axon regrowth in the rat CNS when delivered into the cerebrospinal fluid.[62,63] This is accompanied by a degree of functional recovery, as measured by restoration of several limb reflexes and locomotor function in the rat following spinal injury.[64] Further evidence that CNS myelin components inhibit regeneration comes from the finding that immunization of adult mice with myelin extracts (under conditions that prevent the induction of allergic encephalomyelitis) also allows regeneration in injured white matter tracts.[65] The transition from the permissiveness of the foetal brain for axon growth to the inhibitory nature of the mature brain is probably partly a result of maturational changes in astrocytes[66] and the onset of myelination by oligodendroglia.

The formation of scar tissue, largely due to 'reactive' changes in astrocytes at the site of injury, may also impede central regeneration.[67] When the rat pyramidal tract is cut, leaving blocks of grey matter linking the rostral and caudal ends of the spinal cord, and IN-1 antibody and NT-3 are administered to promote the distalwards regeneration of pyramidal tract axons, the few axons which do grow long distances into the caudal cord avoid the site of section and scar formation, taking instead an indirect route through the grey matter bridges.[68,69] It has also been shown that when small volumes of dissociated adult primary sensory neurons are microinjected into the rat brain, axons extend freely for long distances within white matter tracts, provided the local reaction at the site of injection is minimal. Failure of regeneration is associated with the upregulation of chondroitin sulphate immunoreactivity at the injection site, suggesting that molecules associated with scar formation, such as chondroitin sulphate proteoglycans,[70,71] might be directly inhibitory to axon regeneration at lesion sites. This observation further implies that CNS myelin does not create an absolute barrier for regenerating axons,[72] as shown previously for human forebrain neuroblasts grafted into the adult rat CNS.[73] Neither do reactive astrocytes necessarily create an absolute barrier for axon regeneration, at least in the case of primary sensory axons. These can penetrate the dorsal root entry zone and enter the grey matter of the dorsal horn following rhizotomy, provided they are given added neurotrophic support;[74] they can also regenerate centrally following a dorsal column lesion if the peripheral axon is given a prior conditioning lesion distal to the cell body.[75]

Grafts of fetal spinal cord can be used to bridge gaps in CNS tissue and allow CNS regeneration, perhaps not surprisingly given that axons normally have to grow along the developing spinal cord. However, unless the transplant is into neonatal animals, in which the pyramidal tract is still growing,[76] the axons grow poorly out of the transplant into the cord.[68] Grafts of Schwann cells[77,78] and olfactory glial cells[79,80] have also been shown to promote CNS axon regeneration.

Intrinsic reduction in growth potential

In addition to the non-supportive nature of the CNS environment, it is likely that a proportion of CNS neurons lose some or all of their developmental capacity to support axonal growth, and may be unable to restore it after axotomy. An example is provided by retinal neurons. Cultured retinal ganglion cells extend axons in response to BDNF some 10 times faster if they derive from embryonic animals (E19 rats) compared with postnatal (P8) animals.[56] Expression of the *bcl-2* gene, an important element in the regulation of apoptosis (see Chapter 13), has also been implicated in the regeneration response of retinal axons. After axons have grown into the rat tectum during development, retinal neurons normally downregulate *bcl-2* expression. However, neurons from adult transgenic mice that overexpress *bcl-2* can innervate tectal tissue from foetal rats, something that normal adult ganglion cells cannot do.[81] Neurons so primed are not, however, able to regrow into the adult tectum, so a suitably enhanced cell body appears unable to overcome the local inhibitory factors present in the adult neuropil. Nor does *bcl-2* overexpression in transgenic mice restore regeneration of the crushed optic nerve in adult animals.[82] It is likely, then, that additional genes must be active for the full neonatal growth potential to be restored.

In summary, if successful regrowth of axons over long distances in the CNS of adult mammals is to be achieved, it will be necessary first to provide appropriate neurotrophic factors to prevent nerve cell death following injury, second to activate a vigorous regrowth programme in the cell body, third to overcome inhibitory factors present in white and grey matter and scar tissue, and fourth to provide a suitable pathway from the lesion site to the target.[83,84]

Transplanted neurons

Neurons can be isolated in small blocks of tissue, or enzymatically dissociated from foetal brains at a stage before they have grown extensive processes, and inserted or injected into the adult brain. Some neurons survive under these conditions, provided they acquire an adequate blood supply, and even become incorporated into neural circuits.[85] They do best when placed in young brains of genetically similar strains, which reduces the likelihood of early immune rejection, and if they are close to the region that they normally innervate, especially if it has been deafferented. This technique can restore lost function in experimental animals,[55,86] and has been used in patients with Parkinson's disease to replace degenerated dopaminergic neurons of the substantia nigra. There is some clinical improvement, although ethical and financial issues preclude its use at present as a standard form of therapy.[87]

Stem cells in the adult brain

An important question, with significant implications for promoting functional recovery following CNS injury, is whether the adult CNS contains populations of stem cells or progenitor cells that can continue to divide throughout life. By 'stem' cell is meant a self-renewing multipotential cell that can generate the full repertoire of neurons and glia through symmetric and/or asymmetric divisions, while the term 'progenitor' refers to a precursor cell that can also self-renew but whose phenotypic potential is more restricted. Neurogenesis is known to continue throughout adulthood in certain regions of the avian brain, and is particularly prominent in a region of the forebrain in songbirds, the neostriatal higher vocal centre, where more than 1 per cent of the neuron population can be generated each day.[88–90] It is also known that supporting cells in the epithelia of the inner ear can regenerate lost hair cells in birds, as well as in fish and amphibia, but not in mammals.[91]

Although it has often been stated that the adult mammalian CNS is incapable of stem/progenitor cell renewal, the olfactory bulb[92] has been recognized for some time as an exception to this rule. More recently, moreover, several other regions of the adult mammalian brain have been shown to contain progenitor cells capable of neurogenesis, but the evidence for the existence of a multipotential neural stem cell, equivalent to that seen for the haematopoietic lineage in the bone marrow, is more contentious.

Proliferative cells can be identified by autoradiography after pulse-labelling the adult brain with tritiated thymidine, by bromodeoxyuridine labelling, or by labelling with a replication-defective retrovirus containing the *lacZ* gene. Their differentiated progeny can be seen simultaneously by staining for phenotype-specific markers such as neuron-specific enolase or the glial fibrillary acidic protein (GFAP). These methods have revealed a progenitor population in the granule cell layer of the rat dentate gyrus that generates mature neurons,[93] and a population of cells in the most rostral region of the forebrain subventricular (subependymal) zone in the adult mouse that migrates to the olfactory bulb over long distances (up to 5 mm) before differentiating into olfactory interneurons (see also Chapter 7).[94] Many other areas of the adult CNS, such as the external granular layer of the cerebellum[95] and the spinal cord,[96] are further possible sources of quiescent progenitor cells, and neurogenesis has also been detected in the adult human hippocampus.[97]

The forebrain subventricular zone contains the largest population of constitutively dividing cells in the adult rodent CNS, and many of those that do not migrate to the olfactory bulb appear to divide asymmetrically, one daughter cell dying and the other maintaining the population. Their precise origin in the CNS has proved difficult to establish.[98] They have been shown to derive from a population of relatively quiescent subependymal cells which furnishes neurons and glia when driven *in vitro* by EGF[99,100] or FGF-2.[101] This population can also be expanded in the adult mouse brain *in vivo* by intraventricular infusion of EGF, yielding cells that migrate into the adjacent forebrain parenchyma and differentiate into neurons and glia.[102] Some may originate from subventricular zone astrocytes,[103] but their earlier lineal origins are unclear.[98] One possibility is that the subependymal population derives in turn from the ependymal cells that line the ventricles. When the latter cells are labelled selectively by intraventricular injection of DiI, their progeny can be seen to migrate into the olfactory bulb, and isolated ependymal cells propagated in culture are also capable of differentiation into neurons and glia.[104]

Such cells may satisfy some of the criteria for a stem cell, and are even capable of differentiating into haematopoietic cells when exposed to bone marrow,[105] but how far their normal function extends beyond replacing olfactory bulb neurons is uncertain.[106] In the case of the rodent dentate gyrus, the proliferation and survival of newly-formed neurons can be increased by exposure to an 'enriched' laboratory environment, and exercise has been identified as an important factor in generating this effect.[107] Survival is also increased during hippocampal-dependent learning tasks such as spatial learning in a water maze (see Chapter 16),[108] so newly-formed neurons may contribute to learning mechanisms in this region of the CNS. One further role may concern CNS injury; following experimental spinal cord injury, the spinal cord ependymal cells in the vicinity of the lesion can furnish astrocytes that contribute to the glial scar.[104]

A detailed understanding of the factors that modulate the differentiation of these cells, and of similar cells that can be isolated from the developing CNS, may ultimately provide a useful route to the difficult clinical problem of CNS repair. One strategy under investigation is the transplantation into the injured CNS of immortalized stem and progenitor cells,[109] including the use of human embryonic stem cells.[110] It has been shown, for example, that in rats subjected to ischaemic hippocampal injury, recovery of spatial learning can take place after grafts into the hippocampal CA1 region of conditionally-immortalized cells derived from mouse embryonic hippocampal neuroepithelium.[111] A further approach will be to engineer such cells to express suitable transcription factors, trophic factors and transmitter-related enzymes.[110]

Collateral sprouting

Collateral sprouts are outgrowths from the axons of intact undamaged neurons. They typically appear from undamaged axons in a tissue which has had part of its nerve supply removed, and they can often innervate successfully any cells that have lost some or all of their original synaptic input. This surprising phenomenon was first suspected nearly a hundred years ago, when it was found that partly denervated muscles recovered their full contractile strength and contained few atrophied muscle fibres long before any of the motor axons which had been cut had regenerated. Later histological examination of silver-stained axons in such muscles[112] proved that the denervated cells had indeed become reinnervated by sprouts from the intact axons.

In partly denervated mammalian muscles, sprouting begins 2–3 days after partial denervation. Sprouts emerge from nodes of Ranvier (nodal sprouts) and from the motor nerve terminals (terminal sprouts) (Fig. 17.3).[112] Nodal sprouts leave their own endoneurial sheath and cross into the sheaths vacated by the degenerating axons, where they grow distally and without deviation towards the denervated endplates. Terminal sprouts seem to grow in a more irregular way until they locate an uninnervated endplate, which they rapidly take over. Any one motor neuron can generate enough sprouts to innervate almost five times more muscle fibres than it normally does, but if the original axons regenerate to the endplates, many of these extra branches are eliminated.[113] In small animals such as mice it takes less than two weeks to restore complete innervation to a partly denervated muscle by collateral sprouting.

Similar recovery following partial denervation has been demonstrated in cutaneous sensory nerves[114] and in autonomic ganglia.[115,116] In skin it has been found that only the nociceptive afferents sprout,[117,118] and that the speed of the response is greater if the nociceptive afferents which are sprouting are activated.[119]

Definite proof that collateral sprouting occurs in the CNS has been harder to obtain. It has depended on the use of specific axonal staining by transported labels,[120,121] staining for specific transmitters to observe enlargement of areas innervated by particular sets of axons,[122] electron microscopy to show replacement of degenerating synaptic boutons by recognizably different ones,[123] and electrophysiological evidence for synaptic redistribution on the dendrites and soma.[124] It is now clear that

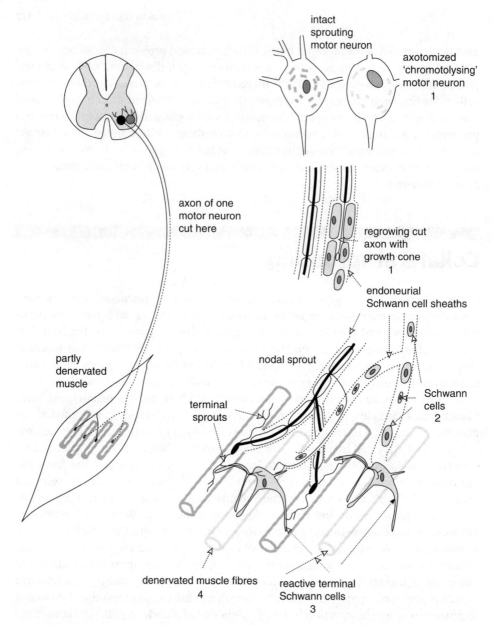

Figure 17.3 Collateral sprouting by intact motor axons is from nodes of Ranvier within the body of the partly denervated muscle (nodal sprouting), and from motor nerve terminals (terminal sprouting). In the magnified views on the right of the diagram some of the factors thought to trigger sprouting are numbered 1–4. (1) Spread of a signal of some sort from axotomized motor neurons, which are reprogrammed to grow new axons, to intact neurons nearby. (2) Schwann cells within the endoneurial sheaths that were formerly occupied by the now-degenerated axons may send a sprouting signal. They are known to support regeneration of cut axons. (3) Schwann cells at the nerve terminal grow long branches which precede the appearance of terminal sprouts, and may stimulate and guide such sprouts. (4) Denervated muscle fibres may release neurotrophic factors, as may fibroblasts within the muscle parenchyma (see Fig. 16.3).

injury-induced sprouting does occur at many but not all CNS loci,[125] and is particularly vigorous in the young developing brain where sprouts can travel long distances.[124] Sprouting in the adult CNS is less vigorous, presumably because of the same factors that limit axon regeneration. Electrophysiological experiments have shown, nevertheless, that some of the synapses formed by sprouts can transmit,[126] and behavioural tests have further shown some restoration of function following sprouting.[127,128] Sprouting may therefore contribute to recovery that may follow various types of damage to the brain. For example, the dementia associated with HIV-1 infection of the brain is partially reversible by the retroviral blocking agent AZT (3'-azido-3'-deoxythymidine). Since the dementia is accompanied by loss of neurons and reduction in dendritic arbors,[129] the clinical improvement accompanying the fall in viral load in brain macrophages must involve repair of some sort, and sprouting could play a part. It should be remembered, however, that CNS sprouting may also lead to abnormal function and sensations, and may be involved in the production of injury-associated clinical states such as spasticity.

Sprouting may also contribute to slow changes in receptive field sizes in various neocortical sensory areas when part of the sensory input is removed by a peripheral nerve lesion, or when part of the sensory input to a cortical area is given undue excitation compared with the rest (see below),[130] although at present there is no anatomical proof of this. Under these circumstances cortical neurons are not denervated, but simply undergo changes in activity levels.

Mechanisms that may stimulate collateral sprouting following injury

The stimuli that cause intact undamaged neurons to grow collateral sprouts have been investigated largely in the PNS. There are several changes in partly denervated tissues and around the neurons which had been innervating them that could be involved (Fig. 17.3).

Breakdown products from degenerating axons and myelin

Sprouting could be stimulated by the release of some breakdown product of degenerating axons or myelin. This has not been directly proved or disproved. Sprouting can be elicited, however, in circumstances where there is no degeneration, so such products are not essential. Degeneration products and inflammation may, nevertheless, be able to assist by triggering changes in nearby cells which help to stimulate axon growth. For example, it is possible to stimulate changes in muscle fibres by inflammation, which are very like those following denervation,[131] and these can in turn elicit motor nerve sprouting.

Production of growth factors by denervated tissue

Trophic factors normally taken up by neurons whose axons have degenerated could become available in partly denervated tissues to any remaining axons, providing them with a surplus and stimulating them to sprout. In addition, the denervated tissue might upregulate its output of trophic factors. Evidence for such a mechanism is the observation that sprouting of cutaneous nociceptive afferents (which are maintained by NGF derived from the skin) is inhibited by antibodies to NGF, and is increased by exogenous NGF injections which can also trigger sprouting in unoperated normal skin.[27,132,133] NGF injections can also induce sprouting of mature uninjured sympathetic axons,[134] and antibodies to NGF can inhibit collateral sprouting of septohippocampal fibres following entorhinal cortex lesions in adult rats.[135]

The nature of the stimulus for motor neuron sprouting is less certain, but when muscles are paralysed by blocking transmitter release, transmitter action or motor nerve impulses, sprouting is stimulated from motor nerve terminals and even from a few nodes of Ranvier.[136–139] Muscle fibres are well known to undergo many changes as a result of inactivity that are almost identical to the changes that follow denervation (see Chapter 16) and the effects on motor axons are most simply explained by the action of a trophic factor released by the paralysed muscle fibres (but see following section on Schwann cells). Support for this view is provided by finding that selective destruction of muscle fibres at the time of partial denervation inhibits nodal sprouting of the remaining axons innervating the muscle.[140] A good candidate for a muscle-derived sprouting factor is insulin-like growth factor (IGF-II), the mRNA for which is expressed in foetal and denervated muscles.[141] Elevated levels of IGFs can induce sprouting in fully innervated adult mouse muscles,[142] and terminal sprouting can be inhibited in paralysed muscles by an IGF binding protein.[143] Motor nerves can also be induced to sprout by injections of CNTF, especially if it is coupled with FGF,[144] but CNTF is not a product of innervated or denervated muscle fibres. Denervated muscle fibres do, however, upregulate BDNF mRNA and it is known that motor neurons express TrkB BDNF receptors and can be rescued from axotomy-induced death by exogenous BDNF.[145] By analogy with NGF and its effects on the sprouting of cutaneous nociceptors, BDNF might therefore be able to evoke sprouting in motor neurons.

Production of growth factors by Schwann cells

Schwann cells have powerfully attractive and supportive effects on regrowing axons (see above), so it would be surprising if they did not play some part in collateral sprouting after partial denervation. Nodal sprouts may be attracted into adjacent, axon-free endoneurial tubes by the 'denervated' Schwann cells in the latter, crossing two layers of basal lamina in the process. The same agents that were suggested to assist in axon regeneration may be involved here. Sensory and motor axon sprouting can indeed be stimulated by anastomosing a length of degenerated nerve by its end to the side of an intact nerve.[146] Motor nerves can also be made to sprout in intact undamaged frog muscle by placing a small piece of isolated peripheral nerve on the muscle surface some distance from the endplates.[147] However, nodal sprouting induced conventionally by partial denervation seems to be confined, at least initially, largely to nodes of Ranvier close to denervated target tissue. This is despite the fact that if tissues are so denervated some way from their target, intact axons at this distance are still exposed to local Schwann cell products in adjacent denervated endoneurial sheaths, yet do not sprout at this position.[148]

Following axotomy, the 'terminal' Schwann cells that previously overlaid the motor nerve ending at the neuromuscular junction upregulate GAP-43 and grow long, axon-like branches that extend up to several hundred micrometres.[149,150] Careful examination suggests that these outgrowths provide a stimulus for motor nerve terminal sprouts to grow from intact to denervated endplates.[151,152] Terminal Schwann cells undergo the same changes in paralysed muscles, so they are probably important in terminal sprouting in paralysed muscles too. Sprouting is poor in neonatal muscles, and this is probably because the terminal Schwann cells die when glial growth factor provided by the motor axon is removed.[153] It is perhaps less likely that glial cells in the CNS are involved in sprouting, given their largely negative actions on regrowth.

Production of stimuli by axotomized neurons

Sprouting, and changes in synaptic effectiveness, can be produced in a muscle on one side of an animal by denervation of a muscle on the animal's other side. This is especially clear in frogs.[154-157] The response is seen only in the equivalent contralateral muscle. It is possible that a growth stimulus present in axotomized neurons can spread across the spinal cord to influence neurons on the other side. In mammalian muscles sprouting is localized to terminals and axons near to denervated muscle fibres.[158,159] This observation makes it unlikely that any significant sprouting stimulus passes from axotomized to intact motor neurons even within a single motor nucleus in the spinal cord. Contralateral effects have nevertheless been reported in mammals.[160]

Cell body reaction and growth-promoting surfaces in collateral sprouting

It has been emphasized that successful axonal regeneration needs both an adequate reaction in the nerve cell body and a supportive local environment for the growth cone. Conventional histological examination surprisingly fails to detect a typical chromatolytic reaction in motor neurons whose axons are sprouting but which have not themselves been axotomized.[161] Nor does there seem to be an upregulation of GAP-43 mRNA on anything like the scale seen after axotomy.[162] Nevertheless, c-jun protein is elevated in sprouting motor neurons, GAP-43 protein is readily detectable in the terminals of sprouting motor neurons,[163] and there is upregulation of GAP-43 mRNA in sprouting DRG cells[164] and of mRNA for $T\alpha 1$ tubulin in sprouting sympathetic neurons.[165] Were GAP-43 to be more vigorously produced, it is likely that collateral sprouting would be greatly improved, as in transgenic mice overexpressing GAP-43 constitutively, sprouting in response to the usual stimuli is dramatic.[34] The trigger for any cell body reaction in uninjured neurons is unknown.

A suitable substrate for growth of terminal sprouts in muscle is NCAM (see Chapter 9), which appears in inactive muscles and on reactive Schwann cells at the endplate. Antibodies to NCAM can partially suppress terminal sprout growth.[166] Nodal sprouts which gain access to denervated endoneurial tubes have the same factors available to them as are presented to regenerating axons.

Activation of 'suppressed synapses'

The idea that the CNS might contain a significant number of structurally normal but physiologically ineffective synapses is relatively recent, and was put forward following experiments on the motor innervation of fish eye muscles. These suggested that foreign motor nerves could innervate the eye muscles but became inactivated (silenced) rather than withdrawn if the correct innervation was restored.[167] Subsequent studies showed this not to be the case.[168,169] Paradoxically, however, there is now considerable evidence for the existence of synapses in the CNS that are normally quiescent but that can be activated by a variety of peripheral nerve lesions that stop sensory impulses reaching the brain. This results in a rapid enlargement of the receptive fields of those neurons still connected to the periphery (Fig. 17.4). There is also evidence that expansion of receptive fields following injury or overuse may be augmented on a slower time scale, possibly by growth of axonal terminal arbors.

Cells in both the dorsal horn and the dorsal column nuclei of the spinal cord rapidly develop new receptive fields if their normal inputs are removed by cutting the appropriate peripheral nerve or dorsal roots.[170,171] Three lines of evidence support the view that these new receptive fields arise from synapses that are already present but are tonically suppressed by activity in the other sensory axons: first, sprouting of the intact afferents cannot be detected;[172,173] second, subliminal inputs can be detected if sensory nerves are electrically stimulated;[174] and third, immediate changes in the shape and size of receptive fields are revealed if the excitability of cells and presynaptic terminals is increased pharmacologically.[175,176] It is possible that decreased 'surround' presynaptic inhibition is responsible for unmasking the synapses.[177]

There are, however, features of the phenomenon that are puzzling. For example, some studies have failed to find any plasticity in the pathway that leads from skin to dorsal horn neurons and then to the spinocervical tract.[178] Also, in pathways that do

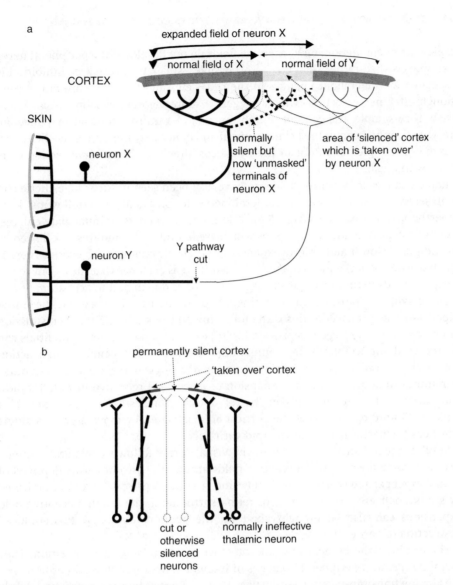

Figure 17.4 Rapid changes in the cortical receptive fields of sensory afferents following injury to peripheral axons innervating nearby areas in the skin may be the result of 'unmasking' of pre-existent, but functionally silent, connections. (Later expansion of receptive fields of intact cutaneous sensory neurons may be the result of collateral sprouting.) Excess activation of one pathway compared with another can also lead to changes in the sizes of the receptive fields, as can blockade of inhibitory cortical networks. A reduction in inhibitory control is one factor that may be important for field expansion following injury, but in the cortex expansion may also need the cooperation of diffuse cholinergic inputs from the basal nucleus of Meynert and the participation of NMDA receptors. Two possible anatomical bases for rapid receptive field expansion are depicted. In (a), silent terminals of individual thalamic axons start to transmit; in (b), thalamic neurons with atypical projections may start to activate successfully cells in the cortex. For simplicity, the pathway to the cortex has been depicted as consisting of only a single axon. In practice, several neurons in series are involved. Reorganization following injury may also occur at relay stations in the spinal cord and thalamus (see reference 182).

display the phenomenon, new receptive fields do not develop if the peripheral nerve is simply crushed rather than cut.[171] A possible explanation is that disinhibition is associated with metabolic changes in the DRG cells, and that these are only strong enough after nerve section, which triggers a more vigorous response than nerve crush. For example, the content of Substance P,[179] a transmitter that may mediate presynaptic inhibition in the normal animal and hence may limit receptive field size, is reduced to a greater extent in the DRG cells after peripheral nerve section compared with crush.

Rapid changes in receptive field size have also been seen in the somaesthetic cortical sensory area following peripheral nerve lesions, and even following local anaesthesia of lumbar roots (Fig. 17.4).[180] In monkeys there is an immediate enlargement of receptive fields of the nerves which are left intact,[181] and this is followed by an additional slower and orderly expansion of their somatotopic projection. There is much debate about the mechanism,[182,183] but there is evidence that the expansion of receptive fields in the cortex, as in the spinal cord, is due in part to activation of preexisting synapses rather than sprouting.[184] In addition to the speed of the initial expansion, the evidence for this is the following: (i) block of inhibitory transmission can give rise to very large receptive fields; (ii) excitatory postsynaptic potentials can be recorded intracellularly by stimulating skin areas that cannot evoke action potentials; (iii) prolonged electrical stimulation of a single nerve can, over the course of minutes to hours, lead to an expansion of its cortical receptive field; (iv) topical application of NGF to the whisker 'barrel' cortex of anaesthetized rats leads to a rapid (< 25 min) expansion of the cortical area activated by movement of a single whisker,[185] whereas BDNF causes rapid shrinkage.

Similar rapid changes can occur in the visual cortex following bilateral symmetrical lesions to the retina.[186] Receptive fields around the area of cortex deprived of retinal input expand in size immediately, and later the deprived area can be activated by stimuli delivered to the region of retina surrounding the lesion. Receptive field expansions can also be brought about in the auditory cortex by toxin-induced destruction of part of the cochlea.[187]

The origin of the branches that become active and take over is uncertain. They might be the most peripheral branches of individual neurons whose other branches are already transmitting successfully (Fig. 17.4a). Alternatively, neurons with slightly atypical projections outside the range of their neighbours might begin to transmit (Fig. 17.4b). There is evidence that a minority of thalamic neurons do have projections outside the normal range of their neighbours.[188] Finally, horizontal connections within the cortex may be needed to explain cortical expansion of receptive fields.[189]

Purpose and mechanism of synaptic repression

'Silent' synapses were first revealed or unmasked after nerve injury, but it has since been discovered that cortical receptive fields in adult animals can also be modified by vigorous changes in the patterns of ascending afferent activity. For example, if two digits are sutured together, novel receptive fields develop in which inputs from the two fingers, which are normally completely separate, are both represented.[190] Similarly, if monkeys are trained to use one digit excessively, the amount of cortical area devoted to it increases.[191] It is probable, therefore, that the functional rearrangements that follow nerve injury, when one input becomes completely silent, are a special case of a more general synaptic mechanism, at work continuously, in which there is competition for effectiveness driven by activity patterns.[130]

The exact mechanisms of synaptic repression and unmasking are still unknown. The most direct mechanism would be mutual repression between synapses sharing an area on the postsynaptic membrane, a phenomenon which has been reported in multiply-innervated muscle fibres[192] but whose cellular basis is unknown. Alternatively, synaptic inhibitory circuits could be involved, in view of the fact that GABA immunoreactivity is reduced in areas of cortex in which field expansion has occurred.[193] There is also evidence that cholinergic inputs to the cortex from the basal forebrain are needed for injury-induced expansion of fields to occur.[194] Finally, there is evidence that many AMPA glutamate receptors may be 'silent', at least in the hippocampus, until they are reactivated during LTP (Chapter 15).[195] There is also evidence that active NMDA receptors are needed for expansion of receptive fields in the somaesthetic cortex,[196] so 'unmasking' of silent synapses maybe similar to LTP in the hippocampus. This is supported by the results of neurotrophin application described above, since neurotrophins are known to influence LTP (see Chapter 15).

The phenomenon of receptive field expansion (and retraction), brought on by altering the balance of activity in partly overlapping sensory pathways, allows the adult brain an important measure of adaptability. The degree of plasticity is considerably less than during the critical period (Chapter 14), probably because the extent of the axonal tree of any one neuron is smaller than during the neonatal period, and the capacity of the neurons to develop new branches is severely limited.

Key points

1 Severed or crushed motor, sensory and autonomic axons in the peripheral nervous systems of mammals can regrow successfully, especially in small animals. The rate of axonal elongation during regrowth is a few millimetres per day.

2 Success depends on: (i) survival of the neuron whose axon has been cut and the reprogramming of its synthetic machinery to produce material needed for axon elongation; (ii) a local pathway for regrowing axons to follow which actively encourages sprout growth (e.g. containing activated Schwann cells); (iii) some means of guidance back to the denervated tissue, such as the pathways provided by intact endoneurial sheaths following crush injuries.

3 Axons regrow successfully in the CNS of some lower vertebrates but very poorly within the CNS of mammals. The poor regrowth is probably a result of several

factors; (i) actively inhibitory molecules in the white and grey matter, and in glial scar tissue; (ii) lack of growth-promoting agents equivalent to those produced by peripheral Schwann cells; (iii) an inadequate cell body response.

4 Most regions of the adult mammalian brain do not generate new neurons, but important exceptions are provided by the olfactory bulb and a population of progenitor cells that remains dormant in the forebrain. This population can be expanded *in vitro* with appropriate growth factors. Foetal neurons can survive if implanted in adult brains, and make functional synaptic connections. To do so they need to be transplanted close to an appropriate, denervated neuronal population.

5 The axons of uninjured neurons grow collateral sprouts in tissues that have been partly denervated. These can successfully innervate vacated synaptic sites and restore function. Sprouting is probably triggered by neurotrophic factors released from denervated cells, including denervated Schwann cells.

6 Injury to peripheral sensory nerves also causes rapid enlargement of the central receptive fields of those sensory axons which remain. This occurs at all levels of the sensory pathways in the CNS. It is likely that the rapid expansion of receptive fields of intact neurons is due partly to activation of previously subthreshold connections. The phenomenon may be an exaggerated example of an alteration in the dynamic balance between overlapping sensory terminal connections. In these, relative rates and amounts of activity seem to control the functional extents of the competing terminal domains.

General reading

- Larner, A. J., Johnson, A. R. and Keynes, R. J. Regeneration in the vertebrate central nervous system: phylogeny, ontogeny, and mechanisms. *Biol. Rev. Camb. Philos. Soc.* **70**, 597–619 (1995).

- Fawcett, J. W. and Asher, R. A. The glial scar and central nervous system repair. *Brain Res. Bull.* **49**, 377–91 (1999).

- Goldberg, J. L. and Barres, B. A. The relationship between neuronal survival and regeneration. *Annu. Rev. Neurosci.* **23**, 579–612 (2000).

References

1. Larner, A. J., Johnson, A. R. and Keynes, R. J. Regeneration in the vertebrate central nervous system: phylogeny, ontogeny, and mechanisms. *Biol. Rev. Camb. Philos. Soc.* **70**, 597–619 (1995).

2. Ramón y Cajal, S. *Degeneration and regeneration of the nervous system* (Oxford University Press, London, 1928).

3. Friede, R. L. and Bischhausen, R. The fine structure of stumps of transected nerve fibers in subserial sections. *J. Neurol. Sci.* **44**, 181–203 (1980).

4. Sunderland, S. *Nerves and nerve injuries* (Churchill-Livingstone, London, 1978).

5. Brown, M. C., Lunn, E. R. and Perry, V. H. Poor growth of mammalian motor and sensory axons

into intact proximal nerve stumps. *Eur. J. Neurosci.* **3**, 1366–9 (1991).

6. Chen, S. and Bisby, M. A. Impaired motor axon regeneration in the C57BL/Ola mouse. *J. Comp. Neurol.* **333**, 449–54 (1993).

7. Brown, M. C., Perry, V. H., Hunt, S. P. and Lapper, S. R. Further studies on motor and sensory nerve regeneration in mice with delayed Wallerian degeneration. *Eur. J. Neurosci.* **6**, 420–8 (1994).

8. Bedi, K. S., Winter, J., Berry, M. and Cohen, J. Adult rat dorsal root ganglion neurons extend neurites on predegenerated but not on normal peripheral nerves *in vitro*. *Eur. J. Neurosci.* **4**, 193–200 (1992).

9. Vidal Sanz, M., Bray, G. M., Villegas Perez, M. P., Thanos, S. and Aguayo, A. J. Axonal regeneration and synapse formation in the superior colliculus by retinal ganglion cells in the adult rat. *J. Neurosci.* **7**, 2894–909 (1987).

10. Richardson, P. M., Issa, V. M. K. and Shemie, S. Regeneration and retrograde degeneration of axons in the rat optic nerve. *J. Neurocytol.* **11**, 949–66 (1982).

11. Doster, S. K., Lozano, A. M., Aguayo, A. J. and Willard, M. B. Expression of the growth-associated protein GAP-43 in adult rat retinal ganglion cells following axon injury. *Neuron* **6**, 635–47 (1991).

12. Villegas Perez, M. P., Vidal Sanz, M., Bray, G. M. and Aguayo, A. J. Influence of peripheral nerve grafts on the survival and regrowth of axotomised retinal ganglion cells in adult rats. *J. Neurosci.* **8**, 265–80 (1988).

13. Nadim, W., Anderson, P. N. and Turmaine, M. The role of Schwann cells and basal lamina tubes in the regeneration of axons through long lengths of freeze-killed nerve grafts. *Neuropathol. Appl. Neurobiol.* **16**, 411–21 (1990).

14. Chong, M. S. *et al.* The downregulation of GAP-43 is not responsible for the failure of regeneration in freeze-killed nerve grafts in the rat. *Exp. Neurol.* **129**, 311–20 (1994).

15. Kuffler, D. P. Isolated satellite cells of a peripheral nerve direct the growth of regenerating frog axons. *J. Comp. Neurol.* **249**, 57–64 (1986).

16. Rath, E. M., Kelly, D., Bouldin, T. W. and Popko, B. Impaired peripheral nerve regeneration in a mutant strain of mice (*Enr*) with a Schwann cell defect. *J. Neurosci.* **15**, 7226–37 (1995).

17. Ide, C., Tohyama, K., Yokota, R., Nitatori, T. and Onodera, S. Schwann cell basal lamina and nerve regeneration. *Brain Res.* **288**, 61–75 (1983).

18. Keynes, R. J., Hopkins, W. G. and Huang, C. L.-H. Regeneration of mouse peripheral nerves in degenerating skeletal muscle: guidance by residual muscle fibre basement membrane. *Brain Res.* **295**, 275–81 (1984).

19. Ide, C., Osawa, T. and Tohyama, K. Nerve regeneration through allogeneic nerve grafts, with special reference to the role of the Schwann cell basal lamina. *Prog. Neurobiol.* **34**, 1–38 (1990).

20. Daniloff, J. K., Levi, G., Grumet, M., Rieger, F. and Edelman, G. M. Altered expression of neuronal cell adhesion molecule induced by nerve injury and repair. *J. Cell Biol.* **103**, 929–45 (1986).

21. Martini, R. and Schachner, M. Immunoelectronmicroscopic localization of neural cell adhesion molecules (L1, N-CAM, and myelin-associated glycoprotein) in regenerating adult mouse sciatic nerve. *J. Cell Biol.* **106**, 1735–44 (1988).

22. Bixby, J. L., Lilien, J. and Reichardt, L. F. Identification of the major proteins that promote neuronal process outgrowth on Schwann cells *in vitro*. *J. Cell Biol.* **107**, 353–61 (1988).

23. Bjerre, B., Bjorklund, A. and Edwards, D. C. Axonal regeneration of peripheral adrenergic neurons; effects of antiserum to NGF in mouse. *Cell Tissue Res.* **148**, 441–76 (1974).

24. Turner, J. E. and Glaze, K. A. Regenerative repair in the severed optic nerve of the newt (*Triturus viridescens*): effect of nerve growth factor. *Exp. Neurol.* **57**, 687–97 (1977).

25. Glaze, K. A. and Turner, J. E. Regenerative repair in the severed optic nerve of the newt (*Triturus viridescens*): effect of nerve growth factor antiserum. *Exp. Neurol.* **58**, 500–10 (1978).

26. Johnson, E. M., Taniuchi, M. and Di Stefano, P. S. Expression and possible function of nerve growth factor receptors on Schwann cells. *Trends Neurosci.* **11**, 299–304 (1988).

27. Diamond, J., Coughlin, M., MacIntyre, L., Holmes, M. and Visheau, B. Evidence that endogenous B nerve growth factor is responsible for the collateral sprouting, but not the regeneration, of nociceptive axons in adult rats. *Proc. Natl. Acad. Sci. USA* **84**, 6596–600 (1987).

28. Kanje, M., Skottner, A., Sjoeberg, J. and Lundborg, G. Insulin-like growth factor I (IGF-I) stimulates regeneration of the rat sciatic nerve. *Brain Res.* **486**, 396–8 (1989).

29. Glazner, G. W., Lupien, S., Miller, J. A. and Ishii, D. N. Insulin-like growth factor II increases the rate of sciatic nerve regeneration in rats. *Neuroscience* **54**, 791–7 (1993).

30. Funakoshi, H. *et al.* Differential expression of mRNAs for neurotrophins and their receptors after axotomy of the sciatic nerve. *J. Cell Biol.* **123**, 455–65 (1993).

31. DiStefano, P. S., Chelsea, D. M., Schick, C. M. and McKelvy, J. F. Involvement of a metalloprotease in low-affinity nerve growth factor receptor truncation: inhibition of truncation *in vitro* and *in vivo*. *J. Neurosci.* **13**, 2405–14 (1993).

32. Ignatius, M. J., Shooter, E. M., Pitas, R. E. and Mahley, R. W. Lipoprotein uptake by neuronal growth cones in vitro. *Science* **236**, 959–62 (1987).

33. Popko, B., Goodrum, J. F., Bouldin, T. W., Zhang, S. H. and Maeda, N. Nerve regeneration occurs in the absence of apolipoprotein E in mice. *J. Neurochem.* **60**, 1155–8 (1993).

34. Aigner, L. *et al.* Overexpression of the neural growth-associated protein GAP-43 induces nerve sprouting in the adult nervous system of transgenic mice. *Cell* **83**, 269–78 (1995).

35. McQuarrie, I. G. The effect of a conditioning lesion on the regeneration of motor axons. *Brain Res.* **152**, 597–602 (1978).

36. Sjoberg, J. and Kanje, M. The initial period of peripheral nerve regeneration and the importance of the local environment for the conditioning lesion effect. *Brain Res.* **529**, 79–84 (1990).

37. Sjoberg, J. and Kanje, M. Effects of repetitive conditioning crush lesions on regeneration of the rat sciatic nerve. *Brain Res.* **530**, 167–9 (1990).

38. Kanje, M., Skottner, A., Lundborg, G. and Sjoeberg, J. Does insulin-like growth factor I (IGF-1) trigger the cell body reaction in the rat sciatic nerve? *Brain Res.* **563**, 285–7 (1991).

39. Turner, J. E., Schwab, M. E. and Thoenen, M. NGF stimulates neurite outgrowth from goldfish retinal explants: the influence of a prior lesion. *Dev. Brain Res.* **4**, 59–86 (1982).

40. Aldskogius, H. and Thomander, L. Selective reinnervation of somatotopically appropriate muscles after facial nerve transection and regeneration in neonatal rats. *Brain Res.* **375**, 126–34 (1986).

41. Hardman, V. J. and Brown, M. C. Accuracy of re-innervation of rat intercostal muscles by their own segmental nerves. *J. Neurosci.* **7**, 1031–6 (1987).

42. Brushart, T. M. E. Motor axons preferentially reinnervate motor pathways. *J. Neurosci.* **13**, 2730–8 (1993).

43. Madison, R. G., Archibald, S. J. and Brushart, T. M. Reinnervation accuracy of the rat femoral nerve by motor and sensory neurons. *J. Neurosci.* **16**, 5698–703 (1996).

44. Fawcett, J. W. and Keynes, R. J. Muscle basal lamina: a new graft material for peripheral nerve repair. *J. Neurosurg.* **65**, 354–63 (1986).

45. Zhao, Q., Dahlin, L. B., Kanje, M. and Lundborg, G. Specificity of muscle reinnervation following repair of the transected sciatic nerve. A comparative study of different repair techniques in the rat. *J. Hand Surg.* **17**, 257–61 (1992).

46. Aldskogius, H., Arvidsson, J. and Grant, G. The reaction of primary sensory neurons to peripheral nerve injury with particular emphasis on transganglionic changes. *Brain Res. Rev.* **10**, 27–46 (1985).

47. Grimm, C. M. An evaluation of myotypic respecification in axolotls. *J. Exp. Zool.* **178**, 479–96 (1971).

48. Devor, M. The pathophysiology of damaged peripheral nerves. In *Textbook of pain* (ed. P. D. Wall and R. Melzack), pp. 63–81 (Churchill-Livingstone, Edinburgh, 1989).

49. Woolf, C. J., Shortland, P. and Coggeshall, R. E. Peripheral nerve injury triggers central sprouting of myelinated afferents. *Nature* **355**, 75–8 (1992).

50. Woolf, C. J., Safieh-Garabedian, B., Ma, Q.-P., Crilly, P. and Winter, J. Nerve growth factor contributes to the generation of inflammatory sensory hypersensitivity. *Neuroscience* **62**, 327–31 (1994).

51. McMahon, S. B., Bennett, D. L. H., Priestley, J. V. and Shelton, D. L. The biological effects of endogenous nerve growth factor on adult sensory neurons revealed by a trkA-IgG fusion molecule. *Nat. Med.* **1**, 774–80 (1995).

52. Richardson, P. M., McGuiness, U. M. and Aguayo, A. J. Axons from CNS neurones regenerate into PNS grafts. *Nature* **284**, 264–5 (1980).

53. Liuzzi, F. J. and Lasek, R. J. Astrocytes block axonal regeneration in mammals by activating the physiological stop pathway. *Science* **237**, 642–5 (1987).

54. Tetzlaff, W., Alexander, S. W., Miller, F. D. and Bisby, M. A. Response of facial and rubrospinal neurons to axotomy: changes in mRNA expression for cytoskeletal proteins and GAP-43. *J. Neurosci.* **11**, 2528–44 (1991).

55. Bjorklund, A. *et al.* Mechanisms of action of intracerebral neural implants: studies on nigral and striatal grafts to the lesioned striatum. *Trends Neurosci.* **10**, 509–16 (1987).

56. Goldberg, J. L. and Barres, B. A. The relationship between neuronal survival and regeneration. *Annu. Rev. Neurosci.* **23**, 579–612 (2000).

57. Fawcett, J. W. and Asher, R. A. The glial scar and central nervous system repair. *Brain Res. Bull.* **49**, 377–91 (1999).

58. Chen, M. S. *et al.* Nogo-A is a myelin-associated neurite outgrowth inhibitor and an antigen for monoclonal antibody IN-1. *Nature* **403**, 434–9 (2000).

59. Keynes, R. J., Johnson, A. R., Picart, C. J., Dunin-Borkowski, O. M. and Cook, G. M. W. A growth cone collapsing activity in chicken gray matter. *Ann. New York Acad. Sci.* **633**, 562 (1991).

60. Bandtlow, C. E., Schmidt, M. F., Hassinger, T. D., Schwab, M. E. and Kater, S. B. Role of intracellular calcium in NI-35-evoked collapse of neuronal growth cones. *Science* **259**, 80–3 (1993).

61. Wanner, M. *et al.* Reevaluation of the growth-permissive substrate properties of goldfish optic nerve myelin and myelin proteins. *J. Neurosci.* **15**, 7500–8 (1995).

62. Caroni, P. and Schwab, M. E. Antibody against myelin- associated inhibitor of neurite growth neutralizes non-permissive substrate properties of CNS white matter. *Neuron* **1**, 85–96 (1988).

63. Schnell, L. and Schwab, M. E. Axonal regeneration in the rat spinal cord produced by an antibody against myelin-associated neurite growth inhibitors. *Nature* **343**, 269–72 (1990).

64. Bregman, B. S. *et al.* Recovery from spinal cord injury mediated by antibodies to neurite growth inhibitors. *Nature* **378**, 498–501 (1995).

65. Huang, D. W., McKerracher, L., Braun, P. E. and David, S. A therapeutic vaccine approach to stimulate axon regeneration in the adult mammalian spinal cord. *Neuron* **24**, 639–47 (1999).

66. Smith, G. M., Rutishauser, U., Silver, J. and Miller, R. H. Maturation of astrocytes *in vitro* alters the extent and molecular basis of neurite outgrowth. *Dev. Biol.* **138**, 377–90 (1990).

67. Reier, P. J. and Houlé, J. D. In *Advances in neurology: functional recovery in neurological disease* (ed. S. G. Waxman), pp. 87–138 (Raven Press, New York, 1988).

68. Schnell, L. and Schwab, M. E. Sprouting and regeneration of lesioned corticospinal tract fibres in the adult rat spinal cord. *Eur. J. Neurosci.* **5**, 1156–71 (1993).

69. Schnell, L., Schneider, R., Kolbeck, R., Barde, Y.-A. and Schwab, M. E. Neurotrophin-3 enhances sprouting of corticospinal tract during development and after adult spinal cord lesion. *Nature* **367**, 170–3 (1994).

70. Levine, J. M. Increased expression of the NG2 chondroitin-sulfate proteoglycan after brain injury. *J. Neurosci.* **14**, 4716–30 (1994).

71. Bovolenta, P., Fernaud-Espinosa, I., Mendez-Otero, R. and Nieto-Sampedro, M. Neurite outgrowth inhibitor of gliotic brain tissue. Mode of action and cellular localization, studied with specific monoclonal antibodies. *Eur. J. Neurosci.* **9**, 977–89 (1997).

72. Davies, S. J. *et al.* Regeneration of adult axons in white matter tracts of the central nervous system. *Nature* **390**, 680–3 (1997).

73. Wictorin, K., Brundin, P., Gustavii, B., Lindvall, O. and Bjorklund, A. Reformation of long axon pathways in adult rat central nervous system by human forebrain neuroblasts. *Nature* **347**, 556–8 (1990).

74. Ramer, M. S., Priestley, J. V. and McMahon, S. B. Functional regeneration of sensory axons into the adult spinal cord. *Nature* **403**, 312–16 (2000).

75. Neumann, S. and Woolf, C. J. Regeneration of dorsal column fibers into and beyond the lesion site following adult spinal cord injury [see comments]. *Neuron* **23**, 83–91 (1999).

76. Iwashita, Y., Kawaguchi, S. and Murata, M. Restoration of function by replacement of spinal cord segments in the rat. *Nature* **367**, 167–70 (1994).

77. Li, Y. and Raisman, G. Schwann cells induce sprouting in motor and sensory axons in the adult rat spinal cord. *J. Neurosci.* **14**, 4050–63 (1994).

78. Brecknell, J. E. *et al.* Bridge grafts of fibroblast growth factor-4-secreting schwannoma cells promote functional axonal regeneration in the nigrostriatal pathway of the adult rat. *Neuroscience* **74**, 775–84 (1996).

79. Li, Y., Field, P. M. and Raisman, G. Repair of adult rat corticospinal tract by transplants of olfactory ensheathing cells. *Science* **277**, 2000–2 (1997).

80. Ramon-Cueto, A., Plant, G. W., Avila, J. and Bunge, M. B. Long-distance axonal regeneration in the transected adult rat spinal cord is promoted by olfactory ensheathing glia transplants. *J. Neurosci.* **18**, 3803–15 (1998).

81. Chen, D. F., Schneider, G. E., Martinou, J. C. and Tonegawa, S. *Bcl-2* promotes regeneration of severed axons in mammalian CNS. *Nature* **385**, 434–9 (1997).

82. Chierzi, S., Strettoi, E., Cenni, M. and Maffei, L. Optic nerve crush: axonal response in wild-type and *bcl-2* transgenic mice. *J. Neurosci.* **19**, 8367–76 (1999).

83. Baehr, M. and Bonhoeffer, F. Perspectives on axonal regeneration in the mammalian CNS. *Trends Neurosci.* **17**, 473–9 (1994).

84. Schwab, M. E. Bridging the gap in spinal cord regeneration. *Nat. Med.* **2**, 976–7 (1996).

85. Gage, F. H. and Fisher, L. J. Intracerebral grafting: a tool for the neurobiologist. *Neuron* **6**, 1–12 (1991).

86. Charleton, H. M., Barclay, A. N. and Williams, A. F. Detection of neuronal tissue from brain grafts with anti-Thy1.1 antibody. *Nature* **305**, 825–7 (1983).

87. Dunnett, S. B. and Bjorklund, A. Prospects for new restorative and neuroprotective treatments in Parkinson's disease. *Nature* **399**, A32–9 (1999).

88. Goldman, S. A. and Nottebohm, F. Neuronal production, migration, and differentiation in a vocal control nucleus of the adult female canary brain. *Proc. Natl. Acad. Sci. USA* **80**, 2390–4 (1983).

89. Alvarez-Buylla, A., Theelen, M. and Nottebohm, F. Proliferation 'hot spots' in adult

avian ventricular zone reveal radial cell division. *Neuron* **5**, 101–9 (1990).

90. Goldman, S. A. and Luskin, M. B. Strategies utilized by migrating neurons of the postnatal vertebrate forebrain. *Trends Neurosci.* **21**, 107–14 (1998).

91. Corwin, J. T. and Oberholtzer, J. C. Fish n' chicks: model recipes for hair-cell regeneration? *Neuron* **19**, 951–4 (1997).

92. Altman, J. Autoradiographic and histological studies of postnatal neurogenesis. IV. Cell proliferation and migration in the anterior forebrain, with special reference to persisting neurogenesis in the olfactory bulb. *J. Comp. Neurol.* **137**, 433–57 (1969).

93. Cameron, H. A., Woolley, C. S., McEwen, B. S. and Gould, E. Differentiation of newly born neurons and glia in the dentate gyrus of the adult rat. *Neuroscience* **56**, 337–44 (1993).

94. Lois, C. and Alvarez-Buylla, A. Long-distance neuronal migration in the adult mammalian brain. *Science* **264**, 1145–8 (1994).

95. Gage, F. H., Ray, J. and Fisher, L. J. Isolation, characterization, and use of stem cells from the CNS. *Annu. Rev. Neurosci.* **18**, 159–92 (1995).

96. Weiss, S. *et al.* Multipotent CNS stem cells are present in the adult mammalian spinal cord and ventricular neuroaxis. *J. Neurosci.* **16**, 7599–609 (1996).

97. Eriksson, P. S. *et al.* Neurogenesis in the adult human hippocampus. *Nat. Med.* **4**, 1313–17 (1998).

98. Barres, B. A. A new role for glia: generation of neurons! *Cell* **97**, 667–70 (1999).

99. Reynolds, B. A. and Weiss, S. Generation of neurons and astrocytes from isolated cells of the adult mammalian central nervous system. *Science* **255**, 1707–10 (1992).

100. Morshead, C. M. *et al.* Neural stem cells in the adult mammalian forebrain: a relatively quiescent subpopulation of subependymal cells. *Neuron* **13**, 1071–82 (1994).

101. Gritti, A. *et al.* Multipotential stem cells from the adult mouse brain proliferate and self-renew in response to basic fibroblast growth factor. *J. Neurosci.* **16**, 1091–100 (1996).

102. Craig, C. G. *et al. In vivo* growth factor expansion of endogenous subependymal neural precursor cell populations in the adult mouse brain. *J. Neurosci.* **16**, 2649–58 (1996).

103. Doetsch, F., Caille, I., Lim, D. A., Garcia-Verdugo, J. M. and Alvarez-Buylla, A. Subventricular zone astrocytes are neural stem cells in the adult mammalian brain. *Cell* **97**, 703–16 (1999).

104. Johansson, C. B. *et al.* Identification of a neural stem cell in the adult mammalian central nervous system. *Cell* **96**, 25–34 (1999).

105. Bjornson, C. R., Rietze, R. L., Reynolds, B. A., Magli, M. C. and Vescovi, A. L. Turning brain into blood: a hematopoietic fate adopted by adult neural stem cells *in vivo. Science* **283**, 534–7 (1999).

106. Weiss, S. *et al.* Is there a neural stem cell in the mammalian forebrain?. *Trends Neurosci.* **19**, 387–93 (1996).

107. van Praag, H., Kempermann, G. and Gage, F. H. Running increases cell proliferation and neurogenesis in the adult mouse dentate gyrus. *Nat. Neurosci.* **2**, 266–70 (1999).

108. Gould, E., Beylin, A., Tanapat, P., Reeves, A. and Shors, T. J. Learning enhances adult neurogenesis in the hippocampal formation. *Nat. Neurosci.* **2**, 260–5 (1999).

109. McKay, R. Stem cells in the central nervous system. *Science* **276**, 66–71 (1997).

110. Svendsen, C. and Smith, A. New prospects for human stem-cell therapy in the nervous system. *Trends Neurosci.* **22**, 357–64 (1999).

111. Sinden, J. D. *et al.* Recovery of spatial learning by grafts of a conditionally immortalized hippocampal neuroepithelial cell line into the ischaemia-lesioned hippocampus. *Neuroscience* **81**, 599–608 (1997).

112. Hoffmann, H. Local re-innervation in partially denervated muscle: a histo-physiological study. *Aust. J. Exp. Biol. Sci.* **28**, 383–97 (1950).

113. Brown, M. C. and Ironton, R. Sprouting and regression of neuromuscular synapses in partially denervated mammalian muscles. *J. Physiol.* **278**, 325–8 (1978).

114. Devor, M., Schonfeld, D., Seltzer, Z. and Wall, P. D. Two modes of cutaneous reinnervation following peripheral nerve injury. *J. Comp. Neurol.* **185**, 211–20 (1979).

115. Murray, J. G. and Thompson, J. W. The occurrence and function of collateral sprouting in the sympathetic nervous system of the cat. *J. Physiol.* **135**, 133–62 (1957).

116. Courtney, K. and Roper, S. Sprouting of synapses after partial denervation of frog cardiac ganglion. *Nature* **259**, 317–19 (1976).

117. Jackson, P. C. and Diamond, J. Failure of intact cutaneous mechanosensory axons to sprout functional collaterals in skin of adult rabbits. *Brain Res.* **273**, 277–84 (1983).

118. Kinnamon, E. and Aldskogius, H. Collateral sprouting of sensory axons in the glabrous skin of the hindpaw after chronic sciatic nerve lesions in

adult and neonatal rats: a morphological study. *Brain Res.* **377**, 73–82 (1986).

119. Doucette, R. and Diamond, J. Normal and precocious sprouting of heat nociceptors in the skin of adult rats. *J. Comp. Neurol.* **261**, 592–603 (1987).

120. Molander, C., Kinnman, E. and Aldskogius, H. Expansion of spinal cord primary sensory afferent projection following combined sciatic nerve resection and saphenous nerve crush: a horseradish peroxidase study in the adult rat. *J. Comp. Neurol.* **276**, 436–41 (1988) [published erratum appears in *J. Comp. Neurol.* **286**, 541 (1989)].

121. McMahon, S. B. and Kett-White, R. Sprouting of peripherally regenerating primary sensory neurones in the adult central nervous system. *J. Comp. Neurol.* **304**, 307–15 (1991).

122. Bjorklund, A. and Stenevi, U. Regeneration of monoaminergic and cholinergic neurons in the mammalian central nervous system. *Physiol. Rev.* **59**, 62–97 (1979).

123. Raisman, G. and Field, P. M. A quantitative investigation of the development of collateral reinnervation after partial deafferentation of septal nuclei. *Brain Res.* **50**, 241–64 (1973).

124. Tsukahara, N. Sprouting and the neuronal basis of learning. *Trends Neurosci.* **4**, 234–7 (1981).

125. Cotman, C. W., Nieto Sampedro, M. and Harris, E. W. Synapse replacement in the nervous system of adult vertebrates. *Physiol. Rev.* **61**, 684–784 (1981).

126. Lynch, G., Deadwyler, S. and Cotman, C. W. Postlesion axonal growth produces permanent functional connections. *Science* **180**, 1364–6 (1973).

127. Goldberger, M. E. Locomotor recovery after unilateral hindlimb deafferentation. *Brain Res.* **123**, 59–74 (1977).

128. Loesche, J. and Steward, D. Behavioural correlates of denervation and reinnervation of the hippocampal formation of the rat: recovery of alternation performance following unilateral entorhinal cortex lesions. *Brain Res. Bull.* **2**, 21–39 (1977).

129. Nottet, H. S. L. M. and Gendelman, H. E. Unraveling the neuroimmune mechanisms of the HIV-1-associated cognitive/motor complex. *Immunol. Today* **16**, 441–8 (1995).

130. Gilbert, C. D. Learning: neuronal dynamics and perceptual learning. *Curr. Biol.* **4**, 627–9 (1994).

131. Jones, R. and Vrbova, G. Two factors responsible for the development of denervation hypersensitivity. *J. Physiol.* **236**, 517P (1974).

132. Diamond, J., Holmes, M. and Coughlin, M. Endogenous NGF and nerve impulses regulate the collateral sprouting of sensory axons in the skin of the adult rat. *J. Neurosci.* **12**, 1454–66 (1992).

133. Diamond, J., Foerster, A., Holmes, M. and Coughlin, M. Sensory nerves in adult rats regenerate and restore sensory function to the skin independently of endogenous NGF. *J. Neurosci.* **12**, 1467–76 (1992).

134. Isaacson, L. G., Saffran, B. N. and Crutcher, K. A. Nerve growth factor-induced sprouting of mature, uninjured sympathetic axons. *J. Comp. Neurol.* **326**, 327–36 (1992).

135. Van der Zee, C. E., Fawcett, J. and Diamond, J. Antibody to NGF inhibits collateral sprouting of septohippocampal fibers following entorhinal cortex lesion in adult rats. *J. Comp. Neurol.* **326**, 91–100 (1992).

136. Duchen, L. and Strich, S. The effects of botulinum toxin on the pattern of innervation of skeletal muscle of the mouse. *Q. J. Exp. Physiol.* **53**, 84–9 (1968).

137. Brown, M. C. and Ironton, R. Motor neurone sprouting induced by prolonged tetrodotoxin block of nerve action potentials. *Nature* **265**, 459–61 (1977).

138. Holland, R. L. and Brown, M. C. Postsynaptic transmission block can cause terminal sprouting of a motor nerve. *Science* **207**, 649–51 (1980).

139. Hopkins, W. G., Brown, M. C. and Keynes, R. J. Nerve growth from nodes of Ranvier in inactive muscle. *Brain Res.* **222**, 125–8 (1981).

140. Keynes, R. J., Hopkins, W. G. and Brown, M. C. Sprouting of mammalian motor neurones at nodes of Ranvier: the role of the denervated motor endplate. *Brain Res.* **264**, 209–13 (1983).

141. Ishii, D. N. Relationship of insulin-like growth factor II gene expression in muscle to synaptogenesis. *Proc. Natl. Acad. Sci. USA* **86**, 2898–902 (1989).

142. Caroni, P. and Grandes, P. Nerve sprouting in innervated adult skeletal muscle induced by exposure to elevated levels of insulin-like growth factors. *J. Cell Biol.* **110**, 1307–17 (1990).

143. Caroni, P., Schneider, C., Kiefer, M. C. and Zapf, J. Role of muscle insulin-like growth factors in nerve sprouting: suppression of terminal sprouting in paralyzed muscle by IGF-binding protein 4. *J. Cell Biol.* **125**, 893–902 (1994).

144. Gurney, M. E., Yamamoto, H. and Kwon, Y. Induction of motor neuron sprouting *in vivo* by ciliary neurotrophic factor and basic fibroblast growth factor. *J. Neurosci.* **12**, 3241–7 (1992).

145. Koliatsos, V. E., Clatterbuck, R. E., Winslow, J. W., Cayouette, M. H. and Price, D. L. Evidence that brain-derived neurotrophic factor is a trophic factor for motor neurons *in vivo*. *Neuron* **10**, 359–67 (1993).

146. Lundborg, G., Zhao, Q., Kanje, M., Danielsen, N. and Kerns, J. M. Can sensory and

motor collateral sprouting be induced from intact peripheral nerve by end-to-side anastomosis? *J. Hand Surg. (Br.)* **19**, 277–82 (1994).

147. Diaz, J. and Pecot-Dechavassine, M. Nerve sprouting induced by a piece of peripheral nerve placed over a normally innervated frog muscle. *J. Physiol. (London)* **421**, 123–33 (1990).

148. Hopkins, W. G. and Brown, M. C. The distribution of nodal sprouts in a paralyzed or partly denervated mouse muscle. *Neuroscience* **7**, 37–44 (1982).

149. Reynolds, M. L. and Woolf, C. J. Terminal Schwann cells elaborate extensive processes following denervation of the motor endplate. *J. Neurocytol.* **21**, 50–66 (1992).

150. Woolf, C. J. *et al.* Denervation of the motor endplate results in the rapid expression by terminal Schwann cells of the growth- associated protein GAP-43. *J. Neurosci.* **12**, 3999–4010 (1992).

151. Son, Y. J. and Thompson, W. J. Nerve sprouting in muscle is induced and guided by processes extended by Schwann cells. *Neuron* **14**, 133–41 (1995).

152. Son, Y. J., Trachtenberg, J. T. and Thompson, W. J. Schwann cells induce and guide sprouting and reinnervation of neuromuscular junctions. *Trends Neurosci* **19**, 280–5 (1996).

153. Trachtenberg, J. T. and Thompson, W. J. Schwann cell apoptosis at developing neuromuscular junctions is regulated by glial growth factor. *Nature* **379**, 174–7 (1996).

154. Rotshenker, S. Synapse formation in intact innervated cutaneous pectoris muscles of the frog following denervation of the opposite muscle. *J. Physiol.* **292**, 535–47 (1979).

155. Herrera, A. and Grinnell, A. Contralateral denervation causes enhanced transmitter release from frog motor nerve terminals. *Nature* **291**, 495–7 (1981).

156. Herrera, A. A., Grinnell, A. D. and Wololwske, B. Ultrastructural correlates of experimentally altered transmitter release efficacy in frog motor nerve terminals. *Neuroscience* **16**, 491–500 (1985).

157. Herrera, A. A. and Scott, D. R. Motor axon sprouting in frog sartorius muscle is not altered by contralateral axotomy. *J. Neurocytol.* **14**, 145–56 (1985).

158. Brown, M. C., Holland, R. L., Hopkins, W. G. and Keynes, R. J. An assessment of the spread of the signal for terminal sprouting within and between muscles. *Brain Res.* **210**, 145–51 (1980).

159. Slack, J. R. and Pockett, S. Terminal sprouting is a local response to a local stimulus. *Brain Res.* **217**, 368–74 (1981).

160. Pachter, B. R. and Eberstein, A. Nerve sprouting and endplate growth induced in normal muscle by contralateral partial denervation of rat plantaris. *Brain Res.* **560**, 311–14 (1991).

161. Pamphlett, R. Axonal sprouting after botulinum toxin does not elicit a histological axon reaction. *J. Neurol. Sci.* **87**, 175–85 (1988).

162. Bisby, M. A., Tetzlaff, W. and Brown, M. C. GAP-43 mRNA in mouse motoneurons undergoing axonal sprouting in response to muscle paralysis or partial denervation. *Eur. J. Neurosci.* **8**, 1240–9 (1996).

163. Mehta, A., Reynolds, M. L. and Woolf, C. J. Partial denervation of the medial gastrocnemius muscle results in growth-associated protein-43 immunoreactivity in sprouting axons and Schwann cells. *Neuroscience* **57**, 433–42 (1993).

164. Mearow, K. M., Kril, Y., Gloster, A. and Diamond, J. Expression of NGF receptor and GAP-43 mRNA in DRG neurons during collateral sprouting and regeneration of dorsal cutaneous nerves. *J. Neurobiol.* **25**, 127–42 (1994).

165. Mathew, T. C. and Miller, F. D. Increased expression of T alpha 1 alpha-tubulin mRNA during collateral and NGF-induced sprouting of sympathetic neurons. *Dev. Biol.* **141**, 84–92 (1990).

166. Booth, C. M., Kemplay, S. and Brown, M. C. An antibody to neural cell adhesion molecule impairs motor nerve terminal sprouting in a mouse muscle locally paralysed with botulinum toxin. *Neuroscience* **35**, 85–91 (1990).

167. Mark, R. F. Chemospecific synaptic repression as a possible memory store. *Nature* **225**, 178–9 (1970).

168. Scott, S. A. Persistence of foreign innervation on reinnervated goldfish extraocular muscles. *Science* **189**, 644–6 (1975).

169. Dennis, M. J. and Yip, J. W. Formation and elimination of foreign synapses on adult salamander muscle. *J. Physiol.* **274**, 299–310 (1978).

170. Dostrovsky, J. O., Millar, J. and Wall, P. D. The immediate shift of afferent drive of dorsal column nucleus cells following deafferentation: a comparison of acute and chronic deafferentation in gracile nucleus and spinal cord. *Exp. Neurol.* **52**, 480–95 (1976).

171. Devor, M. and Wall, P. D. Plasticity in the spinal cord sensory map following peripheral nerve injury in rats. *J. Neurosci.* **1**, 679–84 (1981).

172. Devor, M. and Claman, D. Mapping and plasticity of acid phosphatase afferents in the rat dorsal horn. *Brain Res.* **190**, 17–28 (1980).

173. Selzer, Z. and Devor, M. Effect of nerve section on the spinal distribution of neighbouring nerves. *Brain Res.* **306**, 31–7 (1984).

174. Dostrovsky, J. O., Jabbur, S. and Millar, J. Neurons in cat gracile nucleus with both local and widefield inputs. *J. Physiol.* **278**, 365–75 (1978).

175. Saade, N. E., Banna, N. R., Khoury, A., Jabbur, S. J. and Wall, P. D. Cutaneous receptive field alterations induced by 4-aminopyridine. *Brain Res.* **232**, 177–80 (1982).

176. Markus, H. and Pomeranz, B. Saphenous has weak ineffective synapses in sciatic territory of rat spinal cord: electrical stimulation of the saphenous and application of drugs reveal these somototopically inappropriate synapses. *Brain Res.* **416**, 315–21 (1987).

177. Wall, P. D. and Devor, M. The effect of peripheral nerve injury on dorsal root potentials and on transmission of afferent segments into the spinal cord. *Brain Res.* **209**, 95–111 (1981).

178. Brown, A. G., Fyffe, R. E. W., Noble, R. and Rowe, M. J. Effects of hindlimb nerve sections on lumbosacral dorsal horn neurones in the cat. *J. Physiol.* **354**, 375–94 (1984).

179. Barbut, D., Polak, J. and Wall, P. D. Substance P in spinal cord dorsal horn decreases following peripheral nerve injury. *Brain Res.* **205**, 289–98 (1981).

180. Metzler, J. and Marks, P. J. Functional changes in cat somatic sensorimotor cortex during short term reversible epidural blocks. *Brain Res.* **177**, 379–83 (1979).

181. Kolarik, R. C., Rasey, S. K. and Wall, J. T. The consistency, extent, and locations of early-onset changes in cortical dominance aggregates following injury of nerves to primate hands. *J. Neurosci.* **14**, 4269–88 (1994).

182. Garraghty, P. E. and Kass, J. H. Dynamic features of sensory and motor maps. *Curr. Opin. Neurobiol.* **2**, 522–7 (1992).

183. O'Leary, D. D. M., Ruff, N. L. and Dyck, R. H. Development, critical period plasticity, and adult reorganizations of mammalian somatosensory systems. *Curr. Opin. Neurobiol.* **4**, 535–44 (1994).

184. Merzenich, M. M., Recanzone, G., Jenkins, W. M., Allan, T. T. and Nudo, R. J. Cortical representational plasticity. In *Neurobiology of neocortex* (ed. P. Rakic and W. Singer), pp. 41–67 (Wiley, Chichester 1988).

185. Prakash, N., Cohen-Cory, S. and Frostig, R. D. Rapid and opposite effects of BDNF and NGF on the functional organisation of the adult cortex. *Nature* **381**, 702–6 (1996).

186. Gilbert, C. D. and Wiesel, T. N. Receptive field dynamics in adult primary visual cortex. *Nature* **356**, 150–2 (1992).

187. Schwaber, M. K., Garraghty, P. E. and Kass, J. H. Neuroplasticity of the adult primate auditory cortex following cochlear hearing loss. *Am. J. Otol.* **14**, 252–8 (1993).

188. Rausell, E. and Jones, E. G. Extent of intracortical arborization of thalamocortical axons as a determinant of representational plasticity in monkey somatic sensory cortex. *J. Neurosci.* **15**, 4270–88 (1995).

189. Darian-Smith, C. and Gilbert, C. D. Topographic reorganization in the striate cortex of the adult cat and monkey is cortically mediated. *J. Neurosci.* **15**, 1631–47 (1995).

190. Allard, T., Clark, S. A., Jenkins, W. M. and Merzenich, M. M. Reorganization of somatosensory area 3b representations in adult owl monkeys after digital syndactyly. *J. Neurophysiol.* **66**, 1048–58 (1991).

191. Jenkins, W. M., Merzenich, M. M., Ochs, M. T., Allard, T. and Guic-Robles, E. Functional reorganization of primary somatosensory cortex in adult owl monkeys after behaviourally controlled tactile stimulation. *J. Neurophysiol.* **63**, 82–104 (1990).

192. Trussell, L. D. and Grinnell, A. D. The regulation of synaptic strength within motor units of the frog cutaneous pectoris muscle. *J. Neurosci.* **5**, 243–54 (1985).

193. Garraghty, P. E., LaChica, E. A. and Kaas, J. H. Injury induced reorganization of somatosensory cortex is accompanied by reductions in GABA staining. *Somatosens. Motor Res.* **8**, 347–54 (1991).

194. Juliano, S. L., Ma, W. and Eslin, D. Cholinergic depletion prevents expansion of topographic maps in somatosensory cortex. *Proc. Natl. Acad. Sci. USA* **88**, 780–4 (1991).

195. Isaac, T. R., Nicoll, R. A. and Malenka, R. C. Evidence for silent synapses: implications for the expression of LTP. *Neuron* **15**, 427–34 (1995).

196. Kano, M. and Lino, K. Functional reorganization of adult cat somatosensory cortex is dependent on NMDA receptors. *NeuroReport* **2**, 77–80 (1991).

Index